Neuroanatomy

*An Atlas of Structures,
Sections, and Systems*

SIXTH EDITION

About the cover:

A series of illustrations showing anatomical and clinical (MRI) orientations of the medulla and how the anatomy of this part of the brain directly correlates with that seen in MRI and CT at comparable levels. From Chapter 5.

Neuroanatomy

An Atlas of Structures, Sections, and Systems

SIXTH EDITION

Duane E. Haines, Ph.D.

Professor and Chairman, Department of Anatomy
and Professor of Neurosurgery
at The University of Mississippi Medical Center
Jackson, Mississippi

Special Contributions By:
John A. Lancon, M.D.
Assistant Professor of Neurosurgery
The University of Mississippi Medical Center
Jackson, Mississippi

Illustrator: M.P. Schenk, BS, MSMI
Photographer: G.W. Armstrong, RBP
Typist: K.M. Squires

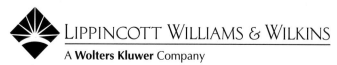

LIPPINCOTT WILLIAMS & WILKINS
A **Wolters Kluwer** Company

Philadelphia • Baltimore • New York • London
Buenos Aires • Hong Kong • Sydney • Tokyo

Editor: Betty Sun
Managing Editor: Dan Pepper
Marketing Manager: Joe Schott
Production Editor: Christina Remsberg
Compositor: Peirce Graphic Services
Printer: RR Donnelley-Willard

Copyright © 2004 Lippincott Williams & Wilkins

351 West Camden Street
Baltimore, Maryland 21201-2436 USA

530 Walnut Street
Philadelphia, Pennsylvania 19106-3621 USA

Printed in the United States

First Edition, 1983
Second Edition, 1987
Third Edition, 1991
Fourth Edition, 1995
Fifth Edition, 2000
Portuguese Edition, 1991
Japanese Editions, 1996, 2000
Chinese Edition (Taiwan), 1997
Chinese Edition (Beijing), 2001

Library of Congress Cataloging-in-Publication Data

Haines, Duane E.
    Neuroanatomy : an atlas of structures, sections, and systems / Duane E. Haines ; special contributions by John A. Lancon ; illustrator, M.P. Schenk ; photographer, G.W. Armstrong.—6th ed.
      p. ; cm.
    Includes bibliographical references and index.
    ISBN 0-7817-4677-9
    1. Neuroanatomy—Atlases.   I. Title.
    [DNLM: 1. Central Nervous System—anatomy & histology—Atlases. WL 17 H153n 2004]
    QM451.H18 2004
    611'.8—dc21

                        2003054519

To purchase additional copies of this book, call our customer service department at (800) 638-3030 or fax orders to (301) 824-7390.

Visit Lippincott Williams & Wilkins on the Internet: http://www.LWW.com. Lippincott Williams & Wilkins customer service representatives are available from 8:30 am to 6:00 pm, EST.

04 05 06
2 3 4 5 6 7 8 9 10

Preface to the Sixth Edition

Previous editions of *Neuroanatomy* have endeavored 1) to provide a structural basis for understanding the function of the central nervous system; 2) to emphasize points of clinical relevance through use of appropriate terminology and examples; and 3) to integrate neuroanatomical and clinical information in a format that will meet the educational needs of the user. The goal of the sixth edition is to continue this philosophy and to present structural information and concepts in an even more clinically useful and relevant format. Information learned in the basic science setting should flow as seamlessly as possible into the clinical setting.

I have received many constructive suggestions and comments from my colleagues and students. This is especially the case for the modifications made in Chapters 2, 5, 7, 8, and 9 in this new edition. The names of the individuals who have provided suggestions or comments are given in the Acknowledgments. This thoughtful and helpful input is greatly appreciated and has influenced the preparation of this new edition.

The major changes made in the sixth edition of *Neuroanatomy* are as follows:

First, recognizing that brain anatomy is seen in clear and elegant detail in MRI and CT, and that this is the primary way the brain is viewed in the health care setting, additional new images have been incorporated into this new edition. Every effort has been made to correlate the MRI or CT with brain or spinal cord anatomy by relating these images on the same page or on facing pages. New MRI or CT have been introduced into chapter 2 (spinal cord, meningeal hemorrhages correlated with the meninges, cisterns, hemorrhage into the brain, hemorrhage into the ventricles correlated with the structure of the ventricles), chapter 5 (spinal cord and brainstem), and chapter 8 (vascular).

Second, the structure of the central nervous system should be available to the student (or the medical professional for that matter) in a format that makes this information immediately accessible, and applicable, to the requirements of the clinical experience. It is commonplace to present brain structure in an anatomical orientation (e.g., the colliculi are "up" in the image and the interpeduncular fossa is "down"). However, when the midbrain is viewed in an axial MRI or CT, the reverse is true: the colliculi are "down" in the image and the interpeduncular fossa is "up". There are many good reasons for making brainstem images available in an anatomical orientation and for teaching this view in the academic setting. These reasons are recognized in this book. On the other hand, the extensive use of MRI or CT in all areas of medicine, not just the clinical neurosciences, requires that students be clearly aware of *how brain and spinal cord structure is viewed, and used, in the clinical environment.* To address this important question, a series of illustrations, including MRI or CT, are introduced in the spinal cord and brainstem sections of chapter 5. These images are arranged to show 1) the small colorized version of the spinal cord or brainstem in an anatomical orientation; 2) the same image flipped bottom-to-top into a clinical orientation; and 3) the clinical orientation of the colorized line drawing followed by T1 and T2 MRI and/or CT at levels comparable to the line drawing and corresponding stained section. This approach retains the inherent strengths of the full-page, colorized line drawing and its companion stained section in the anatomical orientation. At the same time, it introduces, on the same set of pages, the important concept that CNS anatomy, both external and internal, is oriented differently in MRI or CT. It is the clinical orientation issue that will confront the student/clinician in the clinical setting. It is certainly appropriate to introduce, and even stress, this view of the brain and spinal cord in the basic science years.

Third, new images have been included in chapter 8. These include, but are not limited to, new examples of general vessel arrangement in MRA, examples of specific vessels in MRI, and some additional examples of hemorrhage.

Fourth, additional examples of cranial nerves traversing the subarachnoid space are included. In fact, the number of MRI showing cranial nerves has been doubled. In addition, each new plate starts with a gross anatomical view of the nerve (or nerves) shown in the succeeding MRI in that figure.

Fifth, additional clinical information and correlations have been included. These are in the form of new images, new and/or modified figure descriptions, and changes in other portions of the textual elements.

Sixth, in some instances, existing figures have been relocated to improve their correlation with other images. In other instances, existing figures have been repeated and correlated with newly added MRI or CT so as to more clearly illustrate an anatomical-clinical correlation.

Seventh, a new chapter (chapter 9), consisting of approximately 240 study and review questions and answers in the USMLE style, has been added. All of these questions have explained answers keyed to specific pages in the Atlas. Although not designed to be an exhaustive set, this new chapter should give the user of this atlas a unique opportunity for self-assessment.

Two further issues figured prominently in the development of this new edition. First, the question of whether to use eponyms in their possessive form. To paraphrase one of my clinical colleagues "Parkinson did not die of his disease (Parkinson disease), he died of a stroke; it was never his own personal disease." There are rare exceptions, such as Lou Gehrig's disease, but the point is well taken. McKusick (1998a,b) has also made compelling arguments in support of using the non-possessive form of eponyms. It is, however, acknowledged that views differ on this question—much like debating how many angels can dance on the head of a pin. Consultation with my neurology and neurosurgery colleagues, a review of some of the more comprehensive neurology texts (e.g., Rowland, 2000; Victor and Ropper, 2001), and the standards established in The Council of Biology Editors Manual for Authors, Editors, and Publishers (1994) and the American Medical Association's Manual of Style (1998) clearly indicate an overwhelming preference for the non possessive form. Recognizing that many users of this book will enter clinical training, it was deemed appropriate to encourage a contemporary approach. Consequently, the non possessive form of the eponym is used.

The second issue concerns use of the most up-to-date anatomical terminology. With the publication of *Terminologia Anatomica* (Thieme, New York, 1998), a new official international list of anatomical terms for neuroanatomy is available. This new publication, having been adopted by the International Federation of Associations of Anatomists, supersedes *all* previous terminology lists. Every effort has been made to incorporate any applicable new or modified terms into this book. The number of changes is modest and related primarily to directional terms: posterior for dorsal, anterior for ventral, etc. In most cases, the previous term appears in parentheses following the official term, i.e., *posterior (dorsal) cochlear nucleus.* It is almost certain that some changes have eluded detection; these will be caught in subsequent printings.

Last, but certainly not least, the sixth edition is a few pages longer than was the fifth edition. This results exclusively from the inclusion of more MRI and CT, a better integration of anatomical-clinical information, including more clinical examples (text and illustrations), and the inclusion of Study/Review and USMLE style questions with explained answers.

Duane E. Haines
Jackson, Mississippi

References:

Council of Biology Editions Style Manual Committee. *Scientific Style and Format—The CBE Manual for Authors, Editors, and Publishers.* 6th Ed. Cambridge: Cambridge University Press, 1994.

Federative Committee on Anatomical Terminology. *Terminologia Anatomica.* Thieme, Stuttgart and New York, 1998.

Iverson, MA et al. *American Medical Association Manual of Style—A Guide for Authors and Editors.* 9th Ed. Baltimore: Williams & Wilkins, 1998.

McKusick, VA. On the naming of clinical disorders, with particular reference to eponyms. *Medicine* 1998;77: 1–2.

McKusick, VA. *Mendelian Inheritance in Man, A Catalog of Human Genes and Genetic Disorders.* 12th Ed. Baltimore: The Johns Hopkins University Press, 1998.

Rowland, LP. *Merritt's Neurology.* 10th Ed. Baltimore: Lippincott Williams & Wilkins, 2000.

Victor, M and Ropper, AH. *Adams and Victor's Principles of Neurology.* 7th Ed. New York: McGraw-Hill, Medical Publishing Division, 2001.

Preface to the First Edition

This atlas is a reflection of, and a response to, suggestions from professional and graduate students over the years I have taught human neurobiology. Admittedly, some personal philosophy, as regards teaching, has crept into all parts of the work.

The goal of this atlas is to provide a maximal amount of useful information, in the form of photographs and drawings, so that the initial learning experience will be pleasant, logical, and fruitful, and the review process effective and beneficial to longterm professional goals. To this end several guiding principles have been followed. First, the entire anatomy of the central nervous system (CNS), external and internal, has been covered in appropriate detail. Second, a conscientious effort has been made to generate photographs and drawings of the highest quality: illustrations that clearly relay information to the reader. Third, complementary information always appears on facing page. This may take the form of two views of related structures such as brainstem or successive brain slices or a list of abbreviations and description for a full-page figure. Fourth, illustrations of blood supply have been included and integrated into their appropriate chapters. When gross anatomy of the brain is shown, the patterns of blood vessels and relationships of sinuses appear on facing pages. The distribution pattern of blood vessels to internal CNS structures is correlated with internal morphology as seen in stained sections. Including information on external vascular patterns represents a distinct departure from what is available in most atlases, and illustrations of internal vessel distribution are unique to this atlas.

There are other features which, although not unique in themselves, do not usually appear in atlas format. In the chapter containing cross-sections, special effort has been made to provide figures that are accurate, clear, and allow considerable flexibility in how they can be used for both teaching and learning. The use of illustrations that are one-half photograph and one-half drawing is not entirely novel. In this atlas, however, the sections are large, clearly labeled, and the drawing side is a mirror-image of the photograph side. One section of the atlas is devoted to summaries of a variety of major pathways. Including this material in a laboratory atlas represents a distinct departure from the standard approach. However, feedback over the years strongly indicates that this type of information in atlas format is extremely helpful to students in the laboratory and greatly enhances their ability to grasp and retain information on CNS connections. While this atlas does not attempt to teach clinical concepts, a chapter correlating selected views of angiograms and CT scans with morphological relationships of cerebral arteries and internal brain structures is included. These examples illustrate that a clear understanding of normal morphological relationships, as seen in the laboratory, can be directly transposed to clinical situations.

This atlas was not conceived with a particular audience in mind. It was designed to impart a clear and comprehensive understanding of CNS morphology to its readers, whoever they may be. It is most obviously appropriate for human neurobiology courses as taught to medical, dental, and graduate students. In addition, students in nursing, physical therapy, and other allied health curricula, and psychology as well, may also find its contents helpful and applicable to their needs. Inclusion and integration of blood vessel patterns, both external and internal, and the summary pathway drawings may be useful to the individual requiring a succinct, yet comprehensive review before taking board exams in the neurological, neurosurgical, and psychiatric specialties.

The details in some portions of this atlas may exceed that found in comparable parts of other atlases. If one is to err, it seems more judicious to err on the side of greater detail than on the side of inadequate detail. If the student is confronted with more information on a particular point than is needed during the initial learning process, he or she can simply bypass the extra information. However, once the initial learning is completed, the additional information will be there to enhance the review process. If students have inadequate information in front of them it may be difficult, or even impossible, to fill in missing points that may not be part of their repertoire of knowledge. In addition, information may be inserted out of context, and, thereby, hinder the learning experience.

A work such as this is bound to be subject to oversights, and for such foibles, I am solely responsible. I welcome comments, suggestions, and corrections from my colleagues and from students.

Duane E. Haines

Acknowledgments

As was the case in previous editions of this book, my colleagues and students in both medical and graduate programs have been most gracious in offering their suggestions and comments. I greatly appreciate their time and interest in the continuing usefulness of this book.

As changes were being contemplated for this new edition, input on potential modifications was solicited from faculty as well as students in an effort to ascertain how these changes might impact on the usefulness of this Atlas. These individuals went out of their way to review the documents that were provided and to give insightful, and sometimes lengthy, comments on the pros and cons of the ideas being considered. This input was taken into consideration as the initial plans were modified and finalized by the author and then incorporated into this new edition. The faculty who gave generously of their time and energy were Drs. A. Agmon, C. Anderson, R. Baisden, S. Baldwin, J. L. Culberson, B. Hallas, J. B. Hutchins, T. Imig, G. R. Leichnetz, E. Levine, R. C. S. Lin, J. C. Lynch, T. McGraw-Ferguson, G. F. Martin, G. A. Mihailoff, R. L. Norman, R. E. Papka, H. J. Ralston, J. Rho, L. T. Robertson, J. D. Schlag, K. L. Simpson, and C. Stefan. The students who offered helpful and insightful comments were A. Alqueza (medical student, University of Florida at Gainesville), A. S. Bristol (graduate student, University of California at Irvine), L. Simmons (medical student, Vanderbilt University), J. A. Tucker (medical student, The University of Mississippi Medical Center), S. Thomas (graduate student, University of Maryland at College Park), and M. Tomblyn (medical student, Rush Medical College). I greatly appreciate their comments and suggestions.

I would also like to thank my colleagues in the Department of Anatomy at The University of Mississippi Medical Center (UMMC) for their many helpful suggestions and comments. My colleagues in the Department of Neurosurgery at UMMC (Drs. A. Parent [Chairman], L. Harkey, J. Lancon, J. Ross, D. Esposito, and G. Mandybur) and in the Department of Neurology at UMMC (especially Drs. J. Corbett [Chairman], S. Subramony, H. Uschmann, and M. Santiago) have offered valuable input on a range of clinical issues. I am especially indebted to Dr. J. A. Lancon (Neurosurgery) for his significant contributions to this new edition. These include his willingness to participate as co-author of Chapter 9 and his careful review of all new clinical information added to the book. I would also like to thank Ms. Amanda Ellis, B.S.N., for keeping my friend John on track.

I am indebted to the following individuals for their careful review of previous editions of the book: Drs. B. Anderson, R. Borke, Patricia Brown, Paul Brown, T. Castro, B. Chronister, A. Craig, E. Dietrichs, J. Evans, B. Falls, C. Forehand, R. Frederickson, E. Garcis-Rill, G. Grunwald, J. King, A. Lamperti, K. Peusner, C. Phelps, D. Rosene, A. Rosenquist, M. Schwartz, J. Scott, V. Seybold, D. Smith, S. Stensaas, D. Tolbert, F. Walberg, S. Walkley, M. Woodruff, M. Wyss, and B. Yezierski. The stained sections used in this atlas are from the teaching collection in the Department of Anatomy at West Virginia University School of Medicine.

Dr. R. Brent Harrison (former Chairman of Radiology, UMMC), Dr. Robert D. Halpert (current Chairman of Radiology, UMMC) and Dr. Gurmett Dhilon (Neuroradiology) generously continue to give me full access to all their facilities. I would like to express a special thanks to Mr. W. (Eddie) Herrington (Chief CT/MRI Technologist) and Mr. Joe Barnes (Senior MRI Technologist) for their outstanding efforts to supply new images and their special efforts to generate images at specific planes for this new edition. In the same vein, Drs. G. Dhilon and S. Crawford also made special attempts to get specific MRI at special planes. I am also deeply appreciative to several technologists and nurses in the CT/MRI suite, and particularly to Master Johnathan Barnes, for being such cooperative "patients" as we worked to generate scans that matched stained sections in the Atlas as closely as possible.

Modifications, both great and small, to the artwork and labeling scheme, as well as some new renderings, were the work of Mr. Michael Schenk (Director of Biomedical Illustration Services). Mr. Bill Armstrong (Director of Biomedical Photography) produced outstanding photographs of gross specimens and slices, CTs, MRIs, and MRAs. I am very appreciative of the time, effort, and dedication of these individuals to create the very best artwork and photographs possible for this new edition. Ms. Katherine Squires did all the typing for the sixth edition. Her excellent cooperation, patience, and good-natured repartee with the author were key elements in completing the final draft in a timely manner.

This sixth edition would not have been possible without the interest and support of the publisher, Lippincott Williams & Wilkins. I want to express thanks to my editor, Ms. Betty Sun (Acquisitions Editor), to Mr. Dan Pepper (Associate Managing Editor), to Ms. Erica Lukenich (Editorial Assistant), Ms. Jennifer Weir (Associate Production Manager), and to Mr. Joe Scott (Marketing Manager) for their encouragement, continuing interest, and confidence in this project. Their cooperation has given me the opportunity to make the improvements seen herein.

Last, but certainly not least, I would like to express a special thanks to my wife, Gretchen. She put up with me while these revisions were in progress, carefully reviewed all changes in the text and all questions/answers, and was a tangible factor in getting everything done. I dedicate this edition to Gretchen.

Contents

Preface to Sixth Edition v

Preface to the First Edition vii

Acknowledgments ix

Chapter 1   **Introduction and Reader's Guide** 1

        Including Rationale for Labels and Abbreviations 8

Chapter 2   **External Morphology of the Central Nervous System** 9

        The Spinal Cord: Gross Views and Vasculature 10

        The Brain: Lobes, Principle Brodmann Areas, Sensory-Motor Somatotopy 13

        The Brain: Gross Views, Vasculature, and MRI 16

        The Cranial Nerves in MRI 38

        The Insula: Gross View and MRI 45

        The Meninges, Cisterns, and Meningeal and Cisternal Hemorrhages 46

        The Ventricles and Ventricular Hemorrhages 52

Chapter 3   **Dissections of the Central Nervous System** 55

        Lateral, Medial, and Ventral Aspects 56

        Overall Views 59

Chapter 4   **Internal Morphology of the Brain in Slices and MRI** 63

        Brain Slices in the Coronal Plane Correlated with MRI 63

        Brain Slices in the Axial Plane Correlated with MRI 73

Chapter 5   **Internal Morphology of the Spinal Cord and Brain in Stained Sections** 83

        The Spinal Cord with CT and MRI 84

        Arterial Patterns Within the Spinal Cord With Vascular Syndromes 94

        The Degenerated Corticospinal Tract 96

        The Medulla Oblongata with MRI and CT 98

        Arterial Patterns Within the Medulla Oblongata With Vascular Syndromes 110

        The Cerebellar Nuclei 112

        The Pons with MRI and CT 116

        Arterial Patterns Within the Pons With Vascular Syndromes 124

        The Midbrain with MRI and CT 126

        Arterial Patterns Within the Midbrain With Vascular Syndromes 136

        The Diencephalon and Basal Nuclei with MRI 138

        Arterial Patterns Within the Forebrain With Vascular Syndromes 158

Chapter 6   **Internal Morphology of the Brain in Stained Sections:**
Axial–Sagittal Correlations with MRI 161

        Axial–Sagittal Correlations 162

Chapter 7   **Synopsis of Functional Components, Tracts, Pathways, and Systems** 173

        Components of Cranial and Spinal Nerves 174

        Orientation 176

        Sensory Pathways 178

        Motor Pathways 190

        Cerebellum and Basal Nuclei 204

        Optic, Auditory, and Vestibular Systems 220

        Limbic System 232

Chapter 8   **Anatomical–Clinical Correlations: Cerebral Angiogram, MRA, and MRV** 239

Cerebral Angiogram, MRA, and MRV 240

Blood Supply to the Choroid Plexi 251

Overview of Vertebral and Carotid Arteries 252

Chapter 9   **Q&A's: A Sampling of Study and Review Questions, Many in the USMLE Style, All With Explained Answers** 253

Sources and Suggested Readings 297

Index 301

Introduction
and
Reader's Guide

At a time when increasing numbers of atlases and textbooks are becoming available to students and instructors, it is appropriate to briefly outline the approach used in this volume. Most books are the result of 1) the philosophic approach of the author/instructor to the subject matter and 2) students' needs as expressed through their suggestions and opinions. The present atlas is no exception, and as a result, several factors have guided its further development. These include an appreciation of what enhances learning in the laboratory and classroom, the inherent value of correlating structure with function, the clinical value of understanding the blood supply to the central nervous system (CNS), and the essential importance of integrating anatomy with clinical information and examples. The goal is to make it obvious to the user that structure and function in the CNS are integrated elements and not separate entities.

Most neuroanatomic atlases approach the study of the CNS from fundamentally similar viewpoints. These atlases present brain anatomy followed by illustrations of stained sections, in one or more planes. Although variations on this theme exist, the *basic* approach is similar. In addition, most atlases do not make a concerted effort to correlate vascular patterns with external or internal brain structures. Also, most atlases include little or no information on neurotransmitters and do not integrate clinical examples and information with the study of functional systems.

Understanding CNS structure is the basis for learning pathways, neural function, and for developing the skill to diagnose the neurologically impaired patient. Following a brief period devoted to the study of CNS morphology, a significant portion of many courses is spent learning functional systems. This learning experience may take place in the laboratory because it is here that the student deals with images of representative levels of the entire neuraxis. However, few attempts have been made to provide the student with a *comprehensive and integrated guide*—one that correlates, 1) external brain anatomy with MRI and blood supply; 2) meninges and ventricles with examples of meningeal, ventricular, and brain hemorrhage; 3) internal brain anatomy with MRI, blood supply, the organization of tracts and nuclei and selected clinical examples; 4) summaries of clinically relevant pathways with neurotransmitters, numerous clinical correlations, and the essential concept of laterality; and 5) includes a large variety of images such as angiogram, computed tomography (CT), magnetic resonance imaging (MRI), magnetic resonance angiography (MRA), and magnetic resonance venography (MRV).

The present atlas addresses these points. The goal is not only to show external and internal structure per se but also to demonstrate that the relationship between brain anatomy and MRI/CT, the blood supply to specific areas of the CNS and the arrangement of pathways located therein, the neuroactive substances associated with pathways, and examples of clinical deficits are inseparable components of the learning experience. An effort has been made to provide a format that is dynamic and flexible—one that makes the learning experience an interesting and rewarding exercise.

The relationship between blood vessels and specific brain regions (external and/or internal) is extremely important considering that approximately 50% of what goes wrong inside the skull, producing neurological deficits, is vascular-related. To emphasize the value of this information, the distribution pattern of blood vessels is correlated with external spinal cord and brain anatomy (Chapter 2) and with internal structures such as tracts and nuclei (Chapter 5), reviewed in each pathway drawing (Chapter 7), and shown in angiograms, MRAs, and MRVs (Chapter 8). This approach has several advantages: 1) the vascular pattern is *immediately* related to the structures just learned, 2) vascular patterns are shown in the sections of the atlas in which they belong, 3) the reader cannot proceed from one part of the atlas to the next without being reminded of blood supply, and 4) the conceptual importance of the distribution pattern of blood vessels in the CNS is repeatedly reinforced.

The ability to diagnose a neurologically compromised patient is specifically related to a thorough understanding of pathway structure, function, blood supply, and the relationships of this pathway to adjacent structures. To this end Chapter 7 provides a series of semidiagrammatic illustrations of various clinically relevant pathways. *Each figure* shows 1) the trajectory of fibers that comprise the entire pathway; 2) the laterality of fibers comprising the pathway, this being an extremely important concept in diagnosis; 3) the positions and somatotopy of fibers comprising each pathway at representative levels; 4) a review of the blood supply to the entire pathway; 5) important neurotransmitters associated with fibers of the pathway; and 6) examples of deficits seen following lesions of the pathway at various levels throughout the neuraxis. This chapter is designed to be used by itself or integrated with other sections of the atlas; it is designed to provide the reader with the structural and clinical essentials of a given pathway in a single illustration.

The advent and common use of imaging methods (MRI, MRA, and MRV) mandates that such images become an integral part of the educational process when teaching and/or learning clinically applicable neuroscience. To this end, this book contains about 175 MRI and CT images and 12 MRA and MRV. All of these images are *directly* correlated with external brain anatomy such as gyri and sulci, internal structures including pathways and nuclei, cranial nerves and adjacent structures, or they demonstrate examples of hemorrhages related to the meninges and ventricles or the parenchyma of the brain.

Imaging the Brain (CT and MRI): Imaging the brain *in vivo* is now commonplace for the patient with neurological deficits that may indicate a compromise of the central nervous system. Even most rural hospitals have, or have easy access to, CT or MRI. With these facts in mind, it is appropriate to make a few general comments on these imaging techniques and what is routinely seen, or best seen, in each. For details of the methods and techniques of CT and MRI consult sources such as Grossman (1996), Lee et al. (1999), or Buxton (2002).

Computed Tomography (CT): In CT, the patient is passed between a source of x-rays and a series of detectors. Tissue density is measured by the effects of x-rays on atoms within the tissue as these x-rays pass through the tissue. Atoms of higher number have a greater ability to attenuate (stop) x-rays while those with lower numbers are less able to attenuate x-rays. The various attenuation intensities are computerized into numbers (Hounsfield units or CT numbers). Bone is given the value of +1,000 and is white, while air is given a value of −1,000 and is black. Extravascular blood, an enhanced tumor, fat, the brain (grey and white matter), and cerebrospinal fluid form an intervening continuum from white to black. A CT image of a patient with subarachnoid hemorrhage illustrates the various shades seen in a CT (Fig. 1-1). In general, the following table summarizes the white to black intensities seen for selected tissues in CT.

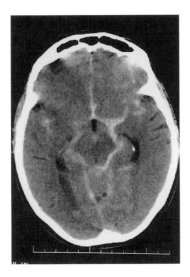

1-1 Computed Tomography (CT) in the axial plane of a patient with subarachnoid hemorrhage. Bone is white, acute blood (white) outlines the subarachnoid space, brain is grey, and cerebrospinal fluid in third and lateral ventricles is black.

The Brain and Related Structures in CT

STRUCTURE/FLUID/SPACE	GREY SCALE
Bone, acute blood	Very white
Enhanced tumor	Very white
Subacute blood	Light grey
Muscle	Light grey
Grey matter	Light grey
White matter	Medium grey
Cerebrospinal fluid	Medium grey to black
Air, Fat	Very black

The advantages of CT are 1) it is rapidly done, which is especially important in trauma; 2) it clearly shows acute and subacute hemorrhages into the meningeal spaces and brain; 3) it shows bone (and skull fractures) to advantage; and 4) it is less expensive than MRI. The disadvantages of CT are 1) it does not clearly show acute or subacute infarcts or ischemia, or brain edema; 2) it does not clearly differentiate white from grey matter within the brain nearly as well as MRI; and 3) it exposes the patient to ionizing radiation.

Magnetic Resonance Imaging (MRI): The tissues of the body contain proportionately large amounts of protons (hydrogen). Protons have a positive nucleus, a shell of negative electrons, and a north and south pole; they function like tiny spinning bar magnets. Normally, these atoms are arranged randomly in relation to each other due to the constantly changing magnetic field produced by the electrons. MRI uses this characteristic of protons to generate images of the brain and body.

When radio waves are sent in short bursts into the magnet containing the patient, they are called a radiofrequency pulse (RP). This pulse may vary in strength. When the frequency of the RP matches the frequency of the spinning proton, the proton will absorb energy from the radio wave (resonance). The effect is two-fold. First, the magnetic effects of some protons are cancelled out and second, the magnetic effects and energy levels in others are increased. When the RP is turned off, the relaxed protons release energy (an "echo") that is received by a coil and computed into an image of that part of the body.

The two major types of MRI images (MRI/T1 and MRI/T2) are related to the effect of RP on protons and the reactions of these protons (relaxation) when the RP is turned off. In general, those cancelled out protons return slowly to their original magnetic strength. The image constructed from this time constant is called T1 (Fig. 1-2). On the other hand, those protons that achieved a higher energy level (were not cancelled-out) lose their energy more rapidly as they return to their original state; the image constructed from this time constant is T2 (Fig. 1-3). The creation of a T1-weighted image versus a T2-weighted image is based on a variation in the times used to receive the "echo" from the relaxed protons.

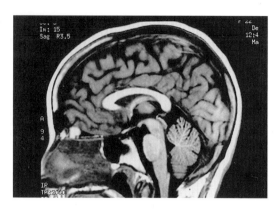

1-2 A sagittal T1 weighted Magnetic Resonance Image (MRI). Brain is grey and cerebrospinal fluid is black.

The following table summarizes the white to black intensities seen in MRI images that are T1-weighted versus T2-weighted. It should be emphasized that a number of variations on these two general MRI themes are routinely seen in the clinical environment.

The advantages of MRI are 1) it can be manipulated to visualize a wide variety of abnormalities or abnormal states within the brain; and 2) it can show great detail of the brain in normal and abnormal states. The disadvantages of MRI are 1) it does not show acute or subacute subarachnoid hemorrhage or hemorrhage into the substance of the brain in any detail; 2) it takes a much longer time to do and, therefore, is not useful in acute situations or in some types of trauma; 3) it is, comparatively, much more expensive than CT, and 4) the scan is extremely loud and may require sedation in children.

The ensuing discussion briefly outlines the salient features of individual chapters. In some sections, considerable flexibility has been designed into the format; at these points, some suggestions are made as to how the atlas can be used. In addition, new clinical correlations and examples have been included and a new chapter of USMLE-style review questions has been added.

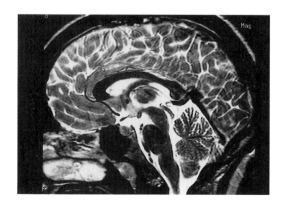

1-3 A sagittal T2 weighted Magnetic Resonance Image (MRI). Brain is grey, blood vessels frequently appear black, and cerebrospinal fluid is white.

The Brain and Related Structures in MRI

NORMAL	T1	T2
Bone	Very black	Very black
Air	Very black	Very black
Muscle	Dark grey	Dark grey
White matter	Light grey	Dark grey
Grey matter	Dark grey	Light grey
Fat	White	Grey
CSF	Very black	Very white

ABNORMAL	T1	T2
Edema	Dark grey	Light grey to white
Tumor	Variable	Variable
Enhanced tumor	White	(Rarely done)
Acute infarct	Dark grey	Light grey to white
Subacute infarct	Dark grey	Light grey to white
Acute ischemia	Dark grey	Light grey to white
Subacute ischemia	Dark grey	Light grey to white

Chapter 2

This chapter presents 1) the gross anatomy of the spinal cord and its principal arteries; 2) the external morphology of the brain, accompanied by MRIs and drawings of the vasculature patterns from the same perspective; 3) cranial nerves as seen in specimens and in MRI; and 4) the meninges and ventricular spaces. Emphasis is placed on correlating external brain and spinal cord anatomy with the respective vascular patterns and on correlating external brain structures and cranial nerves as seen in specimens with how the same structures appear in MRI. Information concerning the organization of the meninges includes clinical correlations, examples of extradural, so-called "subdural", and subarachnoid hemorrhages in CT and examples of cisterns in MRI. The section showing the structure and relations of the ventricular system now includes samples of hemorrhage into lateral, third, and fourth ventricles.

Chapter 3

The dissections in Chapter 3 offer views of some of those brain structures introduced in Chapter 2. Certain structures and/or structural relationships—for example, the orientation of the larger association bundles—are particularly suited to such a presentation. This chapter uses a representative series of dissected views to provide a broader basis for learning human neuroanatomy. Because it is not feasible to illustrate every anatomic feature, the views and structures selected are those that are usually emphasized in medical neurobiology courses. These views provide basic information necessary to make more detailed dissections, if appropriate, in a particular learning situation.

Chapter 4

The study of general morphology of the hemisphere and brainstem is continued in the two sections of Chapter 4. The first section contains a representative series of unstained coronal slices of brain, each of which is accompanied, *on the same page,* by MRIs. The brain slice is labeled (by complete names), and the MRIs are labeled with a corresponding abbreviation. The second section contains a series of unstained brain slices cut in the axial plane, each of which is accompanied, again *on the same page,* by MRIs. Labeling of the axial slices is as done for the coronal slices.

The similarities between the brain slices and the MRIs are remarkable, and this style of presentation closely integrates anatomy in the slice with that as seen in the corresponding MRI. Because the brain, as sectioned at autopsy or in clinical pathologic conferences, is viewed as an unstained specimen, the preference here is to present the material in a format that will most closely parallel what is seen in these clinical situations.

Chapter 5

This chapter has been revised with special emphasis on increasing the correlation between anatomical and clinical information. This new edition retains the quality and inherent strengths of the line drawings and the stained sections being located on facing pages in this chapter. However, an innovative approach (described below) is introduced that allows the use of these images in their classic Anatomical Orientation and, at the same time, their conversion to the Clinical Orientation so universally recognized and used in clinical imaging techniques.

Chapter 5 consists of six sections covering, in sequence, the spinal cord, medulla oblongata, cerebellar nuclei, pons, midbrain, and diencephalon and basal nuclei, all with MRI. In this format, the right-hand page contains a complete image of the stained section. The left-hand page contains a labeled line drawing of the stained section, accompanied by a figure description, and a small orientation drawing. The section part of the line drawing is printed in a 60% screen of black, and the leader lines and labels are printed at 100% black. This gives the illustration a sense of depth and texture, reduces competition between lines, and makes the illustration easy to read at a glance.

Beginning with the first spinal cord level (coccygeal, Figure 5-1), the long tracts that are most essential to understanding how to diagnose the neurologically impaired patient are colored. These tracts are the posterior column–medial lemniscus system, the lateral corticospinal tract, and the anterolateral system. In the brainstem, these tracts are joined by the colorized spinal trigeminal tract, the ventral trigeminothalamic tract, and all of the motor and sensory

nuclei of cranial nerves. This scheme continues rostrally into the caudal nuclei of the dorsal thalamus and the posterior limb of the internal capsule. In addition to the coloring of the artwork, each page has a key that specifies the structure and function of each colored structure. This approach emphasizes anatomical–clinical integration.

Semidiagrammatic representations of the internal blood supply to the spinal cord, medulla, pons, midbrain, and forebrain follow each set of line drawings and stained sections. This allows the immediate, and convenient, correlation of structure with its blood supply as one is studying the internal anatomy of the neuraxis. In addition, *tables that summarize the vascular syndromes of the spinal cord, medulla, pons, midbrain, and forebrain* are located on the pages facing each of these vascular drawings. While learning or reviewing the internal blood supply to these parts of the neuraxis, one can also correlate the deficits seen when the same vessels are occluded. It is essential to successful diagnosis to develop a good understanding of what structure is served by what vessel.

The diencephalon and basal nuclei section of this chapter uses ten cross-sections to illustrate internal anatomy. *It should be emphasized that 8 of these 10 sections (those parallel to each other) are all from the same brain.*

The internal anatomy of the brainstem is commonly taught in an anatomical orientation. That is, posterior structures, such as the vestibular nuclei and colliculi, are "up" in the image, while anterior structures, such as the pyramid and crus cerebri, are "down" in the image. However, when the brainstem is viewed in the clinical setting, as in CT or MRI, this orientation is reversed. In the clinical orientation, posterior structures (4th ventricle, colliculi) are "down" in the image while anterior structures (pyramid, basilar pons, crus cerebri) are "up" in the image.

Recognizing that many users of this book are pursuing a health care career (as a practitioner or teacher of future clinicians), it is essential to introduce MRI and CT of the brainstem into chapter 5. This accomplishes two important points. First, it allows correlation of the size, shape, and configuration of brainstem sections (line drawings and stained slices) with MRI and CT at comparable levels. Second, it offers the user the opportunity to visualize how nuclei, tracts (and their somatotopy) and vascular territories are represented in MRI and CT. Understanding the brain in the Clinical Orientation (as seen in MRI or CT) is extremely important in diagnosis. To successfully introduce MRI and CT in the brainstem portion of chapter 5, a continuum from Anatomical Orientation to Clinical Orientation to MRI needs to be clearly illustrated. This is achieved by 1) placing a small version of the colorized line drawing on the facing page (page with the stained section) in Anatomical Orientation; 2) showing how this image is flipped top to bottom into a Clinical Orientation; and 3) following this flipped image with (usually) T1 and T2 MRIs at levels comparable to the accompanying line drawing and stained section (Fig. 1-4). This approach retains the anatomical strengths of the spinal cord and brainstem sections of chapter 5 but allows the introduction of important concepts regarding how anatomical information is arranged in images utilized in the clinical environment.

Every effort has been made to use MRI and CT that match, as closely as possible, the line drawings and stained sections in the spinal cord and brainstem portions of chapter 5. Recognizing that this match is subject to the vicissitudes of angle and individual variation, special sets of images were used in chapter 5. The first set consisted of T1- and T2-weighted MRI generated from the same individual; these are identified, respectively, as "MRI, T1-weighted" and "MRI, T2-weighted" in chapter 5. The second set consisted of CT images from a patient who had an injection of the radiopaque contrast media Isovue-M^R 200 (iopamidol injection 41 %) into the lumbar cistern. This contrast media diffused throughout the spinal and cranial subarachnoid spaces, outlining the spinal cord and brainstem (Fig. 1-5). Images at spinal levels show neural structures as grey surrounded by a light subarachnoid space; this is a "CT myelogram". A comparable image at brainstem levels (grey brain, light CSF) is a "CT cisternogram". These designations are used in chapter 5. While all matches are not perfect, not all things in life or medicine are, the vast majority of matches between MRI, CT, and drawings/sections are excellent and clearly demonstrate the intended points.

Anatomical orientation   Clinical orientation

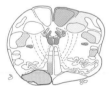

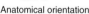

MRI, T1 weighted image

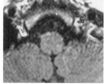

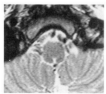

MRI, T2 weighted image

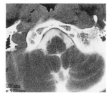

CT cisternogram

1-4 An example showing anatomical and clinical orientations of a brainstem level and the corresponding T1 MRI, T2 MRI, and CT cisternogram. For additional examples and details see chapter 5, pages 84–133.

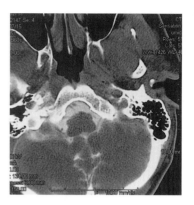

1-5 Computed Tomography (CT) of a patient following injection of a radiopaque contrast media into the lumbar cistern. In this example, at the medullary level (a cisternogram), neural structures appear grey and the subarachnoid space appears light.

The juxtaposition of MRI to stained section extends into the forebrain portion of chapter 5. Many anatomic features seen in the forebrain stained sections are easily identified in the adjacent MRI. These particular MRI are not labeled so as to allow the user to develop and practice his/her interpretive skills. The various subsections of chapter 5 can be used in a variety of ways and will accommodate a wide range of student and/or instructor preferences.

Chapter 6

The three-dimensional anatomy of internal structures in the CNS can also be studied in stained sections that correlate similar structures in different planes. The photographs of stained axial and sagittal sections and of MRIs in Chapter 6 are organized to provide four important levels of information. First, the *general* internal anatomy of brain structures can be easily identified in each photograph. Second, axial photographs are on left-hand pages and arranged from dorsal to ventral (Figures 6-1 to 6-9), whereas sagittal photographs are on right-hand pages and arranged from medial to lateral (Figures 6-2 to 6-10). This setup, in essence, provides complete representation of the brain in *both* planes for use as independent study sets (axial only, sagittal only) or as integrated/correlated sets (compare facing pages). Third, because axial and sagittal sections are on facing pages *and* the plane of section of each is indicated on its companion by a heavy line, the reader can easily visualize the positions of internal structures in more than one plane and develop a clear concept of three-dimensional topography. In other words, one can identify structures dorsal or ventral to the axial plane by comparing them with the sagittal, and structures medial or lateral to the sagittal plane by comparing them with the axial. Such comparisons facilitate a more full understanding of three-dimensional relationships in the brain. Fourth, the inclusion of MRIs with representative axial and sagittal stained sections provides excellent examples of the fact that structures seen in the teaching laboratory are easy to recognize in clinical images.

These MRIs are also not labeled so as to allow the user to develop his/her interpretive skills.

Chapter 7

This chapter provides summaries of a variety of clinically relevant CNS tracts and/or pathways and has four features that enhance student understanding. First, the inclusion of pathway information in atlas format broadens the basis one can use to teach functional neurobiology. This is especially the case when pathways are presented in a style that enhances the development of diagnostic skills. Second, each drawing illustrates, in line color, a given pathway completely, showing its 1) origins, longitudinal extent, course throughout the neuraxis and termination; 2) laterality—an all-important issue in diagnosis; 3) point of decussation, if applicable; 4) position in representative cross sections of the brainstem and spinal cord; and 5) the somatotopic organization of fibers within the pathway, if applicable. The blood supply to each pathway is reviewed on the facing page. Third, a brief summary mentions the main neuroactive substances associated with cells and fibers composing particular segments of the pathway under consideration. The action of the substance, if widely agreed on, is indicated as excitatory (+) or inhibitory (−). *This allows the reader to closely correlate a particular neurotransmitter with a specific population of projection neurons and their terminals.* The limitations of this approach, within the confines of an atlas, are self-evident. The transmitters associated with some pathways are not well known; consequently, such information is not provided for some connections. Also, no attempt is made to identify substances that may be colocalized, to discuss their synthesis or degradation, or to mention *all* neurotransmitters associated with a particular cell group. The goal here is to introduce the reader to selected neurotransmitters and to *integrate* and *correlate* this information with a particular pathway, circuit, or connection. Fourth, *the clinical correlations that accompany each pathway drawing provide examples of deficits resulting from lesions, at various levels in the neuraxis, of the fibers composing that specific pathway.* Also, examples are given of syndromes or diseases in which these deficits are seen. The ways in which these clinical correlations can be used to enrich the learning process are described in Figure 7-3 on page 176.

The drawings in this section were designed to provide the maximum amount of information, to keep the extraneous points to a minimum, and to do it all in a single, easy-to-follow illustration. A complete range of relevant information is contained in each drawing and in its description as explained in the second point above.

Because it is not possible to anticipate *all* pathways that may be taught in a wide range of neurobiology courses, flexibility has been designed into Chapter 7. The last figure in each section is a blank master drawing that follows the same general format as the preceding figures. Photocopies of these blank master drawings can be used by the student for learning and/or review of any pathway and by the instructor to teach additional pathways not included in the atlas or as a substrate for examination questions. The flexibility of information as presented in Chapter 7 extends equally to student and instructor.

Chapter 8

This chapter contains a series of angiograms (arterial and venous phases), magnetic resonance angiography (MRA) images, and magnetic resonance venography (MRV) images. The angiograms are shown in lateral and anterior–posterior projections—some as standard views with corresponding digital subtraction images. MRA and MRV technology are noninvasive methods that allow for the visualization of arteries (MRA) and veins and venous sinuses (MRV). There are, however, many situations when both arteries and veins are seen with either method. Use of MRA and MRV is commonplace, and this technology is an important diagnostic tool. A number of new vascular images have been included in this revised version of Chapter 8.

Chapter 9

A primary goal in the study of functional human neurobiology is to become a competent health care professional. Another, and equally significant, goal is to pass examinations. These may be course examinations, the National Board Subject Exam (some courses require these), or standardized tests, such as the USMLE Step 1 and Step 2, given at key intervals and taken by all students.

The questions comprising chapter 9 were generated in the recognition that examinations are an essential part of the educational process. Whenever possible, and practical, these questions are in the USMLE Step 1 style (single best answer). These questions emphasize 1) anatomical and clinical concepts and correlations; 2) the application of basic human neurobiology to medical practice; and 3) how neurological deficits and diseases relate to damage in specific parts of the nervous system. In general, the questions are grouped by chapter. However, in some instances, questions draw on information provided in more than one chapter. This is sometimes essential in an effort to make appropriate structural/functional/clinical correlations. At the end of each group of questions the correct answers are provided and explained. Included with the explanation is a reference to the page (or pages) containing the answer, be that answer in the text or in a figure. Although not exhaustive, this list of questions should provide the user of this atlas with an excellent opportunity for self-assessment covering a broad range of clinically relevant topics.

Rationale for Labels and Abbreviations

No universally accepted way to identify specific features or structures in drawings or photographs exists. The variety of methods seen in currently available atlases reflects the personal preferences of the authors. Such is the case in the present endeavor. The goal of this atlas is to present basic functional and clinical neuroanatomy in an understandable and useful format.

Among currently available atlases, most figures are labeled with either the complete names of structures or with numbers or letters that are keyed to a list of the complete names. The first method immediately imparts the greatest amount of information; the second method is the most succinct. When using the complete names of structures, one must exercise care to not compromise the quality or size of the illustration, the number of structures labeled, or the size of labels used. Although the use of single letters or numbers results in minimal clutter on the figure, a *major* drawback is the fact that the same number or letter may appear on several different figures and designate different structures in all cases. Consequently, no consistency occurs between numbers and letters and their corresponding meanings as the reader examines different figures. This atlas uses a combination of complete words and abbreviations that are clearly recognized versions of the complete word.

In response to suggestions made by those using this book over the years, the number of abbreviations in the sixth edition has been reduced, and the number of labels using the complete name has been increased. Simultaneously, complete names and abbreviations have been used together in some chapters to the full advantage of each method. For example, structures are labeled on a brain slice by the complete name, but the same structure in the accompanying MRI is labeled with a corresponding abbreviation (see Chapters 2 and 4). This uses the complete word(s) on the larger image of a brain structure while using the shorter abbreviation on the smaller image of the MRI.

The abbreviations used in this atlas do not clutter the illustration; they permit labeling of all relevant structures and are adequately informative while stimulating the thinking–learning process. The abbreviations are, in a very real sense, mnemonics. When learning gyri and sulci of the occipital lobe, for example, one realizes that the abbreviation "LinGy" in the atlas could only mean "lingual gyrus." It could not be confused with other structures in other parts of the nervous system. Regarding the pathways, "RuSp" could mean only "rubrospinal tract" and "LenFas," the "lenticular fasciculus." As the reader learns more and more terminology from lectures and readings, he or she will be able to use these abbreviations with minimal reference to the accompanying list. In addition, a subtle advantage of this method of labeling is that, as the reader looks at the abbreviation and momentarily pauses to ponder its meaning, he or she may form a mental image of the structure *and* the complete word. Because neuroanatomy requires one to conceptualize and form mental images to more clearly understand CNS relationships, this method seems especially useful.

References:

Bruxton, RB. *Introduction to Functional Magnetic Resonance Imaging, Principles and Techniques.* Cambridge: Cambridge University Press, 2002.

Grossman, CB. *Magnetic Resonance Imaging and Computed Tomography of the Head and Spine.* 2nd Ed. Baltimore: Williams & Wilkins, 1996.

Lee, SH, Roa, KCVG, and Zimmerman, RA. *Cranial MRI and CT.* 4th Ed. New York: McGraw-Hill Health Professions Division, 1999.

External Morphology
of the
Central Nervous System

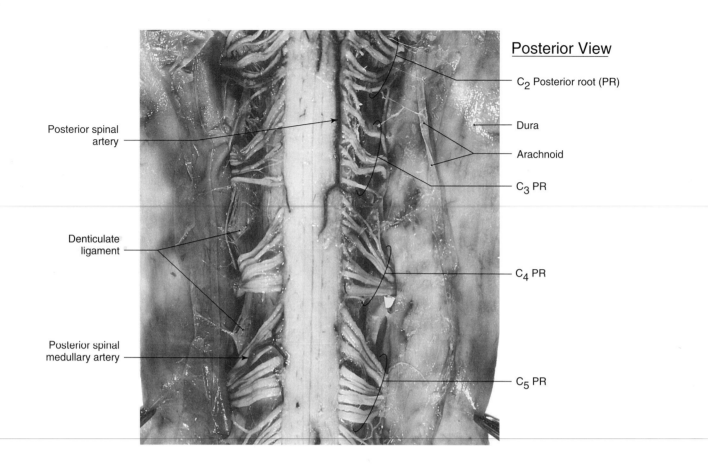

Posterior View

Posterior spinal artery

Denticulate ligament

Posterior spinal medullary artery

C₂ Posterior root (PR)

Dura

Arachnoid

C₃ PR

C₄ PR

C₅ PR

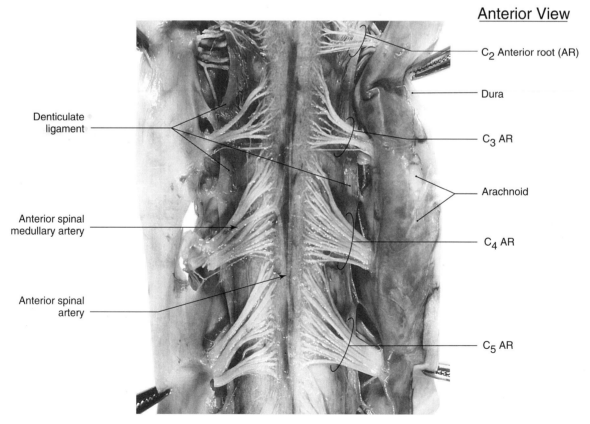

Anterior View

Denticulate ligament

Anterior spinal medullary artery

Anterior spinal artery

C₂ Anterior root (AR)

Dura

C₃ AR

Arachnoid

C₄ AR

C₅ AR

2-1   Posterior (upper) and anterior (lower) views showing the general features of the spinal cord as seen at levels C₂–C₅. The dura and arachnoid are reflected, and the pia is intimately adherent to the spinal cord and rootlets. Posterior and anterior spinal medullary arteries (see Figure 2-3 on facing page) follow their respective roots. The posterior spinal artery is found medial to the entering posterior rootlets (and the dorsolateral sulcus), while the anterior spinal artery is in the anterior median fissure (see also Figure 2-2, facing page).

Posterior View

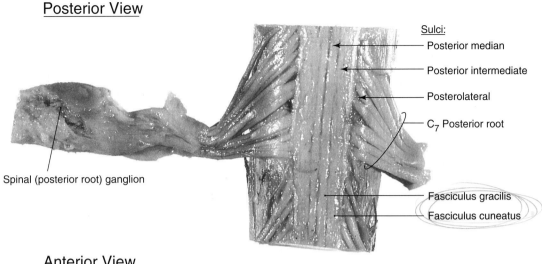

Sulci:
- Posterior median
- Posterior intermediate
- Posterolateral

C_7 Posterior root

Spinal (posterior root) ganglion

Fasciculus gracilis
Fasciculus cuneatus

Anterior View

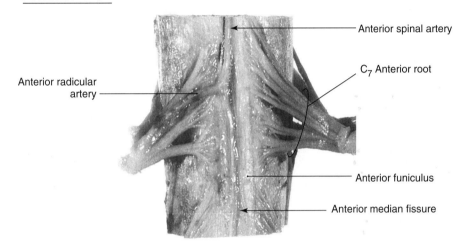

Anterior spinal artery

C_7 Anterior root

Anterior radicular artery

Anterior funiculus

Anterior median fissure

2-2   Posterior (upper) and anterior (lower) views showing details of the spinal cord as seen in the C_7 segment. The posterior (dorsal) root ganglion is partially covered by dura and connective tissue.

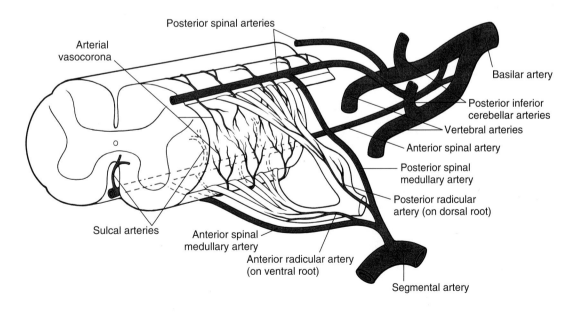

Posterior spinal arteries

Arterial vasocorona

Basilar artery

Posterior inferior cerebellar arteries

Vertebral arteries

Anterior spinal artery

Posterior spinal medullary artery

Posterior radicular artery (on dorsal root)

Sulcal arteries

Anterior spinal medullary artery

Anterior radicular artery (on ventral root)

Segmental artery

2-3   Semidiagrammatic representation showing the origin and general location of principal arteries supplying the spinal cord. The *anterior and posterior radicular arteries* arise at every spinal level and serve their respective roots and ganglion. The *anterior and posterior spinal medullary arteries* (also called medullary feeder arteries or segmental medullary arteries) arise at intermittent levels and serve to augment the blood supply to the spinal cord. The artery of Adamkiewicz is an unusually large spinal medullary artery arising usually on the left in low thoracic or upper lumbar levels (T_9–L_1). The arterial vasocorona is a diffuse anastomotic plexus covering the cord surface.

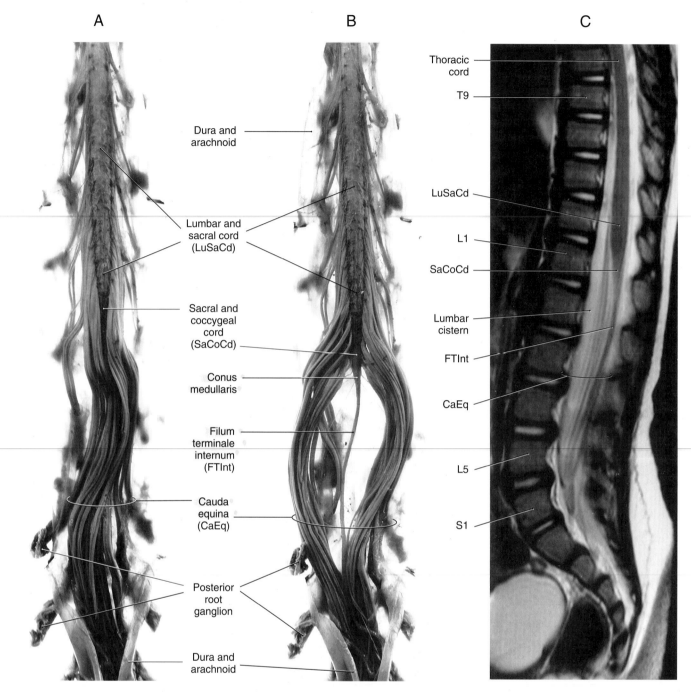

A   B   C

Dura and arachnoid

Lumbar and sacral cord (LuSaCd)

Sacral and coccygeal cord (SaCoCd)

Conus medullaris

Filum terminale internum (FTInt)

Cauda equina (CaEq)

Posterior root ganglion

Dura and arachnoid

Thoracic cord

T9

LuSaCd

L1

SaCoCd

Lumbar cistern

FTInt

CaEq

L5

S1

2-4   Overall posterior (**A,B**) and sagittal MRI (**C,** T2-weighted) views of the lower thoracic, lumbar, sacral, and coccygeal spinal cord segments and the cauda equina. The dura and arachnoid are retracted in **A** and **B.** The cauda equina is shown in situ in **A,** and in **B** the nerve roots of the cauda equina have been spread laterally to expose the conus medullaris and filum terminale internum. This latter structure is also called the pial part of the filum terminale. See Figures 5-1 and 5-2 on pages 84–87 for cross-sectional views of the cauda equina.

In the sagittal MRI (**C**), the lower portions of the cord, the filum terminale internum, and cauda equina are clearly seen. In addition, the intervertebral discs and the bodies of the vertebrae are clear. The lumbar cistern is an enlarged part of the subarachnoid space caudal to the

end of the spinal cord. This space contains the anterior and posterior roots from the lower part of the spinal cord that collectively form the cauda equina. The filum terminale internum also descends from the conus medullaris through the lumbar cistern to attach to the inner surface of the dural sac. The dural sac ends at about the level of the S2 vertebra and is attached to the coccyx by the filum terminale externum (also see Fig. 2-47 on page 47). A lumbar puncture is made by inserting a large gauge needle (18-22 gauge) between the L3 and L4 vertebra or L4 and L5 vertebra and retrieving a sample of cerebrospinal fluid from the lumbar cistern. This sample may be used for a number of diagnostic procedures.

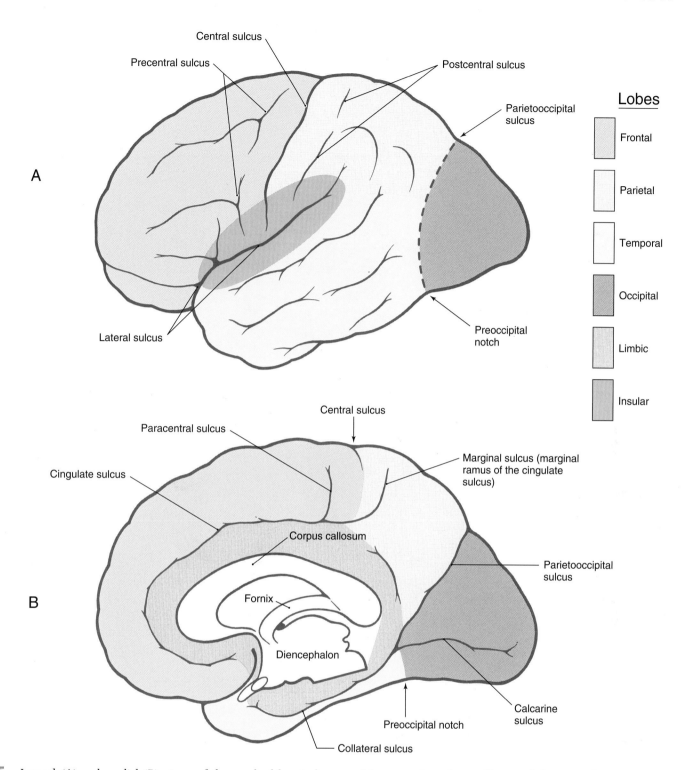

2-5   Lateral (A) and medial (B) views of the cerebral hemisphere showing the landmarks used to divide the cortex into its main lobes.

On the lateral aspect, the central sulcus (of Rolando) separates frontal and parietal lobes. The lateral sulcus (of Sylvius) forms the border between frontal and temporal lobes. The occipital lobe is located caudal to an arbitrary line drawn between the terminus of the parieto-occipital sulcus and the preoccipital notch. A horizontal line drawn from approximately the upper two-thirds of the lateral fissure to the rostral edge of the occipital lobe represents the border between parietal and temporal lobes. The insular cortex (see also Figs. 2-46 on page 45 and 3-1 on page 56) is located internal to the lateral sulcus. This part

of the cortex is made up of long and short gyri that are separated from each other by the central sulcus of the insula. The insula, as a whole, is separated from the adjacent portions of the frontal, parietal, and temporal opercula by the circular sulcus.

On the medial aspect, the cingulate sulcus separates medial portions of frontal and parietal lobes from the limbic lobe. An imaginary continuation of the central sulcus intersects with the cingulate sulcus and forms the border between frontal and parietal lobes. The parieto-occipital sulcus and an arbitrary continuation of this line to the preoccipital notch separate the parietal, limbic, and temporal lobes from the occipital lobe.

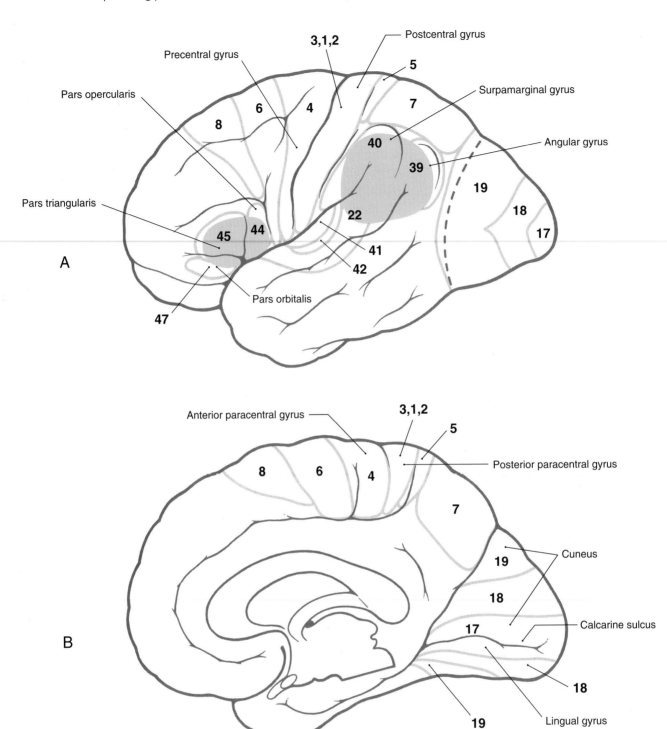

2-6 Lateral **(A)** and medial **(B)** views of the cerebral hemisphere showing the more commonly described Brodmann areas. In general, area 4 comprises the primary somatomotor cortex, areas 3,1, and 2 the primary somatosensory cortex, and area 17 the primary visual cortex. Area 41 is the primary auditory cortex, and the portion of area 6 in the caudal part of the middle frontal gyrus is generally recognized as the frontal eye field.

The inferior frontal gyrus has three portions: a pars opercularis, pars triangularis, and a pars orbitalis. A lesion that is located primarily in areas 44 and 45 (shaded) will give rise to what is called a Broca aphasia, also called expressive or nonfluent aphasia.

The inferior parietal lobule consists of supramarginal (area 40) and angular (area 39) gyri. Lesions in this general area of the cortex (shaded), and sometimes extending into area 22, will give rise to what is known as Wernicke aphasia, also sometimes called receptive or fluent aphasia.

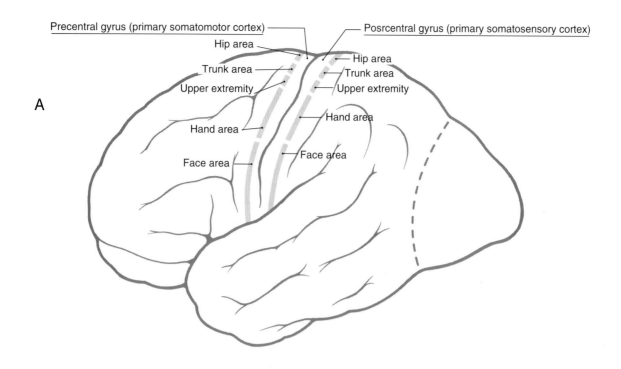

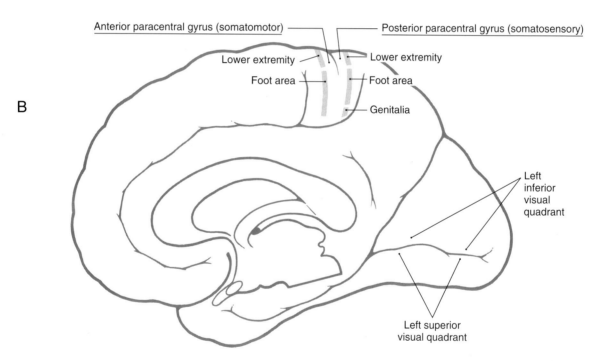

2-7 Lateral **(A)** and medial **(B)** views of the cerebral hemisphere showing the somatotopic organization of the primary somatomotor and somatosensory cortices. The lower extremity and foot areas are located on medial aspects of the hemisphere in the anterior paracentral (motor) and the posterior paracentral (sensory) gyri. The remaining portions of the body extend from the margin of the hemisphere over the convexity to the lateral sulcus in the precentral and postcentral gyri.

In general, the precentral gyrus can be divided into three regions: the lateral third representing the face area, the middle third represent-ing the hand and upper extremity areas, and the medial third representing the trunk and the hip. Lesions of the somatomotor cortex result in motor deficits on the contralateral side of the body while lesions in the somatosensory cortex result in a loss of sensory perception from the contralateral side of the body.

The medial surface of the right hemisphere **(B)** illustrates the position of the left portions of the visual field. The inferior visual quadrant is located in the primary visual cortex above the calcarine sulcus while the superior visual quadrant is found in the cortex below the calcarine sulcus.

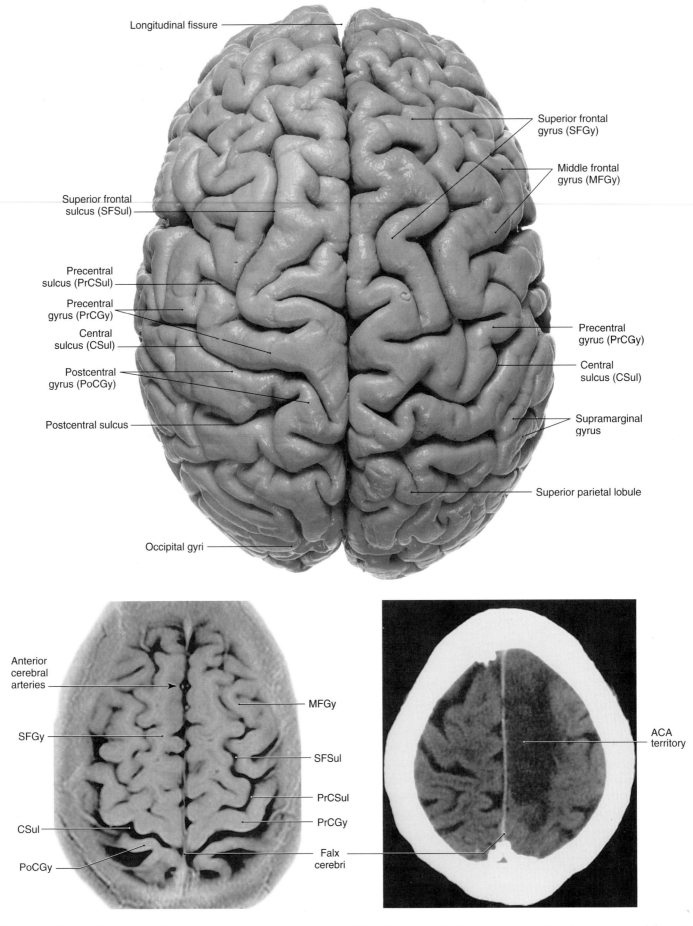

Longitudinal fissure

Superior frontal gyrus (SFGy)

Middle frontal gyrus (MFGy)

Superior frontal sulcus (SFSul)

Precentral sulcus (PrCSul)

Precentral gyrus (PrCGy)

Central sulcus (CSul)

Postcentral gyrus (PoCGy)

Postcentral sulcus

Occipital gyri

Precentral gyrus (PrCGy)

Central sulcus (CSul)

Supramarginal gyrus

Superior parietal lobule

Anterior cerebral arteries

MFGy

SFGy

SFSul

PrCSul

PrCGy

CSul

PoCGy

Falx cerebri

ACA territory

2-8 Dorsal view of the cerebral hemispheres showing the main gyri and sulci and an MRI (inverted inversion recovery—lower left) and a CT (lower right) identifying structures from the same perspective.

Note the area of infarction representing the territory of the anterior cerebral artery (ACA).

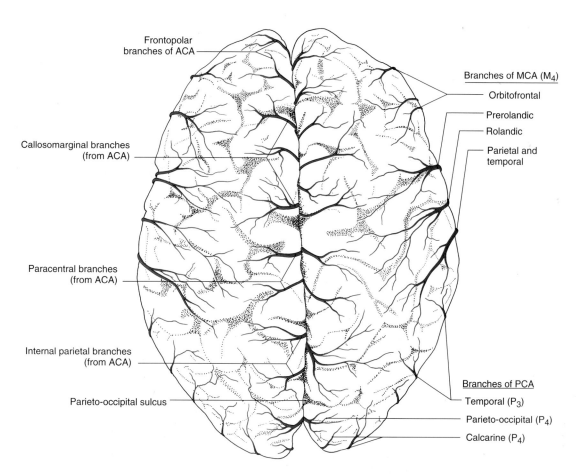

Frontopolar
branches of ACA

Branches of MCA (M₄)

Orbitofrontal

Prerolandic

Rolandic

Parietal and
temporal

Callosomarginal branches
(from ACA)

Paracentral branches
(from ACA)

Internal parietal branches
(from ACA)

Parieto-occipital sulcus

Branches of PCA

Temporal (P₃)

Parieto-occipital (P₄)

Calcarine (P₄)

2-9   Dorsal view of the cerebral hemispheres showing the location and general branching patterns of the anterior (ACA), middle (MCA), and posterior (PCA) cerebral arteries. Gyri and sulci can be identified by a comparison with Figure 2-8 (facing page).

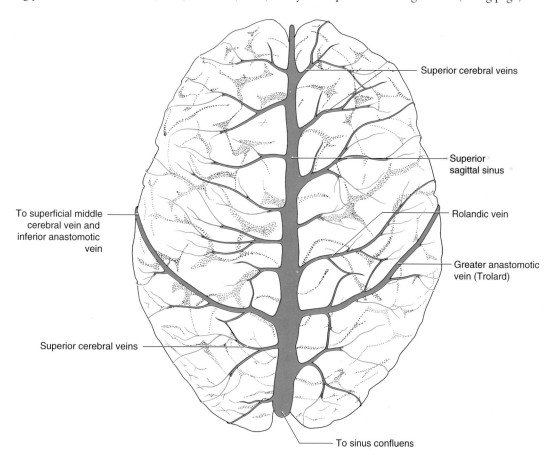

Superior cerebral veins

Superior
sagittal sinus

Rolandic vein

Greater anastomotic
vein (Trolard)

To superficial middle
cerebral vein and
inferior anastomotic
vein

Superior cerebral veins

To sinus confluens

2-10   Dorsal view of the cerebral hemispheres showing the location of the superior sagittal sinus and the locations and general branching patterns of veins. Gyri and sulci can be identified by a comparison with Figure 2-8 (facing page). See Figures 8-4 and 8-5 (pp. 243–244) for comparable angiograms (venous phase) of the superior sagittal sinus.

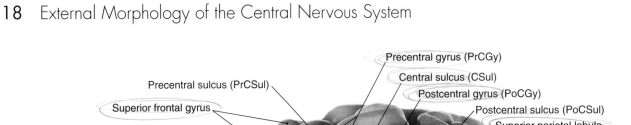

Precentral gyrus (PrCGy)

Central sulcus (CSul)

Postcentral gyrus (PoCGy)

Precentral sulcus (PrCSul)

Postcentral sulcus (PoCSul)

Superior frontal gyrus

Superior parietal lobule

Superior frontal sulcus

Supramarginal gyrus

Interparietal sulcus

Inferior Parietal Lobule

Middle frontal gyrus (MFGy)

Inferior frontal sulcus (IFSul)

Angular gyrus

Inferior frontal gyrus:

Pars opercularis (PoP)

Pars triangularis (PTr)

Pars orbitalis (POrb)

Occipital gyri (OGy)

Lateral sulcus (LatSul)

Superior temporal gyrus (STGy)

Superior temporal sulcus (STSul)

Middle temporal gyrus (MTGy)

Preoccipital notch

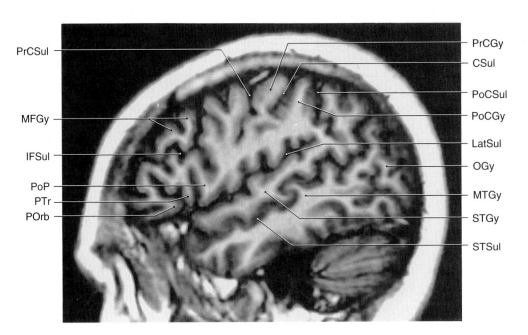

PrCSul

PrCGy

CSul

PoCSul

MFGy

PoCGy

IFSul

LatSul

OGy

PoP

MTGy

PTr

POrb

STGy

STSul

2-11 Lateral view of the left cerebral hemisphere showing the principal gyri and sulci and an MRI (inversion recovery) identifying many of these structures from the same perspective.

All Branches of Middle Cerebral Artery

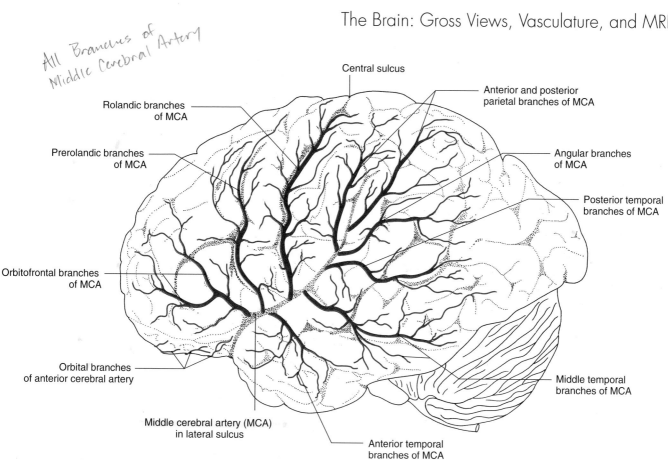

Central sulcus

Rolandic branches of MCA

Anterior and posterior parietal branches of MCA

Prerolandic branches of MCA

Angular branches of MCA

Posterior temporal branches of MCA

Orbitofrontal branches of MCA

Orbital branches of anterior cerebral artery

Middle temporal branches of MCA

Middle cerebral artery (MCA) in lateral sulcus

Anterior temporal branches of MCA

2-12   Lateral view of the right cerebral hemisphere showing the branching pattern of the middle cerebral artery. Gyri and sulci can be identified by comparison with Figure 2-11 (facing page). The middle cerebral artery initially branches in the depths of the lateral sulcus (as M_2 and M_3 segments); these branches seen on the surface of the hemi-sphere represent the M_4 segment. Terminal branches of the posterior and anterior cerebral arteries course over the edges of the temporal and occipital lobes, and parietal and frontal lobes, respectively (see Figure 2-9 on page 17). See Figure 8-1 (p. 240) for a comparable angiogram of the middle and anterior cerebral arteries.

Bridging Vein

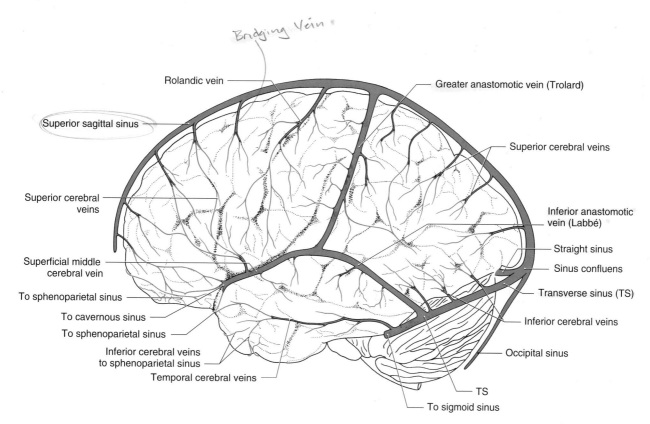

Rolandic vein

Greater anastomotic vein (Trolard)

Superior sagittal sinus

Superior cerebral veins

Superior cerebral veins

Inferior anastomotic vein (Labbé)

Straight sinus

Superficial middle cerebral vein

Sinus confluens

To sphenoparietal sinus

Transverse sinus (TS)

To cavernous sinus

Inferior cerebral veins

To sphenoparietal sinus

Inferior cerebral veins to sphenoparietal sinus

Occipital sinus

Temporal cerebral veins

TS

To sigmoid sinus

2-13   Lateral view of the right cerebral hemisphere showing the lo-cations of sinuses and the locations and general branching patterns of veins. Gyri and sulci can be identified by comparison with Figure 2-11 (facing page). Communications between veins and sinuses or between sinuses are also indicated. See Figures 8-2 (p. 241) and 8-11 (p. 250) for comparable angiogram and MRV of the sinuses and superficial veins.

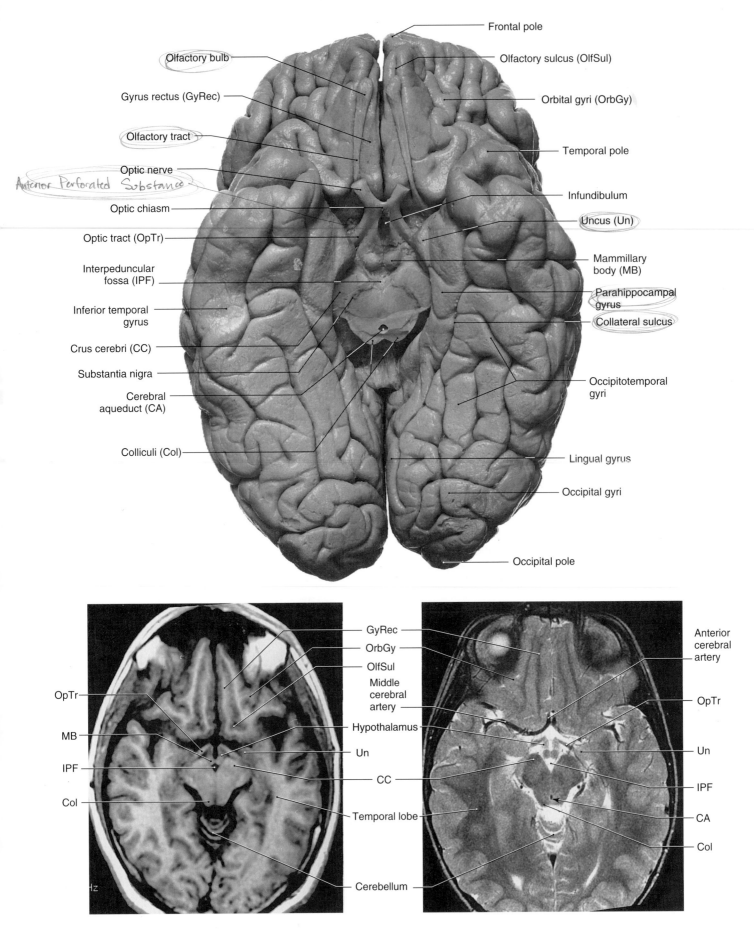

Frontal pole

Olfactory bulb

Olfactory sulcus (OlfSul)

Gyrus rectus (GyRec)

Orbital gyri (OrbGy)

Olfactory tract

Optic nerve

Temporal pole

Anterior Perforated Substance

Infundibulum

Optic chiasm

Uncus (Un)

Optic tract (OpTr)

Mammillary body (MB)

Interpeduncular fossa (IPF)

Parahippocampal gyrus

Inferior temporal gyrus

Collateral sulcus

Crus cerebri (CC)

Substantia nigra

Occipitotemporal gyri

Cerebral aqueduct (CA)

Colliculi (Col)

Lingual gyrus

Occipital gyri

Occipital pole

GyRec

Anterior cerebral artery

OrbGy

OlfSul

Middle cerebral artery

OpTr

Hypothalamus

MB

Un

IPF

Un

CC

CA

Col

Temporal lobe

Col

Cerebellum

OpTr

2-14 Ventral view of the cerebral hemispheres and diencephalon with the brainstem caudal to midbrain removed and two MRIs (inversion recovery—lower left; T2-weighted—lower right) showing many structures from the same perspective.

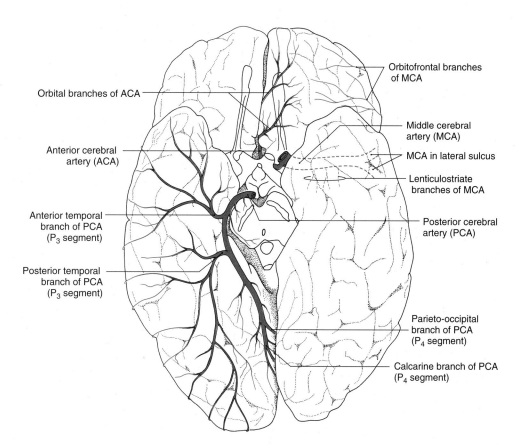

Orbital branches of ACA

Anterior cerebral
artery (ACA)

Anterior temporal
branch of PCA
(P₃ segment)

Posterior temporal
branch of PCA
(P₃ segment)

Orbitofrontal branches
of MCA

Middle cerebral
artery (MCA)

MCA in lateral sulcus

Lenticulostriate
branches of MCA

Posterior cerebral
artery (PCA)

Parieto-occipital
branch of PCA
(P₄ segment)

Calcarine branch of PCA
(P₄ segment)

2-15 Ventral view of the cerebral hemisphere with the brainstem removed, which shows the branching pattern of the posterior cerebral artery (PCA) and some branches of the anterior and middle cerebral arteries. The P₁ and P₂ segments of the PCA are shown on Figure 2-21 on page 25. Shown here are P₃ (origin of temporal arteries) and P₄ (origin of calcarine and parietooccipital arteries) segments. Gyri and sulci can be identified by comparison with Figure 2-14 (facing page).

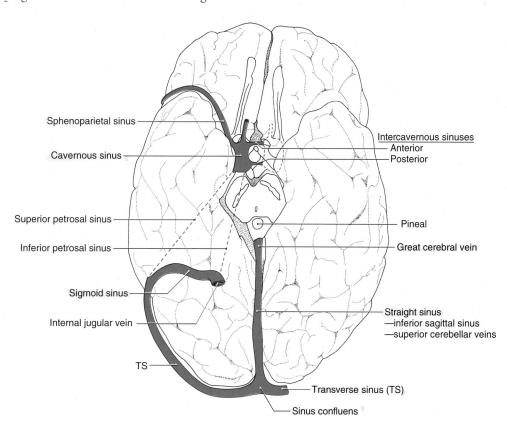

Sphenoparietal sinus

Cavernous sinus

Superior petrosal sinus

Inferior petrosal sinus

Sigmoid sinus

Internal jugular vein

TS

Intercavernous sinuses
Anterior
Posterior

Pineal

Great cerebral vein

Straight sinus
—inferior sagittal sinus
—superior cerebellar veins

Transverse sinus (TS)

Sinus confluens

2-16 Ventral view of the cerebral hemisphere, with brainstem removed, showing the locations and relationships of the main sinuses. Gyri and sulci can be identified by comparison with Figure 2-14 (facing page). The listings preceded by an en-dash (–) under principal sinuses are the main tributaries of that sinus. See Figures 8-5 (p. 245), 8–9 (p. 248), and 8–11 (p. 250) for comparable MRV of the transverse sinus.

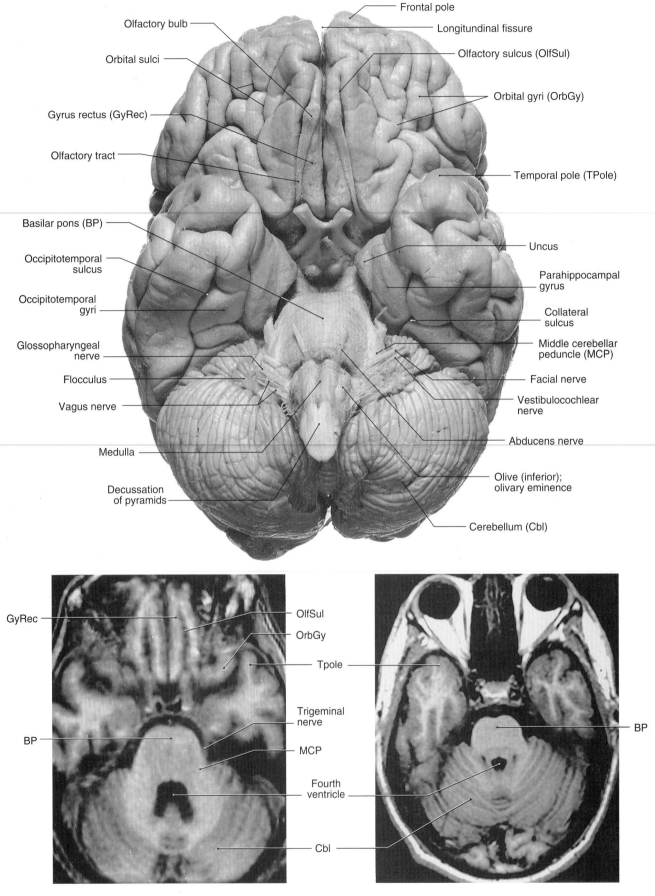

2-17   Ventral view of the cerebral hemispheres, diencephalon, brainstem, and cerebellum and two MRIs (both T1-weighted images) that shows structures from the same perspective. A detailed view of the ventral aspect of the brainstem is seen in Figure 2-20 on page 24.

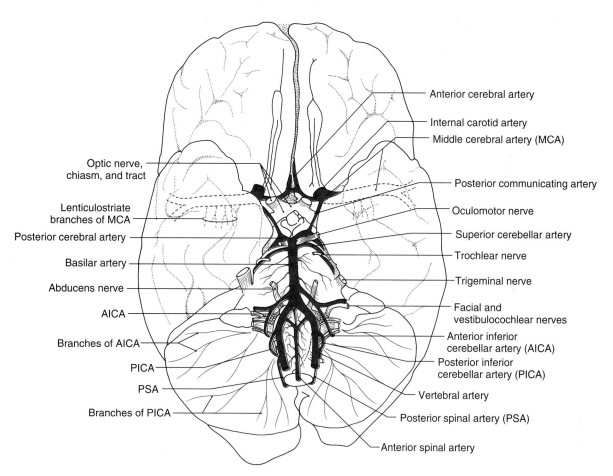

Anterior cerebral artery

Internal carotid artery

Middle cerebral artery (MCA)

Posterior communicating artery

Oculomotor nerve

Superior cerebellar artery

Trochlear nerve

Trigeminal nerve

Facial and
vestibulocochlear nerves

Anterior inferior
cerebellar artery (AICA)

Posterior inferior
cerebellar artery (PICA)

Vertebral artery

Posterior spinal artery (PSA)

Anterior spinal artery

Optic nerve,
chiasm, and tract

Lenticulostriate
branches of MCA

Posterior cerebral artery

Basilar artery

Abducens nerve

AICA

Branches of AICA

PICA

PSA

Branches of PICA

2-18 Ventral view of the cerebral hemispheres, diencephalon, brainstem, and cerebellum, which shows the arterial patterns created by the internal carotid and vertebrobasilar systems. Note the cerebral arterial circle (of Willis). Gyri and sulci can be identified by comparison with Figure 2-17 (facing page). Details of the cerebral arterial circle and the vertebrobasilar arterial pattern are shown in Figure 2-21 on page 25. See Figure 8-9 and 8-10 (pp. 248–249) for comparable MRA of the cerebral arterial circle and its major branches.

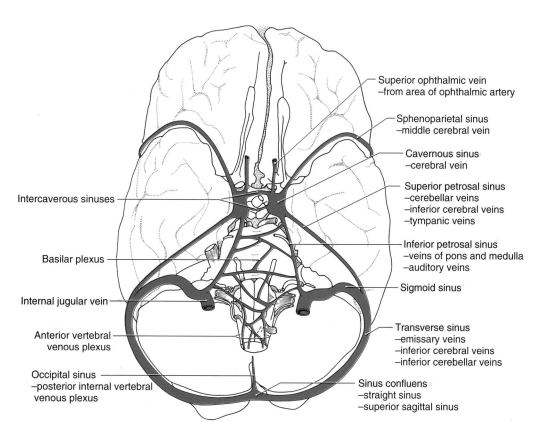

Superior ophthalmic vein
–from area of ophthalmic artery

Sphenoparietal sinus
–middle cerebral vein

Cavernous sinus
–cerebral vein

Superior petrosal sinus
–cerebellar veins
–inferior cerebral veins
–tympanic veins

Inferior petrosal sinus
–veins of pons and medulla
–auditory veins

Sigmoid sinus

Transverse sinus
–emissary veins
–inferior cerebral veins
–inferior cerebellar veins

Sinus confluens
–straight sinus
–superior sagittal sinus

Intercaverous sinuses

Basilar plexus

Internal jugular vein

Anterior vertebral
venous plexus

Occipital sinus
–posterior internal vertebral
venous plexus

2-19 Ventral view of the cerebral hemispheres, diencephalon, brainstem, and cerebellum showing the locations and relationships of principal sinuses and veins. The listings preceded by a dash (–) under principal sinuses are the main tributaries of that sinus.

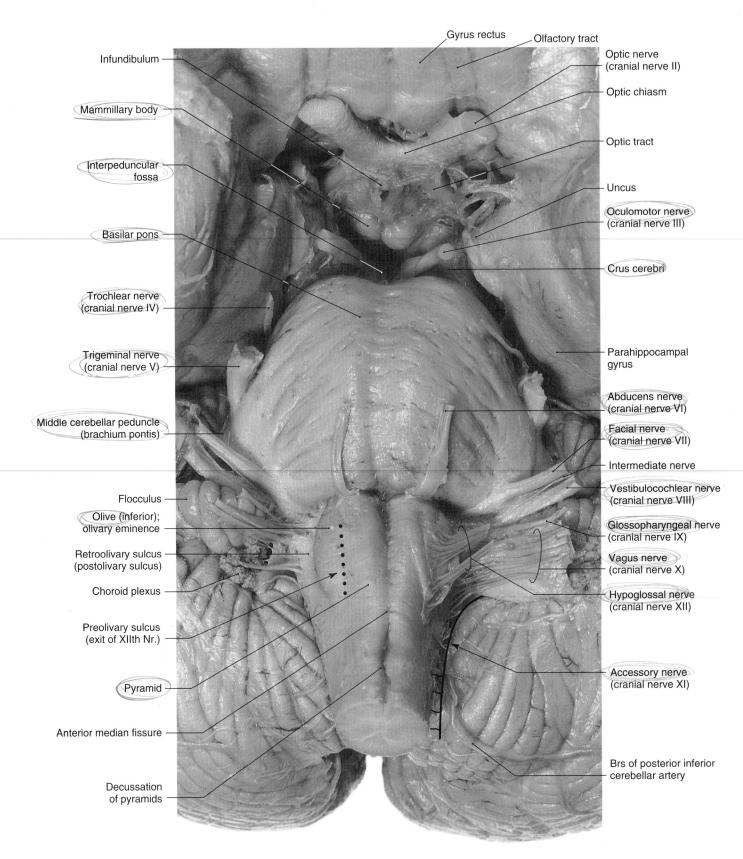

Gyrus rectus

Olfactory tract

Infundibulum

Mammillary body

Interpeduncular fossa

Basilar pons

Trochlear nerve (cranial nerve IV)

Trigeminal nerve (cranial nerve V)

Middle cerebellar peduncle (brachium pontis)

Flocculus

Olive (inferior); olivary eminence

Retroolivary sulcus (postolivary sulcus)

Choroid plexus

Preolivary sulcus (exit of XIIth Nr.)

Pyramid

Anterior median fissure

Decussation of pyramids

Optic nerve (cranial nerve II)

Optic chiasm

Optic tract

Uncus

Oculomotor nerve (cranial nerve III)

Crus cerebri

Parahippocampal gyrus

Abducens nerve (cranial nerve VI)

Facial nerve (cranial nerve VII)

Intermediate nerve

Vestibulocochlear nerve (cranial nerve VIII)

Glossopharyngeal nerve (cranial nerve IX)

Vagus nerve (cranial nerve X)

Hypoglossal nerve (cranial nerve XII)

Accessory nerve (cranial nerve XI)

Brs of posterior inferior cerebellar artery

2-20 Detailed ventral view of the diencephalon and brainstem with particular emphasis on cranial nerves and related structures. The dots on the left side represent the approximate position of the roots of the hypoglossal nerve on that side; the general position of the (spinal) accessory nerve is shown on the right by the dark line.

Vessels

Medial striate artery

Anterior communicating artery

Anterior cerebral artery ⎡ A2
⎣ A1

Posterior communicating artery

Ophthalmic artery

Internal carotid artery

Uncal artery

Anterior and polar temporal arteries

Middle cerebral artery

M1
M2

Lenticulostriate arteries

Anterior choroidal artery

Posterior cerebral artery ⎡ P1
⎣ P2

Posterior choroidal arteries

Quadrigeminal artery

Superior cerebellar artery

Pontine arteries

Basilar artery

Anterior inferior cerebellar artery

Labyrinthine artery

Posterior inferior cerebellar artery

Posterior spinal artery

Vertebral artery

Anterior spinal artery

Structures

Olfactory tract

Optic chiasm

Optic nerve

Anterior perforated substance

Optic tract

Mammillary body

Infundibulum

Crus cerebri

Oculomotor nerve (III)

Trochlear nerve (IV)

Basilar pons

Trigeminal nerve (V)

Abducens nerve (VI)

Facial nerve (VII)

Middle cerebellar peduncle

Vestibulocochlear nerve (VIII)

Choroid plexus

Glossopharyngeal nerve (IX)

Vagus nerve (X)

Accessory nerve (XI)

Hypoglossal nerve (XII)

Olive (inferior); olivary eminence

Cerebellum

Pyramid

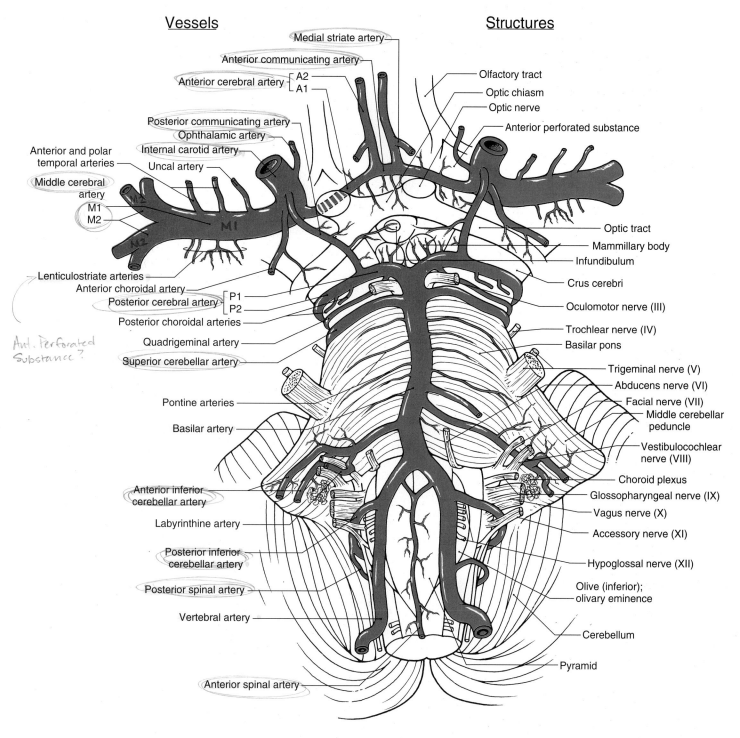

Ant. Perforated Substance?

2-21 Ventral view of the brainstem showing the relationship of brain structures and cranial nerves to the arteries forming the vertebrobasilar system and the cerebral arterial circle (of Willis). The posterior spinal artery usually originates from the posterior inferior cerebellar artery (left), but it may arise from the vertebral (right). Although the labyrinthine artery may occasionally branch from the basilar (right), it most frequently originates from the anterior inferior cerebellar artery (left). Many vessels that arise ventrally course around the brainstem to serve dorsal structures. The anterior cerebral artery consists of A_1 (between the internal carotid bifurcation and the anterior communicating artery) and segments A_2–A_5 which are distal to the anterior communicating artery (see Figure 8-3 on p. 242 for details). Lateral to the internal carotid bifurcation is the M_1 segment of the middle cerebral artery (MCA), which divides and continues as the M_2 segments (branches) on the insular cortex. The M_3 branches of the MCA are those located on the inner surface of the opercula, and the M_4 branches are located on the lateral aspect of the hemisphere. Between the basilar bifurcation and the posterior communicating artery is the P_1 segment of the posterior cerebral artery; P_2 is between the posterior communicator and the first temporal branches. See Figure 8-9, 8-10, and 8-12 (pp. 248, 249, 251) for comparable MRA of the cerebral arterial circle and vertebrobasilar system. See Figure 8-12 on p. 251 for blood supply of the choroid plexus.

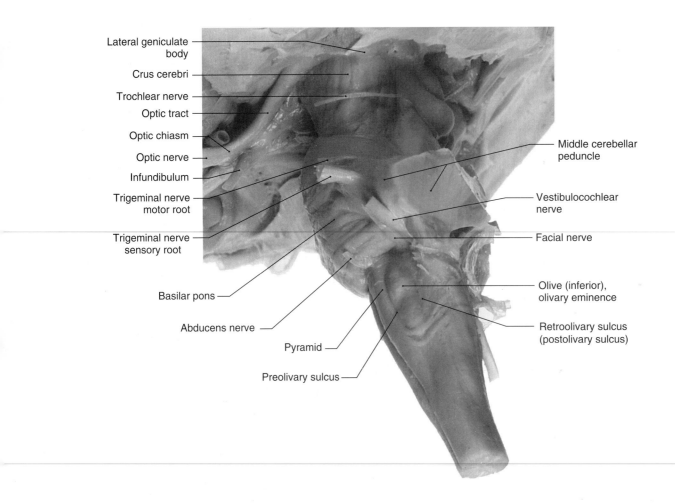

Lateral geniculate body
Crus cerebri
Trochlear nerve
Optic tract
Optic chiasm
Optic nerve
Infundibulum
Trigeminal nerve motor root
Trigeminal nerve sensory root
Basilar pons
Abducens nerve
Pyramid
Preolivary sulcus

Middle cerebellar peduncle
Vestibulocochlear nerve
Facial nerve
Olive (inferior), olivary eminence
Retroolivary sulcus (postolivary sulcus)

2-22   Lateral view of the left side of the brainstem emphasizing structures and cranial nerves on the ventral aspect of the thalamus and brainstem. Compare with Figure 2-24 on the facing page. The cerebellum and portions of the temporal lobe have been removed.

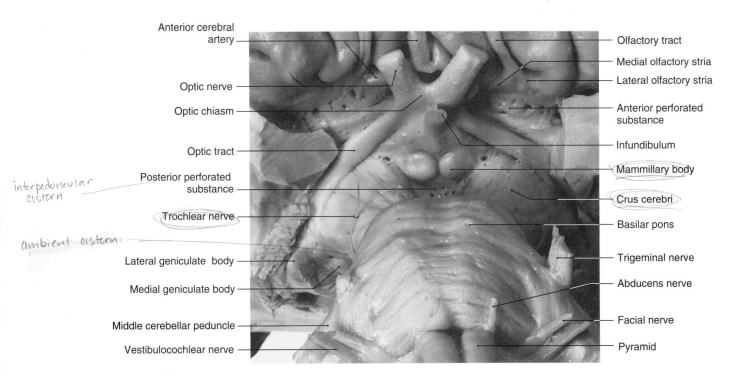

Anterior cerebral artery
Optic nerve
Optic chiasm
Optic tract
Posterior perforated substance
Trochlear nerve
Lateral geniculate body
Medial geniculate body
Middle cerebellar peduncle
Vestibulocochlear nerve

Olfactory tract
Medial olfactory stria
Lateral olfactory stria
Anterior perforated substance
Infundibulum
Mammillary body
Crus cerebri
Basilar pons
Trigeminal nerve
Abducens nerve
Facial nerve
Pyramid

interpeduncular cistern
ambient cistern

2-23   View of the ventral aspect of the diencephalon and part of the brainstem with the medial portions of the temporal lobe removed. Note structures of the hypothalamus, cranial nerves, and optic structures, including the lateral geniculate body.

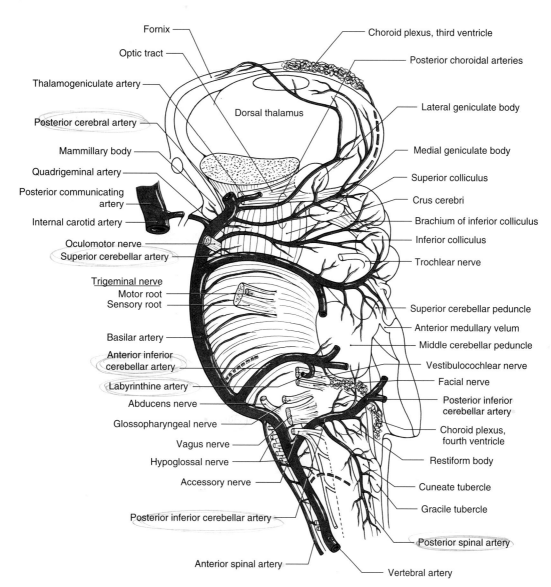

Fornix
Optic tract
Thalamogeniculate artery
Posterior cerebral artery
Mammillary body
Quadrigeminal artery
Posterior communicating artery
Internal carotid artery
Oculomotor nerve
Superior cerebellar artery
Trigeminal nerve
  Motor root
  Sensory root
Basilar artery
Anterior inferior cerebellar artery
Labyrinthine artery
Abducens nerve
Glossopharyngeal nerve
Vagus nerve
Hypoglossal nerve
Accessory nerve
Posterior inferior cerebellar artery
Anterior spinal artery

Dorsal thalamus

Choroid plexus, third ventricle
Posterior choroidal arteries
Lateral geniculate body
Medial geniculate body
Superior colliculus
Crus cerebri
Brachium of inferior colliculus
Inferior colliculus
Trochlear nerve
Superior cerebellar peduncle
Anterior medullary velum
Middle cerebellar peduncle
Vestibulocochlear nerve
Facial nerve
Posterior inferior cerebellar artery
Choroid plexus, fourth ventricle
Restiform body
Cuneate tubercle
Gracile tubercle
Posterior spinal artery
Vertebral artery

2-24   Lateral view of the brainstem and thalamus showing the relationship of structures and cranial nerves to arteries. Arteries that serve dorsal structures originate from ventrally located parent vessels. The approximate positions of the posterior spinal and labyrinthine arteries, when they originate from the vertebral and basilar arteries, respectively, are shown as dashed lines. Compare with Figure 2-22 on the facing page. See Figure 8-7 (p. 246) for comparable angiogram of the vertebrobasilar system. See Figure 8-12 on p. 251 for blood supply of the choroid plexus.

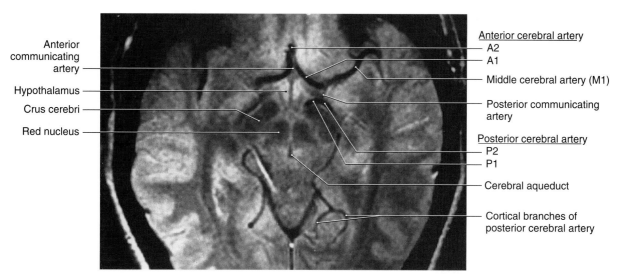

Anterior communicating artery
Hypothalamus
Crus cerebri
Red nucleus

Anterior cerebral artery
  A2
  A1
Middle cerebral artery (M1)
Posterior communicating artery
Posterior cerebral artery
  P2
  P1
Cerebral aqueduct
Cortical branches of posterior cerebral artery

2-25   A proton density MRI through basal regions of the hemisphere and through the midbrain showing several major vessels that form part of the cerebral arterial circle (of Willis). Compare to Figure 2-21 on page 25. See Figure 8-9 and 8-10 (pp. 248–249) for comparable MRA of the cerebral arterial circle.

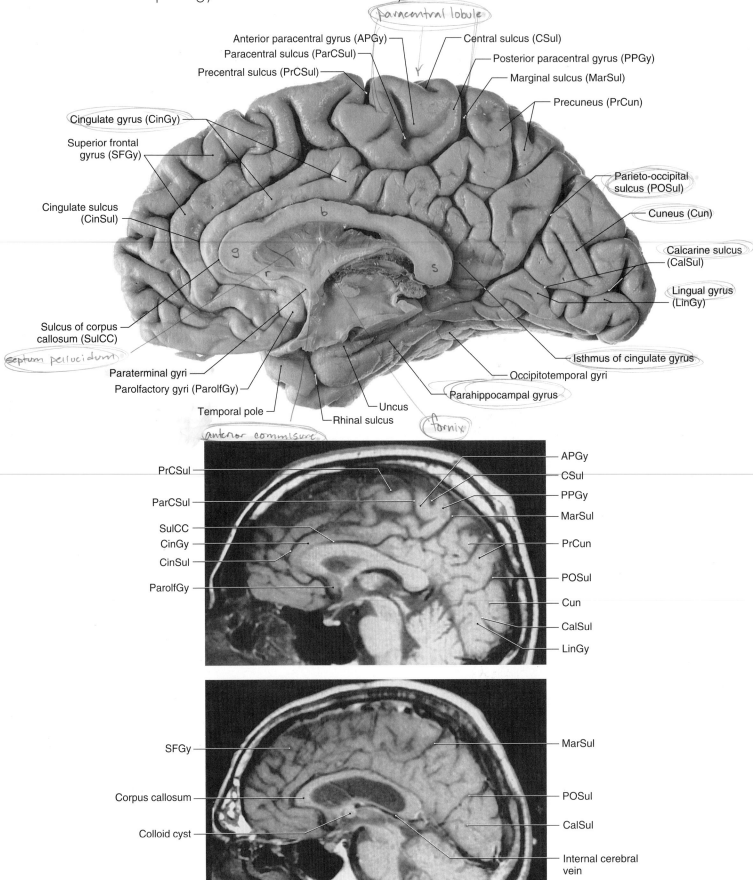

paracentral lobule

Anterior paracentral gyrus (APGy)
Paracentral sulcus (ParCSul)
Precentral sulcus (PrCSul)
Central sulcus (CSul)
Posterior paracentral gyrus (PPGy)
Marginal sulcus (MarSul)
Precuneus (PrCun)
Cingulate gyrus (CinGy)
Superior frontal gyrus (SFGy)
Parieto-occipital sulcus (POSul)
Cingulate sulcus (CinSul)
Cuneus (Cun)
Calcarine sulcus (CalSul)
Lingual gyrus (LinGy)
Sulcus of corpus callosum (SulCC)
septum pellucidum
Paraterminal gyri
Parolfactory gyri (ParolfGy)
Isthmus of cingulate gyrus
Occipitotemporal gyri
Parahippocampal gyrus
Temporal pole
Uncus
Rhinal sulcus
anterior commisure
fornix

PrCSul
ParCSul
SulCC
CinGy
CinSul
ParolfGy

APGy
CSul
PPGy
MarSul
PrCun
POSul
Cun
CalSul
LinGy

SFGy
Corpus callosum
Colloid cyst

MarSul
POSul
CalSul
Internal cerebral vein

2-26 Midsagittal view of the right cerebral hemisphere and diencephalon, with brainstem removed, showing the main gyri and sulci and two MRI (both T1-weighted images) showing these structures from the same perspective. The lower MRI is from a patient with a small colloid cyst in the interventricular foramen. When compared to the upper MRI, note the enlarged lateral ventricle with resultant thinning of the corpus callosum.

A colloid cyst (colloid tumor) is a congenital growth usually discovered in adult life once the flow of CSF through the interventricular foramina is compromised (obstructive hydrocephalus). The patient may have headache, unsteady gait, weakness of the lower extremities, visual or somatosensory disorders, and/or personality changes or confusion. Treatment is usually by surgical removal.

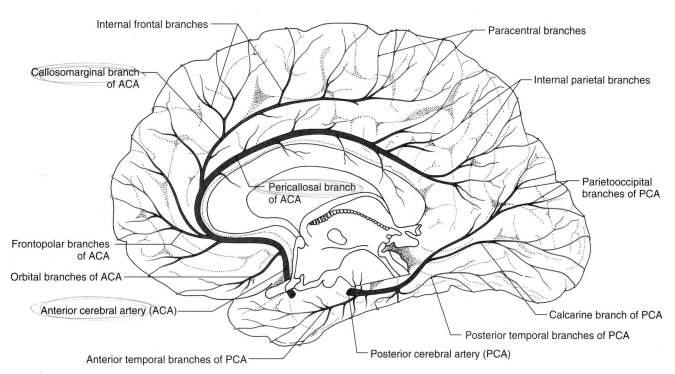

Internal frontal branches

Callosomarginal branch of ACA

Paracentral branches

Internal parietal branches

Pericallosal branch of ACA

Frontopolar branches of ACA

Orbital branches of ACA

Anterior cerebral artery (ACA)

Parietooccipital branches of PCA

Calcarine branch of PCA

Posterior temporal branches of PCA

Anterior temporal branches of PCA

Posterior cerebral artery (PCA)

2-27 Midsagittal view of the cerebral hemisphere and diencephalon showing the locations and branching patterns of anterior and posterior cerebral arteries. The positions of gyri and sulci can be extrapolated from Figure 2-26 (facing page). Terminal branches of the anterior cerebral artery arch laterally over the edge of the hemisphere to serve medial regions of the frontal and parietal lobes, and the same relationship is maintained for the occipital and temporal lobes by branches of the posterior cerebral artery. See Figures 8-1 (p. 240) and 8-7 (p. 246) for comparable angiogram of anterior and posterior cerebral arteries.

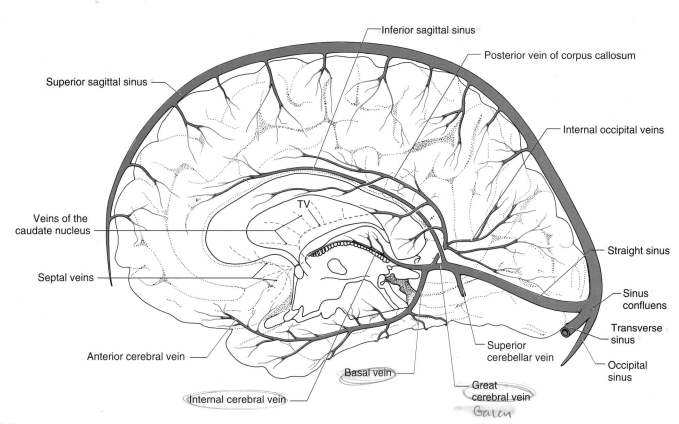

Inferior sagittal sinus

Posterior vein of corpus callosum

Superior sagittal sinus

Internal occipital veins

Veins of the caudate nucleus

TV

Straight sinus

Septal veins

Sinus confluens

Transverse sinus

Anterior cerebral vein

Superior cerebellar vein

Occipital sinus

Basal vein

Great cerebral vein

Internal cerebral vein

Garen

2-28 Midsagittal view of the cerebral hemisphere and diencephalon that shows the locations and relationships of sinuses and the locations and general branching patterns of veins. The position of gyri and sulci can be extrapolated from Figure 2-26 (facing page). TV = Terminal vein (superior thalamostriate vein). See Figures 8-2 (p. 241) and 8-11 (p. 250) for comparable angiogram (venous phase) and MRV showing veins and sinuses.

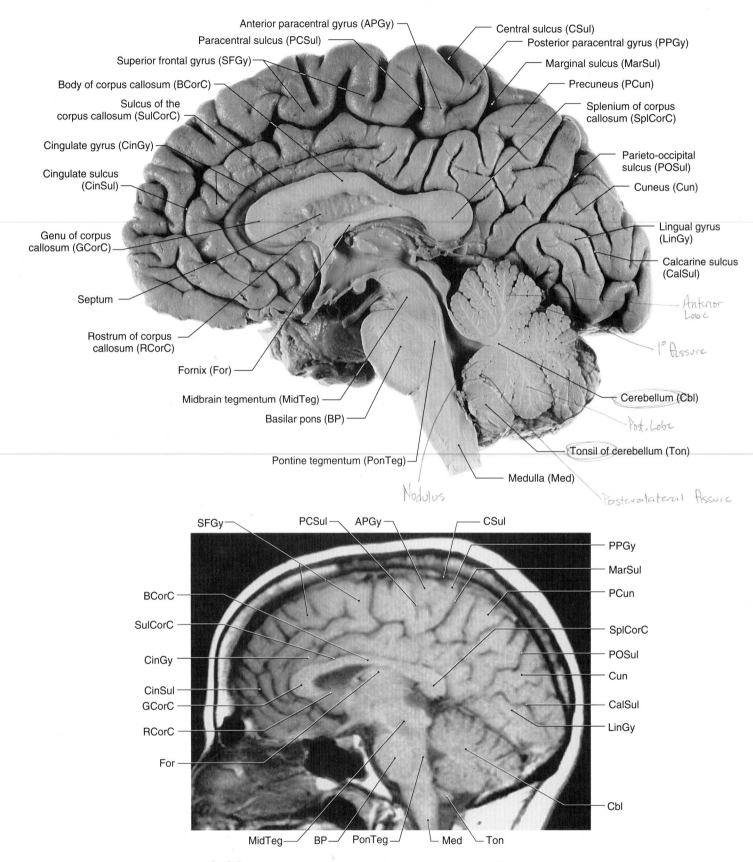

2-29 A midsagittal view of the right cerebral hemisphere and diencephalon with the brainstem and cerebellum *in situ*. The MRI (T1-weighted image) shows many brain structures from the same perspective.

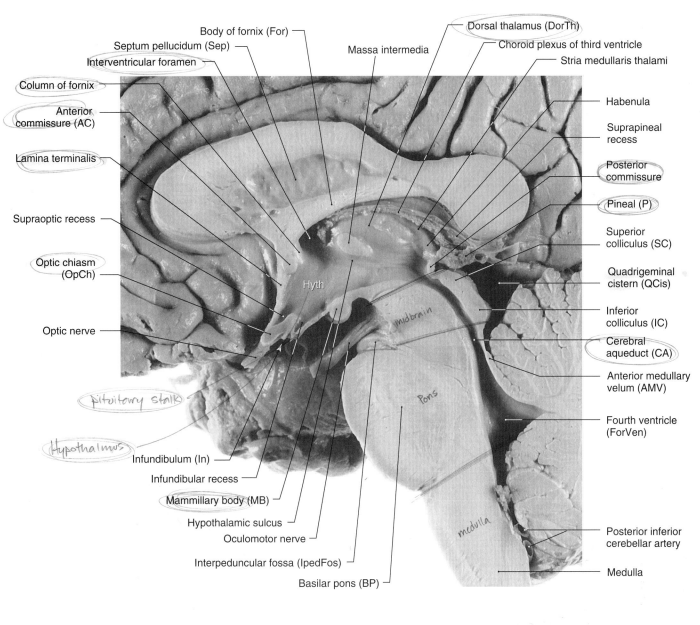

Body of fornix (For)
Septum pellucidum (Sep)
Interventricular foramen
Column of fornix
Anterior commissure (AC)
Lamina terminalis
Supraoptic recess
Optic chiasm (OpCh)
Optic nerve
Pituitary stalk
Hypothalmus
Infundibulum (In)
Infundibular recess
Mammillary body (MB)
Hypothalamic sulcus
Oculomotor nerve
Interpeduncular fossa (IpedFos)
Basilar pons (BP)

Massa intermedia

Dorsal thalamus (DorTh)
Choroid plexus of third ventricle
Stria medullaris thalami
Habenula
Suprapineal recess
Posterior commissure
Pineal (P)
Superior colliculus (SC)
Quadrigeminal cistern (QCis)
Inferior colliculus (IC)
Cerebral aqueduct (CA)
Anterior medullary velum (AMV)
Fourth ventricle (ForVen)
Posterior inferior cerebellar artery
Medulla

Hyth
midbrain
Pons
medulla

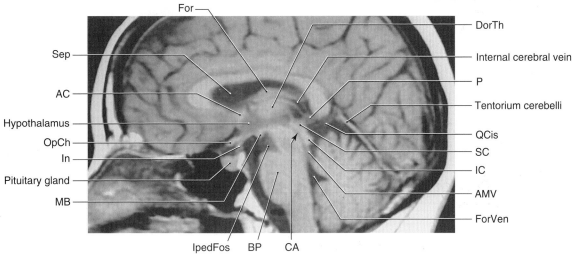

For
Sep
AC
Hypothalamus
OpCh
In
Pituitary gland
MB

DorTh
Internal cerebral vein
P
Tentorium cerebelli
QCis
SC
IC
AMV
ForVen

IpedFos   BP   CA

2-30   A midsagittal view of the right cerebral hemisphere and diencephalon with the brainstem *in situ* focusing on the details primarily related to the diencephalon and third ventricle. The MRI (T1-weighted image) shows these brain structures from the same perspective. Hyth = hypothalamus.

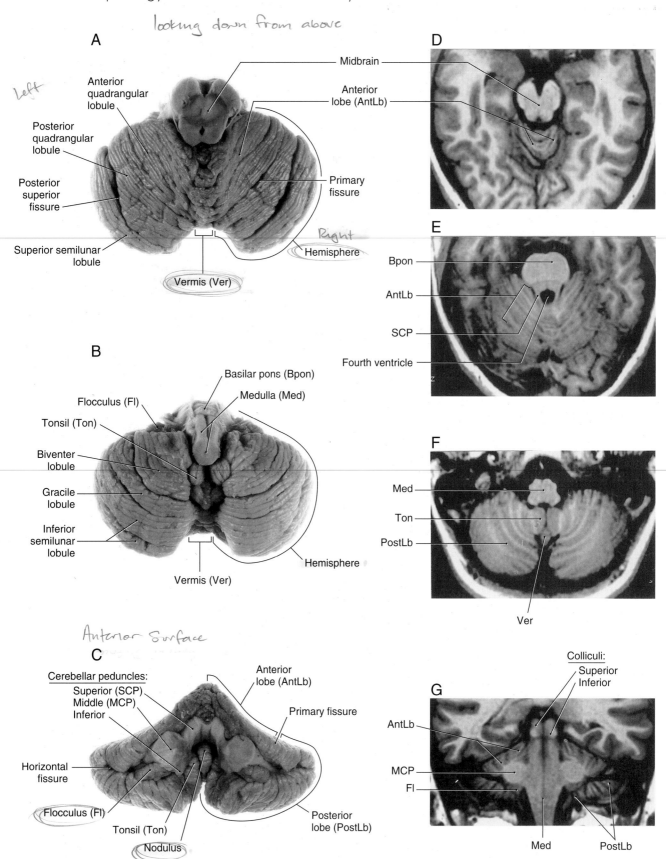

A looking down from above

Left

Midbrain

Anterior quadrangular lobule

Anterior lobe (AntLb)

Posterior quadrangular lobule

Posterior superior fissure

Primary fissure

Superior semilunar lobule

Right

Hemisphere

Vermis (Ver)

B

Basilar pons (Bpon)

Flocculus (Fl)

Medulla (Med)

Tonsil (Ton)

Biventer lobule

Gracile lobule

Inferior semilunar lobule

Hemisphere

Vermis (Ver)

C Anterior Surface

Cerebellar peduncles:
Superior (SCP)
Middle (MCP)
Inferior

Anterior lobe (AntLb)

Primary fissure

Horizontal fissure

Flocculus (Fl)

Tonsil (Ton)

Nodulus

Posterior lobe (PostLb)

D

Midbrain

Anterior lobe (AntLb)

E

Bpon

AntLb

SCP

Fourth ventricle

F

Med

Ton

PostLb

Ver

G

Colliculi:
Superior
Inferior

AntLb

MCP

Fl

Med

PostLb

2-31 Rostral (**A,** superior surface), caudal (**B,** inferior surface), and an inferior view (**C,** inferior aspect) of the cerebellum. The view in **C** shows the aspect of the cerebellum that is continuous into the brainstem via cerebellar peduncles. The view in **C** correlates with superior surface of the brainstem (and middle superior cerebellar peduncles) as shown in Figure 2-34 on page 34.

Note that the superior view of the cerebellum (**A**) correlates closely

with cerebellar structures seen in axial MRIs at comparable levels (**D, E**). Structures seen on the inferior surface of the cerebellum, such as the tonsil (**F**), correlate closely with an axial MRI at a comparable level. In **G**, note the appearance of the margin of the cerebellum, the general appearance and position of the lobes, and the obvious nature of the middle cerebellar peduncle. All MRI images are T1-weighted.

A

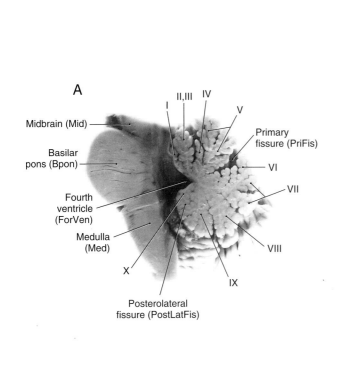

B

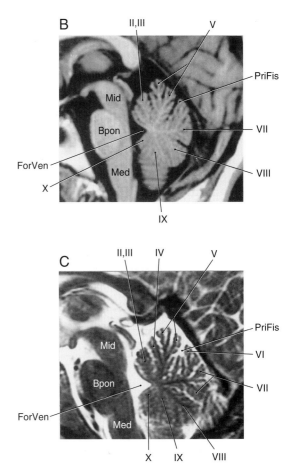

C

2-32   A median sagittal view of the cerebellum (**A**) showing its relationships to the midbrain, pons, and medulla. This view of the cerebellum also illustrates the two main fissures and the vermis portions of lobules I-X. Designation of these lobules follows the method developed by Larsell.

Lobules I-V are the vermis parts of the anterior lobe; lobules VI-IX are the vermis parts of the posterior lobe; and lobule X (the nodulus) is the vermis part of the flocculonodular lobe. Note the striking similarities between the gross specimen (**A**) and a median sagittal view of the cerebellum in a T1-weighted MRI (**B**) and a T2-weighted MRI (**C**).

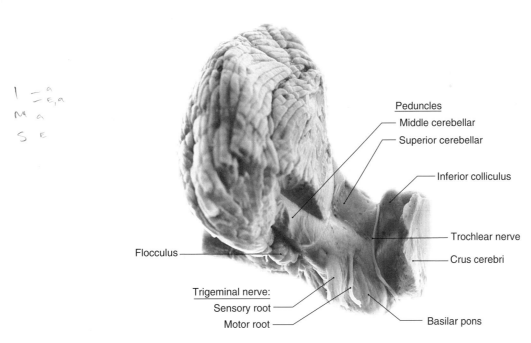

2-33   Lateral and slightly rostral view of the cerebellum and brainstem with the middle and superior cerebellar peduncles exposed. Note the relationship of the trochlear nerve to the inferior colliculus and the relative positions of, and distinction between, motor and sensory roots of the trigeminal nerve. See page 40, Figure 2-41D for an MRI showing the trochlear nerve.

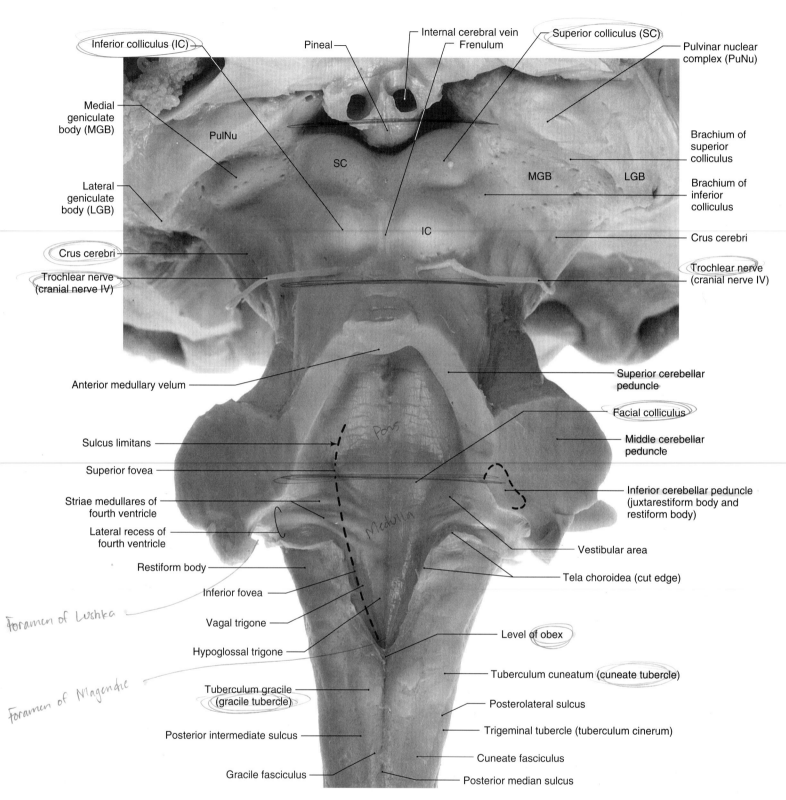

Inferior colliculus (IC)

Pineal

Internal cerebral vein
Frenulum

Superior colliculus (SC)

Pulvinar nuclear
complex (PuNu)

Medial
geniculate
body (MGB)

PulNu

SC

Brachium of
superior
colliculus

MGB

LGB

Lateral
geniculate
body (LGB)

IC

Brachium of
inferior
colliculus

Crus cerebri

Crus cerebri

Crus cerebri

Trochlear nerve
(cranial nerve IV)

Trochlear nerve
(cranial nerve IV)

Anterior medullary velum

Pons

Superior cerebellar
peduncle

Facial colliculus

Sulcus limitans

Middle cerebellar
peduncle

Superior fovea

Striae medullares of
fourth ventricle

Inferior cerebellar peduncle
(juxtarestiform body and
restiform body)

Lateral recess of
fourth ventricle

Medulla

Restiform body

Vestibular area

Inferior fovea

Tela choroidea (cut edge)

Foramen of Lushka

Vagal trigone

Hypoglossal trigone

Level of obex

Tuberculum cuneatum (cuneate tubercle)

Foramen of Magendie

Tuberculum gracile
(gracile tubercle)

Posterolateral sulcus

Trigeminal tubercle (tuberculum cinerum)

Posterior intermediate sulcus

Cuneate fasciculus

Gracile fasciculus

Posterior median sulcus

2-34   Detailed dorsal view of the brainstem, with cerebellum removed, providing a clear view of the rhomboid fossa (and floor of the
fourth ventricle) and contiguous parts of the caudal diencephalon. The
dashed line on the left represents the position of the sulcus limitans and
the area of the inferior cerebellar peduncle is shown on the right. The
tuberculum cinereum is also called the trigeminal tubercle (tuberculum trigeminale) because it is the surface representation of the spinal
trigeminal tract and its underlying nucleus. Figure 3-10 on page 61 also
shows a comparable view of the brainstem and the posterior portions
of the diencephalon.

Vessels

Structures

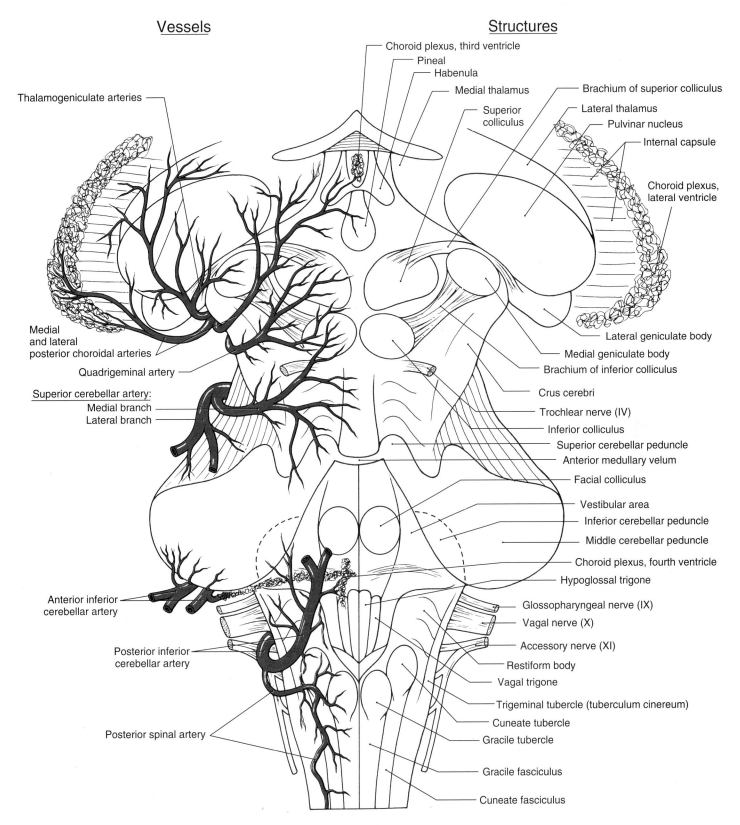

Thalamogeniculate arteries

Medial and lateral posterior choroidal arteries

Quadrigeminal artery

Superior cerebellar artery:
Medial branch
Lateral branch

Anterior inferior cerebellar artery

Posterior inferior cerebellar artery

Posterior spinal artery

Choroid plexus, third ventricle
Pineal
Habenula
Medial thalamus
Superior colliculus
Brachium of superior colliculus
Lateral thalamus
Pulvinar nucleus
Internal capsule
Choroid plexus, lateral ventricle
Lateral geniculate body
Medial geniculate body
Brachium of inferior colliculus
Crus cerebri
Trochlear nerve (IV)
Inferior colliculus
Superior cerebellar peduncle
Anterior medullary velum
Facial colliculus
Vestibular area
Inferior cerebellar peduncle
Middle cerebellar peduncle
Choroid plexus, fourth ventricle
Hypoglossal trigone
Glossopharyngeal nerve (IX)
Vagal nerve (X)
Accessory nerve (XI)
Restiform body
Vagal trigone
Trigeminal tubercle (tuberculum cinereum)
Cuneate tubercle
Gracile tubercle
Gracile fasciculus
Cuneate fasciculus

2-35 Dorsal view of the brainstem and caudal diencephalon show-ing the relationship of structures and some of the cranial nerves to ar-teries. The vessels shown in this view have originated ventrally and wrapped around the brainstem to gain their dorsal positions. In addi-tion to serving the medulla, branches of the posterior inferior cerebel-lar artery also supply the choroid plexus of the fourth ventricle. The tuberculum cinereum is also called the trigeminal tubercle. See Figure 8-12 on p. 251 for blood supply of the choroid plexus.

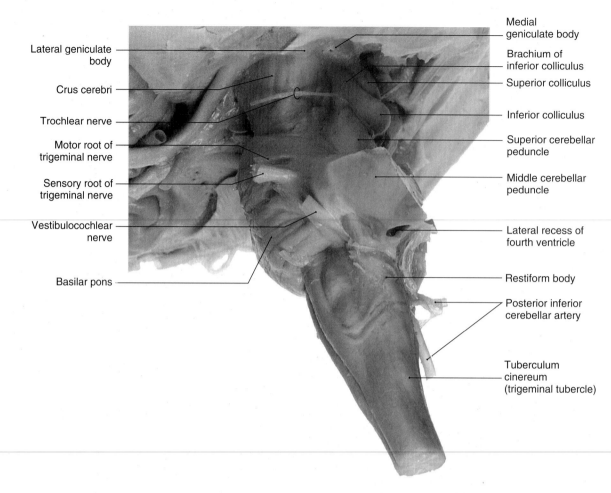

Lateral geniculate body

Crus cerebri

Trochlear nerve

Motor root of trigeminal nerve

Sensory root of trigeminal nerve

Vestibulocochlear nerve

Basilar pons

Medial geniculate body

Brachium of inferior colliculus

Superior colliculus

Inferior colliculus

Superior cerebellar peduncle

Middle cerebellar peduncle

Lateral recess of fourth ventricle

Restiform body

Posterior inferior cerebellar artery

Tuberculum cinereum (trigeminal tubercle)

2-36 Lateral view of the left side of the brainstem emphasizing structures that are located dorsally. The cerebellum and portions of the temporal lobe have been removed. Compare with Figure 2-38 on the facing page.

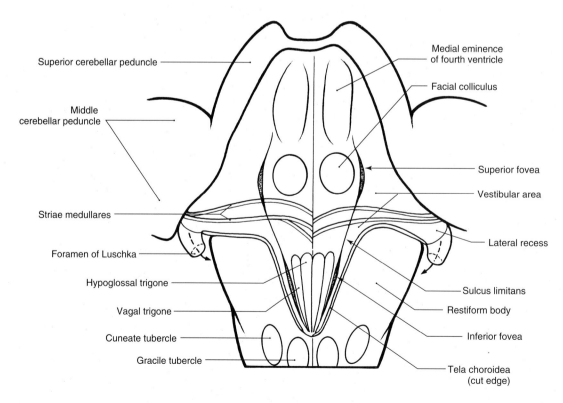

Superior cerebellar peduncle

Middle cerebellar peduncle

Striae medullares

Foramen of Luschka

Hypoglossal trigone

Vagal trigone

Cuneate tubercle

Gracile tubercle

Medial eminence of fourth ventricle

Facial colliculus

Superior fovea

Vestibular area

Lateral recess

Sulcus limitans

Restiform body

Inferior fovea

Tela choroidea (cut edge)

2-37 The floor of the fourth ventricle (rhomboid fossa) and immediately adjacent structures. Also compare with Figure 2-34 on page 34.

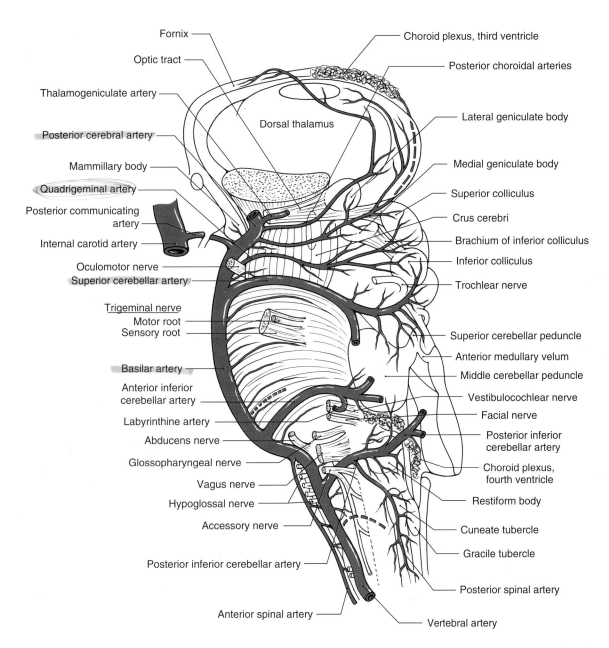

Fornix

Optic tract

Thalamogeniculate artery

Posterior cerebral artery

Mammillary body

Quadrigeminal artery

Posterior communicating artery

Internal carotid artery

Oculomotor nerve

Superior cerebellar artery

Trigeminal nerve
Motor root
Sensory root

Basilar artery

Anterior inferior cerebellar artery

Labyrinthine artery

Abducens nerve

Glossopharyngeal nerve

Vagus nerve

Hypoglossal nerve

Accessory nerve

Posterior inferior cerebellar artery

Anterior spinal artery

Choroid plexus, third ventricle

Posterior choroidal arteries

Dorsal thalamus

Lateral geniculate body

Medial geniculate body

Superior colliculus

Crus cerebri

Brachium of inferior colliculus

Inferior colliculus

Trochlear nerve

Superior cerebellar peduncle

Anterior medullary velum

Middle cerebellar peduncle

Vestibulocochlear nerve

Facial nerve

Posterior inferior cerebellar artery

Choroid plexus, fourth ventricle

Restiform body

Cuneate tubercle

Gracile tubercle

Posterior spinal artery

Vertebral artery

2-38   Lateral view of the brainstem and thalamus, which shows the relationship of structures and cranial nerves to arteries. The approximate positions of the labyrinthine and posterior spinal arteries, when they originate from the basilar and vertebral arteries, respectively, are shown as dashed lines. Arteries that distribute to dorsal structures originate from large ventral vessels. Compare with Figure 2-36 on the facing page.

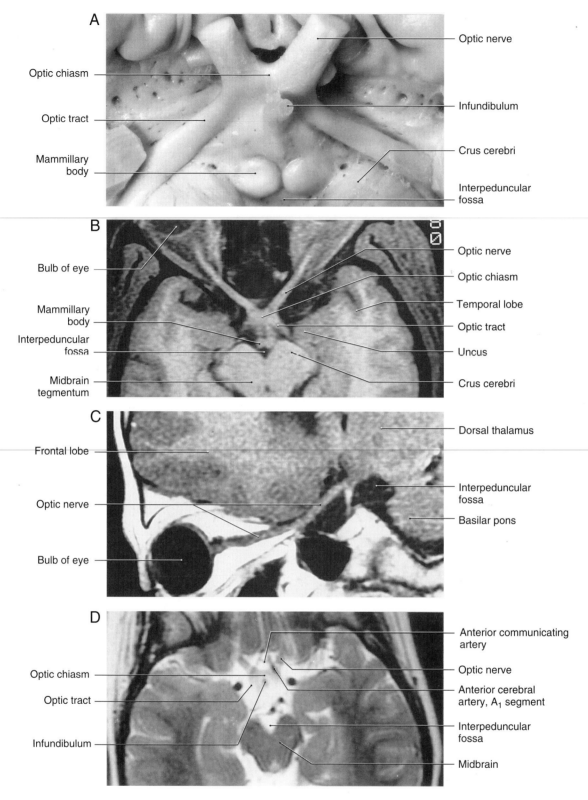

A

Optic chiasm

Optic tract

Mammillary body

Optic nerve

Infundibulum

Crus cerebri

Interpeduncular fossa

B

Bulb of eye

Mammillary body

Interpeduncular fossa

Midbrain tegmentum

Optic nerve

Optic chiasm

Temporal lobe

Optic tract

Uncus

Crus cerebri

C

Frontal lobe

Optic nerve

Bulb of eye

Dorsal thalamus

Interpeduncular fossa

Basilar pons

D

Optic chiasm

Optic tract

Infundibulum

Anterior communicating artery

Optic nerve

Anterior cerebral artery, A₁ segment

Interpeduncular fossa

Midbrain

2-39 Inferior view of the hemisphere showing the optic nerve (II), chiasm, tract, and related structures (**A**). The MRIs of cranial nerve II are shown in axial (**B,** T1-weighted; **D,** T2-weighted) and in oblique sagittal (**C,** T1-weighted) planes. Note the similarity between the axial planes, especially (**B**), and the gross anatomical specimen. In addition, note the relationship between the anterior cerebellar artery, anterior communicating artery, and the structures around the optic chiasm (**D**).

The anterior communicating artery or its junction with the anterior cerebral artery (**D**) is the most common site of supratentorial (carotid system) aneurysms. Rupture of aneurysms at this location is one of the more common causes of spontaneous subarachnoid hemorrhage. The proximity of these vessels to optic structures and the hypothalamus (**D**) explain the variety of visual and hypothalamic disorders experienced by these patients. A lesion of the optic nerve results in blindness in that eye and loss of the afferent limb of the pupillary light reflex. Lesions in, or caudal to, the optic chiasm result in deficits in the visual fields of both eyes.

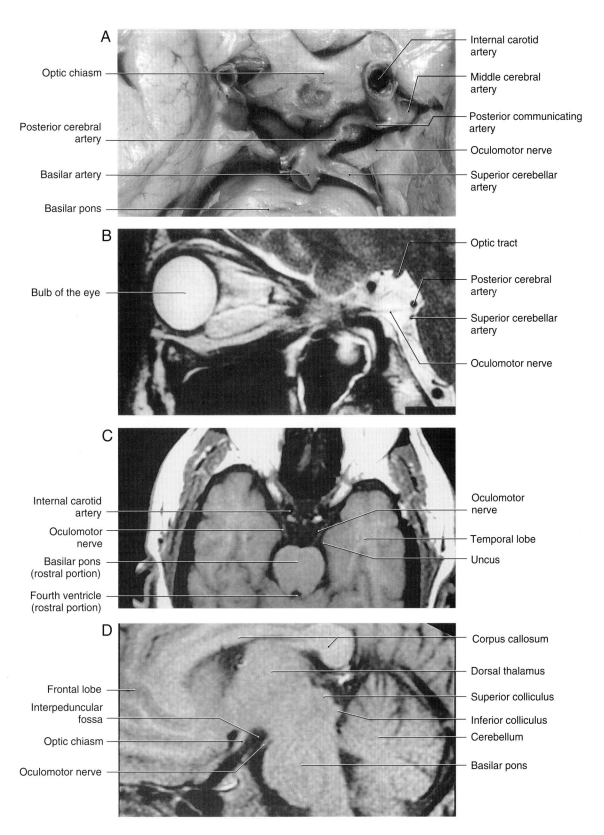

A

Optic chiasm

Posterior cerebral artery

Basilar artery

Basilar pons

Internal carotid artery

Middle cerebral artery

Posterior communicating artery

Oculomotor nerve

Superior cerebellar artery

B

Bulb of the eye

Optic tract

Posterior cerebral artery

Superior cerebellar artery

Oculomotor nerve

C

Internal carotid artery

Oculomotor nerve

Basilar pons (rostral portion)

Fourth ventricle (rostral portion)

Oculomotor nerve

Temporal lobe

Uncus

D

Frontal lobe

Interpeduncular fossa

Optic chiasm

Oculomotor nerve

Corpus callosum

Dorsal thalamus

Superior colliculus

Inferior colliculus

Cerebellum

Basilar pons

2-40   Inferior view of the hemisphere showing the exiting fibers of the oculomotor nerve (III), and their relationship to the posterior cerebral and superior cerebellar arteries (**A**). The MRIs of cranial nerve III are shown in sagittal (**B,** T2-weighted; **D,** T1-weighted) and in axial (**C,** T1-weighted) planes. Note the relationship of the exiting fibers of the oculomotor nerve to the posterior cerebral and superior cerebellar arteries (**A, B**) and the characteristic appearance of the III nerve as it passes through the subarachnoid space toward the superior orbital fissure (**C**). The sagittal section (**D**) is just off the midline and shows the position of the oculomotor nerve in the interpeduncular fossa rostral to the basilar pons and caudal to optic structures.

That portion of the posterior cerebral artery located between the basilar artery and the posterior communicating artery (**A**) is the P_1 segment. The most common site of aneurysms in the infratentorial area (vertebrobasilar system) is at the bifurcation of the basilar artery, also called the basilar tip. Patients with aneurysms at this location may present with eye movement disorders and pupillary dilation due to damage to the root of the third nerve (**A,B**).

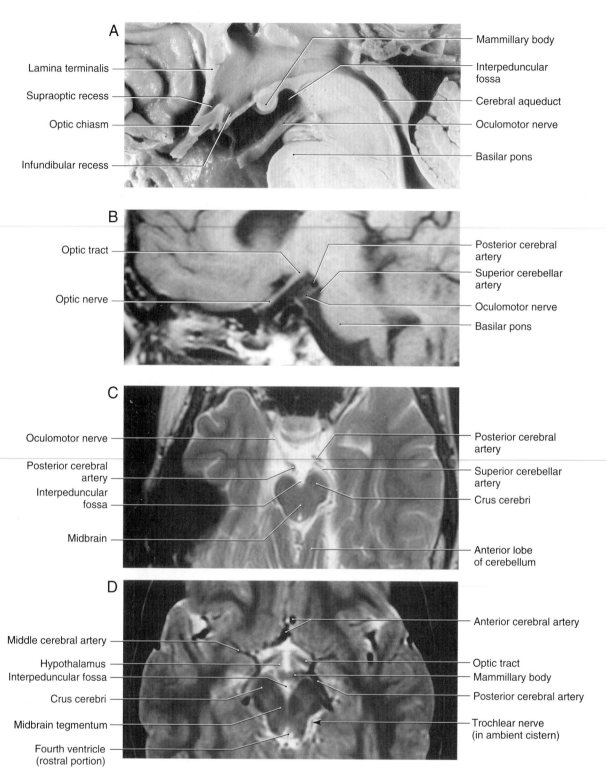

A

Lamina terminalis

Supraoptic recess

Optic chiasm

Infundibular recess

Mammillary body

Interpeduncular fossa

Cerebral aqueduct

Oculomotor nerve

Basilar pons

B

Optic tract

Optic nerve

Posterior cerebral artery

Superior cerebellar artery

Oculomotor nerve

Basilar pons

C

Oculomotor nerve

Posterior cerebral artery

Interpeduncular fossa

Midbrain

Posterior cerebral artery

Superior cerebellar artery

Crus cerebri

Anterior lobe of cerebellum

D

Middle cerebral artery

Hypothalamus

Interpeduncular fossa

Crus cerebri

Midbrain tegmentum

Fourth ventricle (rostral portion)

Anterior cerebral artery

Optic tract

Mammillary body

Posterior cerebral artery

Trochlear nerve (in ambient cistern)

2-41   A median sagittal view of the brainstem and diencephalon (**A**) reveals the position of the oculomotor nerve (III) in relation to adjacent structures. The MRI in **B** and **C** show the position of the oculomotor nerve in sagittal (**B,** T1-weighted) and in axial (**C,** T2-weighted) planes. Note the relationship of the oculomotor nerve to the adjacent posterior cerebral and superior cerebellar arteries (**B, C**). Also compare these images with that of figure 2-40B on page 39. In **D** (T2-weighted), the trochlear nerve is seen passing through the ambient cistern around the lateral aspect of the midbrain (compare with Fig. 2-32 on page 32).

The oculomotor (III) and trochlear (IV) nerves are the cranial nerves of the midbrain. The third nerve exits via the interpeduncular fossa to innervate four major extraocular muscles (see Fig. 7-15 on page 201) and, through the ciliary ganglion, the sphincter pupillae muscles. Damage to the oculomotor nerve may result in paralysis of most eye movement, a dilated pupil, and loss of the efferent limb of the pupillary light reflex, all in the ipsilateral eye. The fourth nerve is unique in that it is the only cranial nerve to exit the posterior (dorsal) aspect of the brainstem and is the only cranial nerve motor nucleus to innervate, exclusively, a muscle on the contralateral side of the midbrain.

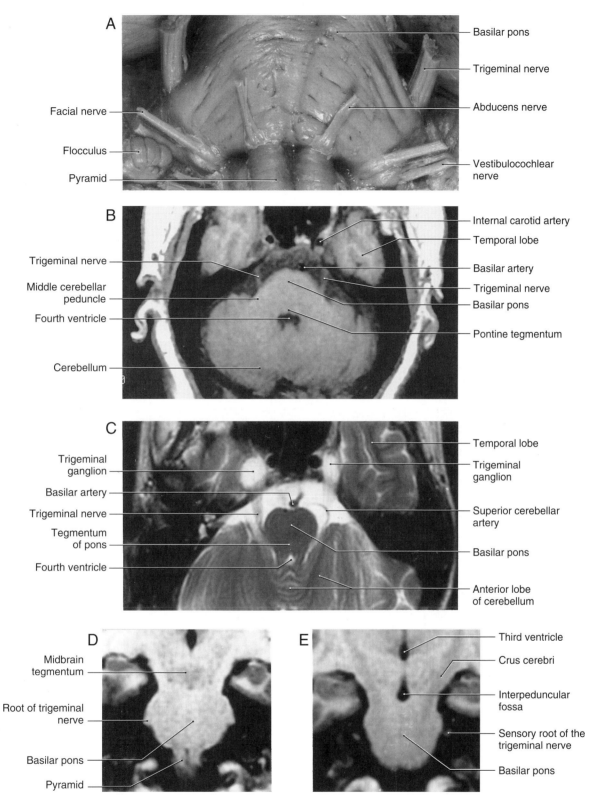

A

Facial nerve

Flocculus

Pyramid

Basilar pons

Trigeminal nerve

Abducens nerve

Vestibulocochlear nerve

B

Trigeminal nerve

Middle cerebellar peduncle

Fourth ventricle

Cerebellum

Internal carotid artery

Temporal lobe

Basilar artery

Trigeminal nerve

Basilar pons

Pontine tegmentum

C

Trigeminal ganglion

Basilar artery

Trigeminal nerve

Tegmentum of pons

Fourth ventricle

Temporal lobe

Trigeminal ganglion

Superior cerebellar artery

Basilar pons

Anterior lobe of cerebellum

D

Midbrain tegmentum

Root of trigeminal nerve

Basilar pons

Pyramid

E

Third ventricle

Crus cerebri

Interpeduncular fossa

Sensory root of the trigeminal nerve

Basilar pons

2-42 The trigeminal nerve (V) is the largest of the cranial nerve roots exiting the brainstem (**A**). It exits at an intermediate position on the lateral aspect of the pons roughly in line with cranial nerves VII, IX, and X. The fifth nerve, and these latter three, are mixed nerves in that they have motor and sensory components. The trigeminal nerve is shown in axial MRI (**B,** T1-weighted; **C,** T2-weighted) and in coronal planes (**D, E,** both T1-weighted images). Note the characteristic appearance of the root of the trigeminal nerve as it traverses the subarachnoid space (**B** and **C**), the origin of the trigeminal nerve, and the position of the sensory root of the nerve at the lateral aspect of the pons

in the coronal plane (**D, E**). In addition, the MRI in **C** clearly illustrates the position of the trigeminal ganglion in the middle cranial fossa.

Trigeminal neuralgia (tic douloureux) is a lancinating paroxysmal pain within the V_2–V_3 territories frequently triggered by stimuli around the corner of the mouth. The causes are probably multiple and may include neurovascular compression by the superior cerebellar artery (see the apposition of this vessel to the nerve root in **C**), multiple sclerosis, tumors, and ephaptic transmission within the nerve or ganglion.

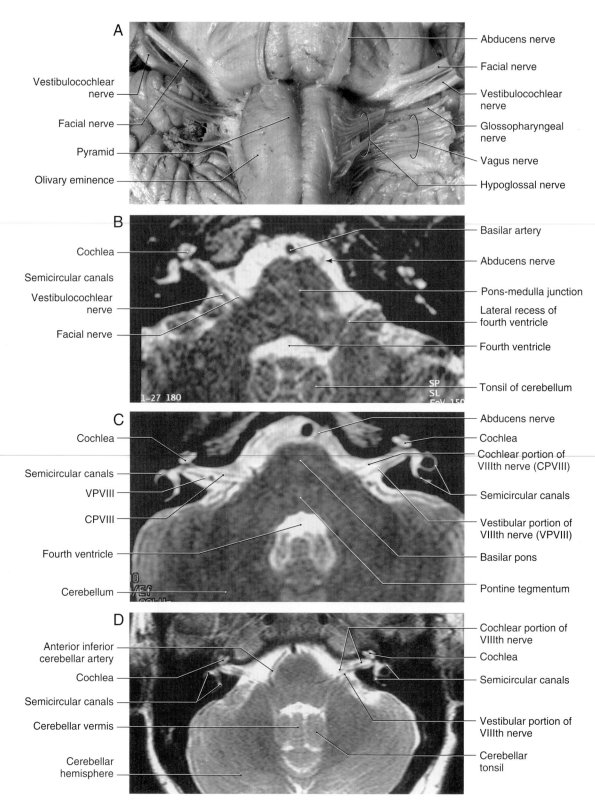

A

Vestibulocochlear nerve
Facial nerve
Pyramid
Olivary eminence

Abducens nerve
Facial nerve
Vestibulocochlear nerve
Glossopharyngeal nerve
Vagus nerve
Hypoglossal nerve

B

Cochlea
Semicircular canals
Vestibulocochlear nerve
Facial nerve

Basilar artery
Abducens nerve
Pons-medulla junction
Lateral recess of fourth ventricle
Fourth ventricle
Tonsil of cerebellum

C

Cochlea
Semicircular canals
VPVIII
CPVIII
Fourth ventricle
Cerebellum

Abducens nerve
Cochlea
Cochlear portion of VIIIth nerve (CPVIII)
Semicircular canals
Vestibular portion of VIIIth nerve (VPVIII)
Basilar pons
Pontine tegmentum

D

Anterior inferior cerebellar artery
Cochlea
Semicircular canals
Cerebellar vermis
Cerebellar hemisphere

Cochlear portion of VIIIth nerve
Cochlea
Semicircular canals
Vestibular portion of VIIIth nerve
Cerebellar tonsil

2-43   The cranial nerves at the pons medulla junction are the abducens (VI), the facial (VII), and the vestibulocochlear (VIII) (**A**). The facial and vestibulocochlear nerves both enter the internal acoustic meatus, the facial nerve distributing eventually to the face through the stylomastoid foramen, and the vestibulocochlear nerve to structures of the inner ear. MRI in the axial plane, **B, C, D,** (all T2-weighted images) show the relationships of the vestibulocochlear root and the facial nerve to the internal acoustic meatus. Also notice the characteristic appearance of the cochlea (**B, C**) and the semicircular canals (**C**). In addition to these two cranial nerves, the labyrinthine branch of the anterior inferior cerebellar artery also enters the internal acoustic meatus.

The so-called acoustic neuroma, a tumor associated with the eighth nerve, is actually a vestibular schwannoma since it arises from the neurilemma sheath of the vestibular root. Most patients with this tumor have hearing loss, tinnitus and equilibrium problems, or vertigo. As the tumor enlarges (to more than about 2 cm) it may cause facial weakness (seventh root), numbness (fifth root), or abnormal corneal reflex (fifth or seventh). Treatment is usually by surgery, radiation therapy, or a combination thereof.

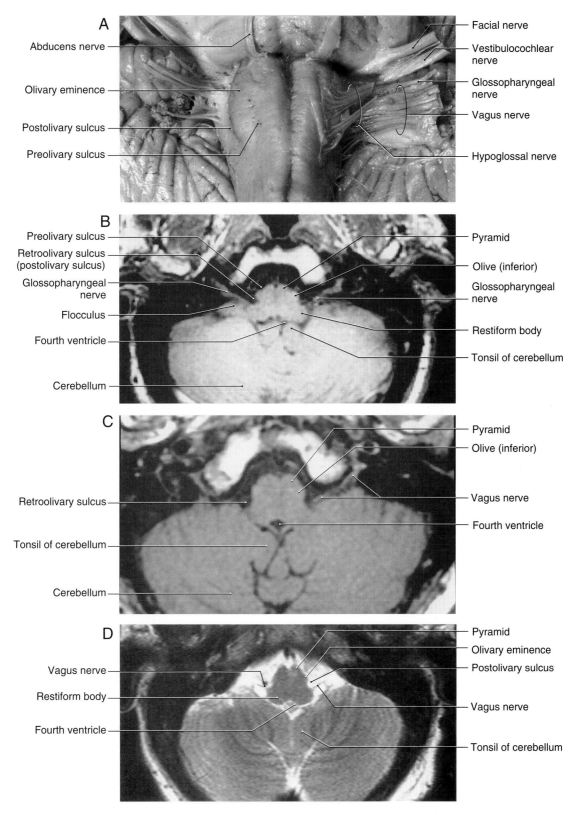

A
Abducens nerve
Olivary eminence
Postolivary sulcus
Preolivary sulcus
Facial nerve
Vestibulocochlear nerve
Glossopharyngeal nerve
Vagus nerve
Hypoglossal nerve

B
Preolivary sulcus
Retroolivary sulcus (postolivary sulcus)
Glossopharyngeal nerve
Flocculus
Fourth ventricle
Cerebellum
Pyramid
Olive (inferior)
Glossopharyngeal nerve
Restiform body
Tonsil of cerebellum

C
Retroolivary sulcus
Tonsil of cerebellum
Cerebellum
Pyramid
Olive (inferior)
Vagus nerve
Fourth ventricle

D
Vagus nerve
Restiform body
Fourth ventricle
Pyramid
Olivary eminence
Postolivary sulcus
Vagus nerve
Tonsil of cerebellum

2-44 The glossopharyngeal (IX) and vagus (X) nerves (**A**) exit the lateral aspect of the medulla via the postolivary sulcus; the ninth nerve exits rostral to the row of rootlets comprising the tenth nerve (**A**). These nerves are generally in line with the exits of the facial and trigeminal nerves; all of these are mixed nerves. The exit of the glossopharyngeal nerve (**A, B**) is close to the pons–medulla junction and correlates with the corresponding shape (more rectangular) of the medulla. The vagus nerve exits at a slightly more caudal position (**A, C, D**); the shape of the medulla is more square and the fourth ventri-

cle is smaller. The ninth and tenth cranial nerves and the spinal portion of the accessory nerve (XI) exit the skull via the jugular foramen.

Glossopharyngeal neuralgia is a lancinating pain originating from the territories served by the ninth and tenth nerves at the base of the tongue and throat. Trigger events may include chewing and swallowing. Lesions of nerves passing through the jugular foramen (IX, X, XI) may result in loss of the gag reflex (motor limb via ninth nerve), and drooping of the ipsilateral shoulder accompanied by an inability to turn the head to the opposite side against resistance (eleventh nerve).

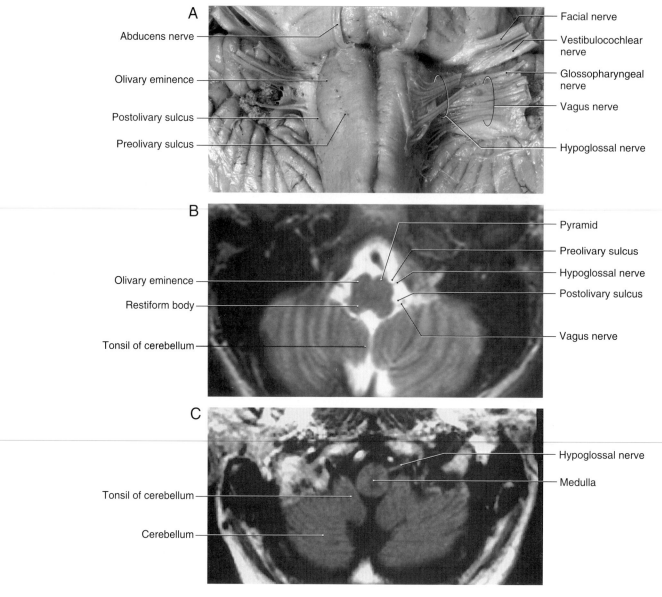

A

Abducens nerve

Olivary eminence

Postolivary sulcus

Preolivary sulcus

Facial nerve

Vestibulocochlear nerve

Glossopharyngeal nerve

Vagus nerve

Hypoglossal nerve

B

Olivary eminence

Restiform body

Tonsil of cerebellum

Pyramid

Preolivary sulcus

Hypoglossal nerve

Postolivary sulcus

Vagus nerve

C

Tonsil of cerebellum

Cerebellum

Hypoglossal nerve

Medulla

2-45   The hypoglossal nerve (XII) (**A**) exits the inferolateral aspect of the medulla via the preolivary sulcus. This cranial nerve exits in line with the abducens nerve found at the pons–medulla junction and in line with the exits of the third and fourth nerves of the midbrain. The twelfth nerve exit is characteristically located laterally adjacent to the pyramid, which contains corticospinal fibers.

In axial MRI (**B,** T2-weighted; **C,** T1-weighted), note the charac-teristic position of the hypoglossal nerve in the subarachnoid space and its relation to the overall shape of the medulla. This shape is indicative of a cranial nerve exiting at more mid-to-caudal medullary levels. In **B,** note its relationship to the preolivary sulcus and olivary eminence. The hypoglossal exits the base of the skull by traversing the hypoglossal canal. A lesion of the hypoglossal nerve results in a deviation of the tongue to the ipsilateral side on attempted protrusion.

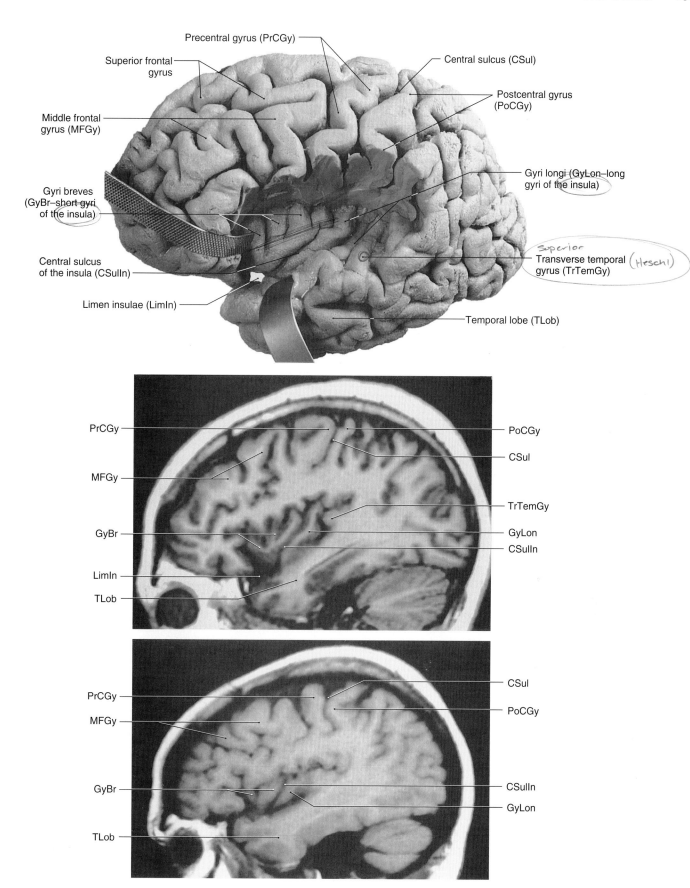

Precentral gyrus (PrCGy)

Superior frontal gyrus

Central sulcus (CSul)

Postcentral gyrus (PoCGy)

Middle frontal gyrus (MFGy)

Gyri longi (GyLon–long gyri of the insula)

Gyri breves (GyBr–short gyri of the insula)

Central sulcus of the insula (CSulIn)

Superior Transverse temporal gyrus (TrTemGy) (Heschl)

Limen insulae (LimIn)

Temporal lobe (TLob)

PrCGy

PoCGy

MFGy

CSul

TrTemGy

GyBr

GyLon

LimIn

CSulIn

TLob

PrCGy

CSul

MFGy

PoCGy

GyBr

CSulIn

GyLon

TLob

2-46   Lateral view of the left cerebral hemisphere with the cortex overlying the insula removed. Structures characteristic of the insular cortex, and immediately adjacent areas, are clearly seen in the two MRIs in the sagittal plane through lateral portions of the hemisphere (inversion recovery—upper; T1-weighted image—lower).

Comparison of Cerebral versus Spinal Meninges

Cerebral	Spinal
Dura	*Dura*
• adherent to inner table of skull (no epidural space)	• separated from vertebrae by epidural space
• composed of two fused layers (periosteal and meningeal), which split to form sinuses	• composed of one layer (spinal dura only; vertebrae have their own periosteum)
Arachnoid (outer part of leptomeninges)	*Arachnoid (outer part of leptomeninges)*
• attached to dura in living condition (no subdural space)	• attached to dura in living condition (no subdural space)
• arachnoid villi (in superior sagittal sinus)	• no arachnoid villi
• arachnoid trabeculae	• few or no arachnoid trabeculae but larger arachnoid septae
• subarachnoid space with many cisterns	• subarachnoid space with one cistern
Pia (inner part of leptomeninges)	*Pia (inner part of leptomeninges)*
• intimately adherent to surface of brain	• intimately adherent to surface of cord
• no pial specializations	• specializations in the form of denticulate ligaments, filum terminale, and linea splendens
• follows vessels as they pierce the cerebral cortex	• follows vessels as they pierce the cord

Meningitis, Meningeal Hemorrhages, Meningioma

A wide variety of disease processes and lesions may involve the meninges; only a few examples are mentioned here.

Bacterial infections of the meninges (***bacterial meningitis***) are commonly called ***leptomeningitis*** because the causative organisms are usually found in the subarachnoid space and involve the pia and arachnoid. The organism seen in about one-half of adult cases is *Streptococcus pneumoniae,* while in neonates and children up to about 1 year it is *Escherichia coli.* The patient becomes acutely ill (i.e., confusion, fever, stiff neck, stupor), may have generalized or focal signs/symptoms, and, if not treated rapidly, will likely die. Treatment is with appropriate antibiotics. Patients with ***viral meningitis*** may become ill over a period of several days, experience headache, confusion, and fever, but, with supportive care, will recover after an acute phase of approximately 1–2 weeks. These patients usually recover with no permanent deficits.

The most common cause of an ***epidural (extradural) hematoma*** is a skull fracture that results in a laceration of a major dural vessel, such as the middle meningeal artery. In approximately 15% of cases, bleeding may come from a venous sinus. The extravasated blood dissects the dura mater off the inner table of the skull; there is no preexisting (extradural) space for the blood to enter. These lesions are frequently large, lens (lenticular) shaped, may appear loculated, and are "short and thick" compared to subdural hematomas (see Fig. 2-48 on page 48). The patient may lapse into a coma and, if the lesion is left untreated, death may result. In some cases, the patient may initially be unconscious followed by a lucid interval (the patient is wide awake), then subsequently deteriorate rapidly and die; this is called "talk and die." Treatment of choice for large lesions is surgical removal of the clot and coagulation of the damaged vessel.

Tearing of bridging veins (veins passing from the brain outward through the arachnoid and dura), usually the result of trauma, is a common cause of ***subdural hematoma.*** This designation is somewhat a misnomer because the extravasated blood actually dissects through a specialized, yet structurally weak, cell layer at the dura-arachnoid interface; this is the dural border cell layer. There is no preexisting "subdural space" in the normal brain. Acute subdural hematomas, more commonly seen in younger patients, are usually detected immediately or within a few hours after the precipitating incident. Chronic subdural hematomas, usually seen in the elderly, are frequently of unknown origin; may take days or weeks to become symptomatic; and cause a progressive change in mental status of the patient. This lesion appears "long and thin," compared to an epidural hematoma, follows the surface of the brain, and may extend for considerable distances (see Fig. 2-48 on p. 48 and Fig. 2-51 on p. 51). Treatment is surgical evacuation (for larger or acute lesions) or close monitoring for small, asymptomatic, or chronic lesions.

The most common cause of ***subarachnoid hemorrhage*** is trauma. In approximately 80% of patients with **spontaneous (*nontraumatic*) *subarachnoid hemorrhage,*** the precipitating event is rupture of an intracranial aneurysm. Symptomatic bleeding from an arteriovenous malformation occurs in approximately 5% of cases. Blood collects in, and percolates through, the subarachnoid space and cisterns (see Fig. 2-51 on page 51). Sometimes, the deficits seen (assuming the patient is not in coma) may be a clue as to location, especially if cranial nerves are nearby. Onset is sudden; the patient complains of an excruciating headache and may remain conscious, become lethargic and disoriented, or may be comatose. Treatment of an aneurysm is to surgically occlude it (by clip or coil), if possible, and to protect against the development of vasospasm. During surgery, some blood in the subarachnoid space and cisterns may be removed.

Tumors of the meninges (***meningiomas***) are classified in different ways but they usually arise from arachnoid cap/stem cells (a small number are dural in origin) around the villi or at places where vessels or cranial nerves penetrate the dura-arachnoid. These tumors grow slowly (symptoms may develop almost imperceptibly over years), are histologically benign, may result in hyperostosis of the overlying skull, and frequently contain calcifications. In decreasing order, meningiomas are found in the following locations: parasagittal area + falx (together 29%), convexity 15%, sella 13%, sphenoid ridge 12%, and olfactory groove 10%. Treatment is primarily by surgical removal, although some meningiomas are treated by radiotherapy.

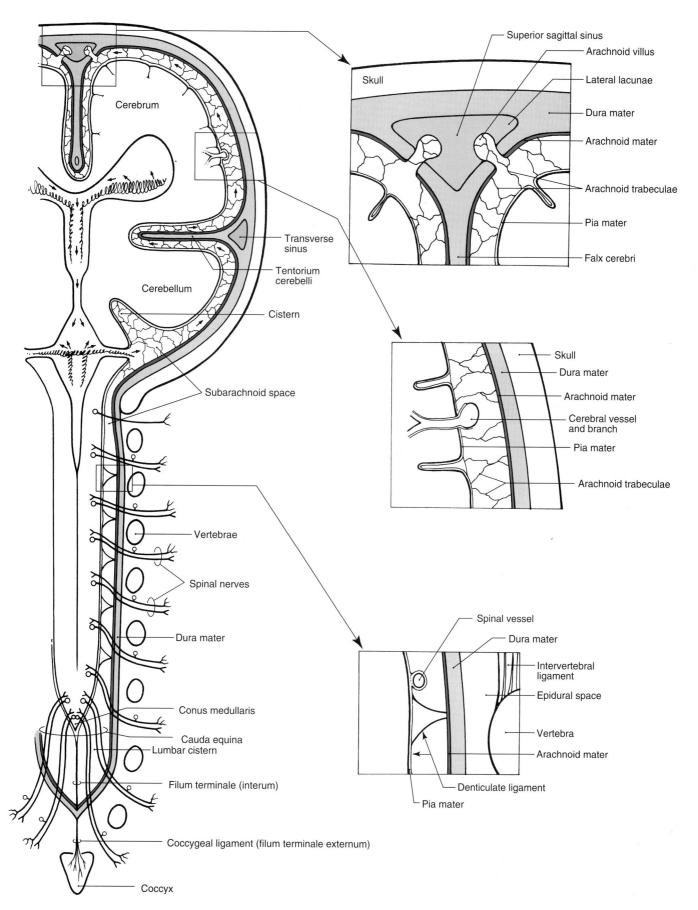

2-47 Semidiagrammatic representation of the central nervous system and its associated meninges. The details show the relationships of the meninges in the area of the superior sagittal sinus, on the lateral aspect of the cerebral hemisphere, and around the spinal cord. Cerebrospinal fluid is produced by the choroid plexi of lateral, third, and fourth ventricles. It circulates through the ventricular system (small arrows) and enters the subarachnoid space via the medial foramen of Magendie and the two lateral foramen of Luschka. In the living situation the arachnoid is attached to the inner surface of the dura. There is no *actual* or *potential* subdural space.

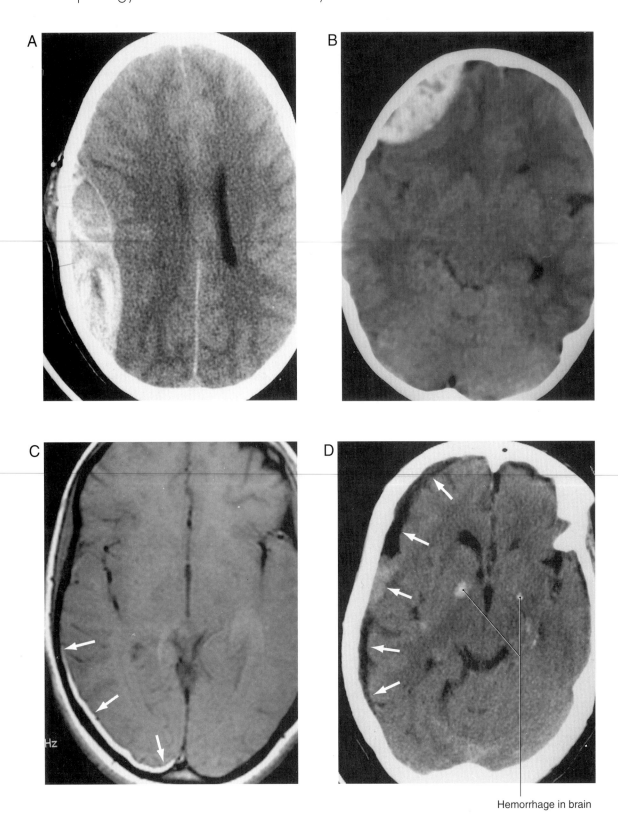

Hemorrhage in brain

2-48 Examples of epidural (extradural) hemorrhages (**A, B**) and of acute (**C**) and subacute (**D**) subdural hematoma. Note the lenticular shape of the epidural lesions (**A, B**), their loculated appearance, and their location external to the substance of the brain. In contrast, the acute subdural lesion (**C**) is quite thin and extends over a longer distance on the cortex.

In **D,** the subdural hematoma has both chronic and subacute phases. The chronic phase is indicated by the upper two and lower two arrows where the blood is replaced by fluid, and the subacute phase by the middle arrow where fresher blood has entered the lesion. Note the extent of this lesion on the surface of the cortex and its narrowness compared to epidural lesions. The patient in **D** also has small hemorrhages into the substance of the brain, the larger of these in the region of the genu of the internal capsule. Images **A–D** are CT. For additional comments on epidural and subdural hemorrhages see page 46.

A

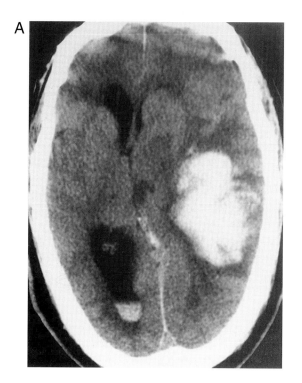

B

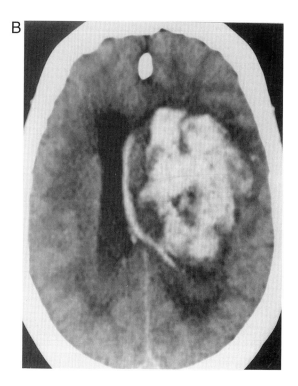

C

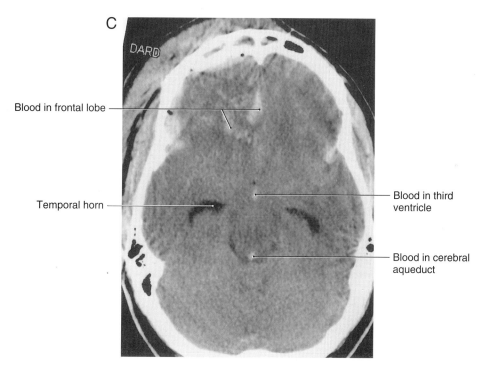

Blood in frontal lobe

Temporal horn

Blood in third ventricle

Blood in cerebral aqueduct

2-49   Examples of hemorrhages into the substance of the brain that, in some cases, have also resulted in blood in the ventricular system. The large hemorrhages into the hemisphere (**A, B**) have resulted in enlargement of the ventricles, a midline shift, and, in the case of **A,** a small amount of blood in the posterior horn of the lateral ventricle. In these examples, the lesion is most likely a result of hemorrhage from lenticulostriate branches of the M_1 segment.

Blood in the substance of the brain and in the ventricular system may also result from trauma (**C**). In this example (**C**), blood is seen in the frontal lobe and in the third ventricle and cerebral aqueduct. The enlarged temporal horns (**C**) of the lateral ventricles are consistent with the interruption of CSF flow through the cerebral aqueduct (noncommunicating hydrocephalus). Images **A–C** are CT.

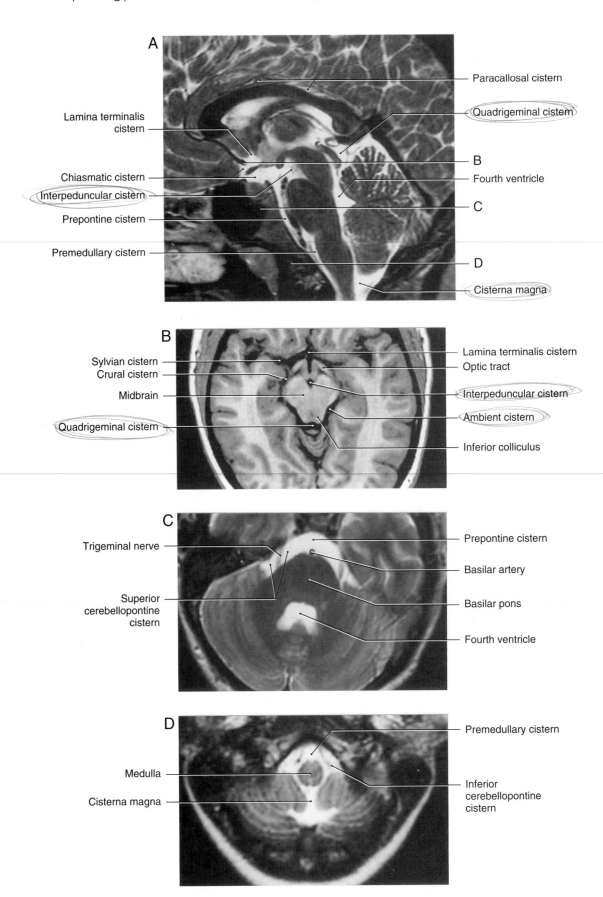

A

Paracallosal cistern

Quadrigeminal cistern

Lamina terminalis cistern

Chiasmatic cistern

Interpeduncular cistern

Prepontine cistern

Premedullary cistern

B

Fourth ventricle

C

D

Cisterna magna

B

Sylvian cistern

Crural cistern

Midbrain

Quadrigeminal cistern

Lamina terminalis cistern

Optic tract

Interpeduncular cistern

Ambient cistern

Inferior colliculus

C

Trigeminal nerve

Superior cerebellopontine cistern

Prepontine cistern

Basilar artery

Basilar pons

Fourth ventricle

D

Medulla

Cisterna magna

Premedullary cistern

Inferior cerebellopontine cistern

2-50 A median sagittal MRI (**A,** T2-weighted) of the brain showing the positions of the major cisterns associated with midline structures. Axial views of the midbrain (**B,** T1-weighted), pons (**C,** T2-weighted), and medulla (**D,** T2-weighted) represent the corresponding planes indicated in the sagittal view (**A**).

Cisterns are the enlarged portions of the subarachnoid space that contain arteries and veins, roots of cranial nerves, and, of course, cerebrospinal fluid. Consequently, the subarachnoid space and cisterns are continuous one with the other. In addition, the subarachnoid space around the brain is continuous with that around the spinal cord. Compare these cisterns with blood-filled parts of the subarachnoid space and cisterns in Figure 2-51 on the facing page.

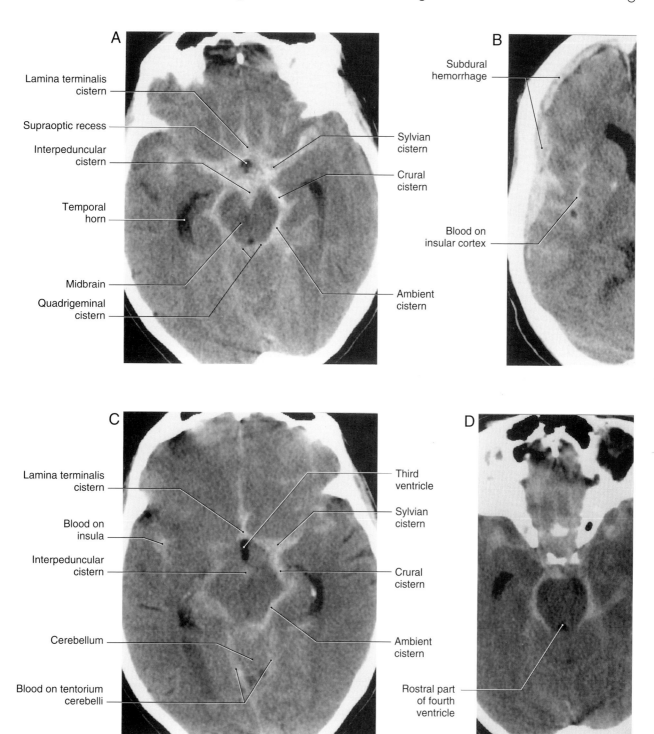

A

Lamina terminalis cistern

Supraoptic recess

Interpeduncular cistern

Temporal horn

Midbrain

Quadrigeminal cistern

Sylvian cistern

Crural cistern

Ambient cistern

B

Subdural hemorrhage

Blood on insular cortex

C

Lamina terminalis cistern

Blood on insula

Interpeduncular cistern

Cerebellum

Blood on tentorium cerebelli

Third ventricle

Sylvian cistern

Crural cistern

Ambient cistern

D

Rostral part of fourth ventricle

2-51   Blood in the subarachnoid space and cisterns. In these CT examples, blood occupies the subarachnoid space and cisterns, outlining these areas in white. Consequently, the shape of the cisterns is indicated by the configuration of the white area, the white area representing blood.

Around the base of the brain (**A**), it is easy to identify the cisterns related to the midbrain, the supraoptic recess which is devoid of blood, and blood extending laterally into the Sylvian cistern. In some cases (**B**), subdural hemorrhage may penetrate the arachnoid membrane and result in blood infiltrating between gyri, such as this example with blood on the cortex of the insula. In **C**, the blood is located around the midbrain (crural and ambient cisterns), extends into the Sylvian cistern, and into the cistern of the lamina terminalis. The sharp interface between the lamina terminalis cistern (containing blood) and the third ventricle (devoid of blood) represents the position of the lamina terminalis. In **D**, blood is located in cisterns around the pons but avoids the rostral part of the fourth ventricle. Compare these images with the locations of some of the comparable cisterns as seen in Figure 2-50 on the facing page. Images **A–D** are CT.

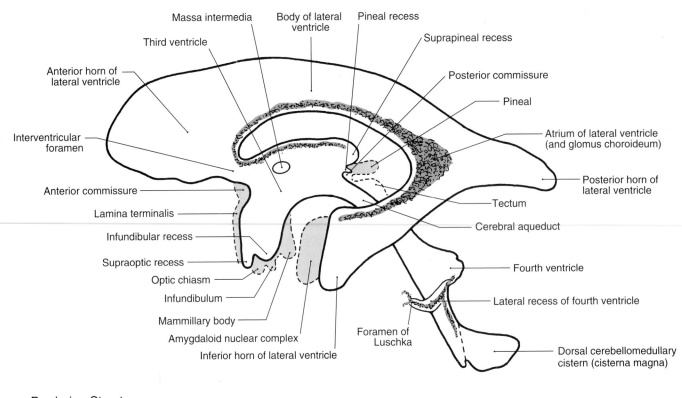

Massa intermedia

Body of lateral ventricle

Pineal recess

Third ventricle

Suprapineal recess

Anterior horn of lateral ventricle

Posterior commissure

Pineal

Interventricular foramen

Atrium of lateral ventricle (and glomus choroideum)

Posterior horn of lateral ventricle

Anterior commissure

Tectum

Lamina terminalis

Cerebral aqueduct

Infundibular recess

Supraoptic recess

Fourth ventricle

Optic chiasm

Lateral recess of fourth ventricle

Infundibulum

Mammillary body

Foramen of Luschka

Amygdaloid nuclear complex

Dorsal cerebellomedullary cistern (cisterna magna)

Inferior horn of lateral ventricle

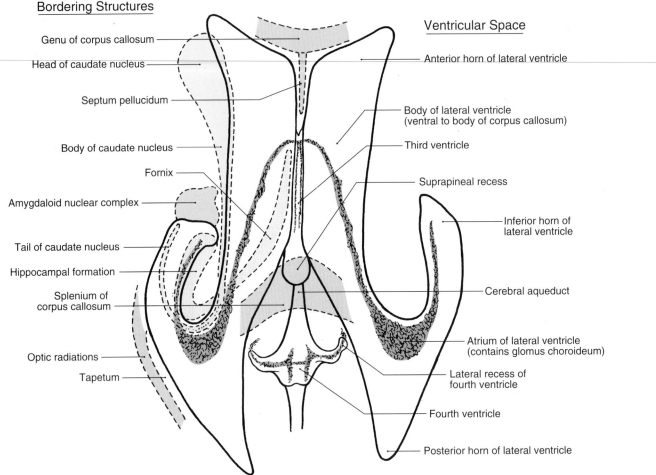

Bordering Structures

Ventricular Space

Genu of corpus callosum

Head of caudate nucleus

Anterior horn of lateral ventricle

Septum pellucidum

Body of lateral ventricle (ventral to body of corpus callosum)

Body of caudate nucleus

Third ventricle

Fornix

Suprapineal recess

Amygdaloid nuclear complex

Tail of caudate nucleus

Inferior horn of lateral ventricle

Hippocampal formation

Splenium of corpus callosum

Cerebral aqueduct

Optic radiations

Atrium of lateral ventricle (contains glomus choroideum)

Tapetum

Lateral recess of fourth ventricle

Fourth ventricle

Posterior horn of lateral ventricle

2-52 Lateral (above) and dorsal (below) views of the ventricles and the choroid plexus. The dashed lines show the approximate positions of some of the important structures that border on the ventricular space. The choroid plexus is shown in red and structures bordering on the various portions of the ventricular spaces are color-coded; these colors are continued in Figure 2-53 on the facing page. Note the relationships between the choroid plexus and various parts of the ventricular system. The large expanded portion of the choroid plexus found in the area of the atrium is the glomus (glomus choroideum). See Figure 8-12 on p. 251 for details of blood supply to the choroid plexus.

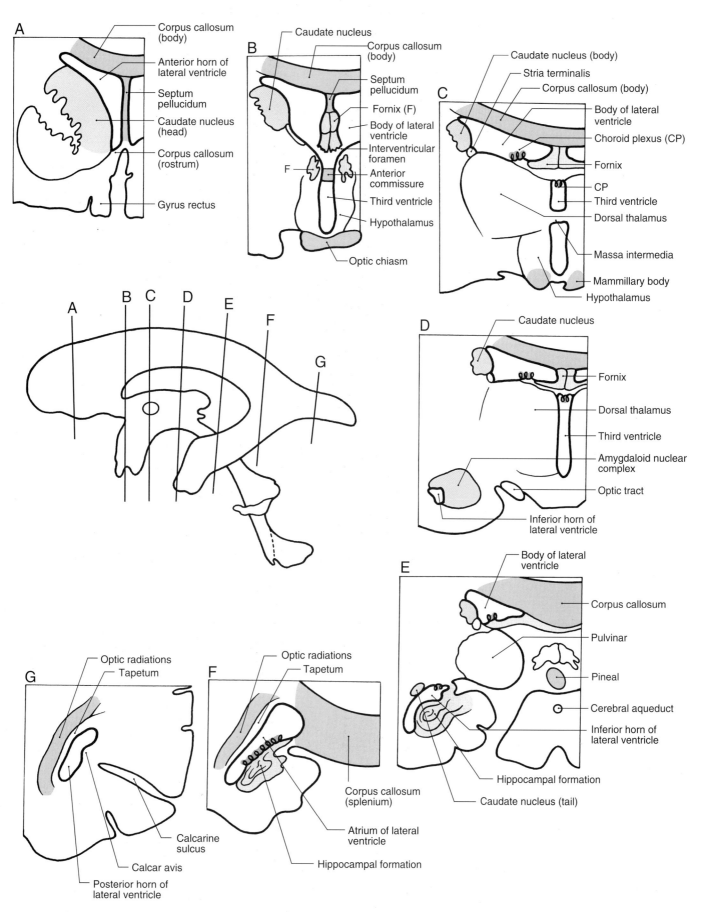

A
- Corpus callosum (body)
- Anterior horn of lateral ventricle
- Septum pellucidum
- Caudate nucleus (head)
- Corpus callosum (rostrum)
- Gyrus rectus

B
- Caudate nucleus
- Corpus callosum (body)
- Septum pellucidum
- Fornix (F)
- Body of lateral ventricle
- Interventricular foramen
- Anterior commissure
- Third ventricle
- Hypothalamus
- Optic chiasm
- F

C
- Caudate nucleus (body)
- Stria terminalis
- Corpus callosum (body)
- Body of lateral ventricle
- Choroid plexus (CP)
- Fornix
- CP
- Third ventricle
- Dorsal thalamus
- Massa intermedia
- Mammillary body
- Hypothalamus

D
- Caudate nucleus
- Fornix
- Dorsal thalamus
- Third ventricle
- Amygdaloid nuclear complex
- Optic tract
- Inferior horn of lateral ventricle

E
- Body of lateral ventricle
- Corpus callosum
- Pulvinar
- Pineal
- Cerebral aqueduct
- Inferior horn of lateral ventricle
- Hippocampal formation
- Caudate nucleus (tail)

F
- Optic radiations
- Tapetum
- Corpus callosum (splenium)
- Atrium of lateral ventricle
- Hippocampal formation

G
- Optic radiations
- Tapetum
- Calcarine sulcus
- Calcar avis
- Posterior horn of lateral ventricle

2-53   Lateral view of the ventricular system and corresponding semidiagrammatic cross-sectional representations from rostral **(A)** to caudal **(G)** identifying specific structures that border on the ventricular space. In the cross-sections, the ventricle is outlined by a heavy line, and the majority of structures labeled have some direct relevance to the ventricular space at that particular level. The color-coding corresponds to that shown in Figure 2-52 on the facing page.

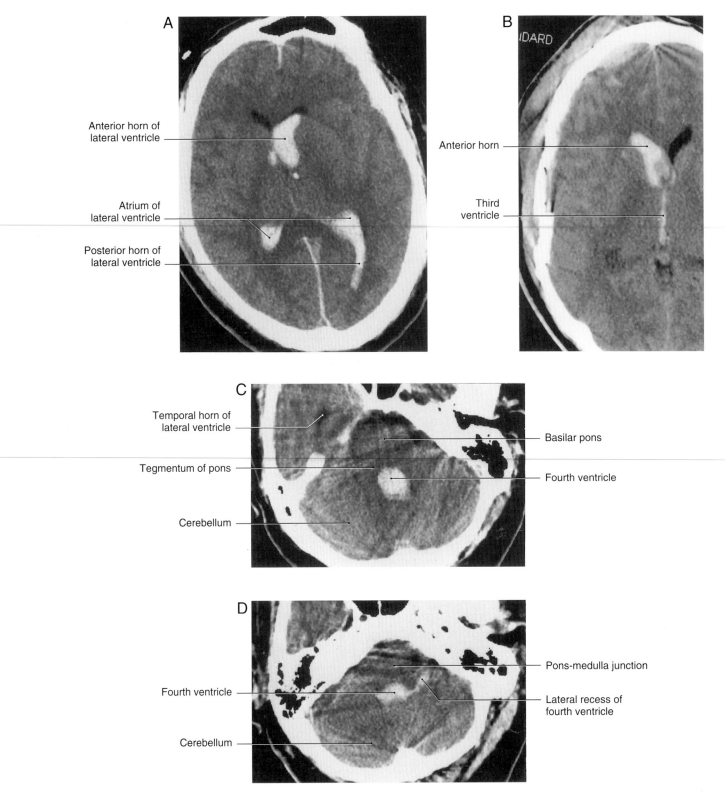

2-54   Examples of hemorrhage occupying portions of the ventricular system (ventricular hemorrhage). In these CT images, blood appears white within the ventricles. Consequently, the shape of the ventricular system is outlined by the white area, and the specific portion of the ventricular system is correspondingly labeled.

Note blood in the anterior horn, atrium, and posterior horn of the lateral ventricles (**A, B**), and blood clearly outlining the shape of the third ventricle (**B**). Blood also clearly outlines central portions of the fourth ventricle (**C**) and caudal portions of the fourth ventricle (**D**), including an extension of blood into the left lateral recess of the fourth ventricle. In addition to these images, Figure 2-49 on page 49 shows blood in the cerebral aqueduct and in the most inferior portions of the third ventricle. Images **A–D** are CT.

Dissections of the
Central Nervous System

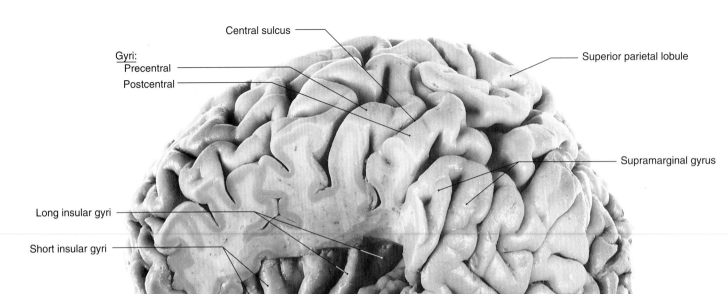

Central sulcus

Gyri:
Precentral
Postcentral

Superior parietal lobule

Supramarginal gyrus

Long insular gyri

Short insular gyri

Central sulcus of insula

Gyri:
Transverse temporal
Superior temporal

Superior temporal sulcus

3-1   Lateral view of the right cerebral hemisphere with the inferior and parts of the middle frontal gyri and precentral and postcentral gyri removed to show the insular cortex, transverse temporal gyri, and related structures.

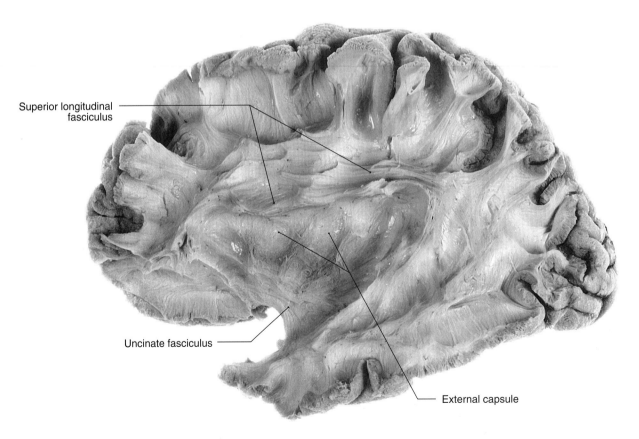

Superior longitudinal fasciculus

Uncinate fasciculus

External capsule

3-2   Dissection of the lateral aspect of the right cerebral hemisphere showing the locations and relationships of some of the main bundles of subcortical white matter. This dissection is deep to that shown in Figure 3-1 (above) and superficial to that shown in Figure 3-3 on page 57.

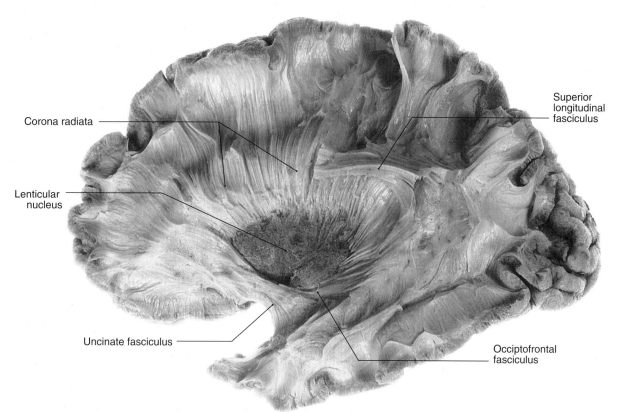

Corona radiata

Lenticular nucleus

Uncinate fasciculus

Superior longitudinal fasciculus

Occiptofrontal fasciculus

3-3   Dissection of the lateral aspect of the right cerebral hemisphere showing the relationship between fibers radiating from the internal capsule (corona radiata) and those of the superior longitudinal fasciculus. The lenticular nucleus is shown in situ, lateral to the internal capsule. This is a deeper dissection of the specimen shown in Figure 3-2 on page 56.

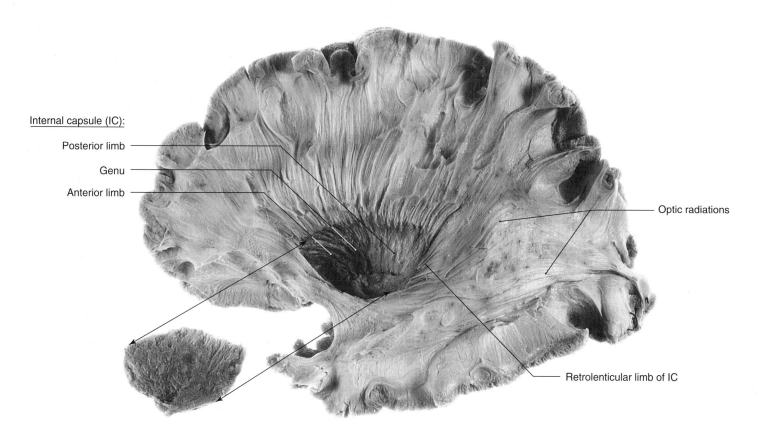

Internal capsule (IC):

Posterior limb

Genu

Anterior limb

Optic radiations

Retrolenticular limb of IC

3-4   Dissection of the lateral aspect of the right cerebral hemisphere showing the internal capsule and the concavity left by removal of the lenticular nucleus. Note the other bundles of subcortical white matter. This is a deeper dissection of the specimen shown in Figure 3-3 (above).

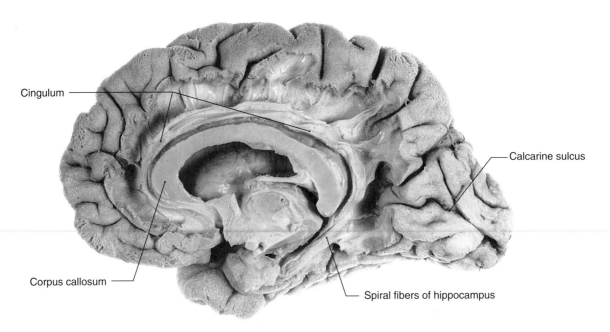

Cingulum

Calcarine sulcus

Corpus callosum

Spiral fibers of hippocampus

3-5 Dissection of the medial aspect of the left cerebral hemisphere showing the cingulum and spiral fibers of the hippocampus.

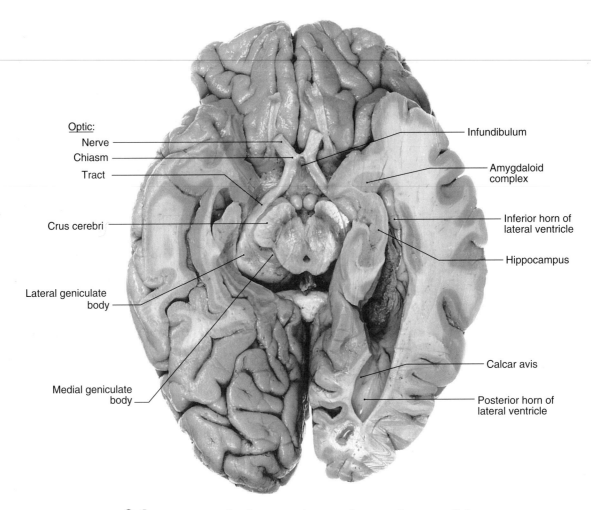

Optic:
Nerve
Chiasm
Tract

Infundibulum

Amygdaloid complex

Crus cerebri

Inferior horn of lateral ventricle

Hippocampus

Lateral geniculate body

Medial geniculate body

Calcar avis

Posterior horn of lateral ventricle

3-6 Overview of a dissection showing the ventral aspect of the cerebral hemispheres. Note the structures related to ventricular spaces and the structures located at the mesencephalon–diencephalon interface. A number of structures in addition to those labeled can be identified.

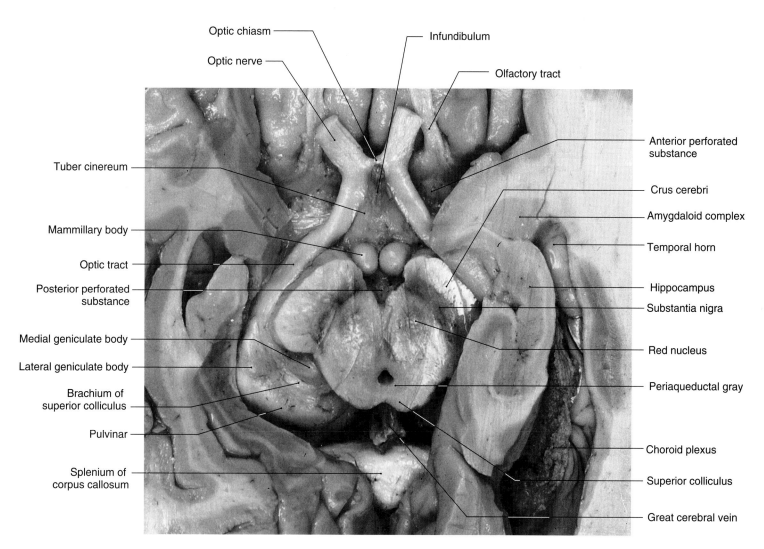

Optic chiasm

Optic nerve

Infundibulum

Olfactory tract

Anterior perforated substance

Tuber cinereum

Crus cerebri

Amygdaloid complex

Mammillary body

Temporal horn

Optic tract

Posterior perforated substance

Hippocampus

Substantia nigra

Medial geniculate body

Lateral geniculate body

Red nucleus

Brachium of superior colliculus

Periaqueductal gray

Pulvinar

Splenium of corpus callosum

Choroid plexus

Superior colliculus

Great cerebral vein

3-7 Detailed view of a dissection showing the ventral aspects of the cerebral hemispheres; this is of the same specimen shown in Figure 3-6 on page 58. Note the continuum of optic nerve, chiasm, and tract to the lateral geniculate body; the relationship of the optic tract to the crus cerebri; and the relationship of hypothalamic structures on the ventral aspect of the brain. In addition to those labeled, other structures can be identified.

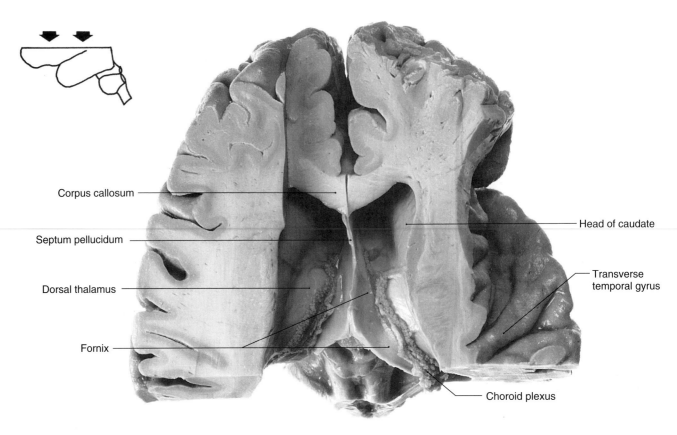

Corpus callosum

Septum pellucidum

Dorsal thalamus

Fornix

Head of caudate

Transverse temporal gyrus

Choroid plexus

3-8 Dissected view of the brain from the dorsal aspect showing structures associated with the lateral ventricles. Note the appearance of insular and transverse temporal gyri, the fornix, and other structures in addition to those labeled.

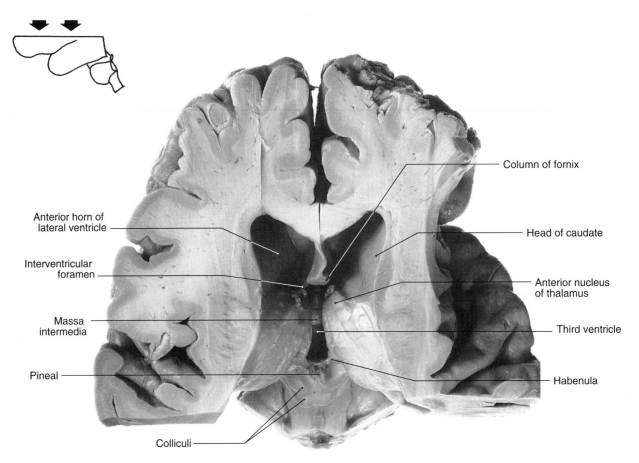

Anterior horn of lateral ventricle

Interventricular foramen

Massa intermedia

Pineal

Column of fornix

Head of caudate

Anterior nucleus of thalamus

Third ventricle

Habenula

Colliculi

3-9 Dissected view of the brain from the dorsal aspect showing lateral and third ventricles, the dorsal surface of the diencephalon, the insula and transverse temporal gyri, and the colliculi. The majority of the fornix and the roof of the third ventricle have been removed. The small tufts of choroid plexus identify the locations of the interventricular foramina. Note the massa intermedia traversing the third ventricle and other structures in addition to those labeled.

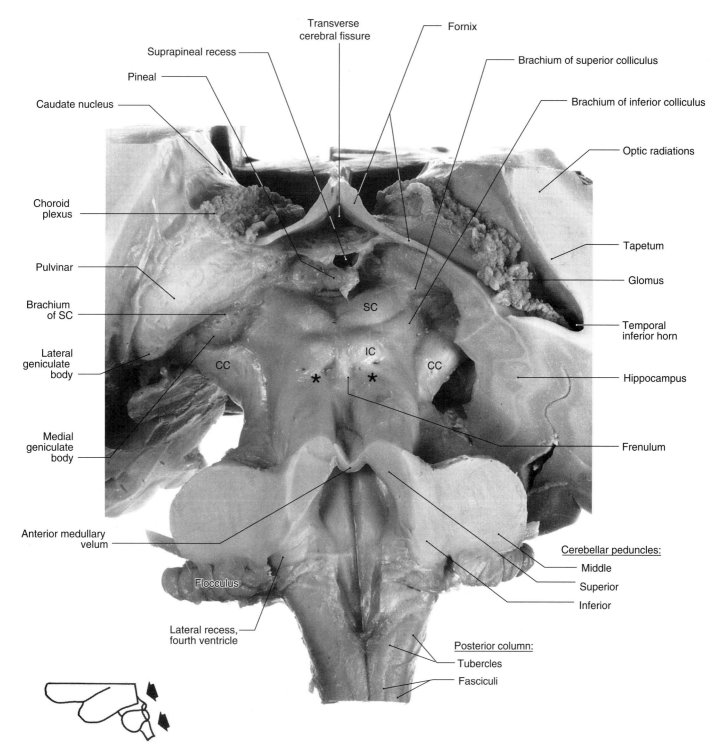

Transverse
cerebral fissure

Fornix

Suprapineal recess

Brachium of superior colliculus

Pineal

Brachium of inferior colliculus

Caudate nucleus

Optic radiations

Choroid
plexus

Tapetum

Pulvinar

Glomus

Brachium
of SC

Temporal
inferior horn

Lateral
geniculate
body

Hippocampus

Medial
geniculate
body

Frenulum

SC

IC

CC

CC

Anterior medullary
velum

Cerebellar peduncles:

Middle

Flocculus

Superior

Inferior

Lateral recess,
fourth ventricle

Posterior column:

Tubercles

Fasciculi

3-10   A dissection showing caudal diencephalic structures, several telencephalic structures, and the interface of the mesencephalon with caudal parts of the thalamus. On the right side, note the continuation between the fornix and hippocampus; on the left, these structures have been removed to expose the underlying pulvinar. The superior colli-culi (SC), the inferior colliculi (IC), and the crus cerebri (CC), as seen from the dorsal aspect, are identified. The asterisks represent the exit points of the trochlear nerves. For further details of the dorsal brain-stem, see Figure 2-34 on page 34. Note structures in addition to those labeled.

4

Internal Morphology
of the Brain in
Slices and MRI

Brain Slices in the Coronal Plane with MRI

Orientation to Coronal MRIs: When looking at a coronal MRI image, you are viewing the image as if you are looking at the face of the patient. Consequently, the observer's right is the left side of the brain in the MRI and the left side of the patient's brain. Obviously, the concept of what is the left side versus what is the right side of the patient's brain is enormously important when using MRI (or CT) to diagnose a neurologically impaired individual.

To reinforce this concept, the rostral surface of each coronal brain slice was photographed. So, when looking at the slice, the observer's right field of view is the left side of the brain slice. This view of the slice correlates exactly with the orientation of the brain as seen in the accompanying coronal MRIs.

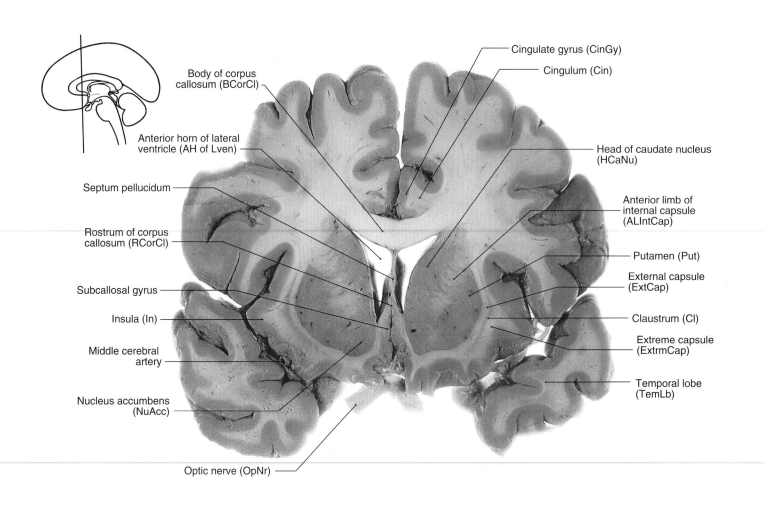

Cingulate gyrus (CinGy)

Cingulum (Cin)

Body of corpus callosum (BCorCl)

Anterior horn of lateral ventricle (AH of Lven)

Head of caudate nucleus (HCaNu)

Septum pellucidum

Anterior limb of internal capsule (ALIntCap)

Rostrum of corpus callosum (RCorCl)

Putamen (Put)

External capsule (ExtCap)

Subcallosal gyrus

Claustrum (Cl)

Insula (In)

Extreme capsule (ExtrmCap)

Middle cerebral artery

Temporal lobe (TemLb)

Nucleus accumbens (NuAcc)

Optic nerve (OpNr)

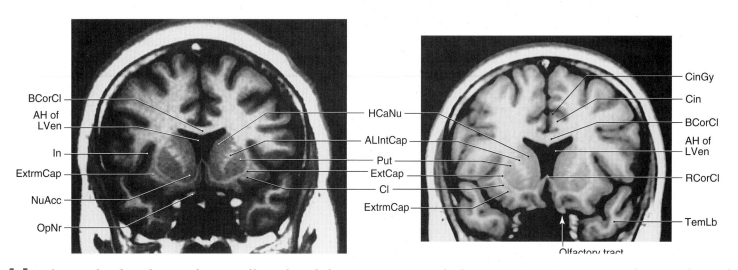

BCorCl

AH of LVen

In

ExtrmCap

NuAcc

OpNr

HCaNu

ALIntCap

Put

ExtCap

Cl

ExtrmCap

CinGy

Cin

BCorCl

AH of LVen

RCorCl

TemLb

Olfactory tract

4-1 The rostral surface of a coronal section of brain through the *anterior limb of the internal capsule* and the *head of the caudate nucleus*. The two MRI images (both are inversion recovery) are at the same plane and show many of the structures identified in the brain slice.

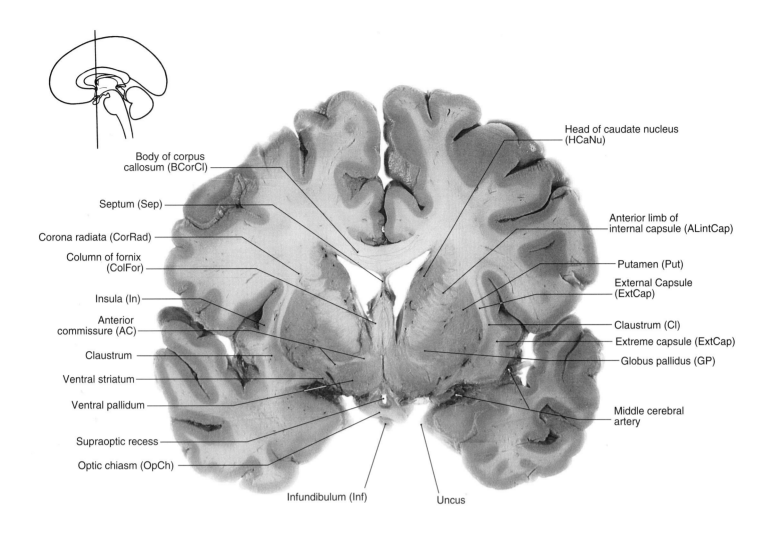

Body of corpus callosum (BCorCl)

Septum (Sep)

Corona radiata (CorRad)

Column of fornix (ColFor)

Insula (In)

Anterior commissure (AC)

Claustrum

Ventral striatum

Ventral pallidum

Supraoptic recess

Optic chiasm (OpCh)

Head of caudate nucleus (HCaNu)

Anterior limb of internal capsule (ALintCap)

Putamen (Put)

External Capsule (ExtCap)

Claustrum (Cl)

Extreme capsule (ExtCap)

Globus pallidus (GP)

Middle cerebral artery

Infundibulum (Inf)

Uncus

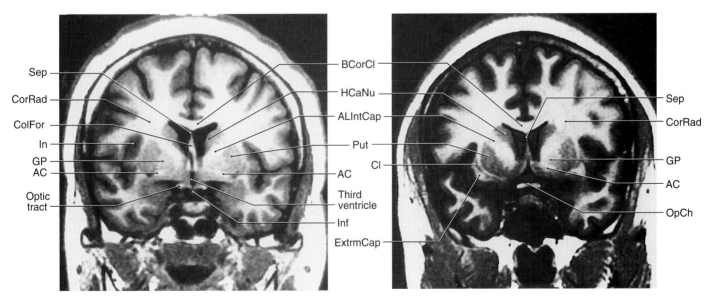

Sep

CorRad

ColFor

In

GP

AC

Optic tract

BCorCl

HCaNu

ALIntCap

Put

AC

Third ventricle

Inf

ExtrmCap

Sep

CorRad

GP

AC

OpCh

Cl

4-2   The rostral surface of a coronal section of brain through the level of the *anterior commissure* and the *column of the fornix*. The two MRI im-ages (both are inversion recovery) are at the same plane and show many of the structures identified in the brain slice.

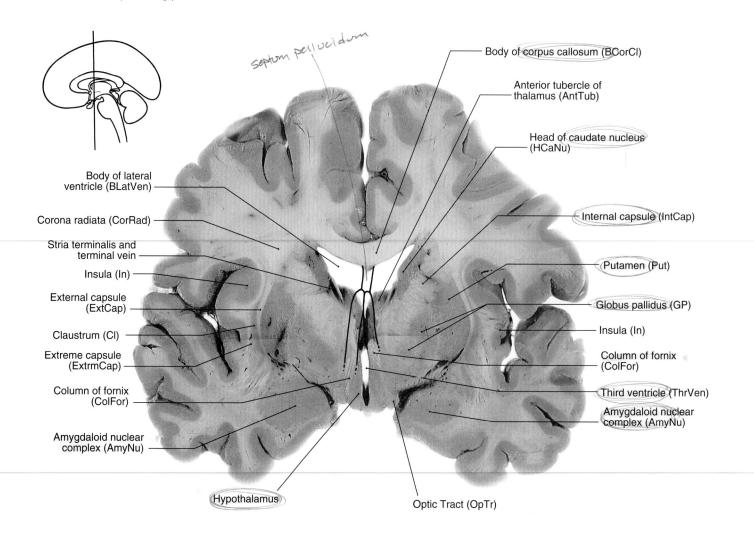

septum pellucidum

Body of corpus callosum (BCorCl)

Anterior tubercle of thalamus (AntTub)

Head of caudate nucleus (HCaNu)

Internal capsule (IntCap)

Putamen (Put)

Globus pallidus (GP)

Insula (In)

Column of fornix (ColFor)

Third ventricle (ThrVen)

Amygdaloid nuclear complex (AmyNu)

Body of lateral ventricle (BLatVen)

Corona radiata (CorRad)

Stria terminalis and terminal vein

Insula (In)

External capsule (ExtCap)

Claustrum (Cl)

Extreme capsule (ExtrmCap)

Column of fornix (ColFor)

Amygdaloid nuclear complex (AmyNu)

Hypothalamus

Optic Tract (OpTr)

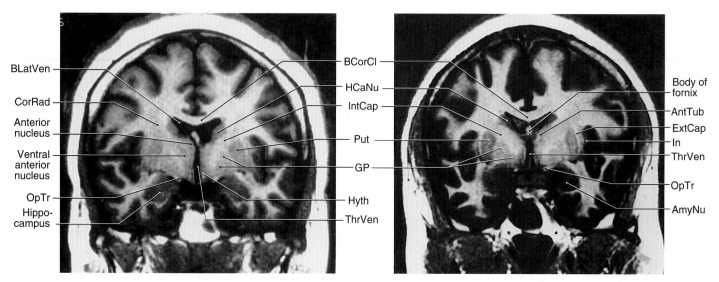

BLatVen

CorRad

Anterior nucleus

Ventral anterior nucleus

OpTr

Hippo-campus

BCorCl

HCaNu

IntCap

Put

GP

Hyth

ThrVen

Body of fornix

AntTub

ExtCap

In

ThrVen

OpTr

AmyNu

4-3   The rostral surface of a coronal section of brain through the level of the *anterior tubercle of the thalamus* and the *column of the fornix* just caudal to the anterior commissure. Portions of the columns of the fornix and the septum (drawn in as black lines) were removed to more ade-quately expose the anterior tubercles of the thalamus. The terminal vein is also called the superior thalamostriate vein. The two MRI images (both are inversion recovery) are at the same plane and show many of the structures identified in the brain slice.

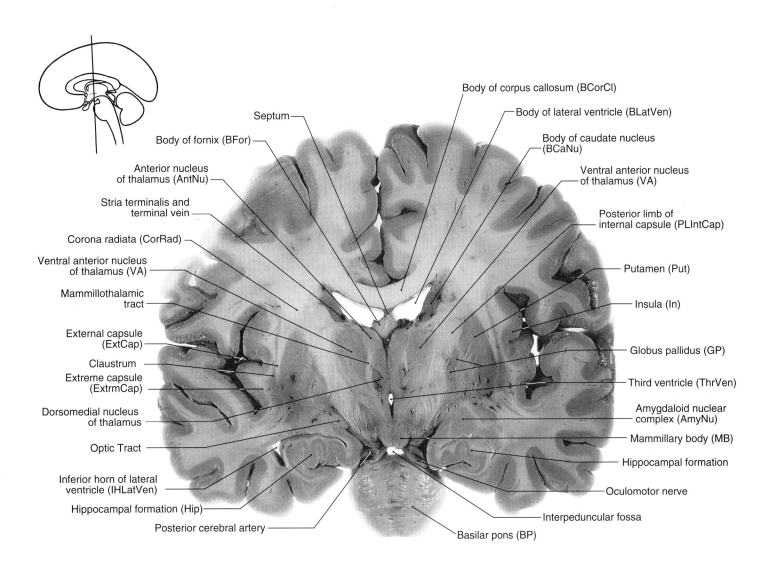

Body of corpus callosum (BCorCl)

Body of lateral ventricle (BLatVen)

Body of caudate nucleus (BCaNu)

Septum

Body of fornix (BFor)

Anterior nucleus of thalamus (AntNu)

Ventral anterior nucleus of thalamus (VA)

Stria terminalis and terminal vein

Posterior limb of internal capsule (PLIntCap)

Corona radiata (CorRad)

Ventral anterior nucleus of thalamus (VA)

Putamen (Put)

Mammillothalamic tract

Insula (In)

External capsule (ExtCap)

Globus pallidus (GP)

Claustrum

Extreme capsule (ExtrmCap)

Third ventricle (ThrVen)

Dorsomedial nucleus of thalamus

Amygdaloid nuclear complex (AmyNu)

Optic Tract

Mammillary body (MB)

Hippocampal formation

Inferior horn of lateral ventricle (IHLatVen)

Oculomotor nerve

Hippocampal formation (Hip)

Interpeduncular fossa

Posterior cerebral artery

Basilar pons (BP)

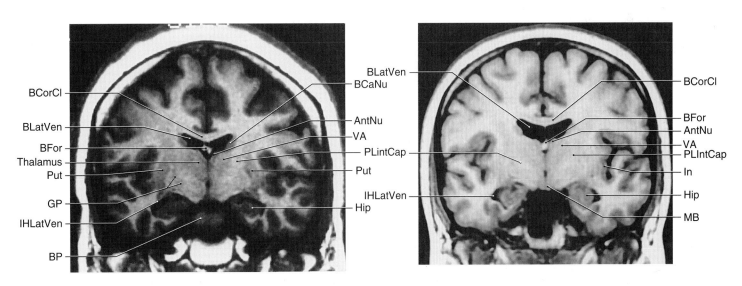

BCorCl

BLatVen

BFor

Thalamus

Put

GP

IHLatVen

BP

BLatVen

BCaNu

AntNu

VA

PLintCap

Put

IHLatVen

Hip

BLatVen

BCorCl

BFor

AntNu

VA

PLIntCap

In

Hip

MB

4-4   The rostral surface of a section of brain through the *anterior nucleus of the thalamus, mammillothalamic tract,* and *mammillary bodies.* The two MRI images (both are inversion recovery) are at the same plane and show many of the structures identified in the brain slice. The globus pallidus is clearly divided into its lateral and medial segments in the brain slice. Additionally, the terminal vein is also called the superior thalamostriate vein.

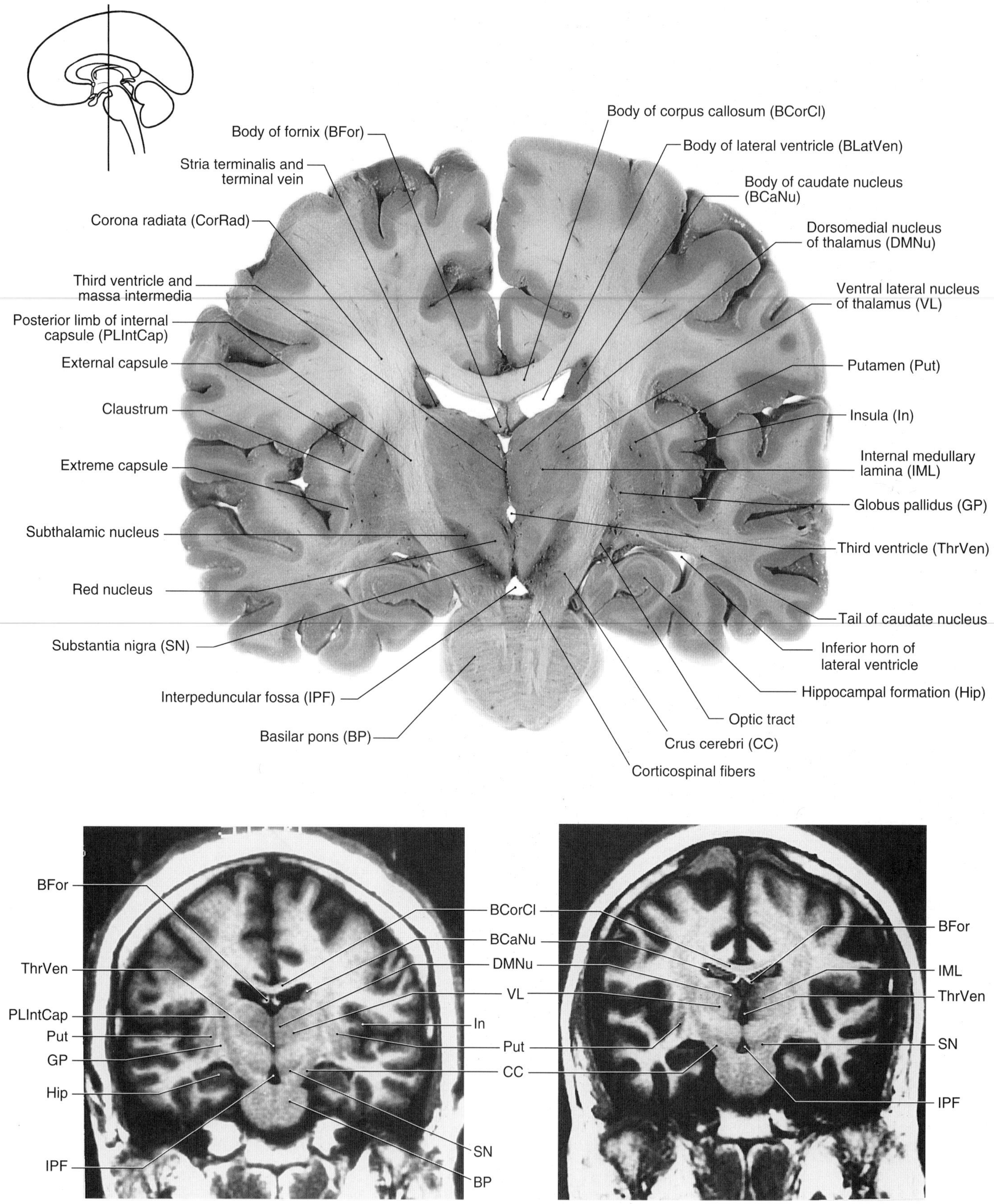

Body of corpus callosum (BCorCl)

Body of fornix (BFor)

Body of lateral ventricle (BLatVen)

Stria terminalis and
terminal vein

Body of caudate nucleus
(BCaNu)

Corona radiata (CorRad)

Dorsomedial nucleus
of thalamus (DMNu)

Third ventricle and
massa intermedia

Ventral lateral nucleus
of thalamus (VL)

Posterior limb of internal
capsule (PLIntCap)

External capsule

Putamen (Put)

Claustrum

Insula (In)

Extreme capsule

Internal medullary
lamina (IML)

Globus pallidus (GP)

Subthalamic nucleus

Third ventricle (ThrVen)

Red nucleus

Tail of caudate nucleus

Substantia nigra (SN)

Inferior horn of
lateral ventricle

Interpeduncular fossa (IPF)

Hippocampal formation (Hip)

Optic tract

Basilar pons (BP)

Crus cerebri (CC)

Corticospinal fibers

BFor

BCorCl

BFor

BCaNu

ThrVen

DMNu

IML

VL

ThrVen

PLIntCap

In

Put

SN

GP

Put

CC

Hip

IPF

IPF

SN

BP

4-5   The rostral surface of a coronal section of brain through caudal parts of the *ventral lateral nucleus*, the *massa intermedia*, the *subthalamic nucleus*, and *basilar pons*. The two MRI images (both are inversion recovery) are at the same plane and show many of the structures identified in the brain slice. The terminal vein is also called the superior thalamostriate vein.

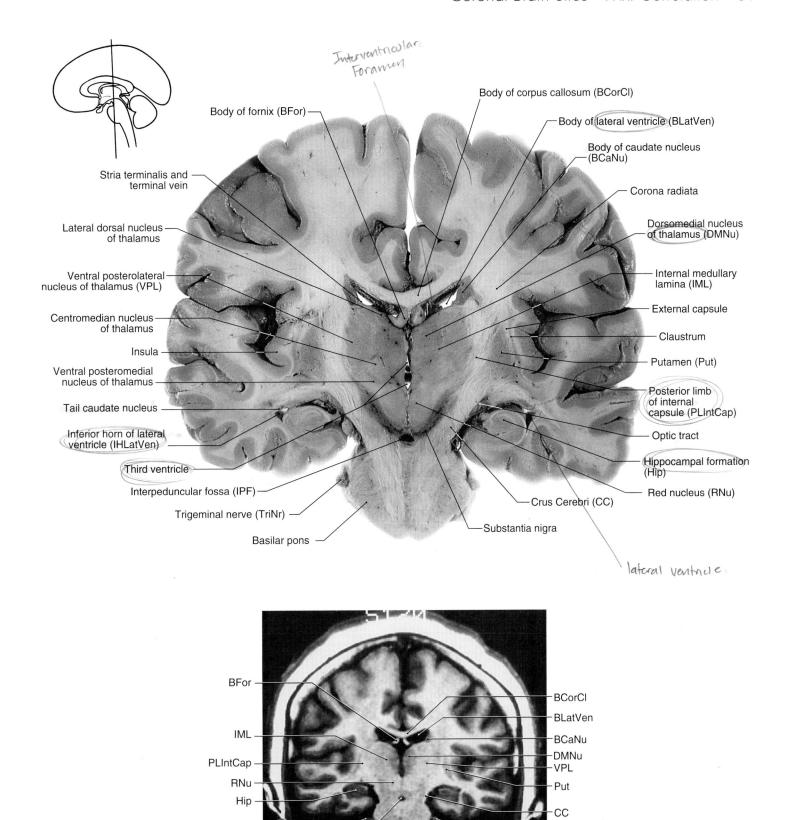

Interventricular Foramen

Body of fornix (BFor)

Body of corpus callosum (BCorCl)

Body of lateral ventricle (BLatVen)

Body of caudate nucleus (BCaNu)

Stria terminalis and terminal vein

Corona radiata

Dorsomedial nucleus of thalamus (DMNu)

Lateral dorsal nucleus of thalamus

Internal medullary lamina (IML)

Ventral posterolateral nucleus of thalamus (VPL)

External capsule

Centromedian nucleus of thalamus

Claustrum

Insula

Putamen (Put)

Ventral posteromedial nucleus of thalamus

Posterior limb of internal capsule (PLIntCap)

Tail caudate nucleus

Optic tract

Inferior horn of lateral ventricle (IHLatVen)

Hippocampal formation (Hip)

Third ventricle

Red nucleus (RNu)

Interpeduncular fossa (IPF)

Crus Cerebri (CC)

Trigeminal nerve (TriNr)

Substantia nigra

Basilar pons

lateral ventricle

BFor

BCorCl

BLatVen

IML

BCaNu

PLIntCap

DMNu

RNu

VPL

Hip

Put

TriNr

CC

IPF

TriNr

BP

4-6   The rostral surface of a coronal section of brain through the *lateral dorsal* and *centromedian nuclei*, rostral midbrain (*red nucleus*), and corticospinal fibers in the *basilar pons*. The MRI image (inversion recovery) is at the same plane and shows many of the structures identified in the brain slice. The terminal vein is also called the superior thalamostriate vein.

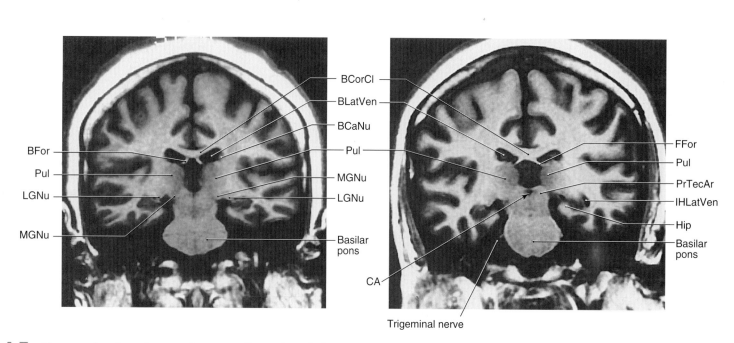

Body of corpus callosum (BCorCl)

Body of fornix (BFor)

Body of lateral ventricle (BLatVen)

Fimbria of fornix (FFor)

Body of caudate nucleus (BCaNu)

Stria terminalis and terminal vein

Pulvinar (Pul)

Pulvinar (Pul)

Retrolenticular limb of internal capsule

Medial geniculate nucleus (MGNu)

Posterior commissure

Lateral geniculate nucleus (LGNu)

Tail of caudate nucleus

Inferior horn of lateral ventricle (HLatVen)

Lateral geniculate nucleus (LGNu)

Hippocampal formation (Hip)

Pretectal area (PrTecAr)

Cerebral aqueduct (CA)

Periaqueductal gray

Decussation of superior cerebellar peduncle

Middle cerebellar peduncle (MCP)

Pyramid

BCorCl

BLatVen

BCaNu

BFor

Pul

Pul

MGNu

Pul

LGNu

PrTecAr

MGNu

LGNu

IHLatVen

Basilar pons

Hip

Basilar pons

CA

Trigeminal nerve

4-7   The rostral surface of a coronal section of brain through the *pulvinar, medial, and lateral geniculate nuclei,* the *basilar pons,* and *middle cerebellar peduncle.* The two MRI images (both inversion recovery) are at the same plane and show many of the structures in the brain slices. The terminal vein is also called the superior thalamostriate vein. For details of the cerebellum see Figures 2-31 to 2-33 on pp. 32 and 33.

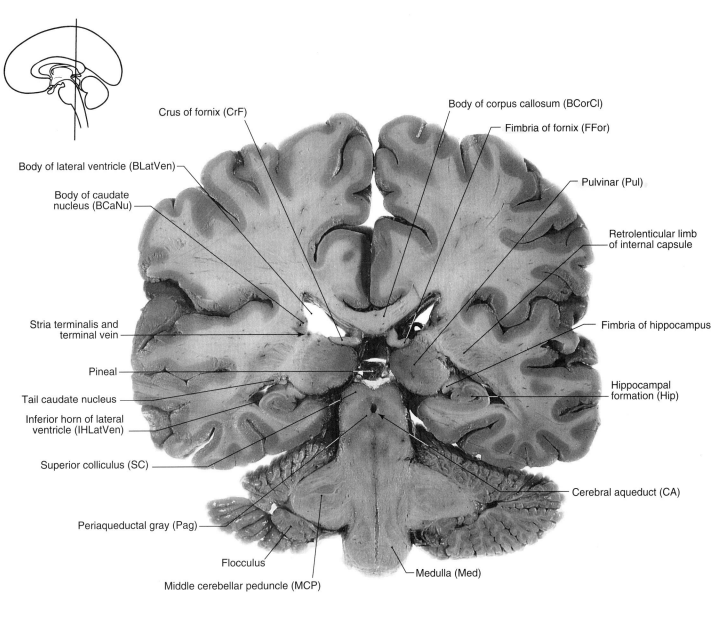

Crus of fornix (CrF)

Body of corpus callosum (BCorCl)

Fimbria of fornix (FFor)

Body of lateral ventricle (BLatVen)

Body of caudate nucleus (BCaNu)

Pulvinar (Pul)

Retrolenticular limb of internal capsule

Stria terminalis and terminal vein

Fimbria of hippocampus

Pineal

Tail caudate nucleus

Hippocampal formation (Hip)

Inferior horn of lateral ventricle (IHLatVen)

Superior colliculus (SC)

Cerebral aqueduct (CA)

Periaqueductal gray (Pag)

Flocculus

Medulla (Med)

Middle cerebellar peduncle (MCP)

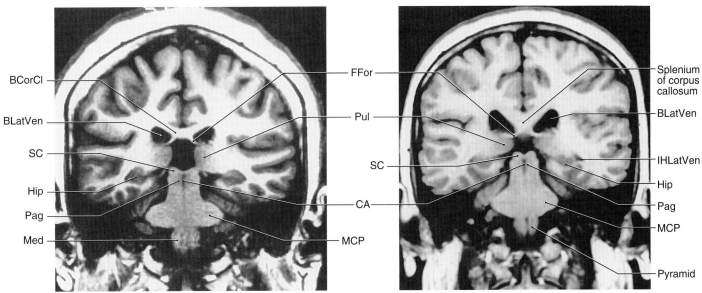

BCorCl

BLatVen

SC

Hip

Pag

Med

FFor

Pul

SC

CA

MCP

Splenium of corpus callosum

BLatVen

IHLatVen

Hip

Pag

MCP

Pyramid

4-8 The rostral surface of a coronal section of brain through the *pulvinar nucleus,* the *superior colliculus,* the *middle cerebellar peduncle,* and the rostral portion of the *medulla oblongata.* The two MRI images (both are inversion recovery) are at the same plane and show many of the structures identified in the brain slice. The terminal vein is also called the superior thalamostriate vein. For details of the cerebellum see Figures 2-31 to 2-33 on pp. 32 and 33.

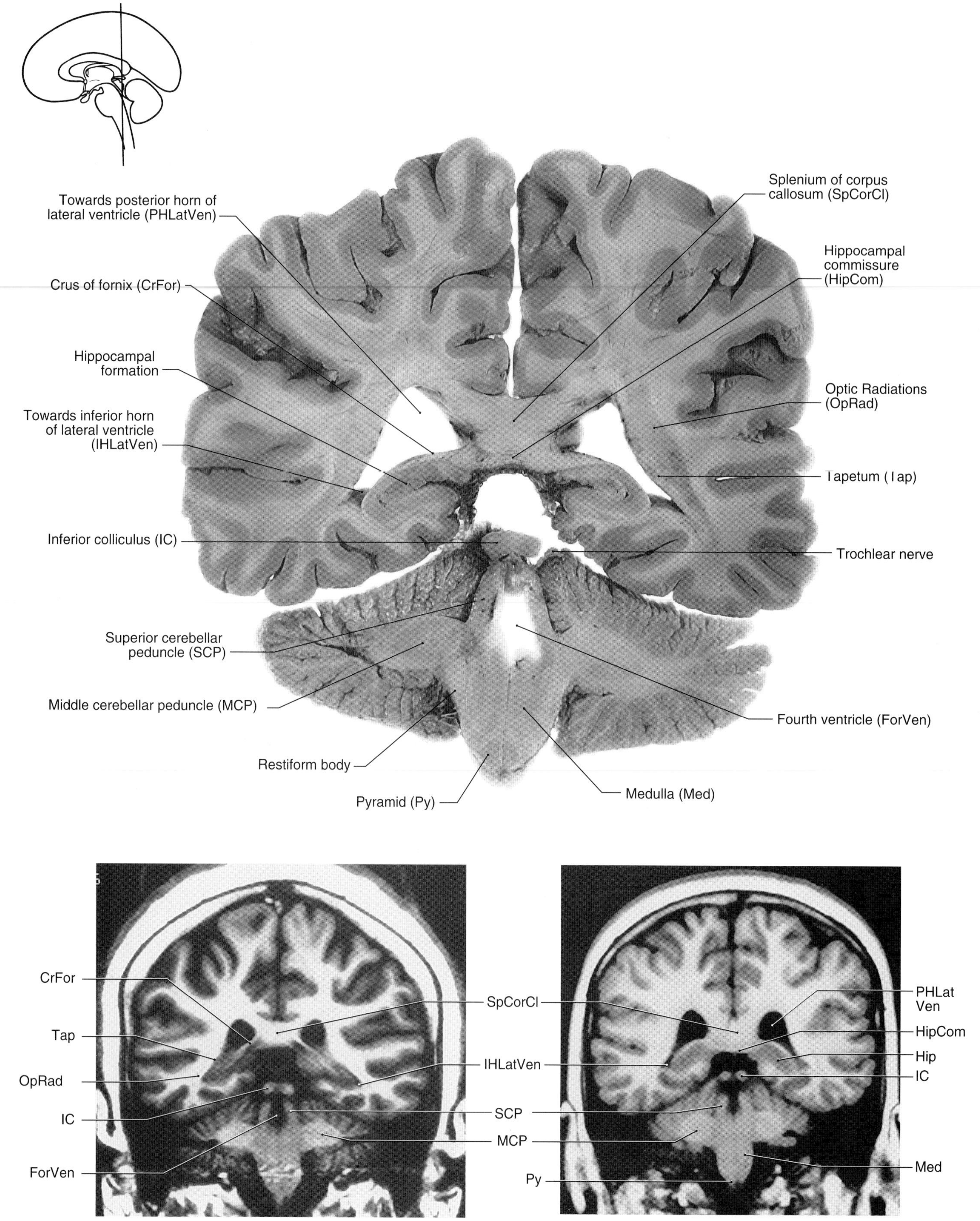

Towards posterior horn of
lateral ventricle (PHLatVen)

Crus of fornix (CrFor)

Hippocampal
formation

Towards inferior horn
of lateral ventricle
(IHLatVen)

Inferior colliculus (IC)

Superior cerebellar
peduncle (SCP)

Middle cerebellar peduncle (MCP)

Restiform body

Pyramid (Py)

Splenium of corpus
callosum (SpCorCl)

Hippocampal
commissure
(HipCom)

Optic Radiations
(OpRad)

Tapetum (Tap)

Trochlear nerve

Fourth ventricle (ForVen)

Medulla (Med)

CrFor

Tap

OpRad

IC

ForVen

SpCorCl

IHLatVen

SCP

MCP

Py

PHLat
Ven

HipCom

Hip

IC

Med

4-9   The rostral surface of a coronal section of brain through the *splenium of corpus callosum,* the *inferior colliculus,* the middle cerebellar peduncle in the base of the cerebellum, and the rostral portion of the medulla oblongata. The plane of the section is also through the atrium of the lateral ventricles. The two MRI images (both are inversion recovery) are at the same plane and show many of the structures identified in the brain slice. For details of the cerebellum see Figures 2-31 to 2-33 on pp. 32 and 33.

Internal Morphology
of the Brain in
Slices and MRI

Brain Slices in the Axial Plane with MRI

Orientation to Axial MRIs: When looking at an axial MRI image, you are viewing the image as if standing at the patient's feet and looking toward his or her head while the patient is lying on his or her back. Consequently, and as is the case in coronal images, the observer's right is the left side of the brain in the MRI and the left side of the patient's brain. It is absolutely essential to have a clear understanding of this right-versus-left concept when using MRI (or CT) in the diagnosis of the neurologically impaired patient.

To reinforce this concept, the ventral surface of each axial slice was photographed. So, when looking at the slice, the observer's right is the left side of the brain slice. This view of the slice correlates exactly with the orientation of the brain as seen in the accompanying axial MRIs.

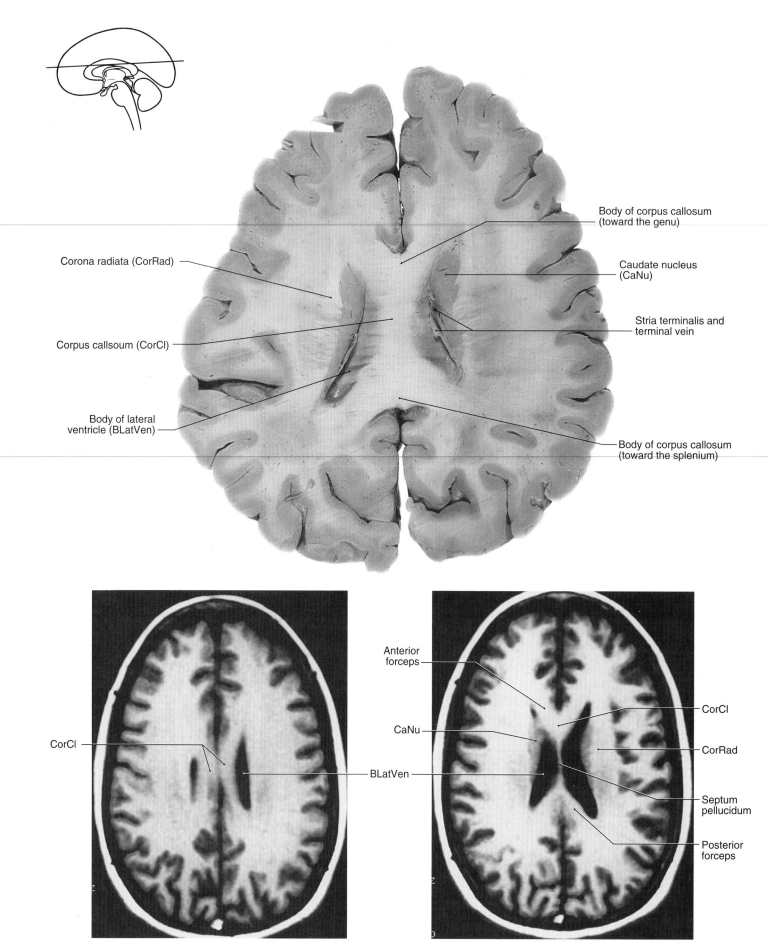

Corona radiata (CorRad)

Corpus callsoum (CorCl)

Body of lateral ventricle (BLatVen)

Body of corpus callosum (toward the genu)

Caudate nucleus (CaNu)

Stria terminalis and terminal vein

Body of corpus callosum (toward the splenium)

CorCl

Anterior forceps

CaNu

BLatVen

CorCl

CorRad

Septum pellucidum

Posterior forceps

4-10 Ventral surface of an axial section of brain through dorsal portions of *corpus callosum*. The plane of the section just touches the upper portion of *the body of caudate nucleus*. The two MRI images (both inversion recovery) are at a similar plane and show some of the structures identified in the brain slice. The terminal vein is also called the superior thalamostriate vein.

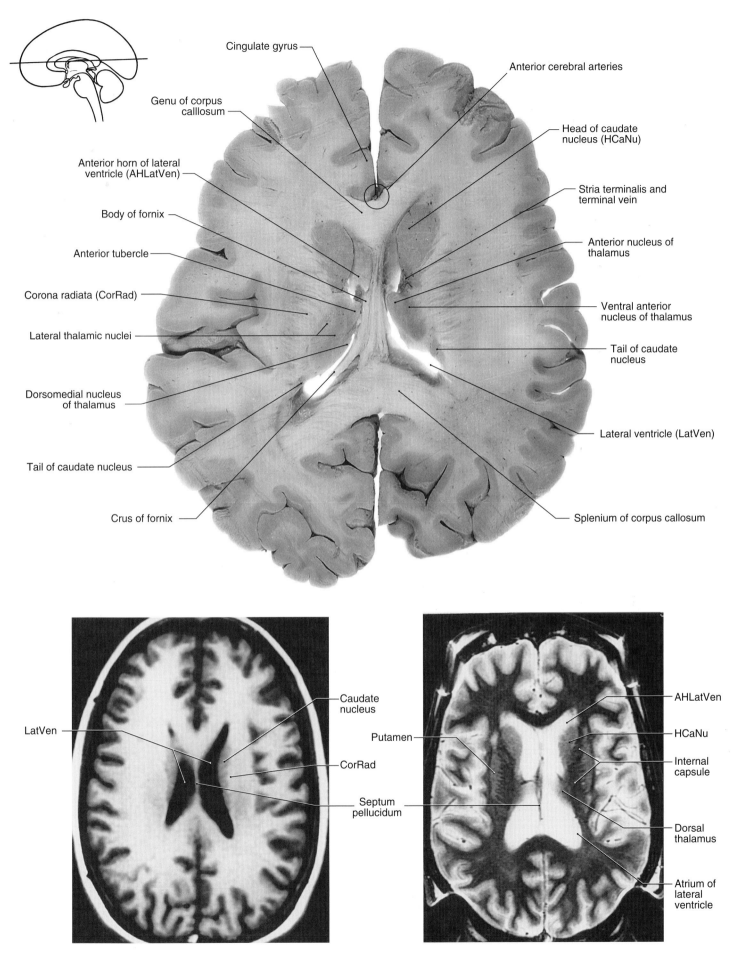

Cingulate gyrus

Genu of corpus callosum

Anterior horn of lateral ventricle (AHLatVen)

Body of fornix

Anterior tubercle

Corona radiata (CorRad)

Lateral thalamic nuclei

Dorsomedial nucleus of thalamus

Tail of caudate nucleus

Crus of fornix

Anterior cerebral arteries

Head of caudate nucleus (HCaNu)

Stria terminalis and terminal vein

Anterior nucleus of thalamus

Ventral anterior nucleus of thalamus

Tail of caudate nucleus

Lateral ventricle (LatVen)

Splenium of corpus callosum

LatVen

Caudate nucleus

CorRad

Septum pellucidum

Putamen

AHLatVen

HCaNu

Internal capsule

Dorsal thalamus

Atrium of lateral ventricle

4-11 Ventral surface of an axial section of brain through the *splenium of corpus callosum* and the *head of the caudate nucleus*. This plane includes only a small portion of the *dorsal thalamus*. The two MRI images (inversion recovery—left; T2-weighted—right) are at a comparable plane and show some of the structures identified in the brain slice. The terminal vein is also called the superior thalamostriate vein.

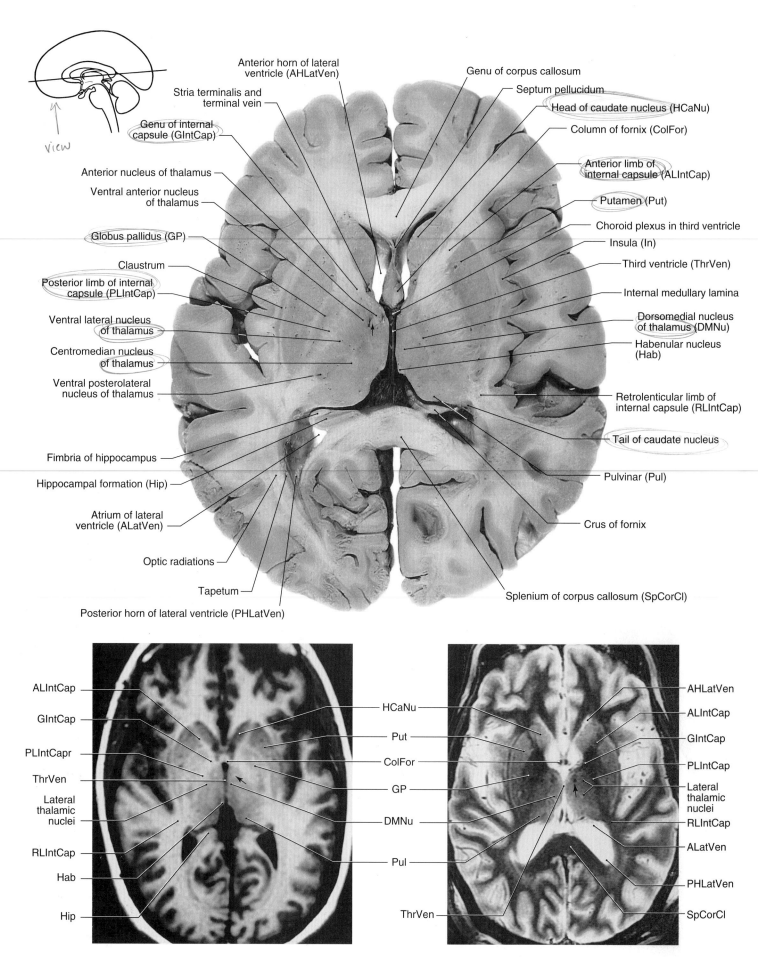

Anterior horn of lateral ventricle (AHLatVen)

Stria terminalis and terminal vein

Genu of internal capsule (GIntCap)

Anterior nucleus of thalamus

Ventral anterior nucleus of thalamus

Globus pallidus (GP)

Claustrum

Posterior limb of internal capsule (PLIntCap)

Ventral lateral nucleus of thalamus

Centromedian nucleus of thalamus

Ventral posterolateral nucleus of thalamus

Fimbria of hippocampus

Hippocampal formation (Hip)

Atrium of lateral ventricle (ALatVen)

Optic radiations

Tapetum

Posterior horn of lateral ventricle (PHLatVen)

Genu of corpus callosum

Septum pellucidum

Head of caudate nucleus (HCaNu)

Column of fornix (ColFor)

Anterior limb of internal capsule (ALIntCap)

Putamen (Put)

Choroid plexus in third ventricle

Insula (In)

Third ventricle (ThrVen)

Internal medullary lamina

Dorsomedial nucleus of thalamus (DMNu)

Habenular nucleus (Hab)

Retrolenticular limb of internal capsule (RLIntCap)

Tail of caudate nucleus

Pulvinar (Pul)

Crus of fornix

Splenium of corpus callosum (SpCorCl)

ALIntCap
GIntCap
PLIntCapr
ThrVen
Lateral thalamic nuclei
RLIntCap
Hab
Hip

HCaNu
Put
ColFor
GP
DMNu
Pul

AHLatVen
ALIntCap
GIntCap
PLIntCap
Lateral thalamic nuclei
RLIntCap
ALatVen
PHLatVen
SpCorCl

ThrVen

4-12 Ventral surface of an axial section of brain through the *genu of the corpus callosum, head of caudate nucleus, centromedian nucleus,* and *dorsal portions of the pulvinar.* The two MRI images (inversion recovery—left; T2-weighted—right) are at the same plane and show many of the structures identified in the brain slice. The arrowheads in the brain slice and in the MRIs are pointing to the mammillothalamic tract. The terminal vein is also called the superior thalamostriate vein.

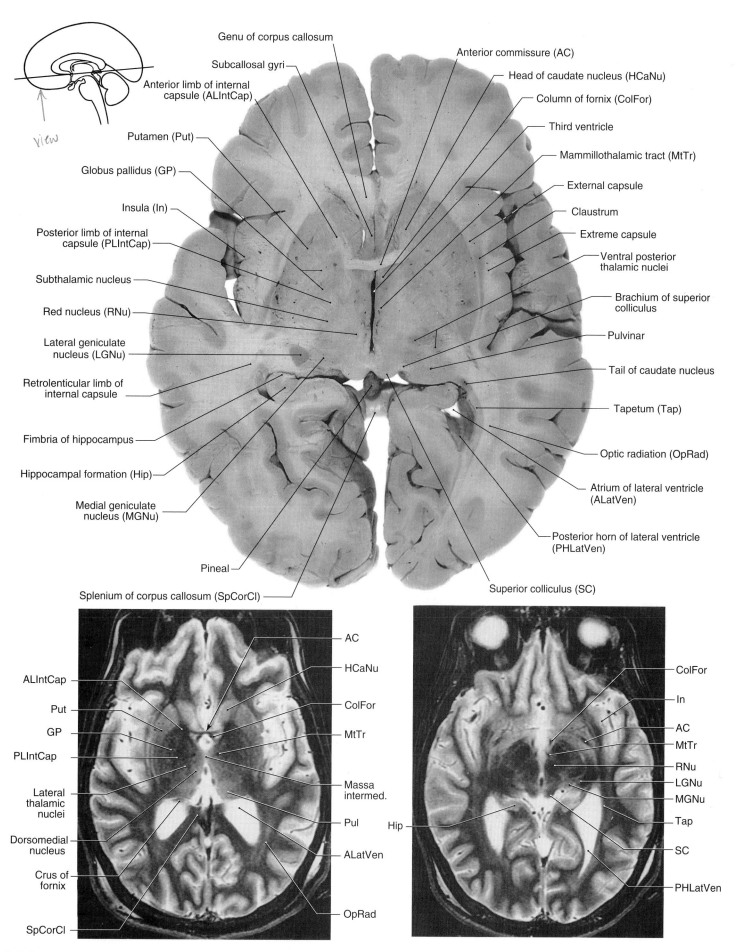

View

Genu of corpus callosum

Subcallosal gyri

Anterior limb of internal capsule (ALIntCap)

Putamen (Put)

Globus pallidus (GP)

Insula (In)

Posterior limb of internal capsule (PLIntCap)

Subthalamic nucleus

Red nucleus (RNu)

Lateral geniculate nucleus (LGNu)

Retrolenticular limb of internal capsule

Fimbria of hippocampus

Hippocampal formation (Hip)

Medial geniculate nucleus (MGNu)

Pineal

Splenium of corpus callosum (SpCorCl)

Anterior commissure (AC)

Head of caudate nucleus (HCaNu)

Column of fornix (ColFor)

Third ventricle

Mammillothalamic tract (MtTr)

External capsule

Claustrum

Extreme capsule

Ventral posterior thalamic nuclei

Brachium of superior colliculus

Pulvinar

Tail of caudate nucleus

Tapetum (Tap)

Optic radiation (OpRad)

Atrium of lateral ventricle (ALatVen)

Posterior horn of lateral ventricle (PHLatVen)

Superior colliculus (SC)

ALIntCap

Put

GP

PLIntCap

Lateral thalamic nuclei

Dorsomedial nucleus

Crus of fornix

SpCorCl

AC

HCaNu

ColFor

MtTr

Massa intermed.

Pul

ALatVen

OpRad

ColFor

In

AC

MtTr

RNu

LGNu

MGNu

Tap

SC

PHLatVen

Hip

4-13 Ventral surface of an axial section of brain through the *anterior commissure, column of fornix, medial and lateral geniculate nuclei,* and *superior colliculus.* The *medial* and *lateral segments* of the globus pallidus are visible on the slice. The lateral and medial segments of the globus pallidus can be discerned on the right side of the brain. The MRI images (both T2-weighted) are at approximately the same plane and show many of the structures identified in the brain slice.

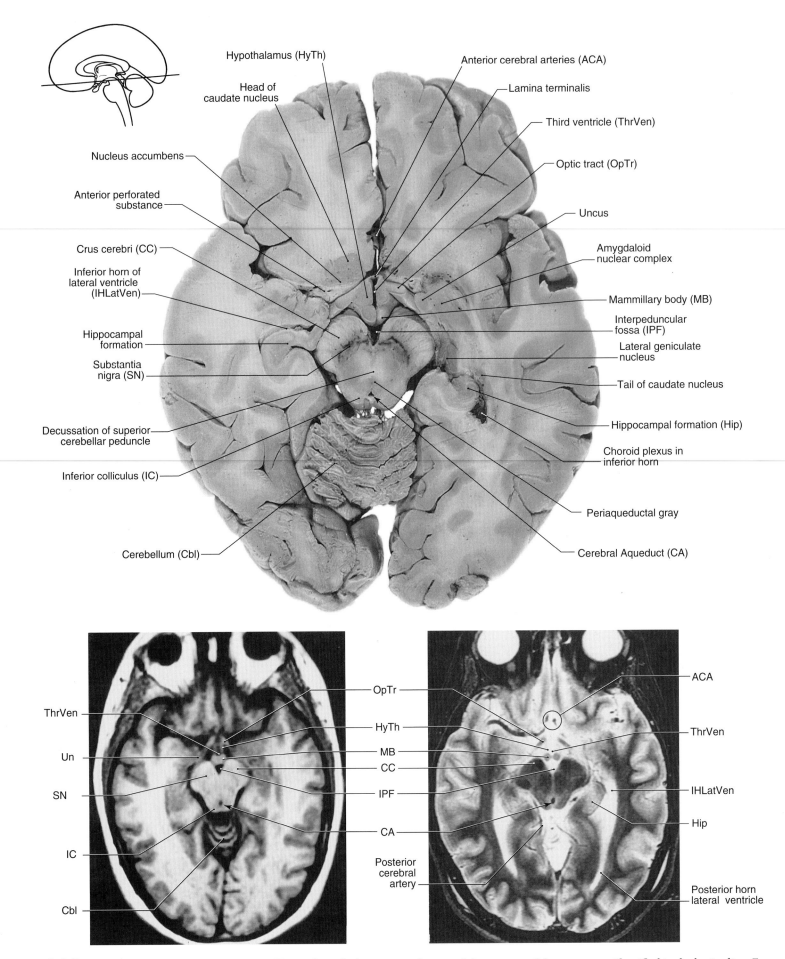

Hypothalamus (HyTh)

Head of caudate nucleus

Anterior cerebral arteries (ACA)

Lamina terminalis

Third ventricle (ThrVen)

Nucleus accumbens

Optic tract (OpTr)

Anterior perforated substance

Uncus

Crus cerebri (CC)

Amygdaloid nuclear complex

Inferior horn of lateral ventricle (IHLatVen)

Mammillary body (MB)

Interpeduncular fossa (IPF)

Hippocampal formation

Lateral geniculate nucleus

Substantia nigra (SN)

Tail of caudate nucleus

Hippocampal formation (Hip)

Decussation of superior cerebellar peduncle

Choroid plexus in inferior horn

Inferior colliculus (IC)

Periaqueductal gray

Cerebellum (Cbl)

Cerebral Aqueduct (CA)

ThrVen

OpTr

ACA

Un

HyTh

ThrVen

SN

MB

CC

IHLatVen

IC

IPF

Hip

Cbl

CA

Posterior cerebral artery

Posterior horn lateral ventricle

4-14 Ventral surface of an axial section of brain through the *hypothalamus, mammillary body, crus cerebri,* and *inferior colliculus.* The two MRI images (inversion recovery—left; T2-weighted—right) are at similar planes and show many of the structures identified in the brain slice. For details of the cerebellum see Figures 2-31 to 2-33 on pp. 32 and 33.

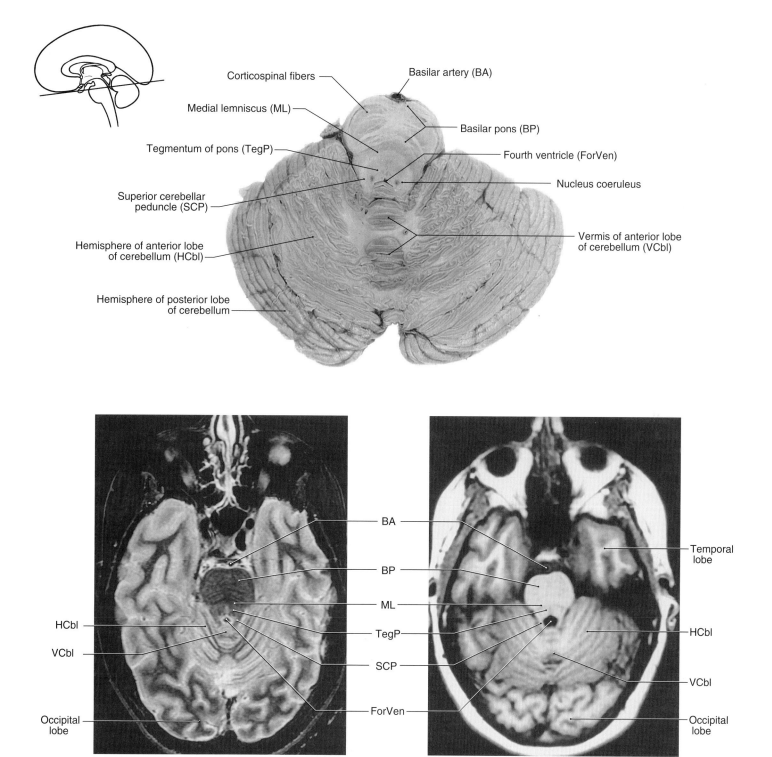

4-15 Ventral surface of an axial section of brain through rostral parts of the *basilar pons* and the *anterior lobe of the cerebellum*. The two MRI images (T2-weighted—left; inversion recovery—right) are at the same plane and show many of the structures identified in the brain slice. For details of the cerebellum see Figures 2-31 to 2-33 on pp. 32 and 33.

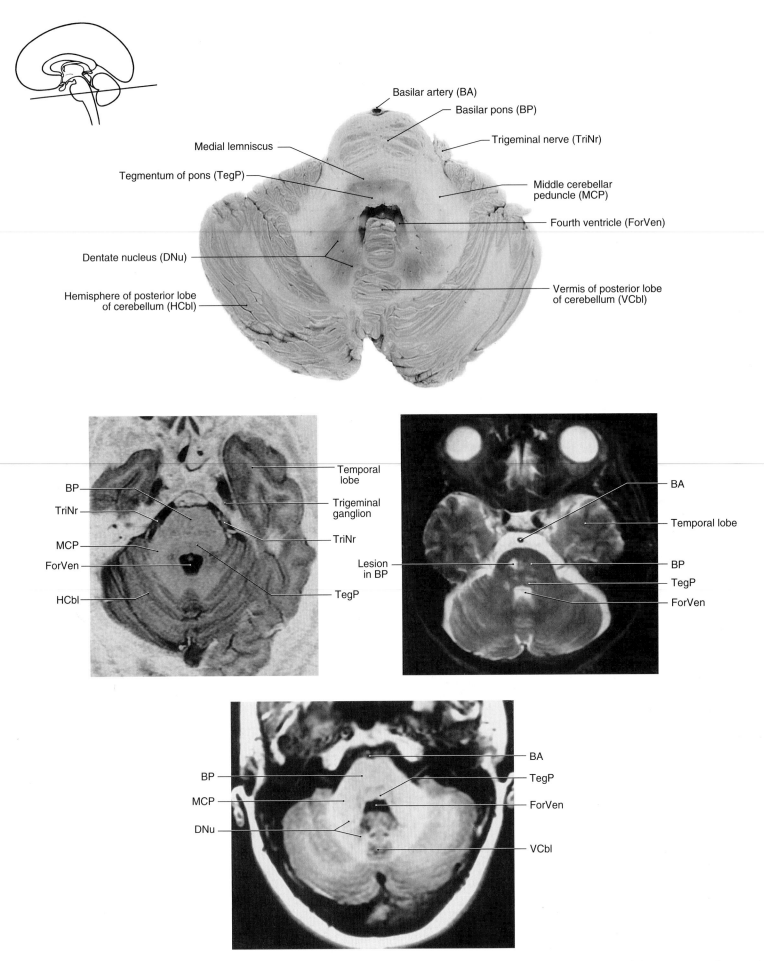

Basilar artery (BA)

Basilar pons (BP)

Trigeminal nerve (TriNr)

Medial lemniscus

Tegmentum of pons (TegP)

Middle cerebellar peduncle (MCP)

Fourth ventricle (ForVen)

Dentate nucleus (DNu)

Hemisphere of posterior lobe of cerebellum (HCbl)

Vermis of posterior lobe of cerebellum (VCbl)

BP
TriNr
MCP
ForVen
HCbl

Temporal lobe

Trigeminal ganglion

TriNr

TegP

BA

Temporal lobe

Lesion in BP

BP

TegP

ForVen

BP
MCP
DNu

BA

TegP

ForVen

VCbl

4-16 Ventral surface of an axial section of brain through the middle regions of the *basilar pons,* the *exit of the trigeminal nerve,* the *fourth ventricle,* and the cerebellar nuclei. The three MRI images (inverted inversion recovery—upper left; T2-weighted—upper right; T1-weighted—lower) are at the same planes and show many of the structures identified in the brain slice. Note the lesion in the basilar pons (upper right). For details of the cerebellum see Figures 2-31 to 2-33 on pp. 32 and 33.

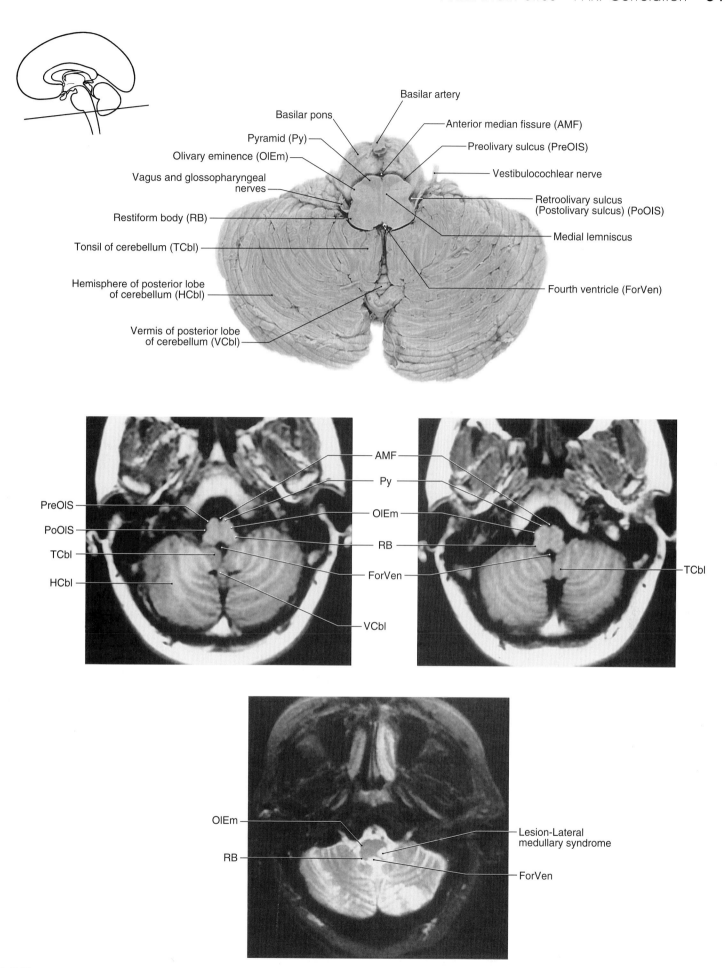

4-17 Ventral surface of an axial section of brain through portions of the *medulla oblongata,* just caudal to the pons–medulla junction and the *posterior lobe* of the cerebellum. The three MRI images (T1-weighted— upper left and right; T2-weighted—lower) are at the same plane and show many of the structures identified in the brain slice. Note the lateral medullary lesion (lower), also known as the posterior inferior artery syndrome or the lateral medullary syndrome (of Wallenberg). For details of the cerebellum see Figures 2-31 to 2-33 on pp. 32 and 33.

Internal Morphology of the Spinal Cord and Brain in Stained Sections

Basic concepts that are essential when one is *initially* learning how to diagnose the neurologically impaired patient include 1) an understanding of cranial nerve nuclei and 2) how these structures relate to long tracts. The importance of these relationships is clearly seen in the combinations of deficits that generally characterize lesions at different levels of the neuraxis. First, deficits of only the body that may present as motor or sensory losses (long tracts) on the same, or opposite, sides are indicative of spinal cord lesions (e.g., Brown-Sequard syndrome). Spinal cord injuries characteristically have *motor and sensory levels;* these are the *lowest functional levels* remaining in the compromised patient. Second, cranial nerve deficits (on one side of the head) in combination with long tract signs (on the opposite side of the body) characterize lesions in the brainstem (e.g., lateral medullary or Weber syndromes). These patterns of loss are frequently called *alternating* or *crossed deficits.* In these examples cranial nerve signs are better *localizing signs* than are long tract signs. A *localizing sign* can be defined as an objective neurologic abnormality that correlates with a lesion (or lesions) at a specific neuroanatomical location (or locations). Third, motor and sensory deficits on the same side of the head and body are usually indicative of a lesion in the forebrain.

Color Coded Cranial Nerve Nuclei and Long Tracts: Cranial nerve nuclei are coded by their function: pink, sensory; red, motor. These structures are colored bilaterally to make it easy to correlate cranial nerve and long tract function on both sides of the midline. For example, one can easily correlate damage to the hypoglossal nerve root and the adjacent corticospinal fibers on one side while comparing this pattern with the clinical picture of a lateral medullary syndrome on the other side.

Long tracts are color-coded beginning at the most caudal spinal cord levels (e.g., see Figures 5-1 and 5-2), with these colors extending into the dorsal thalamus (see Figure 5-30) and the posterior limb of the internal capsule (see Figures 5-31 and 5-32). The colorized spinal tracts are the fasciculus gracilis (dark blue), the fasciculus cuneatus (light blue)*, the anterolateral system (dark green),

and the lateral corticospinal tract (grey). In the brainstem, these spinal tracts are joined by the spinal trigeminal tract and ventral trigeminothalamic fibers (both are light green). The long tracts are color-coded on one side only, to emphasize 1) laterality of function and dysfunction, 2) points at which fibers in these tracts may decussate, and 3) the relationship of these tracts to cranial nerves.

A color key appears on each page. This key identifies the various tracts and nuclei by their color and specifies the function of each structure on each page. This approach not only emphasizes anatomical and clinical concepts, but also lends itself to a variety of instructional settings.

Correlation of MRI and CT with Spinal Cord and Brainstem: As one is learning basic anatomical concepts it is essential to consider how this information may be used in the clinical environment. To this end, MRI (T1- and T2-weighted) and CT (myelogram/cisternogram) images are introduced into the spinal cord and brainstem sections of this chapter (see also Chapter 1). To show the relationship between basic anatomy and how MRI and CT are viewed, a series of self-explanatory illustrations are provided on each set of facing pages in these sections. This continuum of visual information consists of (1) a small version of the colorized line drawing in an Anatomical Orientation, (2) a top-to-bottom flip of this illustration that brings it into a Clinical Orientation, and (3) a CT (spinal cord) or MRI and CT (brainstem) that follows this clinically oriented image. Every effort is made to identify and use MRI and CT that correlate, as closely as possible, with their corresponding line drawing and stained section. This approach recognizes and retains the strength of the anatomical approach, introduces essential clinical concepts while at the same time allowing the user to customize the material to suit a range of educational applications.

---

*The dark and light blue colors represent information originating from lower and upper portions of the body, respectively.

5-1 Transverse section of the spinal cord showing the characteristics of a sacral level. The gray matter occupies most of the cross-section; its H-shaped appearance is not especially obvious at sacral–coccygeal levels. The white matter is a comparatively thin mantle. The sacral cord, although small, appears round in the CT myelogram. Note the appearance of the sacral spinal cord surrounded by the upper portion of the cauda equina (left) and the cauda equina as it appears caudal to the conus medullaris in the lumbar cistern (right). Compare with Figure 2-4 on page 12.

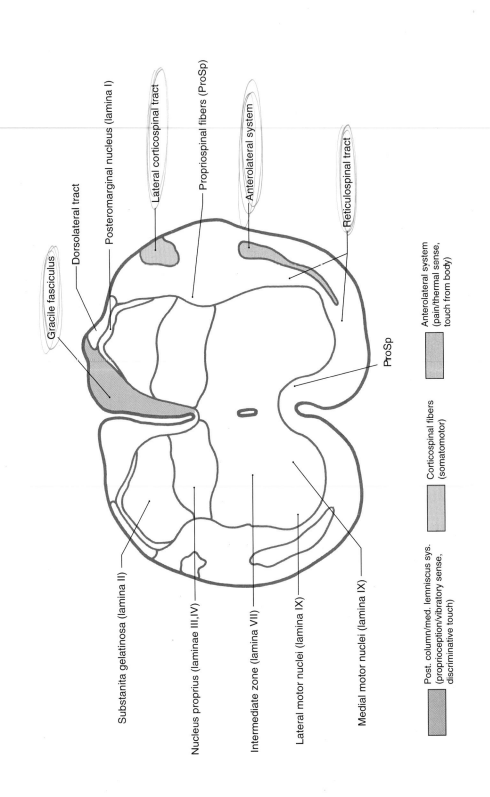

Gracile fasciculus

Dorsolateral tract

Posteromarginal nucleus (lamina I)

Lateral corticospinal tract

Propriospinal fibers (ProSp)

Anterolateral system

Reticulospinal tract

ProSp

Substanita gelatinosa (lamina II)

Nucleus proprius (laminae III,IV)

Intermediate zone (lamina VII)

Lateral motor nuclei (lamina IX)

Medial motor nuclei (lamina IX)

Post. column/med. lemniscus sys. (proprioception/vibratory sense, discriminative touch)

Corticospinal fibers (somatomotor)

Anterolateral system (pain/thermal sense, touch from body)

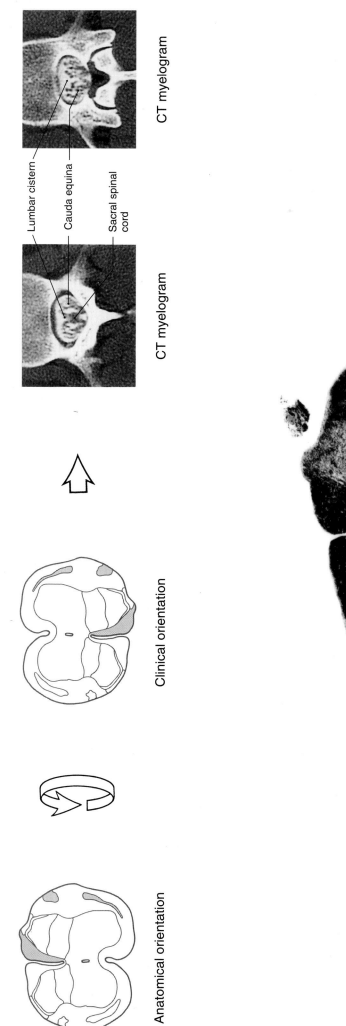

CT myelogram

CT myelogram

Lumbar cistern

Cauda equina

Sacral spinal cord

Clinical orientation

Anatomical orientation

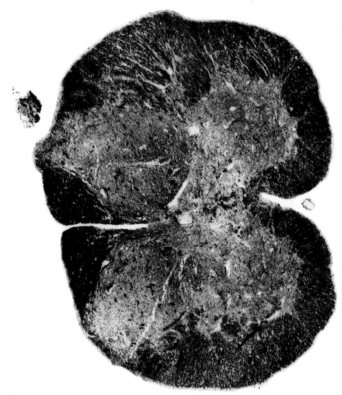

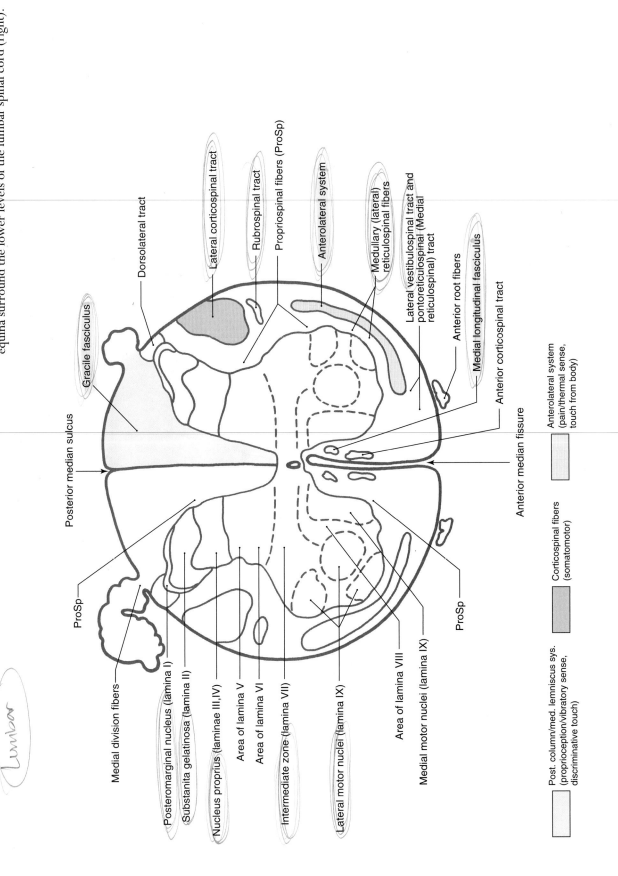

5-2   Transverse section of the spinal cord showing its characteristic appearance at lumbar levels (L4). Posterior and anterior horns are large in relation to a modest amount of white matter, and the general shape of the cord is round. Fibers of the medial division of the posterior root directly enter the gracile fasciculus. The lumbar spinal cord appears round in the CT myelogram. The roots of upper portions of the cauda equina surround the lower levels of the lumbar spinal cord (right).

Gracile fasciculus

Posterior median sulcus

Dorsolateral tract

Lateral corticospinal tract

Rubrospinal tract

Propriospinal fibers (ProSp)

Anterolateral system

Medullary (lateral) reticulospinal fibers

Lateral vestibulospinal tract and pontoreticulospinal (Medial reticulospinal) tract

Anterior root fibers

Medial longitudinal fasciculus

Anterior corticospinal tract

Anterior median fissure

ProSp

Medial division fibers

Posteromarginal nucleus (lamina I)

Substanita gelatinosa (lamina II)

Nucleus proprius (laminae III,IV)

Area of lamina V

Area of lamina VI

Intermediate zone (lamina VII)

Lateral motor nuclei (lamina IX)

Area of lamina VIII

Medial motor nuclei (lamina IX)

ProSp

Post. column/med. lemniscus sys. (proprioception/vibratory sense, discriminative touch)

Corticospinal fibers (somatomotor)

Anterolateral system (pain/thermal sense, touch from body)

Test
Cervical
Thorac
Lumbar

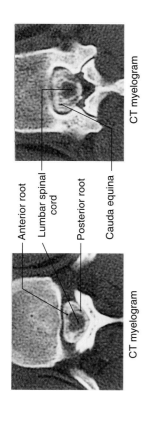

CT myelogram

Anterior root
Lumbar spinal cord
Posterior root
Cauda equina

CT myelogram

Clinical orientation

Anatomical orientation

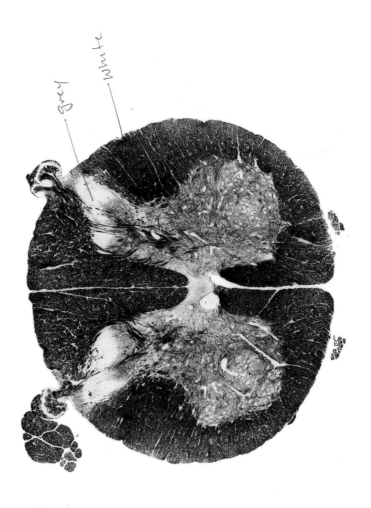

grey

white

white

5-3   Transverse section of the spinal cord showing its characteristic appearance at thoracic levels (T4). The white matter appears large in relation to the rather diminutive amount of gray matter. Posterior and anterior horns are small, especially when compared to low cervical levels and to lumbar levels. The overall shape of the cord is round. The thoracic spinal cord appears round in CT myelogram.

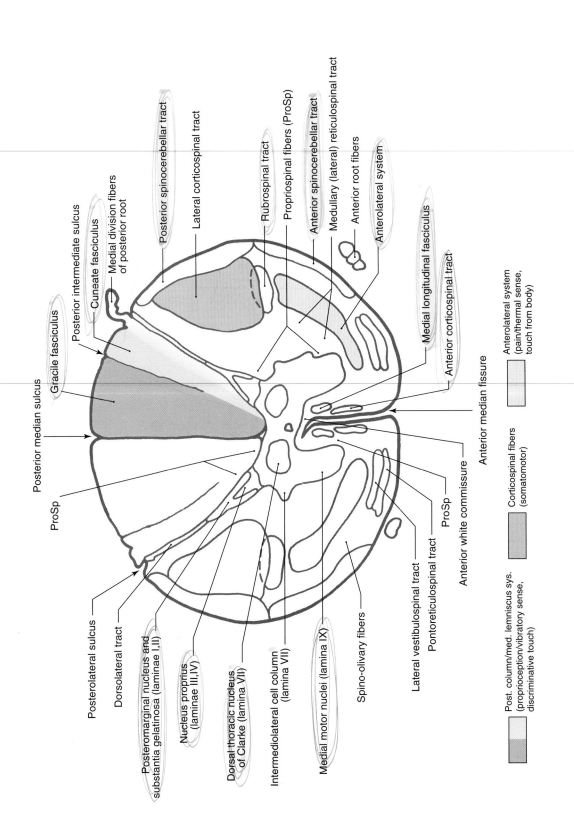

Posterior spinocerebellar tract

Lateral corticospinal tract

Rubrospinal tract

Propriospinal fibers (ProSp)

Anterior spinocerebellar tract

Medullary (lateral) reticulospinal tract

Anterior root fibers

Anterolateral system

Medial longitudinal fasciculus

Anterior corticospinal tract

Medial division fibers of posterior root

Cuneate fasciculus

Posterior intermediate sulcus

Gracile fasciculus

Posterior median sulcus

ProSp

Posterolateral sulcus

Dorsolateral tract

Posteromarginal nucleus and substantia gelatinosa (laminae I,II)

Nucleus proprius (laminae III,IV)

Dorsal thoracic nucleus of Clarke (lamina VII)

Intermediolateral cell column (lamina VII)

Medial motor nuclei (lamina IX)

Spino-olivary fibers

Lateral vestibulospinal tract

Pontoreticulospinal tract

ProSp

Anterior white commissure

Anterior median fissure

Post. column/med. lemniscus sys. (proprioception/vibratory sense, discriminative touch)

Corticospinal fibers (somatomotor)

Anterolateral system (pain/thermal sense, touch from body)

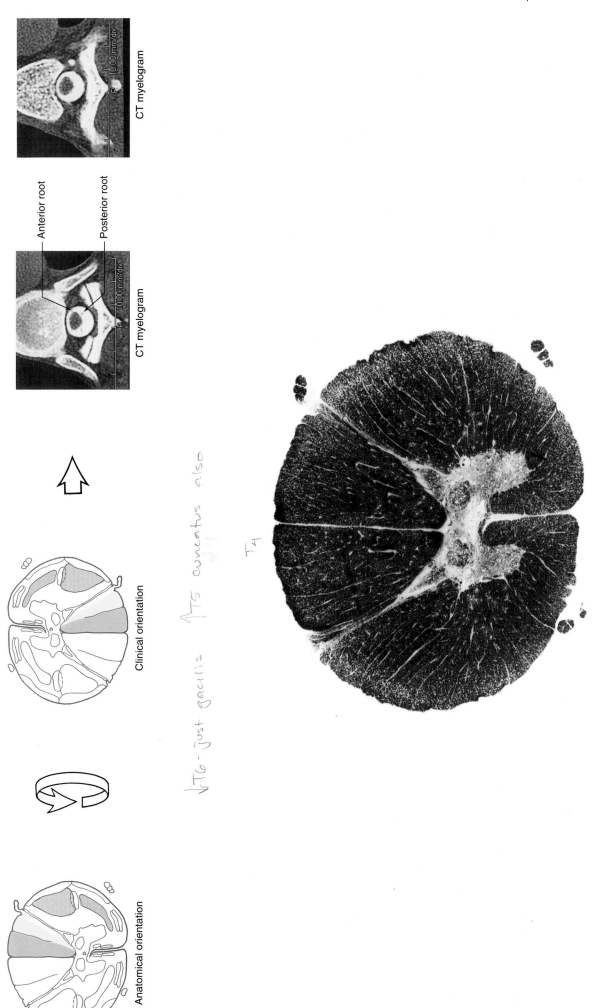

CT myelogram

CT myelogram

Anterior root

Posterior root

Clinical orientation

Anatomical orientation

↓T6 - just gracilis   ↑T5 cuneatus also

T4

5-4 Transverse section of the spinal cord showing its characteristic appearance at lower cervical levels (C7). The anterior horn is large, and there is—proportionally and absolutely—a large amount of white matter. The overall shape of the cord is oval. The lower portions of the cervical spinal cord appears oval in MRI (left) and in CT myelogram (center and right).

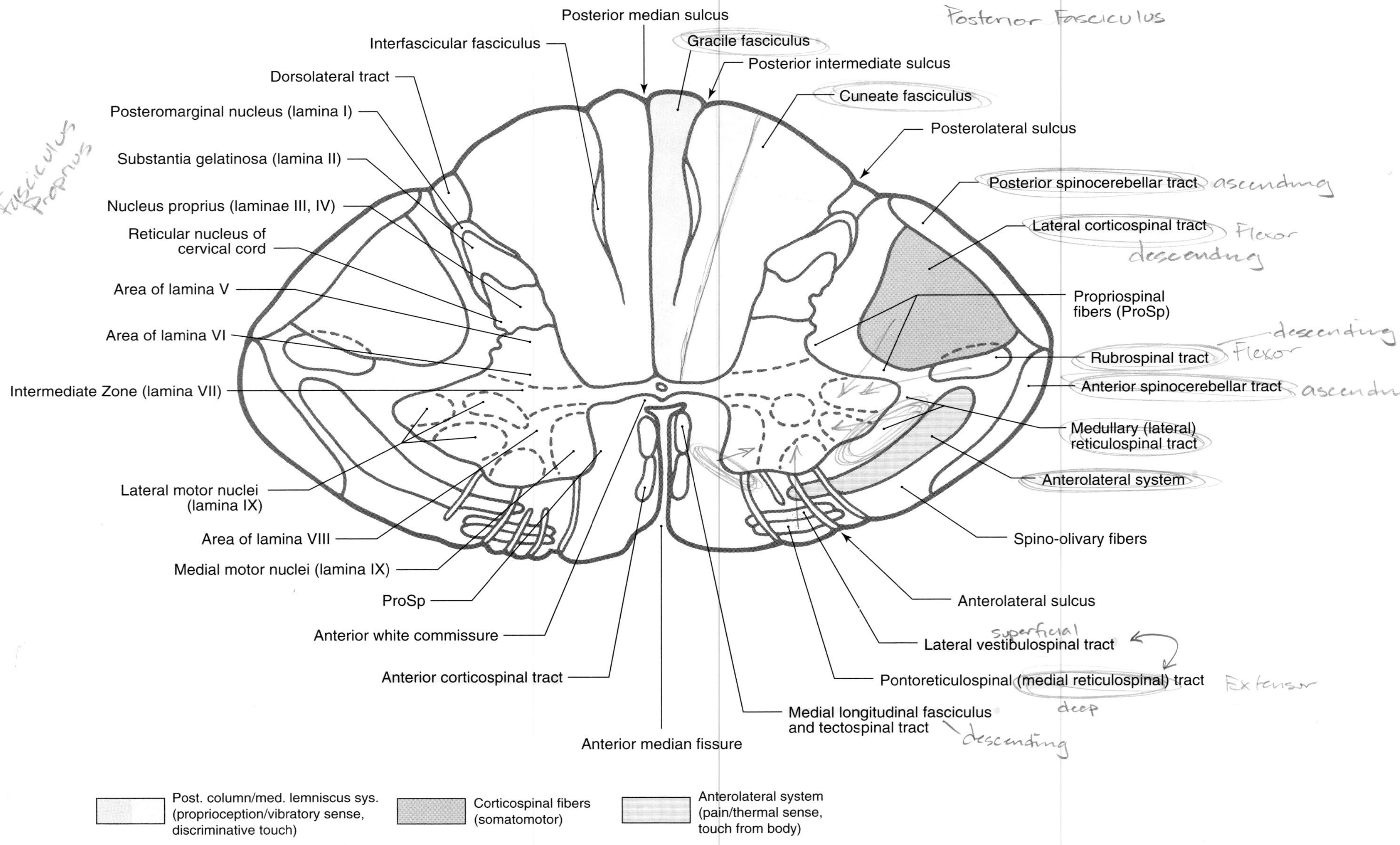

Posterior Fasciculus

Posterior median sulcus

Gracile fasciculus

Posterior intermediate sulcus

Cuneate fasciculus

Posterolateral sulcus

Posterior spinocerebellar tract   ascending

Lateral corticospinal tract   ascending   Flexor   descending

Propriospinal fibers (ProSp)   descending   Flexor

Rubrospinal tract

Anterior spinocerebellar tract   ascending

Medullary (lateral) reticulospinal tract

Anterolateral system

Spino-olivary fibers

Anterolateral sulcus

Lateral vestibulospinal tract   superficial

Pontoreticulospinal (medial reticulospinal) tract   deep   Extensor   descending

Medial longitudinal fasciculus and tectospinal tract

Anterior median fissure

Anterior corticospinal tract

Anterior white commissure

ProSp

Medial motor nuclei (lamina IX)

Area of lamina VIII

Lateral motor nuclei (lamina IX)

Intermediate Zone (lamina VII)

Area of lamina VI

Area of lamina V

Reticular nucleus of cervical cord

Nucleus proprius (laminae III, IV)

Substantia gelatinosa (lamina II)

Posteromarginal nucleus (lamina I)

Dorsolateral tract

Interfascicular fasciculus

Fasciculus proprius

Posterior median sulcus

Anterolateral system (pain/thermal sense, touch from body)

Corticospinal fibers (somatomotor)

Post. column/med. lemniscus sys. (proprioception/vibratory sense, discriminative touch)

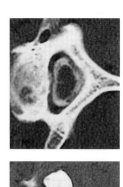

CT myelogram

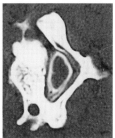

CT myelogram

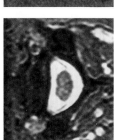

MRI, T2 weighted image

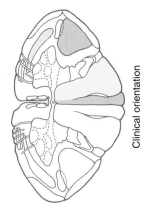

Clinical orientation

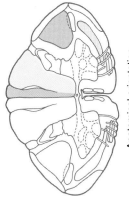

Anatomical orientation

Exam Picture ①

lower Cervical

only place to
ask white matter
tracts.

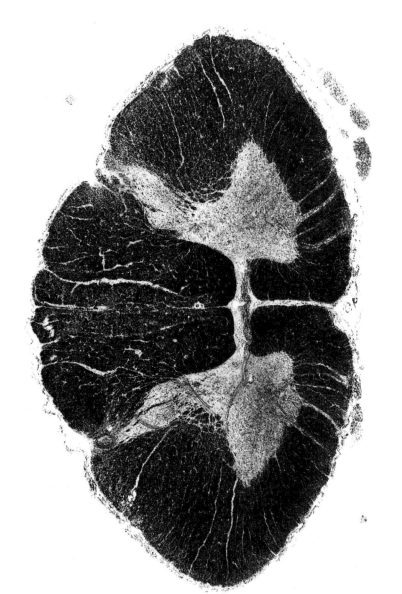

5-5 Transverse section of the spinal cord at the C1 level. Lateral corticospinal fibers are now located medially toward the decussation of the corticospinal fibers, also called the motor decussation or pyramidal decussation (see also Figure 5-8, page 98). At this level, fibers of the spinal trigeminal tract are interdigitated with those of the dorsolateral tract. The spinal cord at C$_1$ and C$_2$ levels appear round in CT myelogram when compared to low cervical levels (see Figure 5-4).

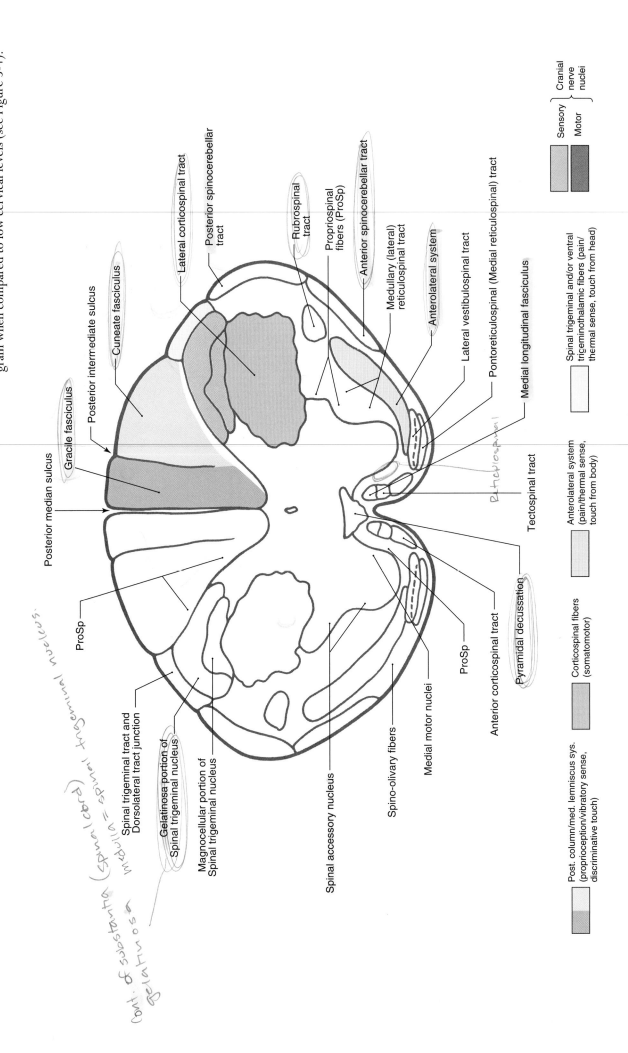

Lateral corticospinal tract

Posterior spinocerebellar tract

Cuneate fasciculus

Posterior intermediate sulcus

Gracile fasciculus

Posterior median sulcus

Rubrospinal tract

Propriospinal fibers (ProSp)

Anterior spinocerebellar tract

Medullary (lateral) reticulospinal tract

Anterolateral system

Lateral vestibulospinal tract

Pontoreticulospinal (Medial reticulospinal) tract

Medial longitudinal fasciculus

ProSp

Tectospinal tract

Reticulospinal

ProSp

Pyramidal decussation

Anterior corticospinal tract

Medial motor nuclei

Spino-olivary fibers

Spinal accessory nucleus

Magnocellular portion of Spinal trigeminal nucleus

Gelatinosa portion of Spinal trigeminal nucleus

Spinal trigeminal tract and Dorsolateral tract junction

cont. of substantia gelatinosa (spinal nucleus = spinal trigeminal nucleus) in medulla

(ProSp = spinal trigeminal nucleus)

anterior trigeminal nucleus

Post. column/med. lemniscus sys. (proprioception/vibratory sense, discriminative touch)

Corticospinal fibers (somatomotor)

Anterolateral system (pain/thermal sense, touch from body)

Spinal trigeminal and/or ventral trigeminothalamic fibers (pain/ thermal sense, touch from head)

Sensory ⎫
Motor ⎬ Cranial nerve nuclei

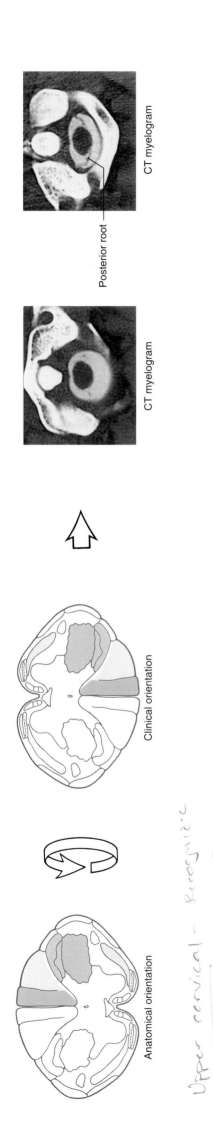

Posterior root

CT myelogram

CT myelogram

Clinical orientation

Anatomical orientation

Upper cervical - Recognize
— Largest Corticospinal Tract.

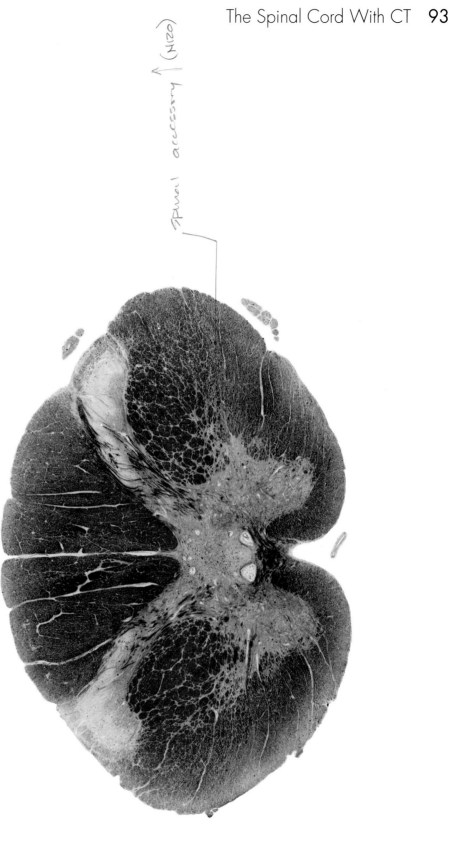

Spinal accessory (N120)

Vascular Syndromes or Lesions of the Spinal Cord

Acute Central Cervical Spinal Cord Syndrome: Results from occlusion of the anterior spinal artery.

Deficit	Structure Damage
• Bilateral paresis or flaccid paralysis of upper extremities	• Medial portions of both lateral corticospinal tracts; ventral grey horns at cervical levels
• Irregular loss of pain and temperature sensations bilaterally over body below lesion	• Anterolateral system fibers (partial involvement bilaterally)

Comment: Hyperextension of the neck may cause damage to the vertebral arteries (which give rise to the anterior spinal artery), or it may directly damage the anterior spinal artery, causing a spasm. This vascular damage leads to a temporary or permanent interruption of blood supply. Deficits may resolve within a few hours or may be permanent, depending on the extent of vascular complication. Sparing of the dorsal columns (proprioception, vibratory sense) is a hallmark; approximately the anterior two-thirds of the spinal cord is ischemic.

Thrombosis of Anterior Spinal Artery: This may occur in a hypotensive crisis, as a result of trauma resulting from a dissecting aortic aneurysm, or in patients with atherosclerosis. It may occur at all spinal levels but is more frequently seen in thoracic and lumbosacral levels unless trauma is the primary cause. Results are *bilateral flaccid paraplegia* (if lesion is below cervical levels) or *quadriplegia* (if lesion is in cervical levels), *urinary retention, and loss of pain and temperature sensation*. Flaccid muscles may become spastic over a period of a day to weeks, with *hyperactive deep tendon reflexes and extensor plantar (Babinski) reflexes*. In addition, lesions at high cervical levels may also result in paralysis of respiratory muscles. The artery of Adamkiewicz (an especially large spinal medullary artery) is usually located at spinal levels T_{12}–L_1 and more frequently arises on the left side. Occlusion of this vessel may infarct lumbosacral levels of the spinal cord.

Hemorrhage in the spinal cord: This is *rarely* seen but may result from trauma or bleeding from congenital vascular lesions. Symptoms may develop rapidly or gradually in stepwise fashion, and blood is usually present in the cerebrospinal fluid.

Arteriovenous malformation in spinal cord: More frequently found in lower cord levels. Symptoms (*micturition problems are seen early, motor deficits, lower back pain*) may appear over time and may seem to resolve then recur (get better then worse). These lesions are usually found external to the cord (extramedullary) and can be surgically treated, especially when the major feeding vessels are few in number and easily identified. *Foix-Alajouanine syndrome* is an inflammation of spinal veins with subsequent occlusion that results in infarct of the spinal cord and a necrotic myelitis. The symptoms are *ascending pain and a flaccid paralysis*.

Brown-Sequard syndrome: This syndrome is a hemisection of the spinal cord that may result from trauma, compression of the spinal cord by tumors or hematomas, or significant protrusion of an intervertebral disc. The deficits depend on the level of the causative lesion. The classic signs are (1) a loss of pain and thermal sensation on the contralateral side of the body beginning about 1–2 segments below the level of the lesion (*damage to anterolateral system fibers*), (2) a loss of discriminative touch and proprioception on the ipsilateral side of the body below the lesion (*interruption of posterior column fibers*), and (3) a paralysis on the ipsilateral side of the body below the lesion (*damage to lateral corticospinal fibers*). This syndrome is classified as an *incomplete spinal cord injury* (see below) and the majority of patients with this lesion will regain some type of motor and sensory function. Compression of the spinal cord may result in some, but not all, of the signs and symptoms of the syndrome.

Syringomyelia: This condition is cavitation of central portion of the spinal cord. A cavitation of the central canal with an ependymal cell lining is *hydromyelia*. A syrinx may originate in central portions of the spinal cord, may communicate with the central canal, and is most commonly seen in cervical levels of the spinal cord. The most common deficits are a *bilateral loss of pain and thermal sensation due to damage to the anterior white commissure*: the loss reflects the levels of the spinal cord damaged (e.g., a cape distribution over the shoulder and upper extremities). The other commonly seen deficit results from extension of the cavity into the anterior horn(s). The result is *unilateral or bilateral paralysis of the upper extremities* (cervical levels) or *lower extremities* (lumbosacral levels) due to damage to the anterior motor neuron cells. This paralysis is characteristically a lower motor neuron deficit. A syrinx in the spinal cord, particularly in cervical levels, may be associated with a variety of other developmental defects in the nervous system.

Spinal Cord Lesions: *A complete spinal cord lesion is characterized by a bilateral and complete loss of motor and sensory function below the level of lesion persisting for more than 24 hours*. The vast majority of the patients with complete lesions (95%+) will suffer some permanent deficits. *Incomplete spinal cord lesions are those with preservation of sacral cord function at presentation*. The above described cases are examples of incomplete spinal cord lesions.

5-6 Semidiagrammatic representation of the internal blood supply to the spinal cord. This is a tracing of a C4 level, with the positions of principal tracts superimposed on the left and the general pattern of blood vessels superimposed on the right.

Abbreviations

A	Representation of arm fibers
AH	Anterior (ventral) horn
AWCom	Anterior white commissure
CenC	Central canal
IZ	Intermediate zone
L	Representation of leg fibers
N	Representation of neck fibers
PH	Posterior (dorsal) horn
S	Representation of sacral fibers
T	Representation of truck fibers

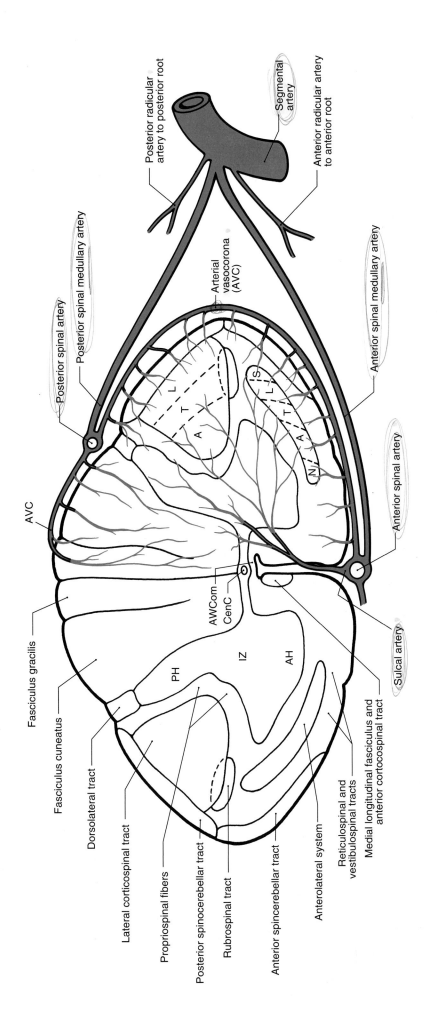

5-7 All of the brainstem sections used in Figures 5-9 through 5-13 (medulla), 5-17 through 5-20 (pons), and 5-22 through 5-25 (midbrain) are from an individual who had an infarct (green in drawing) in the posterior limb of the internal capsule. This lesion damaged corticospinal fibers (grey in drawing), resulting in a contralateral hemiplegia of the arm and leg, and damaged sensory radiations that travel from thalamic nuclei to the somatosensory cortex through the posterior limb of the internal capsule. Although the patient survived the initial episode, corticospinal fibers (grey) distal to the lesion (green) underwent degenerative changes and largely disappeared. This Wallerian (anterograde) degeneration takes place because the capsular infarct effectively separates the descending corticospinal fibers from their cell bodies in the cerebral cortex. Consequently, the location of corticospinal fibers in the middle one-third of the crus cerebri of the midbrain, in the basilar pons, and in the pyramid of the medulla is characterized by the obvious lack of myelinated axons in these structures when compared to the opposite side. In the brainstem, these degenerated fibers are ipsilateral to their cells of origin but are contralateral to their destination in the spinal cord—hence, the contralateral motor deficit. These photographs give the user the unique opportunity of seeing where corticospinal fibers are located at all levels of the human brainstem. Also, one is constantly reminded of 1) the relationship of corticospinal fibers to other structures, 2) the deficits one can expect to see at representative levels due to this lesion, and 3) the general appearance of degenerated fibers in the human central nervous system. These images can be adapted to a wide range of instructional formats.

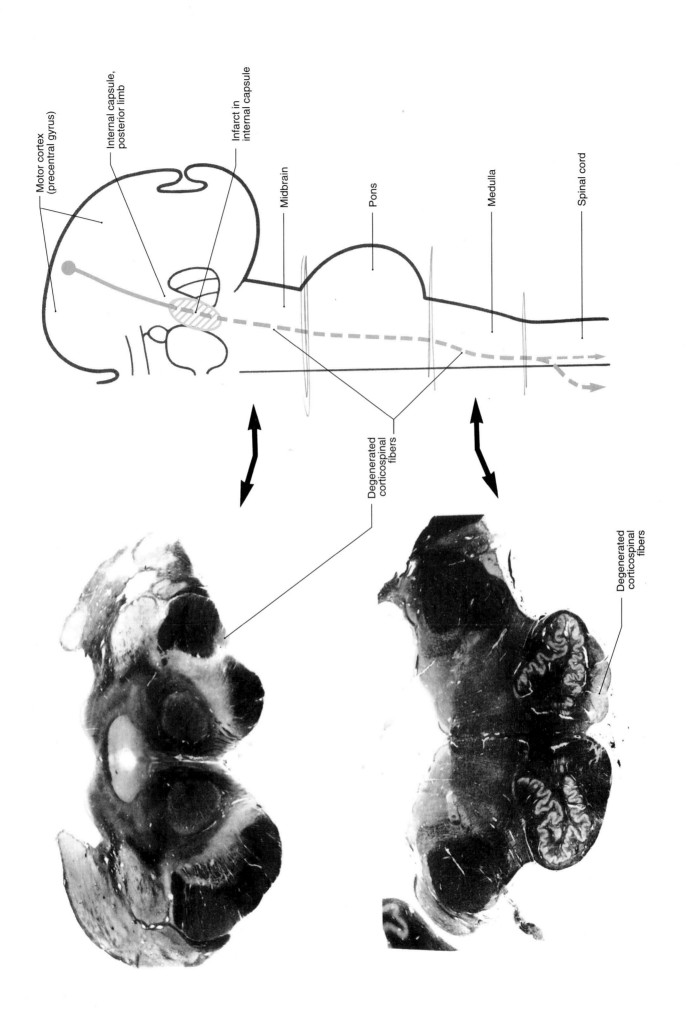

Motor cortex (precentral gyrus)

Internal capsule, posterior limb

Infarct in internal capsule

Midbrain

Pons

Medulla

Spinal cord

Degenerated corticospinal fibers

Degenerated corticospinal fibers

5-8 Transverse section of the medulla through the *decussation of the pyramids* (motor decussation, pyramidal decussation, crossing of corticospinal fibers). This is the level of the spinal cord–medulla transition. The corticospinal fibers have moved from their location in the lateral funiculus to the motor decussation and will cross to form the pyramid on the opposite side.

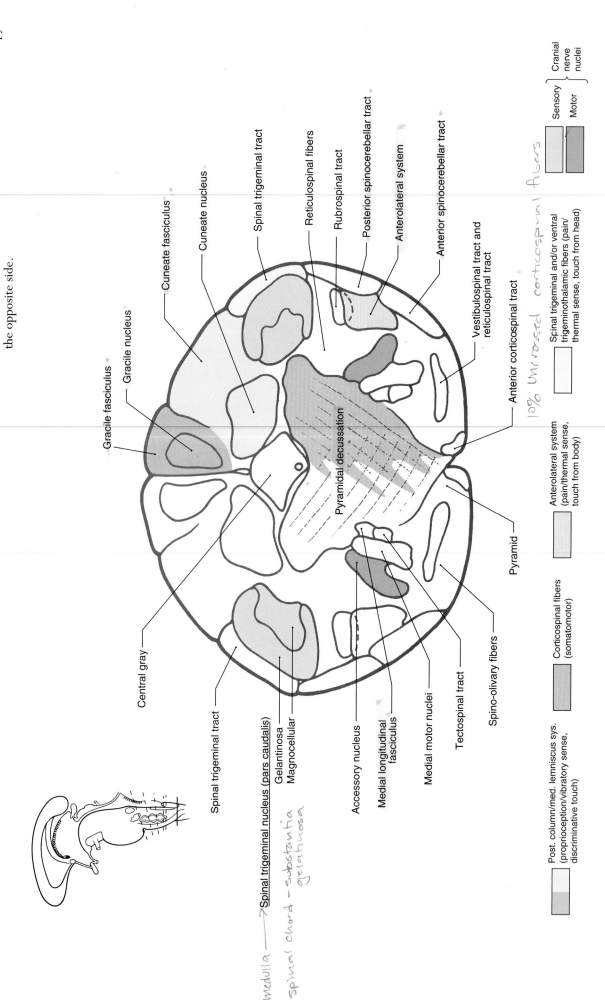

Medulla

Spinal chord → substantia gelatinosa

Spinal trigeminal nucleus (pars caudalis)

Gracile fasciculus

Gracile nucleus

Cuneate fasciculus

Cuneate nucleus

Spinal trigeminal tract

Reticulospinal fibers

Rubrospinal tract

Posterior spinocerebellar tract

Anterolateral system

Anterior spinocerebellar tract

Vestibulospinal tract and reticulospinal tract

Anterior corticospinal tract

10% Uncrossed corticospinal fibers

Pyramid

Spino-olivary fibers

Tectospinal tract

Medial motor nuclei

Medial longitudinal fasciculus

Accessory nucleus

Magnocellular

Gelantinosa

Central gray

Spinal trigeminal tract

Pyramidal decussation

Post. column/med. lemniscus sys. (proprioception/vibratory sense, discriminative touch)

Corticospinal fibers (somatomotor)

Anterolateral system (pain/thermal sense, touch from body)

Spinal trigeminal and/or ventral trigeminothalamic fibers (pain/ thermal sense, touch from head)

Sensory   Cranial nerve nuclei
Motor

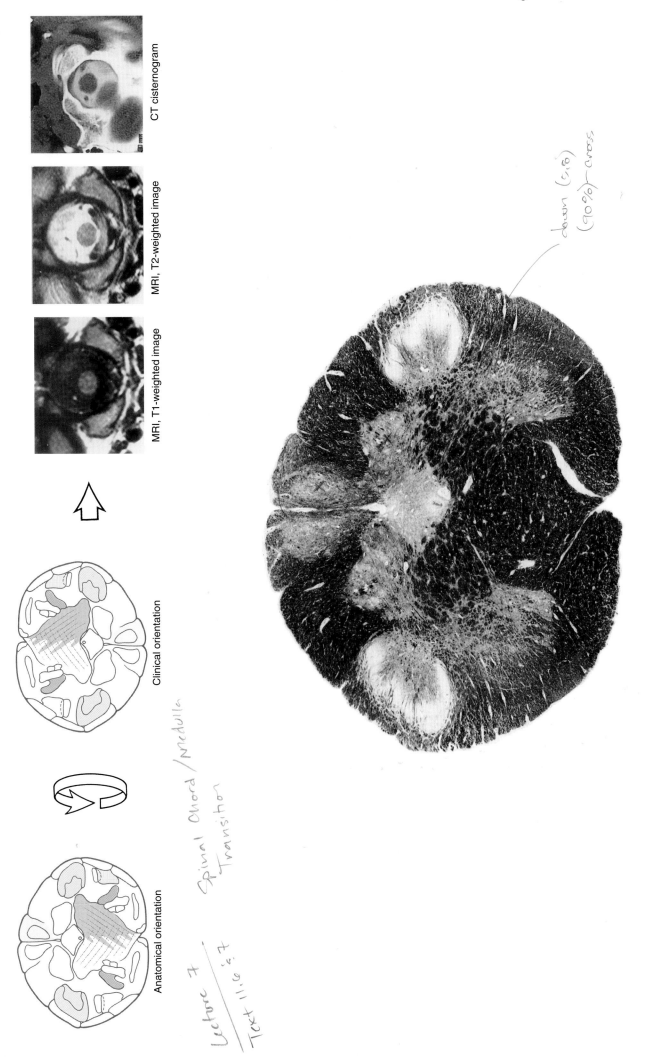

CT cisternogram

MRI, T2-weighted image

MRI, T1-weighted image

Clinical orientation

Anatomical orientation

down (c.o)
(90%) cross

Lecture 7   Spinal Chord / Medulla
                        Transition
Text 11.6 '27

5-9 Transverse section of the medulla through the *dorsal column nuclei* (nucleus gracilis and nucleus cuneatus), caudal portions of the *hypoglossal nucleus*, caudal end of the *principal olivary nucleus*, and middle portions of the *sensory decussation* (crossing of internal arcuate fibers).

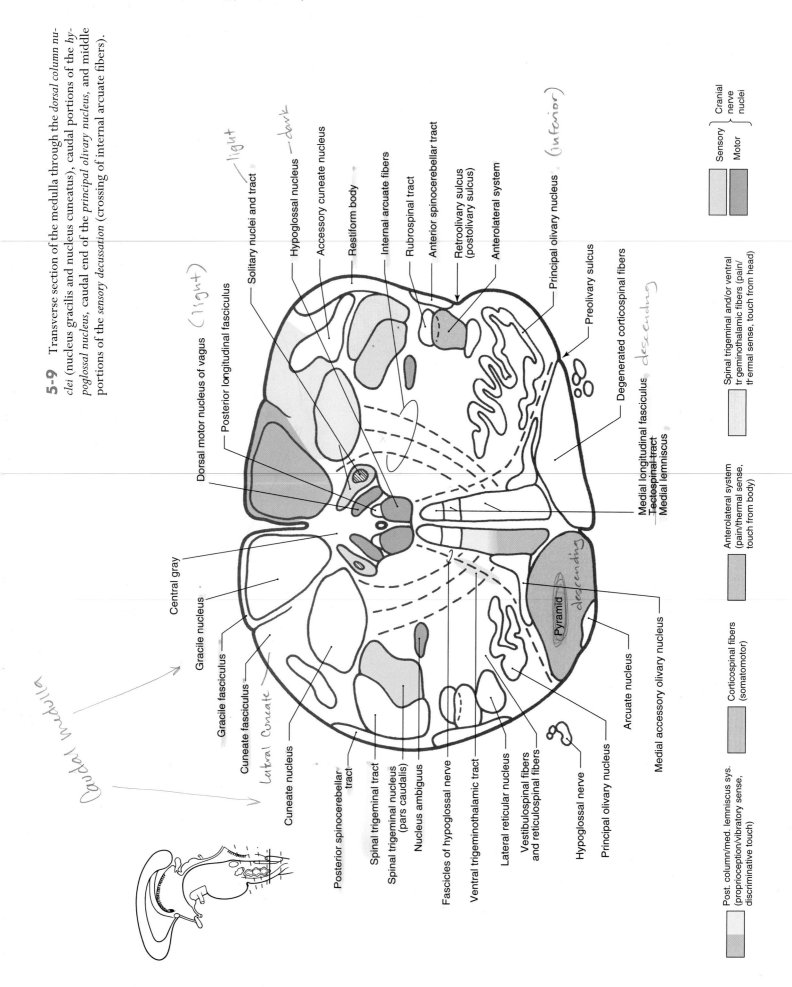

Solitary nuclei and tract

Hypoglossal nucleus — dark

Accessory cuneate nucleus

Restiform body

Internal arcuate fibers

Rubrospinal tract

Anterior spinocerebellar tract

Retroolivary sulcus (postolivary sulcus)

Anterolateral system

Principal olivary nucleus · (inferior)

Preolivary sulcus

Degenerated corticospinal fibers

Medial longitudinal fasciculus · descending
Tectospinal tract
Medial lemniscus

light

Posterior longitudinal fasciculus (light)

Dorsal motor nucleus of vagus (light)

Central gray

Gracile nucleus

Gracile fasciculus

Cuneate fasciculus

Lateral Cuneate

Cuneate nucleus

Caudal Medulla

Posterior spinocerebellar tract

Spinal trigeminal tract

Spinal trigeminal nucleus (pars caudalis)

Nucleus ambiguus

Fascicles of hypoglossal nerve

Ventral trigeminothalamic tract

Lateral reticular nucleus

Vestibulospinal fibers and reticulospinal fibers

Hypoglossal nerve

Principal olivary nucleus

Medial accessory olivary nucleus

Arcuate nucleus

Pyramid · descending

Sensory } Cranial
Motor } nerve nuclei

Post. column/med. lemniscus sys. (proprioception/vibratory sense, discriminative touch)

Corticospinal fibers (somatomotor)

Anterolateral system (pain/thermal sense, touch from body)

Spinal trigeminal and/or ventral tr geminothalamic fibers (pain/ thermal sense, touch from head)

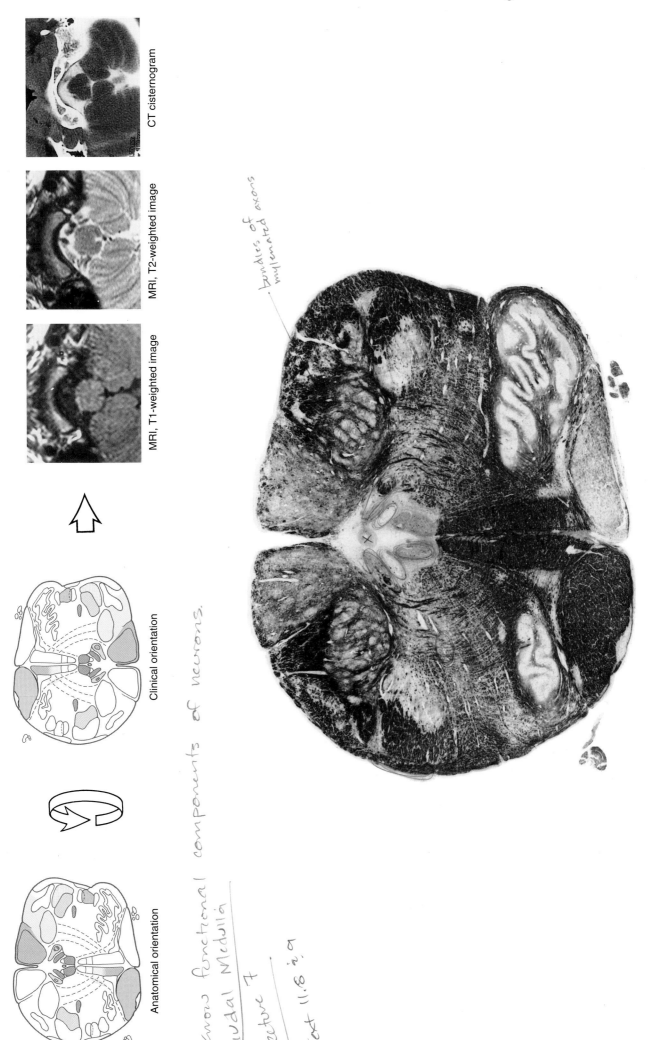

CT cisternogram

MRI, T2-weighted image

MRI, T1-weighted image

Clinical orientation

Anatomical orientation

bundles of myelinated axons

Know functional components of neurons.

Caudal Medulla

Lecture 7

Text 11.8.2.a

5-10   Transverse section of the medulla through rostral portions of the sensory decussation (*crossing of internal arcuate fibers*), *obex*, and the caudal one-third of the *hypoglossal* and *principal olivary nuclei*.

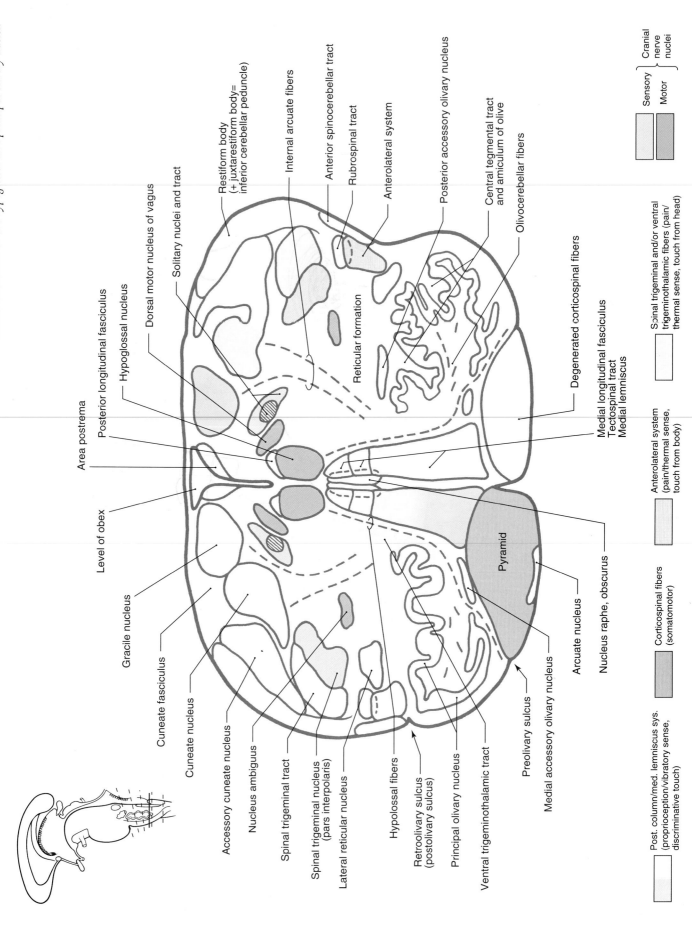

Area postrema

Posterior longitudinal fasciculus

Hypoglossal nucleus

Dorsal motor nucleus of vagus

Solitary nuclei and tract

Restiform body
(+ juxtarestiform body=
inferior cerebellar peduncle)

Internal arcuate fibers

Anterior spinocerebellar tract

Rubrospinal tract

Anterolateral system

Posterior accessory olivary nucleus

Central tegmental tract
and amiculum of olive

Olivocerebellar fibers

Degenerated corticospinal fibers

Reticular formation

Medial longitudinal fasciculus
Tectospinal tract
Medial lemniscus

Level of obex

Gracile nucleus

Cuneate fasciculus

Cuneate nucleus

Accessory cuneate nucleus

Nucleus ambiguus

Spinal trigeminal tract

Spinal trigeminal nucleus
(pars interpolaris)

Lateral reticular nucleus

Hypolossal fibers

Retroolivary sulcus
(postolivary sulcus)

Principal olivary nucleus

Ventral trigeminothalamic tract

Preolivary sulcus

Medial accessory olivary nucleus

Arcuate nucleus

Nucleus raphe, obscurus

Pyramid

Sensory ⎤ Cranial
Motor ⎦ nerve nuclei

Post. column/med. lemniscus sys.
(proprioception/vibratory sense,
discriminative touch)

Corticospinal fibers
(somatomotor)

Anterolateral system
(pain/thermal sense,
touch from body)

Ssinal trigeminal and/or ventral
trigeminothalamic fibers (pain/
thermal sense, touch from head)

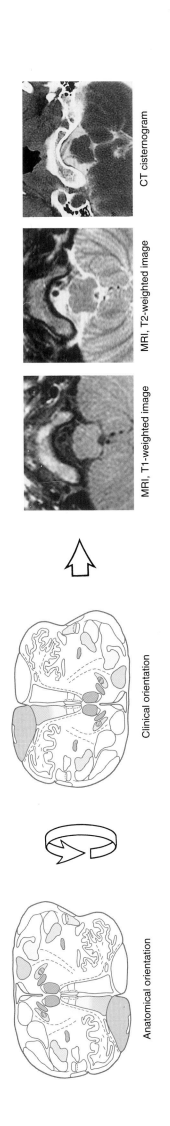

CT cisternogram

MRI, T2-weighted image

MRI, T1-weighted image

Clinical orientation

Anatomical orientation

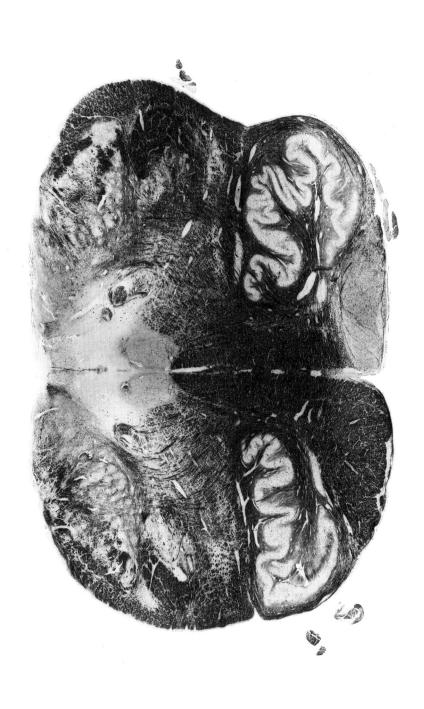

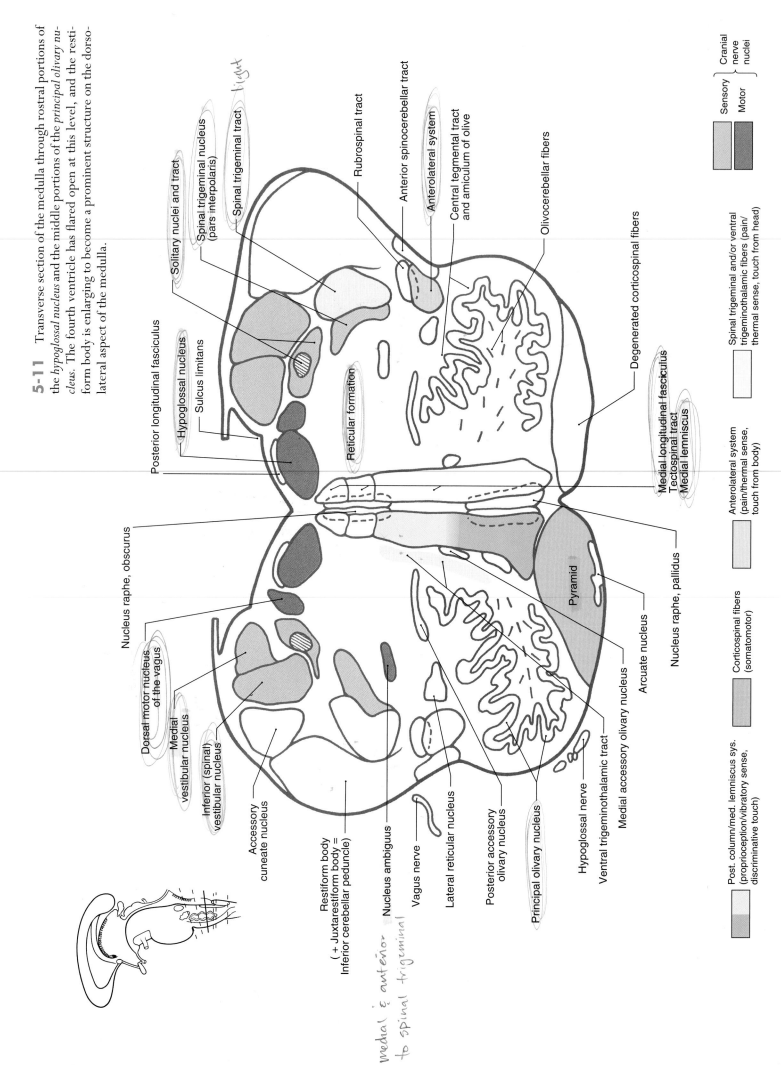

5-11 Transverse section of the medulla through rostral portions of the *hypoglossal nucleus* and the middle portions of the *principal olivary nucleus*. The fourth ventricle has flared open at this level, and the restiform body is enlarging to become a prominent structure on the dorsolateral aspect of the medulla.

Posterior longitudinal fasciculus
Hypoglossal nucleus
Sulcus limitans
Solitary nuclei and tract
Spinal trigeminal nucleus (pars interpolaris)
Spinal trigeminal tract
Rubrospinal tract
Anterior spinocerebellar tract
Anterolateral system
Central tegmental tract and amiculum of olive
Olivocerebellar fibers
Degenerated corticospinal fibers
Medial longitudinal fasciculus
Tectospinal tract
Medial lemniscus
Reticular formation

Nucleus raphe, obscurus
Dorsal motor nucleus of the vagus
Medial vestibular nucleus
Inferior (spinal) vestibular nucleus
Accessory cuneate nucleus
Restiform body (+ Juxtarestiform body = Inferior cerebellar peduncle)
Nucleus ambiguus
Vagus nerve
Lateral reticular nucleus
Posterior accessory olivary nucleus
Principal olivary nucleus
Hypoglossal nerve
Ventral trigeminothalamic tract
Medial accessory olivary nucleus
Arcuate nucleus
Nucleus raphe, pallidus
Pyramid

Post. column/med. lemniscus sys. (proprioception/vibratory sense, discriminative touch)
Corticospinal fibers (somatomotor)
Anterolateral system (pain/thermal sense, touch from body)
Spinal trigeminal and/or ventral trigeminothalamic fibers (pain/thermal sense, touch from head)
Sensory / Motor Cranial nerve nuclei

medial & anterior to spinal trigeminal

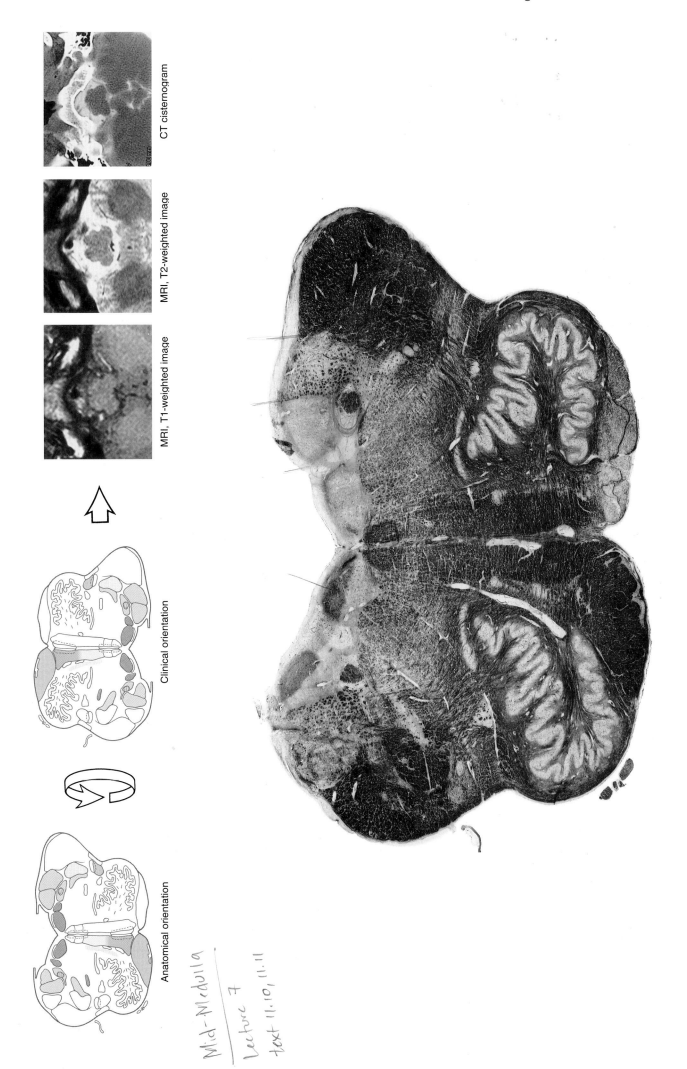

CT cisternogram

MRI, T2-weighted image

MRI, T1-weighted image

Clinical orientation

Anatomical orientation

Mid-Medulla
Lecture 7
text 11.10, 11.11

5-12   Transverse section of the medulla through the *posterior (dorsal)* and *anterior (ventral) cochlear nuclei* and *root of the glossopharyngeal nerve.* This corresponds to approximately the rostral third to fourth of the *principal olivary nucleus.*

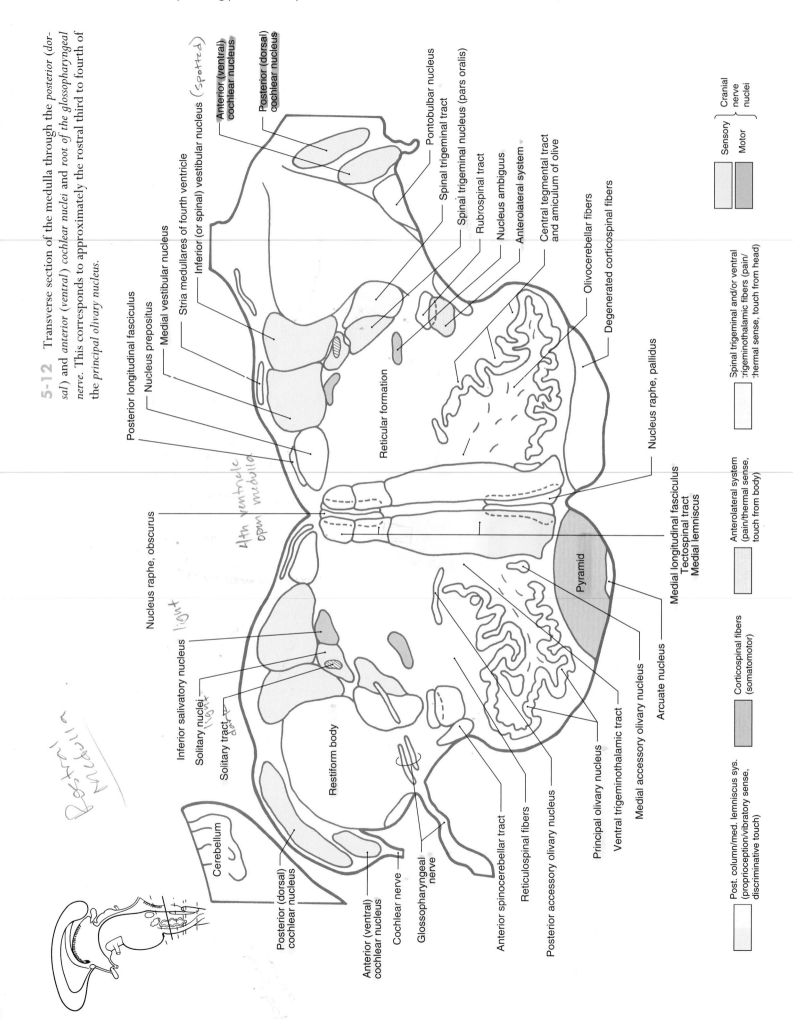

Anterior (ventral) cochlear nucleus

Posterior (dorsal) cochlear nucleus (spotted)

Inferior (or spinal) vestibular nucleus (spotted)

Stria medullares of fourth ventricle

Medial vestibular nucleus

Nucleus prepositus

Posterior longitudinal fasciculus

Pontobulbar nucleus

Spinal trigeminal tract

Spinal trigeminal nucleus (pars oralis)

Rubrospinal tract

Nucleus ambiguus

Anterolateral system

Central tegmental tract and amiculum of olive

Olivocerebellar fibers

Degenerated corticospinal fibers

Reticular formation

4th ventricle open medulla

Nucleus raphe, obscurus

Nucleus raphe, light

Inferior salivatory nucleus

Solitary nuclei light

Solitary tract dark

Restiform body

Cerebellum

Posterior (dorsal) cochlear nucleus

Anterior (ventral) cochlear nucleus

Cochlear nerve

Glossopharyngeal nerve

Anterior spinocerebellar tract

Reticulospinal fibers

Posterior accessory olivary nucleus

Principal olivary nucleus

Ventral trigeminothalamic tract

Medial accessory olivary nucleus

Arcuate nucleus

Nucleus raphe, pallidus

Medial longitudinal fasciculus
Tectospinal tract
Medial lemniscus

Pyramid

Posterior Medulla

Sensory ⎫ Cranial
Motor ⎬ nerve
       ⎭ nuclei

Post. column/ventral. lemniscus sys. (proprioception/vibratory sense, discriminative touch)

Corticospinal fibers (somatomotor)

Anterolateral system (pain/thermal sense, touch from body)

Spinal trigeminal and/or ventral trigeminothalamic fibers (pain/thermal sense, touch from head)

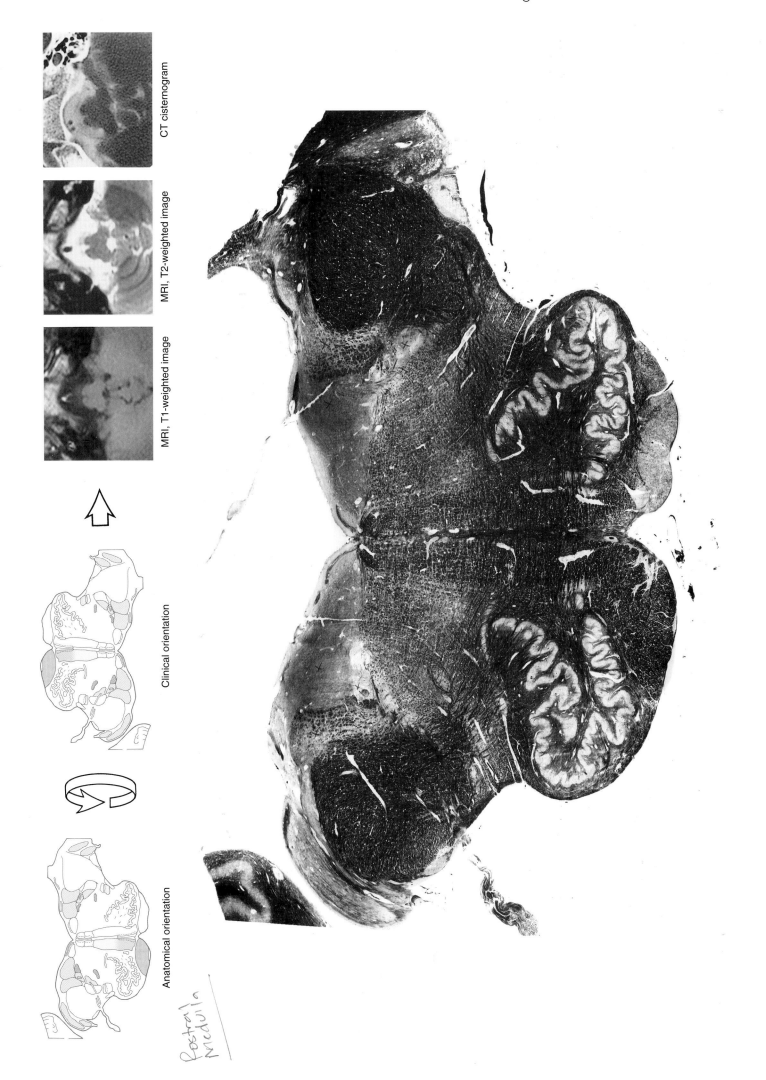

CT cisternogram

MRI, T2-weighted image

MRI, T1-weighted image

Clinical orientation

Anatomical orientation

Rostral
Medulla

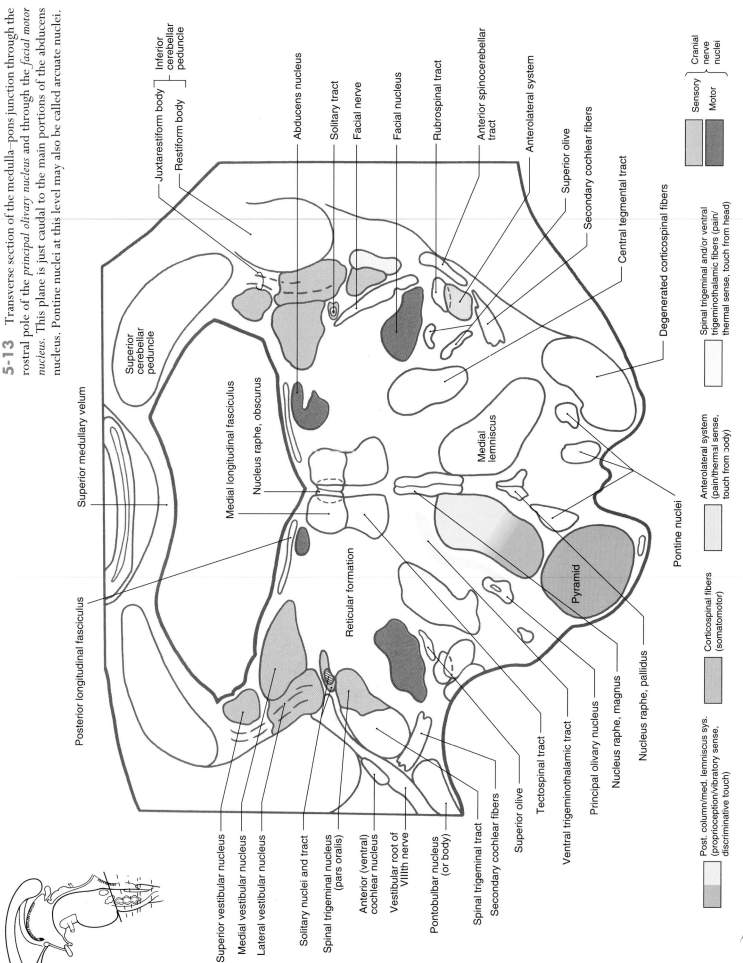

5-13 Transverse section of the medulla–pons junction through the rostral pole of the *principal olivary nucleus* and through the *facial motor nucleus.* This plane is just caudal to the main portions of the abducens nucleus. Pontine nuclei at this level may also be called arcuate nuclei.

Juxtarestiform body ⎫
Restiform body ⎭ Inferior cerebellar peduncle

Abducens nucleus
Solitary tract
Facial nerve
Facial nucleus
Rubrospinal tract
Anterior spinocerebellar tract
Anterolateral system
Superior olive
Secondary cochlear fibers
Central tegmental tract
Degenerated corticospinal fibers

Superior cerebellar peduncle
Superior medullary velum

Medial longitudinal fasciculus
Nucleus raphe, obscurus
Medial lemniscus
Posterior longitudinal fasciculus
Reticular formation
Pyramid
Pontine nuclei

Superior vestibular nucleus
Medial vestibular nucleus
Lateral vestibular nucleus
Solitary nuclei and tract
Spinal trigeminal nucleus (pars oralis)
Anterior (ventral) cochlear nucleus
Vestibular root of VIIIth nerve
Pontobulbar nucleus (or body)
Spinal trigeminal tract
Secondary cochlear fibers
Superior olive
Tectospinal tract
Ventral trigeminothalamic tract
Principal olivary nucleus
Nucleus raphe, magnus
Nucleus raphe, pallidus

Sensory ⎫ Cranial
Motor ⎭ nerve nuclei

Post. column/med. lemniscus sys. (proprioception/vibratory sense, discriminative touch)

Corticospinal fibers (somatomotor)

Anterolateral system (pain/thermal sense, touch from body)

Spinal trigeminal and/or ventral trigeminothalamic fibers (pain/thermal sense, touch from head)

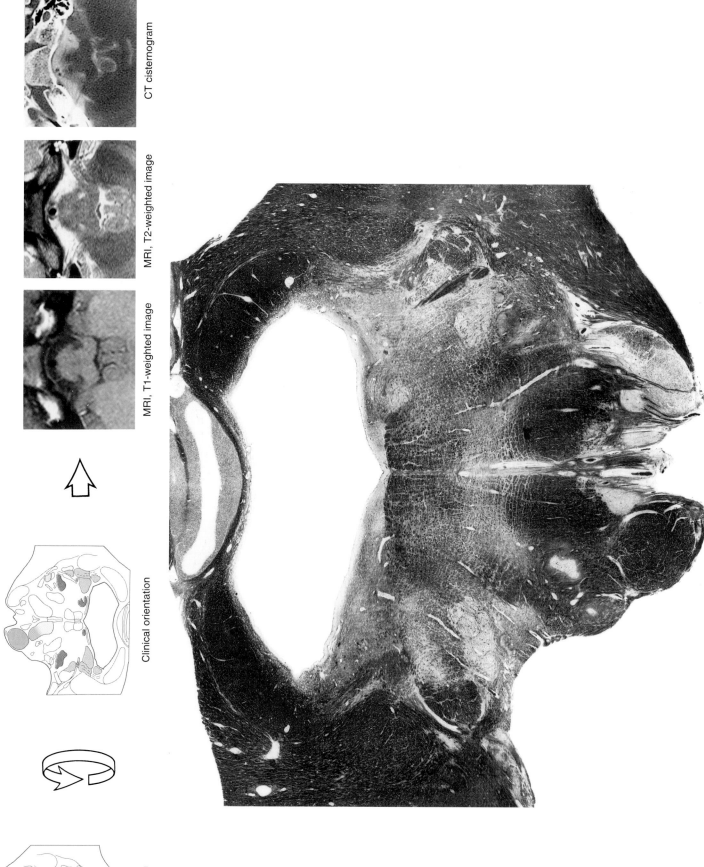

CT cisternogram

MRI, T2-weighted image

MRI, T1-weighted image

Clinical orientation

Anatomical orientation

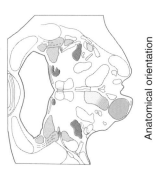

5-14 Semidiagrammatic representation of the internal distribution of arteries in the medulla oblongata. Selected main structures are labeled primarily on the left side of each section and the general pattern of arterial distribution overlies these structures on the right side. The general distribution patterns of arteries in the medulla as illustrated here may vary from patient to patient. For example, the territories served by adjacent vessels may overlap to differing degrees at their margins or the territory of a particular vessel may be smaller or larger than seen in the typical pattern.

Abbreviations

FCu	Cuneate fasciculus
FGr	Gracile fasciculus
ML	Medial lemniscus
NuCu	Cuneate nucleus
NuGr	Gracile nucleus
Py	Pyramid
RB	Restiform body (+ juxtarestiform body = inferior cerebellar peduncle)
RetF	Reticular formation

Vascular Syndromes or Lesions of the Medulla Oblongata

Medial Medullary Syndrome: Results from occlusion of branches of anterior spinal artery.

Deficits	Structure Damaged
Contralateral hemiplegia of arm and leg	Pyramid (cortico-spinal fibers)
Contralateral loss of position sense, vibratory sense and discriminative touch	Medial lemniscus
Deviation of tongue to ipsilateral side when protruded; muscle atrophy and fasciculations	Hypoglossal nerve in medulla or hypoglossal nucleus

Comment: The medial medullary syndrome is rare compared to the more common occurence of the lateral medullary syndrome. *Nystagmus* may result if the lesion involves the medial longitudinal fasciculus or the nucleus prepositus hypoglossi. The lesion may involve ventral trigeminothalamic fibers, but diminished pain and thermal sense from the contralateral side of the face is rarely seen. The combination of a contralateral hemiplegia and ipsilateral deviation of the tongue is called an *inferior alternating hemiplegia* when the lesion is at this level.

Lateral Medullary Syndrome: Results from occulsion of posterior inferior cerebellar artery or branches of PICA to dorsolateral medulla (PICA syndrome, Wallenberg syndrome). In many cases the lateral medullary syndrome frequently results from occlusion of the vertebral artery with consequent loss of flow into PICA.

Deficits	Structure Damaged
Contralateral loss of pain and thermal sense on body	Anterolateral system fibers
Ipsilateral loss of pain and thermal sense on face	Spinal trigeminal tract and nucleus
Dysphagia, soft palate paralysis, hoarseness, diminished gag reflex	Nucleus ambiguus, roots of 9th and 10th nerves
Ipsilateral Horner syndrome (miosis, ptosis, anhidrosis, flushing of face)	Descending hypothalamospinal fibers
Nausea, diplopia, tendency to fall to ipsilateral side, nystagmus, vertigo	Vestibular nuclei (mainly inferior and medial)
Ataxia to the ipsilateral side	Restiform body and spinocerebellar fibers

Comment: In addition to the above, involvement of the solitary tract and nucleus may (rarely) cause *dysgeusia*. *Dyspnea* and *tachycardia* may be seen in patients with damage to the dorsal motor nucleus of the vagus. It is also possible that damage to respiratory centers in the reticular formation or to the vagal motor nucleus may result in hiccup (*singultus*). Bilateral medullary damage may cause the syndrome of "Ondine's curse," an inability to breathe without willing it or "thinking about it."

Tonsillar Herniation: Although the cerebellar tonsil is not part of the medulla, the herniation of this structure (*tonsillar herniation*) down through the foramen magnum has serious consequences for function of the medulla. The coning of the cerebellar tonsils into, and through, the foramen magnum may compress the medulla resulting in *cardiac and respiratory arrest*. This is due to a combination of pressure on the medulla and the occlusion of small vessels serving cardiac and respiratory centers in the lateral area of the medulla. Patients experiencing a sudden herniation of the cerebellar tonsils may lose consciousness rapidly and die.

Syringobulbia: A cavitation within the brainstem (*syringobulbia*) may exist with syringomyelia, be independent of syringomyelia, or in some cases both may exist and communicate with each other. The cavity in syringobulbia is usually on one side of the midline of the medulla. Signs and symptoms of syringobulbia may include *weakness of tongue muscles* (hypoglossal nucleus or nerve), *weakness of pharyngeal, palatal, and vocal musculature* (ambiguus nucleus), *nystagmus* (vestibular nuclei), and *loss of pain and thermal sensation on the ipsilateral side of the face* (spinal trigeminal tract and nucleus or crossing of trigeminothalamic fibers).

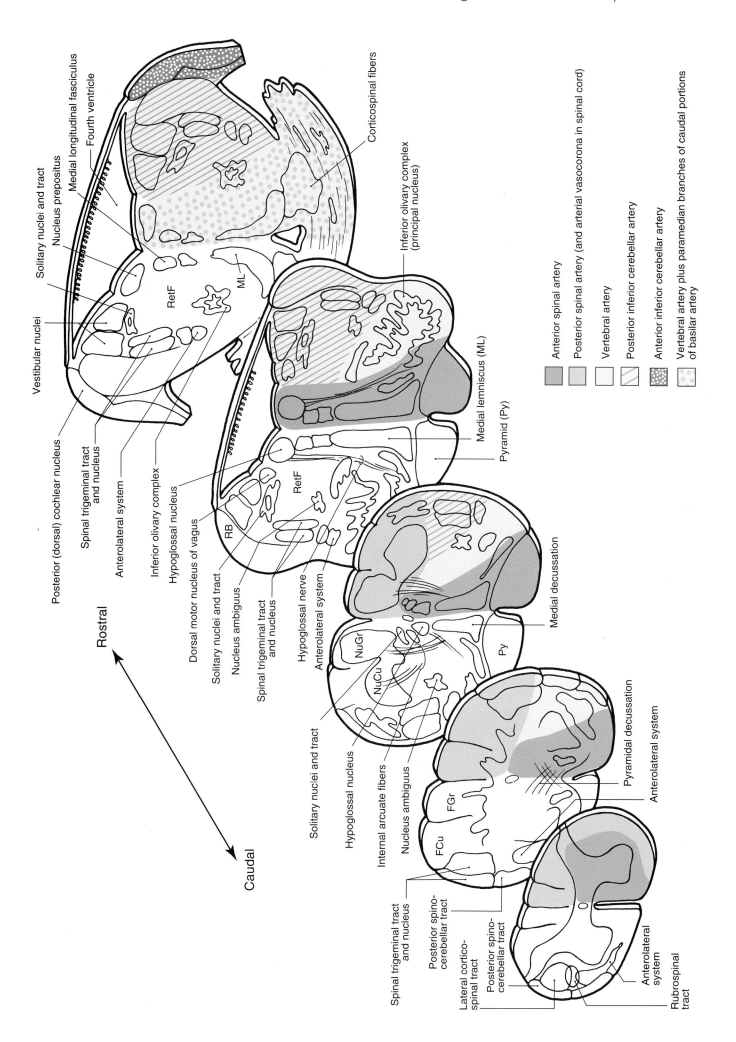

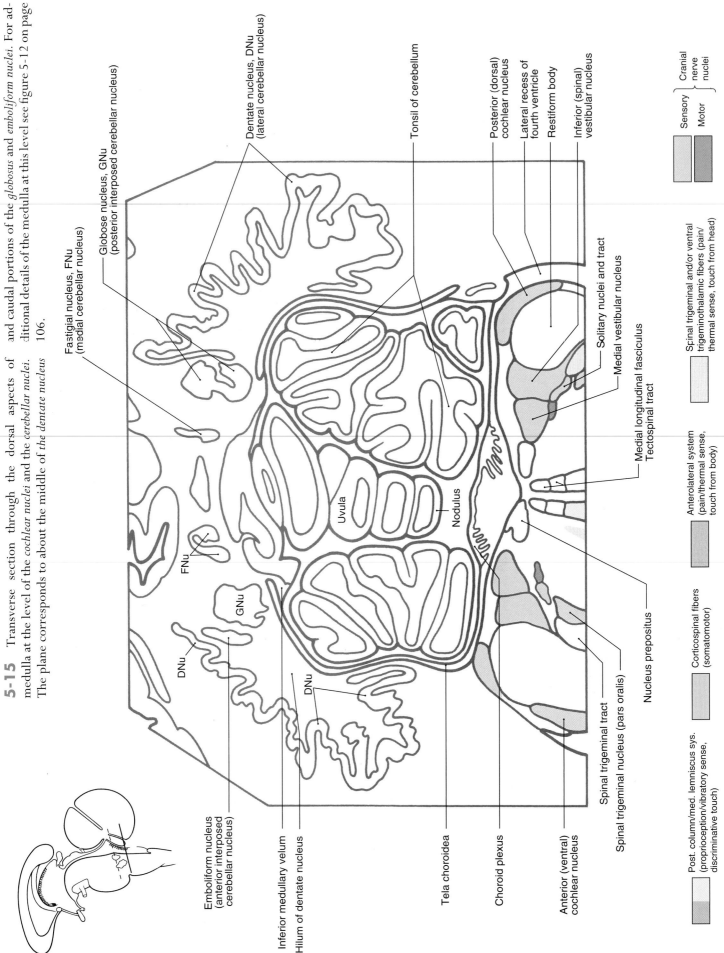

5-15 Transverse section through the dorsal aspects of medulla at the level of the *cochlear nuclei* and the *cerebellar nuclei*. The plane corresponds to about the middle of *the dentate nucleus* and caudal portions of the *globosus* and *emboliform nuclei*. For additional details of the medulla at this level see figure 5-12 on page 106.

Fastigial nucleus, FNu (medial cerebellar nucleus)

Globose nucleus, GNu (posterior interposed cerebellar nucleus)

Dentate nucleus, DNu (lateral cerebellar nucleus)

Tonsil of cerebellum

Posterior (dorsal) cochlear nucleus

Lateral recess of fourth ventricle

Restiform body

Inferior (spinal) vestibular nucleus

Solitary nuclei and tract

Medial vestibular nucleus

Medial longitudinal fasciculus
Tectospinal tract

Uvula

Nodulus

FNu

GNu

DNu

DNu

Embolilorm nucleus (anterior interposed cerebellar nucleus)

Inferior medullary velum

Hilum of dentate nucleus

Tela choroidea

Choroid plexus

Anterior (ventral) cochlear nucleus

Nucleus prepositus

Spinal trigeminal nucleus (pars oralis)

Spinal trigeminal tract

Cranial nerve nuclei

Sensory

Motor

Post. column/med. lemniscus sys. (proprioception/vibratory sense, discriminative touch)

Corticospinal fibers (somatomotor)

Anterolateral system (pain/thermal sense, touch from body)

Spinal trigeminal and/or ventral trigeminothalamic fibers (pain/ thermal sense, touch from head)

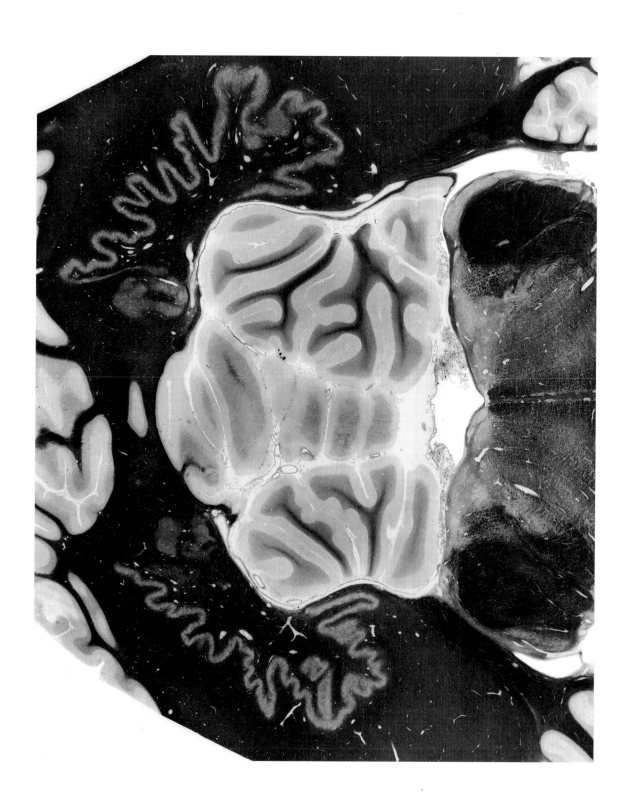

5-16   Transverse section through dorsal portions of pons at the level of the *abducens nucleus* (and *facial colliculus*) and through rostral portions of the *cerebellar nuclei*. For additional details of the pons at this level see Figure 5-17 on page 116.

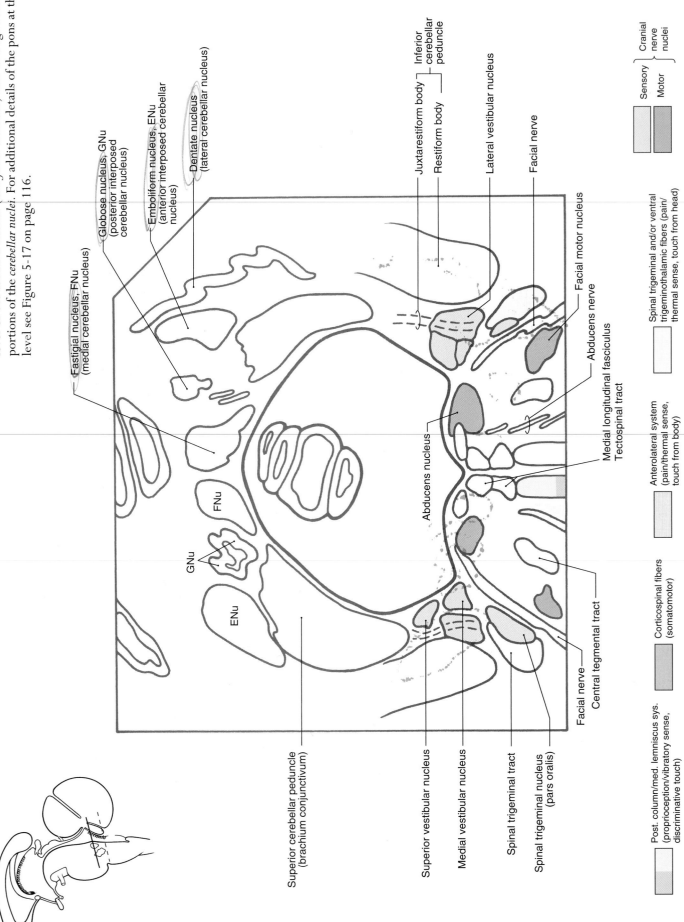

Fastigial nucleus, FNu (medial cerebellar nucleus)

Globose nucleus, GNu (posterior interposed cerebellar nucleus)

Emboliform nucleus, ENu (anterior interposed cerebellar nucleus)

Dentate nucleus (lateral cerebellar nucleus)

Juxtarestiform body

Restiform body

Inferior cerebellar peduncle

Lateral vestibular nucleus

Facial nerve

Facial motor nucleus

Abducens nerve

Abducens nucleus

Medial longitudinal fasciculus

Tectospinal tract

Facial nerve

Central tegmental tract

GNu

FNu

ENu

Superior cerebellar peduncle (brachium conjunctivum)

Superior vestibular nucleus

Medial vestibular nucleus

Spinal trigeminal tract

Spinal trigeminal nucleus (pars oralis)

Sensory ⎱ Cranial
Motor ⎰ nerve nuclei

Post. column/med. lemniscus sys. (proprioception/vibratory sense, discriminative touch)

Corticospinal fibers (somatomotor)

Anterolateral system (pain/thermal sense, touch from body)

Spinal trigeminal and/or ventral trigeminothalamic fibers (pain/ thermal sense, touch from head)

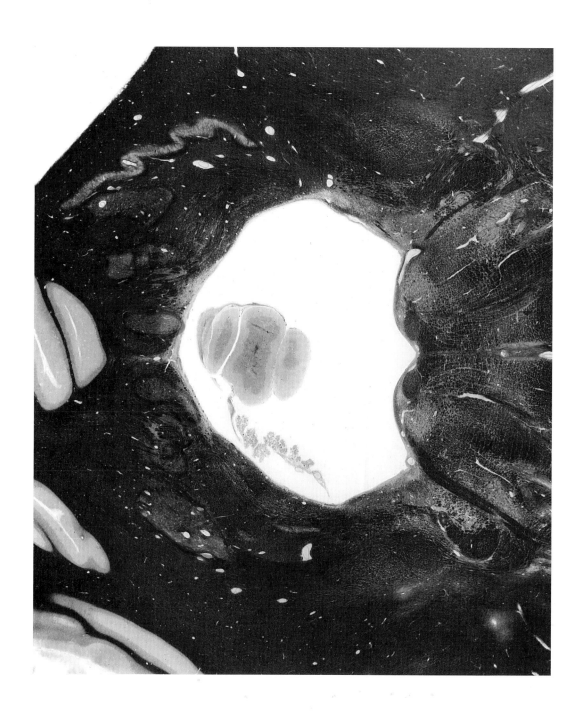

5-17 Transverse section of the caudal pons through the *facial motor nucleus, abducens nucleus* (and *facial colliculus*), and the intramedullary course of fibers of *facial* and *abducens nerves.*

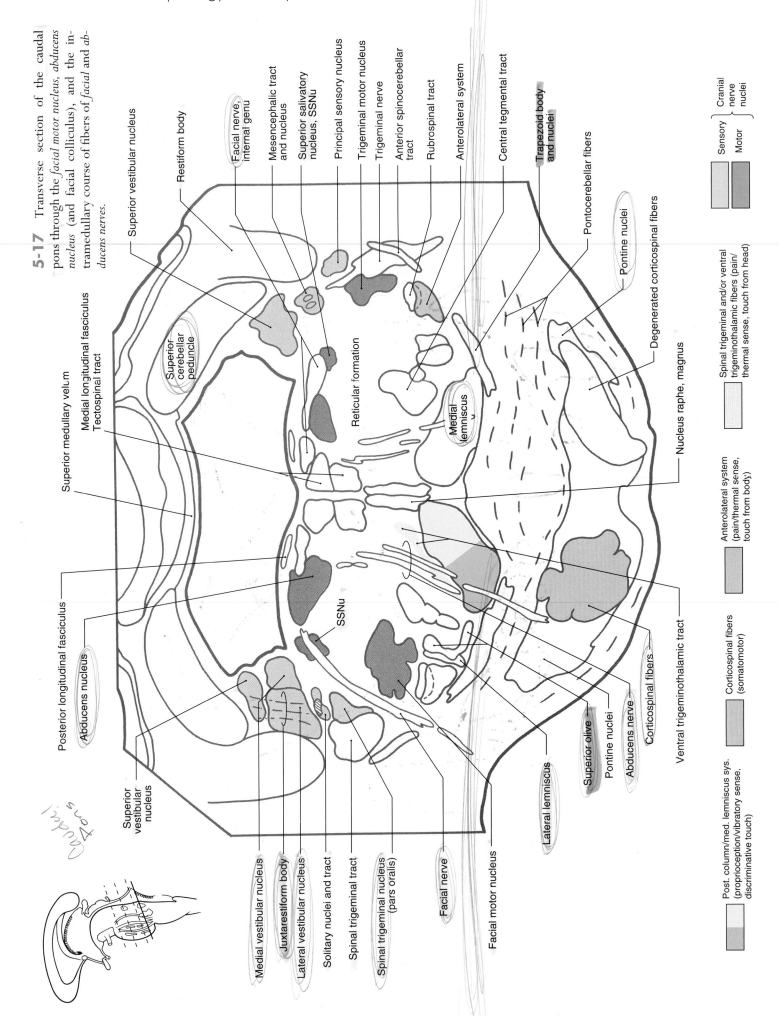

Superior vestibular nucleus

Restiform body

Facial nerve, internal genu

Mesencephalic tract and nucleus

Superior salivatory nucleus, SSNu

Principal sensory nucleus

Trigeminal motor nucleus

Trigeminal nerve

Anterior spinocerebellar tract

Rubrospinal tract

Anterolateral system

Central tegmental tract

Trapezoid body and nuclei

Pontocerebellar fibers

Pontine nuclei

Degenerated corticospinal fibers

Nucleus raphe, magnus

Ventral trigeminothalamic tract

Corticospinal fibers

Abducens nerve

Pontine nuclei

Superior olive

Lateral lemniscus

Facial motor nucleus

Facial nerve

Spinal trigeminal nucleus (pars oralis)

Spinal trigeminal tract

Solitary nuclei and tract

Lateral vestibular nucleus

Juxtarestiform body

Medial vestibular nucleus

Superior vestibular nucleus

Abducens nucleus

Posterior longitudinal fasciculus

Superior medullary velum

Medial longitudinal fasciculus
Tectospinal tract

Superior cerebellar peduncle

Reticular formation

SSNu

Medial lemniscus

Sensory ⎱ Cranial
Motor ⎰ nerve nuclei

Post. column/med. lemniscus sys. (proprioception/vibratory sense, discriminative touch)

Corticospinal fibers (somatomotor)

Anterolateral system (pain/thermal sense, touch from body)

Spinal trigeminal and/or ventral trigeminothalamic fibers (pain/ thermal sense, touch from head)

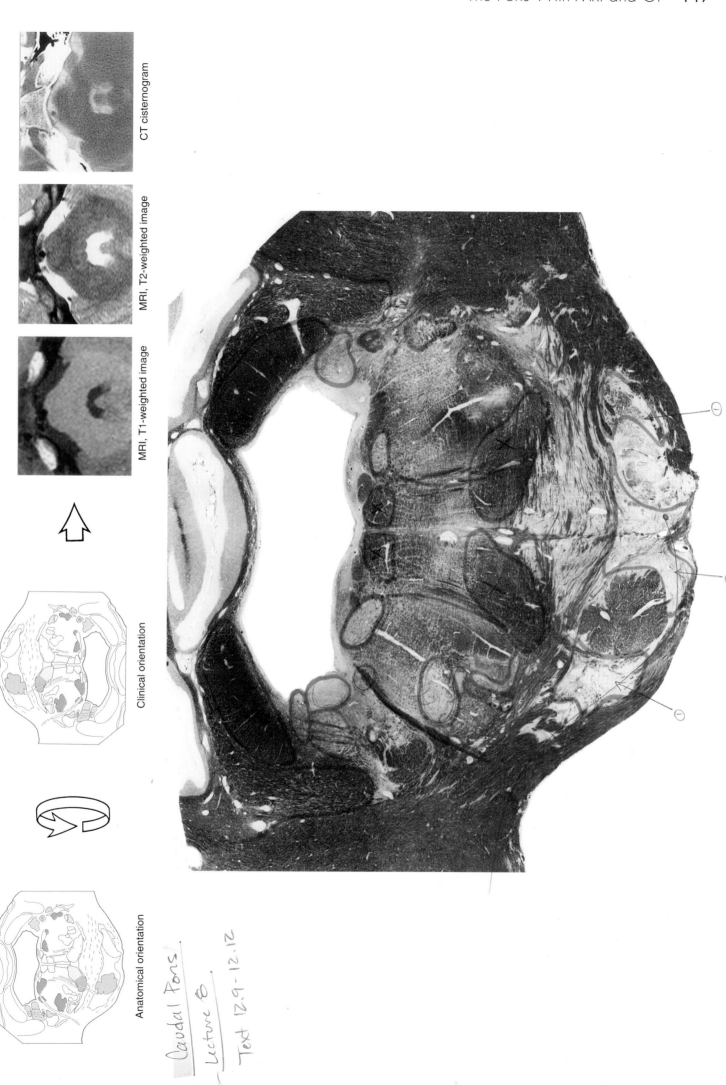

CT cisternogram

MRI, T2-weighted image

MRI, T1-weighted image

Clinical orientation

Anatomical orientation

Caudal Pons

Lecture 8

Text 12.9 - 12.12

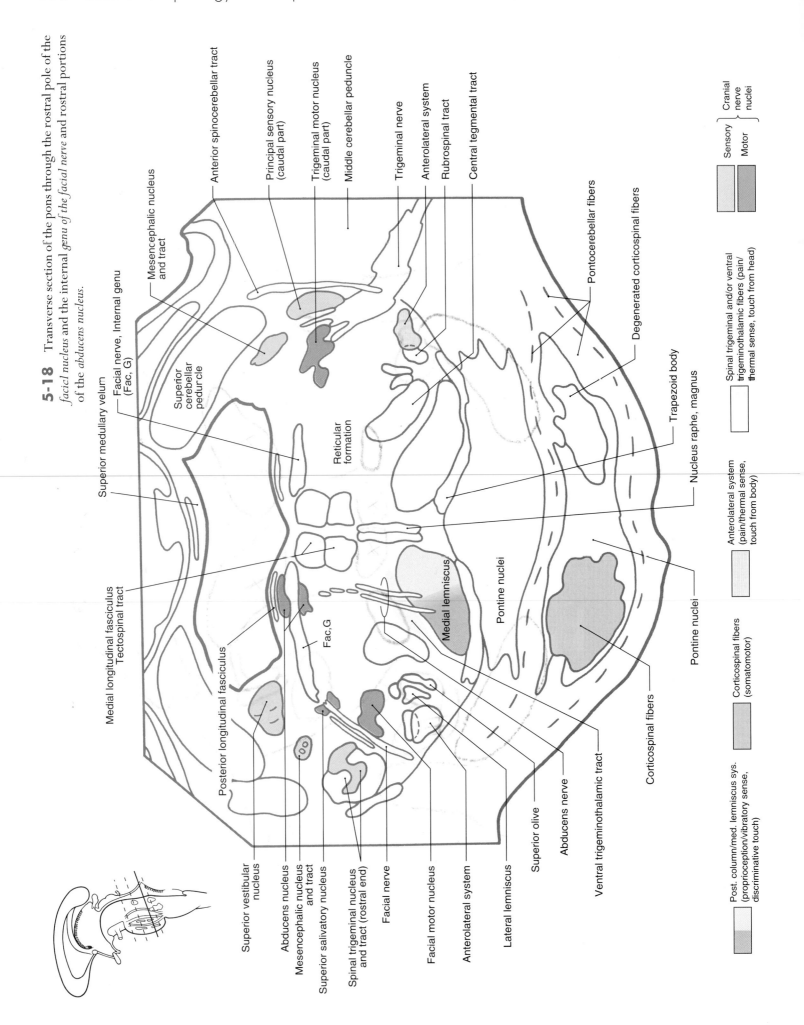

5-18   Transverse section of the pons through the rostral pole of the *facial nucleus* and the internal *genu of the facial nerve* and rostral portions of the *abducens nucleus.*

Mesencephalic nucleus and tract

Anterior spinocerebellar tract

Principal sensory nucleus (cauda part)

Trigeminal motor nucleus (caudal part)

Middle cerebellar peduncle

Trigeminal nerve

Anterolateral system

Rubrospinal tract

Central tegmental tract

Pontocerebellar fibers

Degenerated corticospinal fibers

Facial nerve, Internal genu (Fac, G)

Superior cerebellar peduncle

Superior medullary velum

Reticular formation

Trapezoid body

Nucleus raphe, magnus

Medial longitudinal fasciculus
Tectospinal tract

Posterior longitudinal fasciculus

Fac, G

Medial lemniscus

Pontine nuclei

Pontine nuclei

Superior vestibular nucleus

Abducens nucleus

Mesencephalic nucleus and tract

Superior salivatory nucleus

Spinal trigeminal nucleus and tract (rostral end)

Facial nerve

Facial motor nucleus

Anterolateral system

Lateral lemniscus

Superior olive

Abducens nerve

Ventral trigeminothalamic tract

Corticospinal fibers

Sensory ⎫ Cranial
Motor ⎬ nerve
      ⎭ nuclei

Post. column/med. lemniscus sys. (proprioception/vibratory sense, discriminative touch)

Corticospinal fibers (somatomotor)

Anterolateral system (pain/thermal sense, touch from body)

Spinal trigeminal and/or ventral trigeminothalamic fibers (pain/ thermal sense, touch from head)

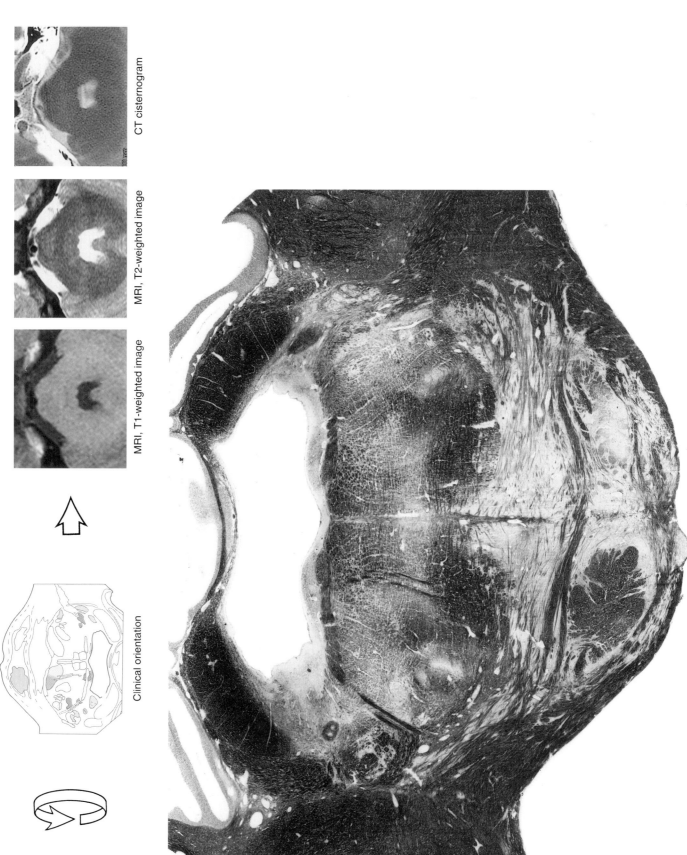

CT cisternogram

MRI, T2-weighted image

MRI, T1-weighted image

Clinical orientation

Anatomical orientation

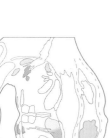

5-19 Transverse section of the pons through the *principal sensory nucleus and motor nucleus of the trigeminal nerve.*

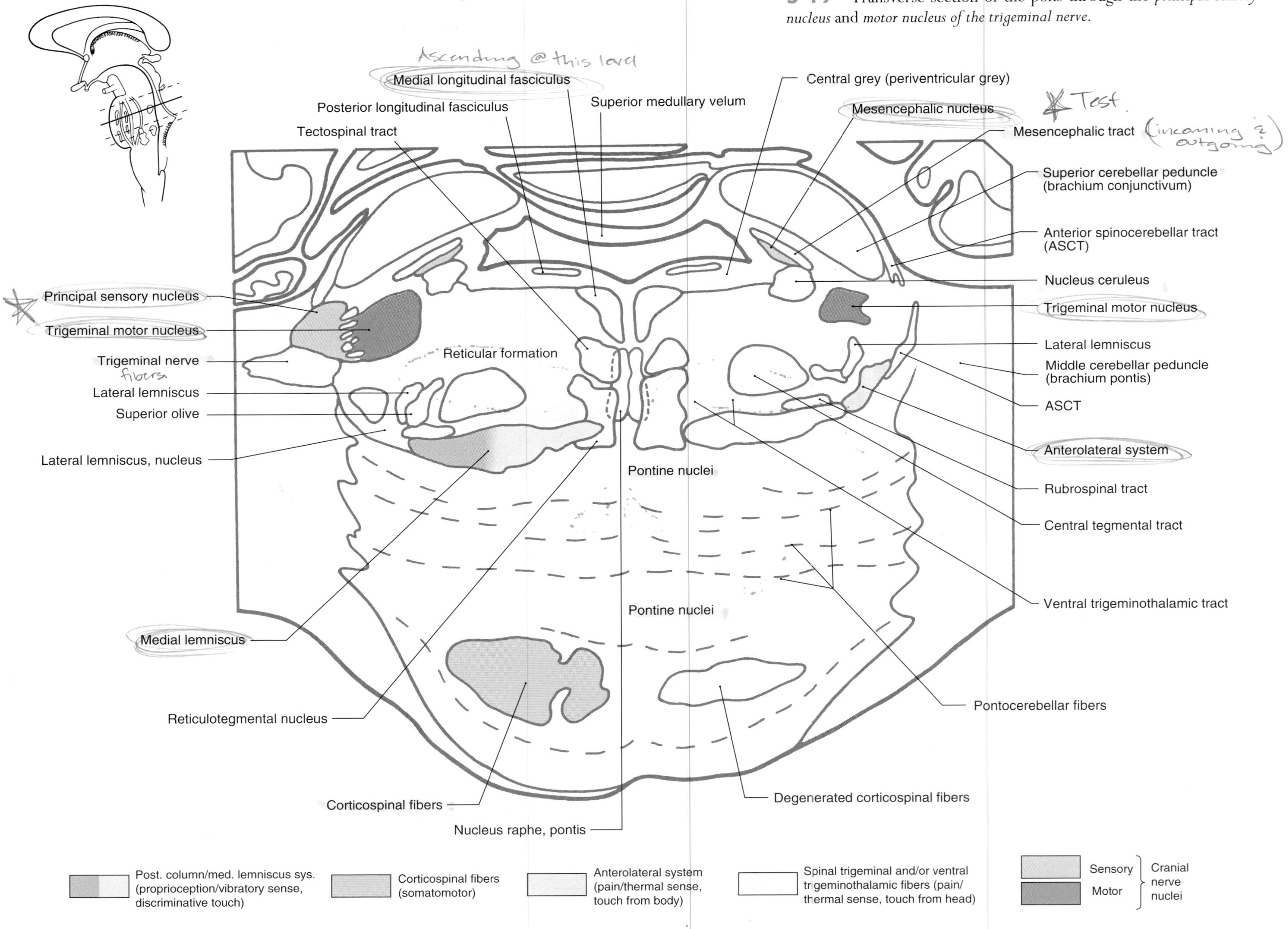

Central grey (periventricular grey)

Mesencephalic tract (incoming + outgoing)

Test

Mesencephalic nucleus

Superior cerebellar peduncle (brachium conjunctivum)

Anterior spinocerebellar tract (ASCT)

Nucleus ceruleus

Trigeminal motor nucleus

Lateral lemniscus

Middle cerebellar peduncle (brachium pontis)

ASCT

Anterolateral system

Rubrospinal tract

Central tegmental tract

Ventral trigeminothalamic tract

Pontocerebellar fibers

Degenerated corticospinal fibers

Superior medullary velum

Ascending @ this level

Medial longitudinal fasciculus

Posterior longitudinal fasciculus

Tectospinal tract

Reticular formation

Pontine nuclei

Pontine nuclei

Nucleus raphe, pontis

Corticospinal fibers

Reticulotegmental nucleus

Principal sensory nucleus

Trigeminal motor nucleus

Trigeminal nerve fibers

Lateral lemniscus

Superior olive

Lateral lemniscus, nucleus

Medial lemniscus

Sensory Cranial nerve nuclei
Motor

Spinal trigeminal and/or ventral trigeminothalamic fibers (pain/thermal sense, touch from head)

Anterolateral system (pain/thermal sense, touch from body)

Corticospinal fibers (somatomotor)

Post. column/med. lemniscus sys. (proprioception/vibratory sense, discriminative touch)

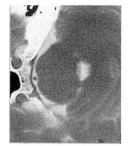

CT cisternogram

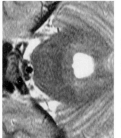

MRI, T2-weighted image

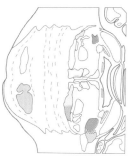

MRI, T1-weighted image

Clinical orientation

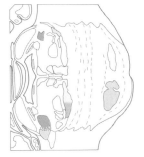

Anatomical orientation

Mid-Pontine Level

Lecture 8

Text 12.14 - 12.15

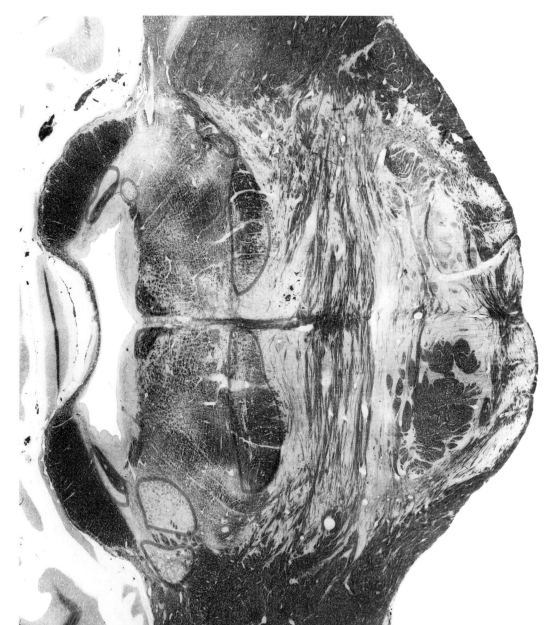

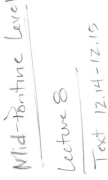

lateral lemniscus

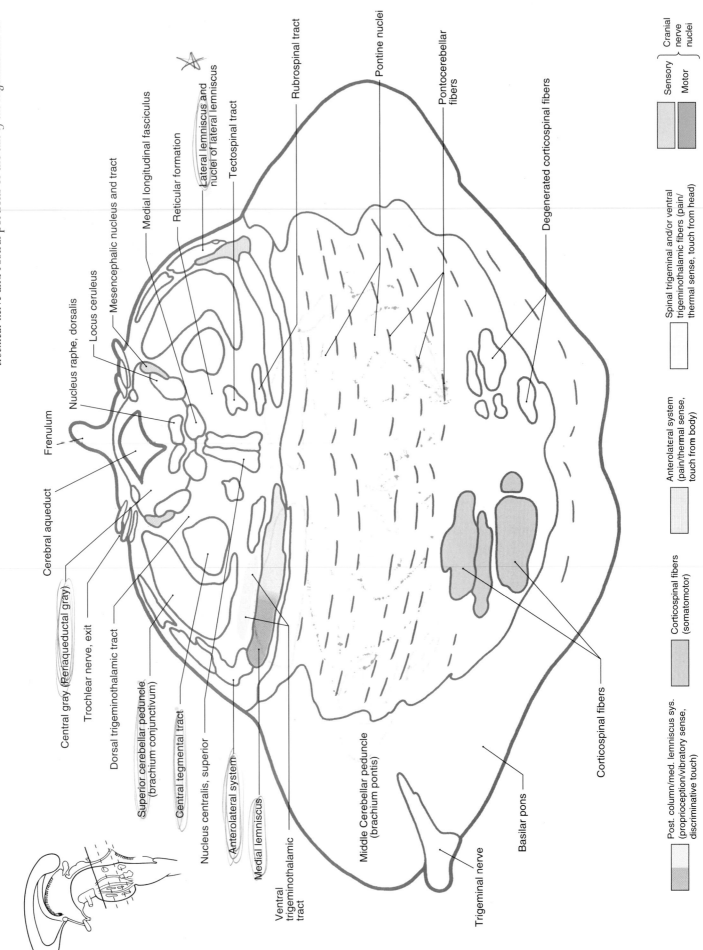

5-20 Transverse section of the rostral pons through the *exit of the trochlear nerve* and rostral portions of the *exit of the trigeminal nerve.*

Cerebral aqueduct

Frenulum

Nucleus raphe, dorsalis

Locus ceruleus

Mesencephalic nucleus and tract

Medial longitudinal fasciculus

Reticular formation

Lateral lemniscus and nuclei of lateral lemniscus

Tectospinal tract

Rubrospinal tract

Pontine nuclei

Pontocerebellar fibers

Degenerated corticospinal fibers

Central gray (Periaqueductal gray)

Trochlear nerve, exit

Dorsal trigeminothalamic tract

Superior cerebellar peduncle (brachium conjunctivum)

Central tegmental tract

Nucleus centralis, superior

Anterolateral system

Medial lemniscus

Ventral trigeminothalamic tract

Middle Cerebellar peduncle (brachium pontis)

Basilar pons

Trigeminal nerve

Corticospinal fibers

Corticospinal fibers

Post. column/med. lemniscus sys. (proprioception/vibratory sense, discriminative touch)

Corticospinal fibers (somatomotor)

Anterolateral system (pain/thermal sense, touch from body)

Spinal trigeminal and/or ventral trigeminothalamic fibers (pain/ thermal sense, touch from head)

Sensory ⎤ Cranial
        ⎥ nerve
Motor ⎦ nuclei

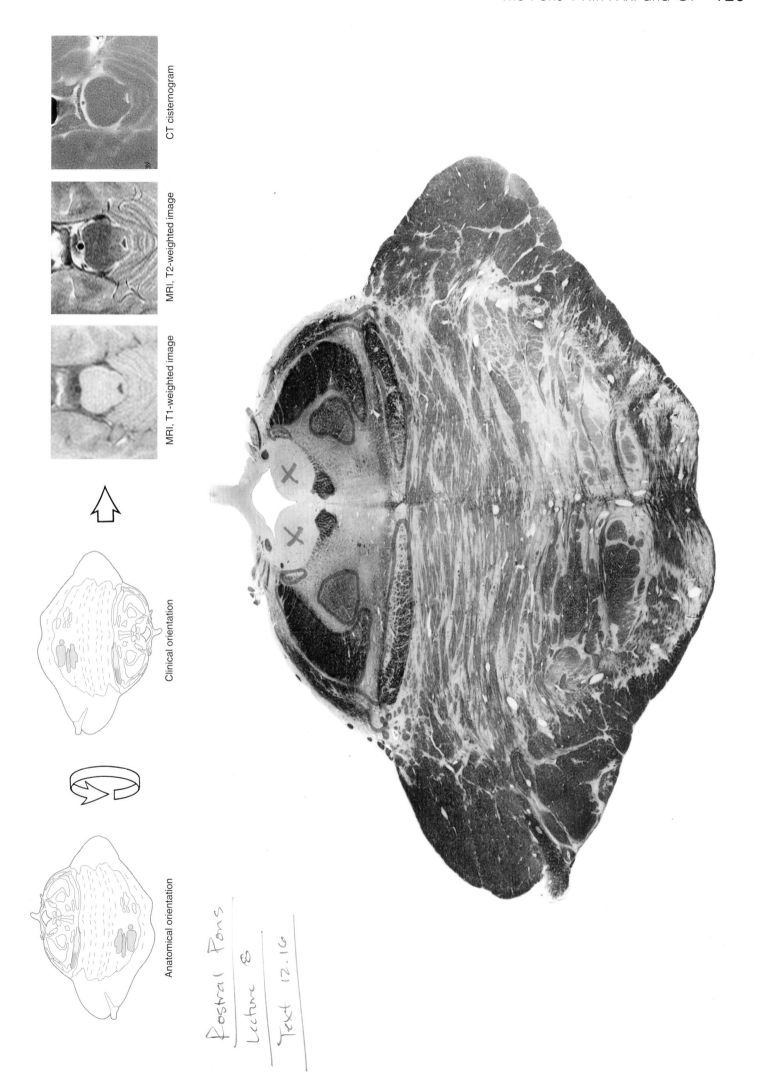

CT cisternogram

MRI, T2-weighted image

MRI, T1-weighted image

Clinical orientation

Anatomical orientation

Rostral Pons

Lecture 8

Text 12.16

5-21 Semidiagrammatic representation of the internal distribution of arteries in the pons. Selected main structures are labeled on the left side of each section; the general pattern of arterial distribution overlies these structures on the right side. Some patients may have variations of the general distribution patterns of arteries to the pons as shown here. For example, the adjacent territories served by vessels may overlap to differing degrees at their margins or the territory of a particular vessel may be smaller or larger than seen in the general pattern.

Abbreviations

BP	Basilar pons
CSp	Corticospinal fibers
CTT	Central tegmental tract
MCP	Middle cerebellar peduncle (brachium pontis)
ML	Medial lemniscus
MLF	Medial longitudinal fasciculus
RB	Restiform body (+juxtarestiform body = inferior cerebellar)
RetF	Reticular formation
SCP	Superior cerebellar peduncle (brachium conjunctivum)

Vascular Syndromes or Lesions of the Pons

Medial Pontine Syndrome: Results from occlusion of paramedian branches of basilar artery.

Deficits	Structure Damaged
• Contralateral hemiplegia of arm and leg	• Corticospinal fibers in basilar pons
• Contralateral loss or decrease of position and vibratory sense and discriminative touch (arm and leg)	• Medial lemniscus
• Ipsilateral lateral rectus muscle paralysis	• Abducens nerve fibers or nucleus
• Paralysis of conjugate gaze toward side of lesion	• Paramedian pontine reticular formation (pontine gaze center)

Comment: The combination of corticospinal deficits on one side of the body coupled with a cranial nerve motor deficit on the opposite is called a *middle alternating hemiplegia* when the lesion is at this level. *Diplopia* will result (abducens nerve lesion) on gaze toward the side of the lesion. Involvement of the abducens nucleus may also result in an inability to adduct the contralateral medial rectus muscle (damage to abducens internuclear neurons).

At caudal levels the lesion may extend lateral to involve the lateral lemniscus (*hypacusis*), parts of the middle cerebellar peduncle (some *ataxia*), the facial motor nucleus (*ipsilateral facial paralysis*), the spinal trigeminal tract and nucleus (*ipsilateral loss of pain and thermal sensation from the face*), and the anterolateral system (*contralateral loss of pain and thermal sensation from the body*). At rostral pontine levels the lesion may extend into the medial lemniscus or may involve only the arm fibers within this structure (*contralateral loss of vibratory sense, proprioception, and discriminative touch*), the motor nucleus of the trigeminal nerve (*ipsilateral paralysis of masticatory muscles*), or may damage the anterolateral system and rostral portions of the spinal trigeminal tract and nucleus (*loss of pain and thermal sensation from the body* [contralateral] *and from the face* [ipsilateral]).

Lateral Pontine Syndrome: Results from occlusion of long circumferential branches of basilar artery.

Deficit	Structure Damaged
• Ataxia, unsteady gait, fall toward side of lesion	• Middle and superior cerebellar peduncles (caudal and rostral levels)
• Vertigo, nausea, nystagmus, deafness, tinnitus, vomiting (at caudal levels)	• Vestibular and cochlear nerves and nuclei
• Ipsilateral paralysis of facial muscles	• Facial motor nucleus (caudal levels)
• Ipsilateral paralysis of masticatory muscles	• Trigeminal motor nucleus (midpontine levels)
• Ipsilateral Horner syndrome	• Descending hypothalamospinal fibers
• Ipsilateral loss of pain and thermal sense from face	• Spinal trigeminal tract and nucleus
• Contralateral loss of pain and thermal sense from body	• Anterolateral system
• Paralysis of conjugate horizontal gaze	• Paramedian pontine reticular formation (at mid to caudal levels)

Comment: The various combinations of these deficits may vary depending on whether the lesion is located in lateral pontine areas at caudal levels versus lateral pontine areas at rostral levels. As noted above lesions located in lateral portions of the pontine tegmentine may also extend medial at either caudal or rostral levels and give rise to some of the deficits discussed above in the section on medial pontine syndrome.

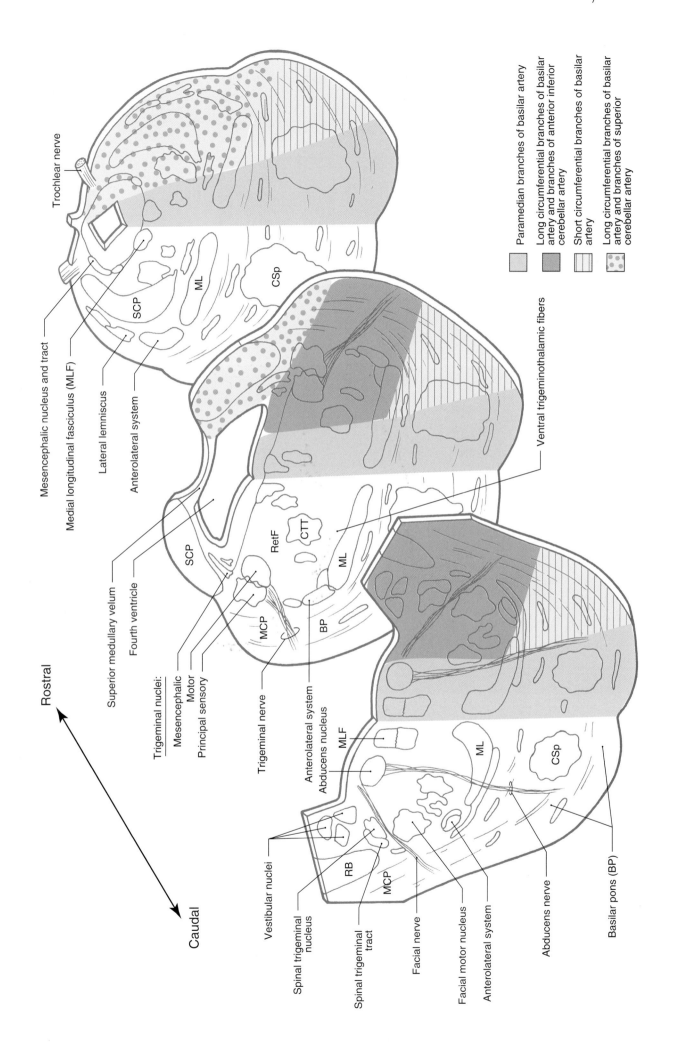

Rostral

Caudal

Trochlear nerve

Mesencephalic nucleus and tract

Medial longitudinal fasciculus (MLF)

Lateral lemniscus

Anterolateral system

Superior medullary velum

Fourth ventricle

Trigeminal nuclei:
Mesencephalic
Motor
Principal sensory

Trigeminal nerve

Anterolateral system

Abducens nucleus

Vestibular nuclei

Spinal trigeminal nucleus

Spinal trigeminal tract

Facial nerve

Facial motor nucleus

Anterolateral system

Abducens nerve

Basilar pons (BP)

Ventral trigeminothalamic fibers

SCP

ML

CSp

RetF

CTT

ML

SCP

MCP

BP

MLF

ML

CSp

RB

MCP

Paramedian branches of basilar artery

Long circumferential branches of basilar artery and branches of anterior inferior cerebellar artery

Short circumferential branches of basilar artery

Long circumferential branches of basilar artery and branches of superior cerebellar artery

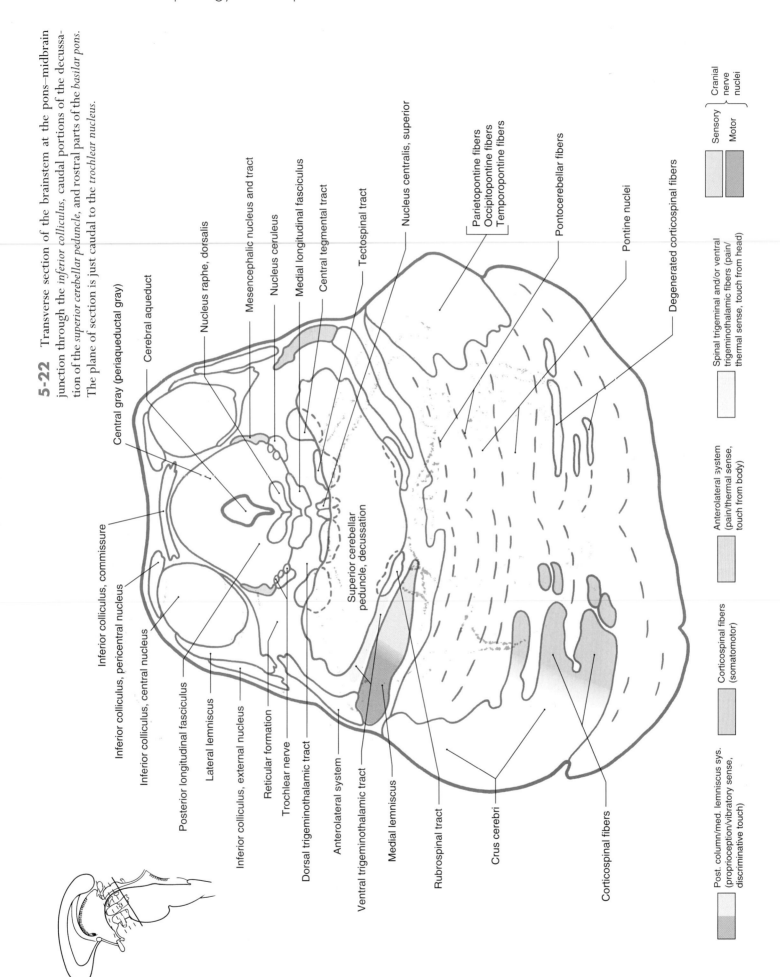

5-22   Transverse section of the brainstem at the pons–midbrain junction through the *inferior colliculus*, caudal portions of the decussation of the *superior cerebellar peduncle*, and rostral parts of the *basilar pons*. The plane of section is just caudal to the *trochlear nucleus*.

Central gray (periaqueductal gray)

Cerebral aqueduct

Nucleus raphe, dorsalis

Mesencephalic nucleus and tract

Nucleus ceruleus

Medial longitudinal fasciculus

Central tegmental tract

Tectospinal tract

Nucleus centralis, superior

Parietopontine fibers
Occipitopontine fibers
Temporopontine fibers

Pontocerebellar fibers

Pontine nuclei

Degenerated corticospinal fibers

Inferior colliculus, commissure

Inferior colliculus, pericentral nucleus

Inferior colliculus, central nucleus

Posterior longitudinal fasciculus

Lateral lemniscus

Inferior colliculus, external nucleus

Reticular formation

Trochlear nerve

Dorsal trigeminothalamic tract

Anterolateral system

Ventral trigeminothalamic tract

Medial lemniscus

Rubrospinal tract

Crus cerebri

Corticospinal fibers

Superior cerebellar peduncle, decussation

Sensory ⎤ Cranial
Motor ⎦ nerve nuclei

Spinal trigeminal and/or ventral trigeminothalamic fibers (pain/thermal sense, touch from head)

Anterolateral system (pain/thermal sense, touch from body)

Corticospinal fibers (somatomotor)

Post. column/med. lemniscus sys. (proprioception/vibratory sense, discriminative touch)

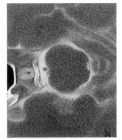

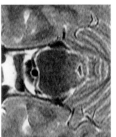

MRI, T2-weighted image

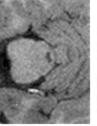

MRI, T1-weighted image

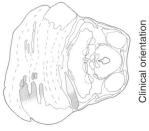

Clinical orientation

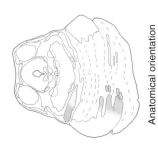

Anatomical orientation

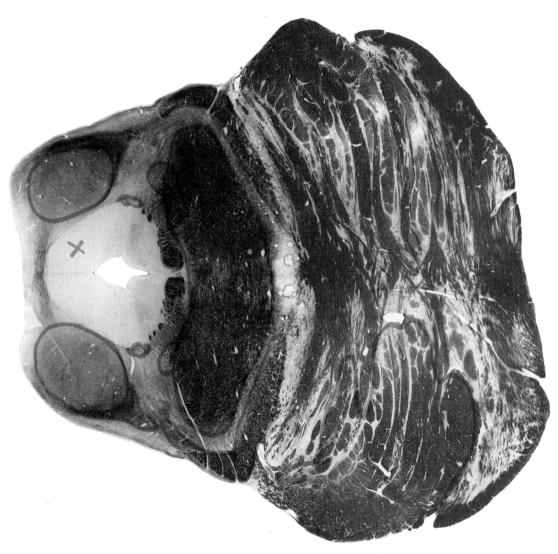

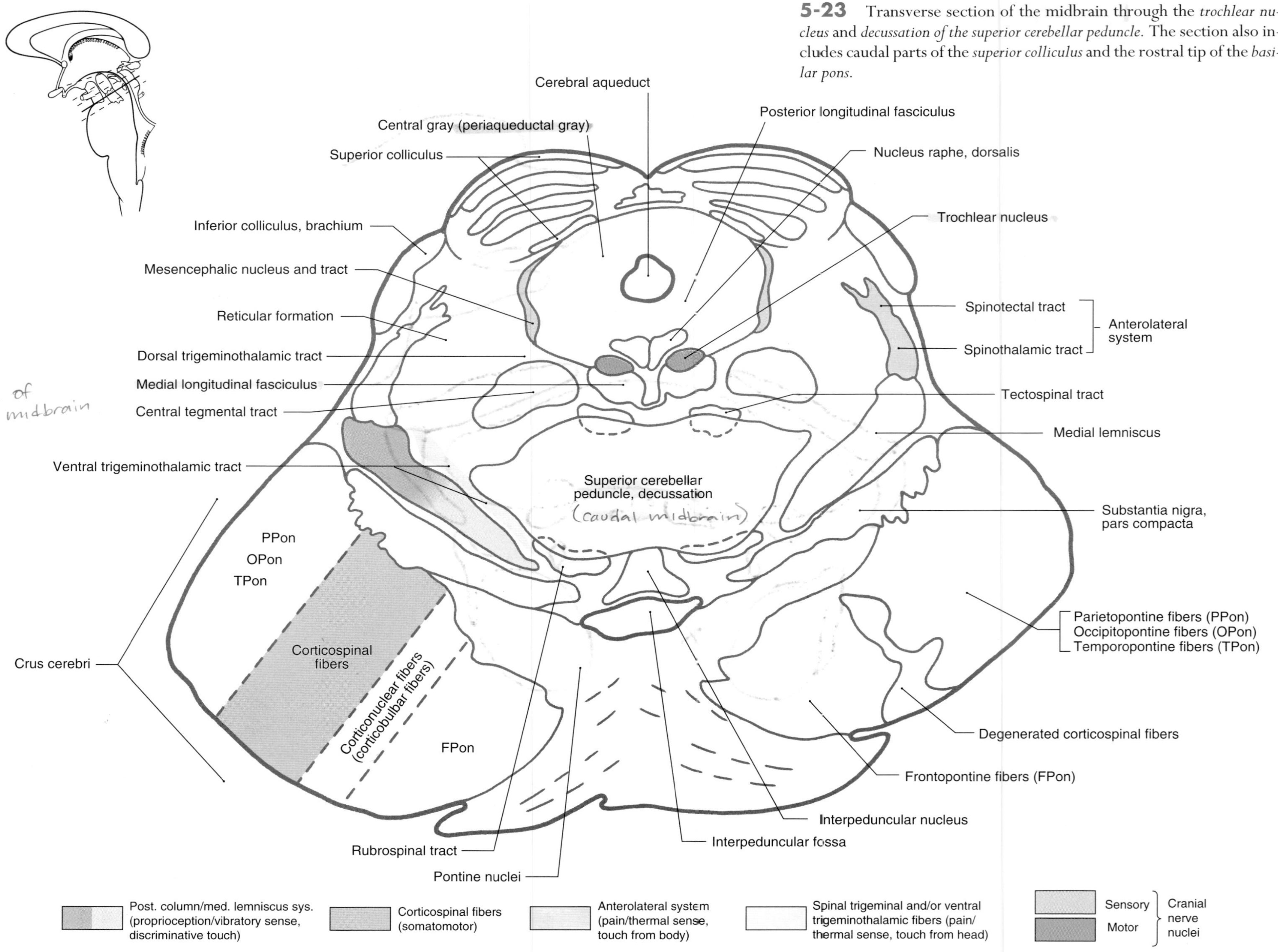

5-23   Transverse section of the midbrain through the *trochlear nucleus and decussation of the superior cerebellar peduncle*. The section also includes caudal parts of the *superior colliculus* and the rostral tip of the *basilar pons*.

Cerebral aqueduct

Central gray (periaqueductal gray)

Superior colliculus

Inferior colliculus, brachium

Mesencephalic nucleus and tract

Reticular formation

Dorsal trigeminothalamic tract

Medial longitudinal fasciculus

Central tegmental tract

Ventral trigeminothalamic tract

Posterior longitudinal fasciculus

Nucleus raphe, dorsalis

Trochlear nucleus

Spinotectal tract

Anterolateral system

Spinothalamic tract

Tectospinal tract

Medial lemniscus

Substantia nigra, pars compacta

Parietopontine fibers (PPon)
Occipitopontine fibers (OPon)
Temporopontine fibers (TPon)

Degenerated corticospinal fibers

Frontopontine fibers (FPon)

Interpeduncular nucleus

Interpeduncular fossa

Pontine nuclei

Rubrospinal tract

Crus cerebri

Corticospinal fibers

Corticonuclear fibers (corticobulbar fibers)

FPon

PPon
OPon
TPon

Superior cerebellar peduncle, decussation (caudal midbrain)

(indicative of caudal midbrain)

Sensory ⎤ Cranial
Motor ⎦ nerve nuclei

Post. column/med. lemniscus sys. (proprioception/vibratory sense, discriminative touch)

Corticospinal fibers (somatomotor)

Anterolateral system (pain/thermal sense, touch from body)

Spinal trigeminal and/or ventral trigeminothalamic fibers (pain/thermal sense, touch from head)

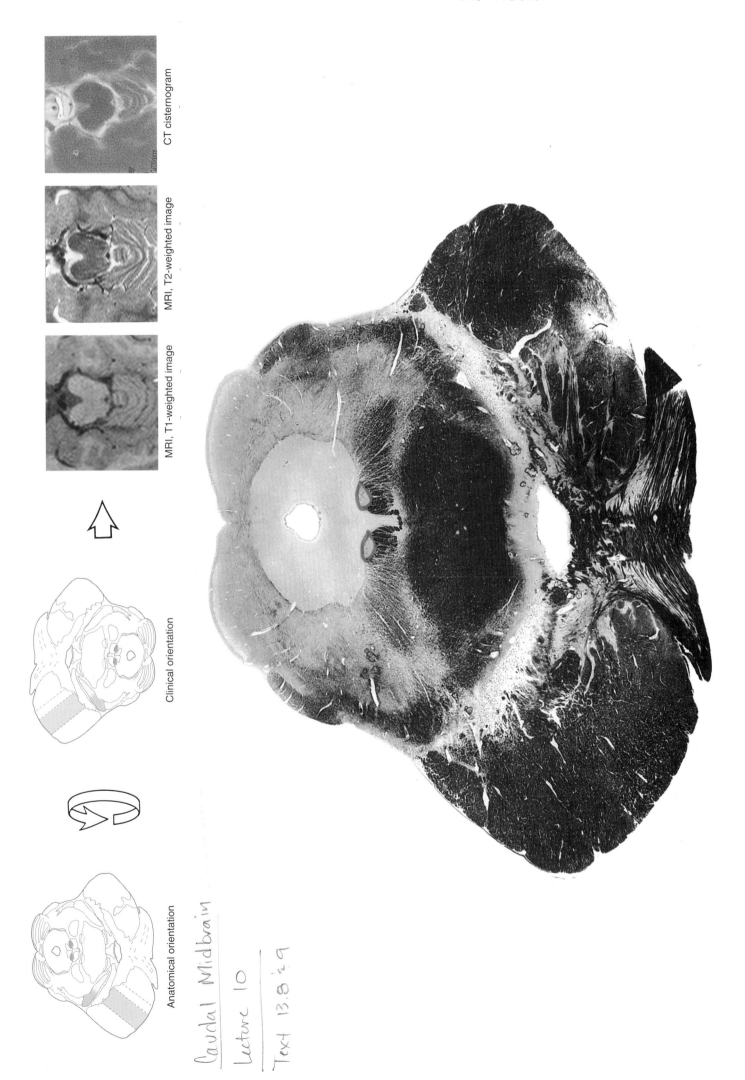

CT cisternogram

MRI, T2-weighted image

MRI, T1-weighted image

Clinical orientation

Anatomical orientation

Caudal Midbrain

Lecture 10

Text 13.8 : 9

5-24   Transverse section of the midbrain through the *superior col-liculus*, caudal parts of the *oculomotor nucleus*, and caudal parts of the *red nucleus*. The plane of section is caudal to the *Edinger-Westphal nucleus* but includes rostral portions of the *decussation of the superior cerebellar pe-duncle*, which, at this level, are intermingled with the caudal part of the red nucleus. Leg = lower extremity; Arm = upper extremity.

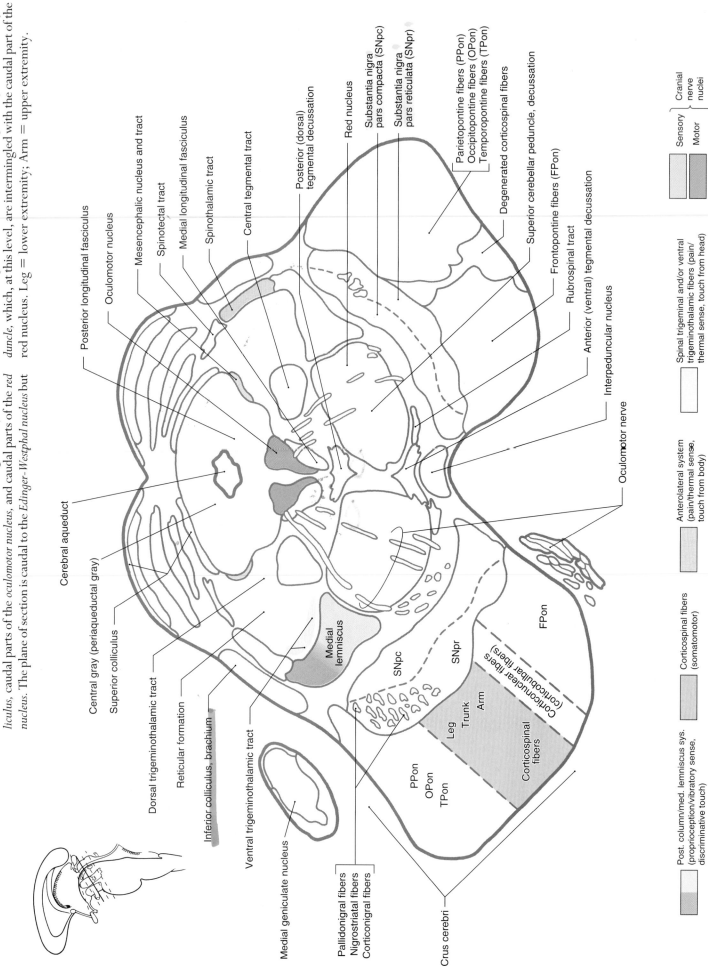

Posterior longitudinal fasciculus
Oculomotor nucleus
Mesencephalic nucleus and tract
Spinotectal tract
Medial longitudinal fasciculus
Spinothalamic tract
Central tegmental tract
Posterior (dorsal) tegmental decussation
Red nucleus
Substantia nigra pars compacta (SNpc)
Substantia nigra pars reticulata (SNpr)
Parietopontine fibers (PPon)
Occipitopontine fibers (OPon)
Temporopontine fibers (TPon)
Degenerated corticospinal fibers
Superior cerebellar peduncle, decussation
Frontopontine fibers (FPon)
Rubrospinal tract
Anterior (ventral) tegmental decussation
Interpeduncular nucleus
Oculomotor nerve

Cerebral aqueduct
Central gray (periaqueductal gray)
Superior colliculus
Dorsal trigeminothalamic tract
Reticular formation
Inferior colliculus, brachium
Ventral trigeminothalamic tract
Medial geniculate nucleus
Pallidonigral fibers
Nigrostriatal fibers
Corticonigral fibers
Crus cerebri

Medial lemniscus
SNpc
SNpr
Corticonuclear fibers (corticobulbar fibers)
Leg
Trunk
Arm
Corticospinal fibers
FPon
PPon
OPon
TPon

Post. column/med. lemniscus sys. (proprioception/vibratory sense, discriminative touch)

Anterolateral system (pain/thermal sense, touch from body)

Corticospinal fibers (somatomotor)

Spinal trigeminal and/or ventral trigeminothalamic fibers (pain/thermal sense, touch from head)

Sensory
Motor
Cranial nerve nuclei

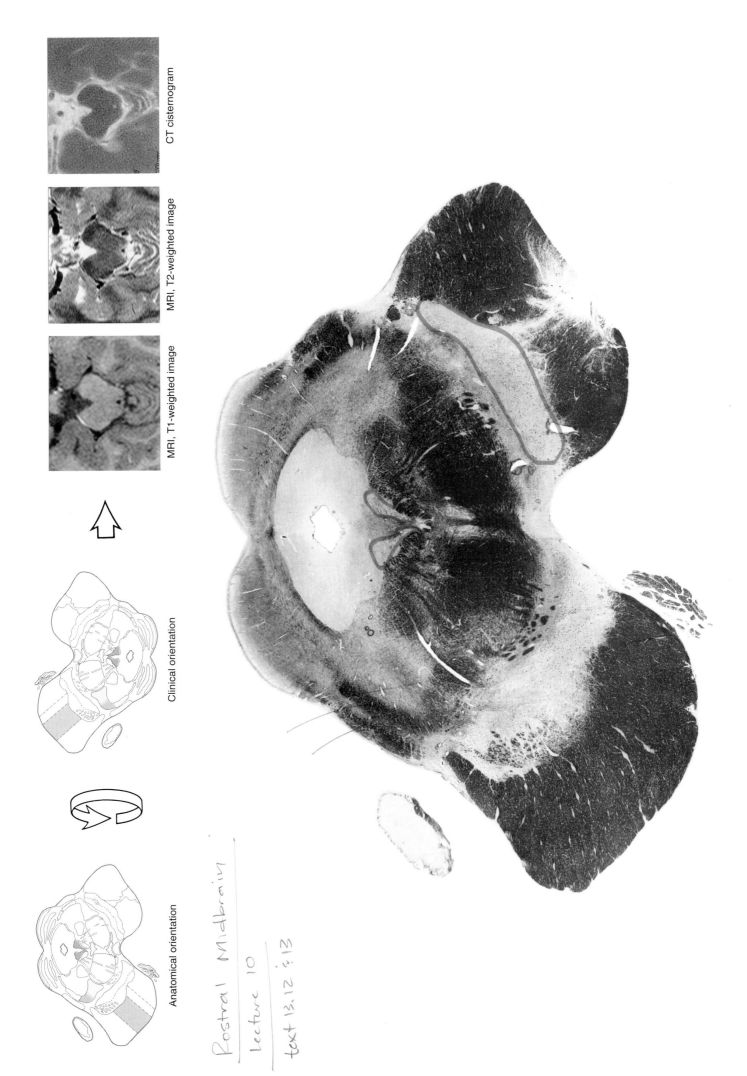

CT cisternogram

MRI, T2-weighted image

MRI, T1-weighted image

Clinical orientation

Anatomical orientation

Rostral Midbrain

Lecture 10

text 13.12 § .13

5-25   Transverse section of the midbrain through the *superior colliculus*, rostral portions of the *oculomotor nucleus*, including the *Edinger-Westphal nucleus*, and the exiting fibers of the *oculomotor nerve*. The plane of this section is also through caudal portions of the diencephalon including the *pulvinar nuclear complex* and the *medial* and *lateral geniculate nuclei*. Leg = lower extremity; Arm = upper extremity.

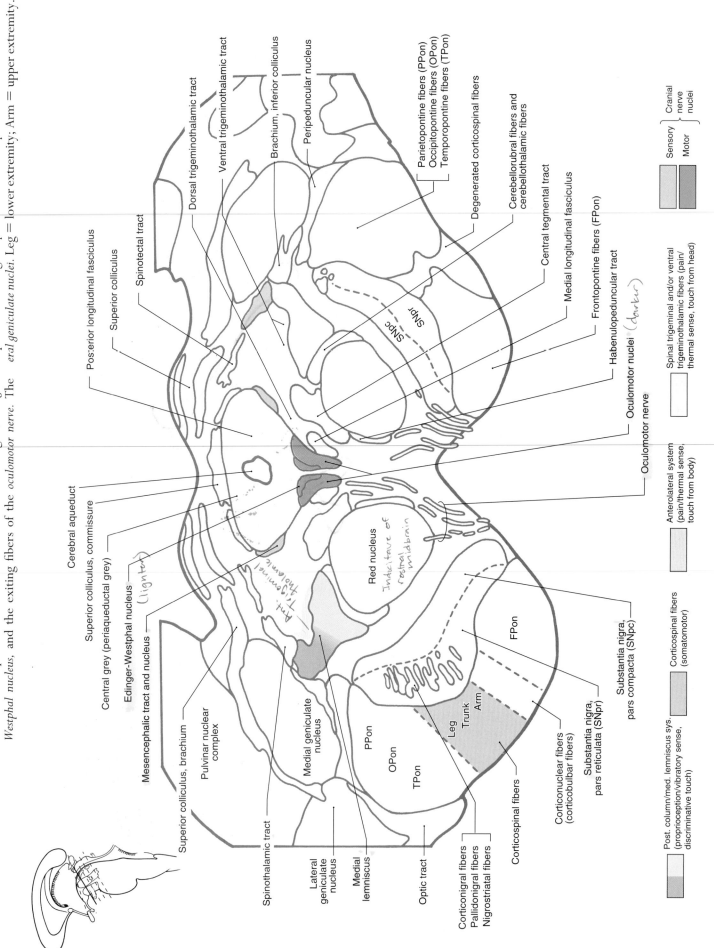

Posterior longitudinal fasciculus

Superior colliculus

Spinotectal tract

Dorsal trigeminothalamic tract

Ventral trigeminothalamic tract

Brachium, inferior colliculus

Peripeduncular nucleus

Parietopontine fibers (PPon)
Occipitopontine fibers (OPon)
Temporopontine fibers (TPon)

Degenerated corticospinal fibers

Cerebellorubral fibers and
cerebellothalamic fibers

Central tegmental tract

Medial longitudinal fasciculus

Frontopontine fibers (FPon)

Habenulopeduncular tract

Oculomotor nuclei (darker)

Oculomotor nerve

SNpr

SNpc

Cerebral aqueduct

Superior colliculus, commissure

Central grey (periaqueductal grey)

Edinger-Westphal nucleus (lighter)

Mesencephalic tract and nucleus

Superior colliculus, brachium

Pulvinar nuclear complex

Medial geniculate nucleus

Lateral geniculate nucleus

Medial lemniscus

Optic tract

Corticonigral fibers
Pallidonigral fibers
Nigrostriatal fibers

Corticospinal fibers

Corticonuclear fibers
(corticobulbar fibers)

Substantia nigra,
pars reticulata (SNpr)

Substantia nigra,
pars compacta (SNpc)

Architecture of rostral midbrain

Ant. Trigeminal thalamic

Red nucleus

Leg
Trunk
Arm

FPon

PPon

OPon

TPon

Spinothalamic tract

Post. column/med. lemniscus sys.
(proprioception/vibratory sense,
discriminative touch)

Anterolateral system
(pain/thermal sense,
touch from body)

Corticospinal fibers
(somatomotor)

Spinal trigeminal and/or ventral
trigeminothalamic fibers (pain/
thermal sense, touch from head)

Sensory ⎱ Cranial
Motor ⎰ nerve
          nuclei

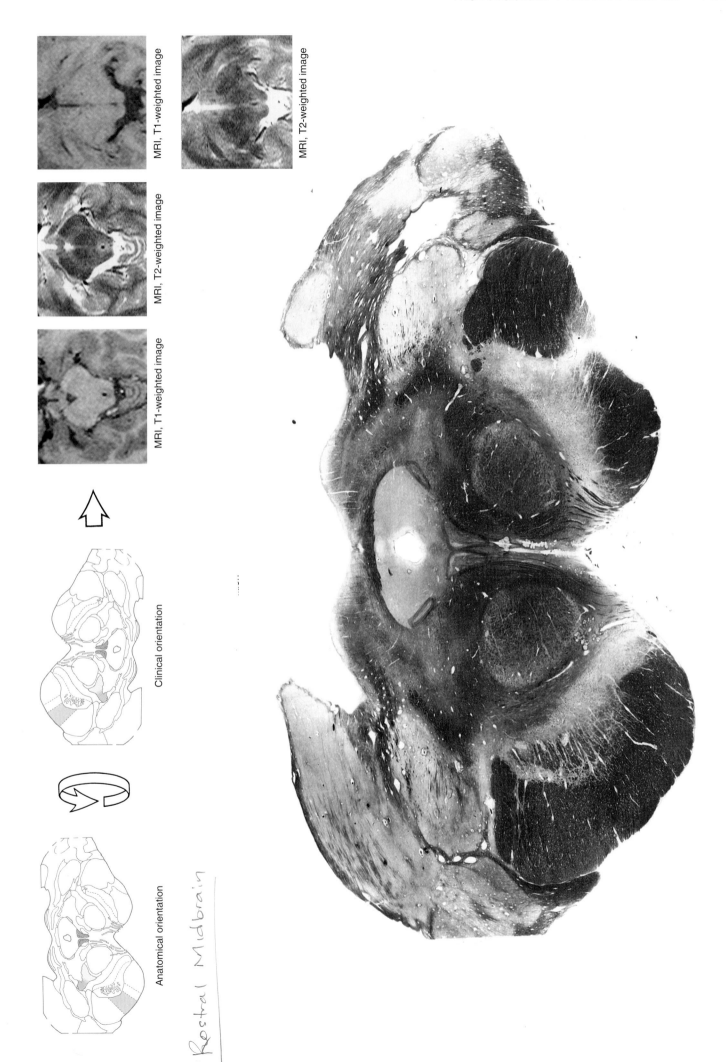

MRI, T1-weighted image

MRI, T2-weighted image

MRI, T2-weighted image

MRI, T1-weighted image

Clinical orientation

Anatomical orientation

Rostral Midbrain

5-26 Slightly oblique section through the midbrain–diencephalon junction. The section passes through the *posterior commissure*, the rostral end of the *red nucleus*, and ends just dorsal to the *mammillary body*. At this level, the structure labeled *mammillothalamic tract* probably also contains some *mammillotegmental fibers*. Structures at the midbrain-thalamus junction are best seen in an MRI angled to accommodate that specific plane. To make the transition from drawing to stained section to MRI easy, selected structures in the MRI are labeled.

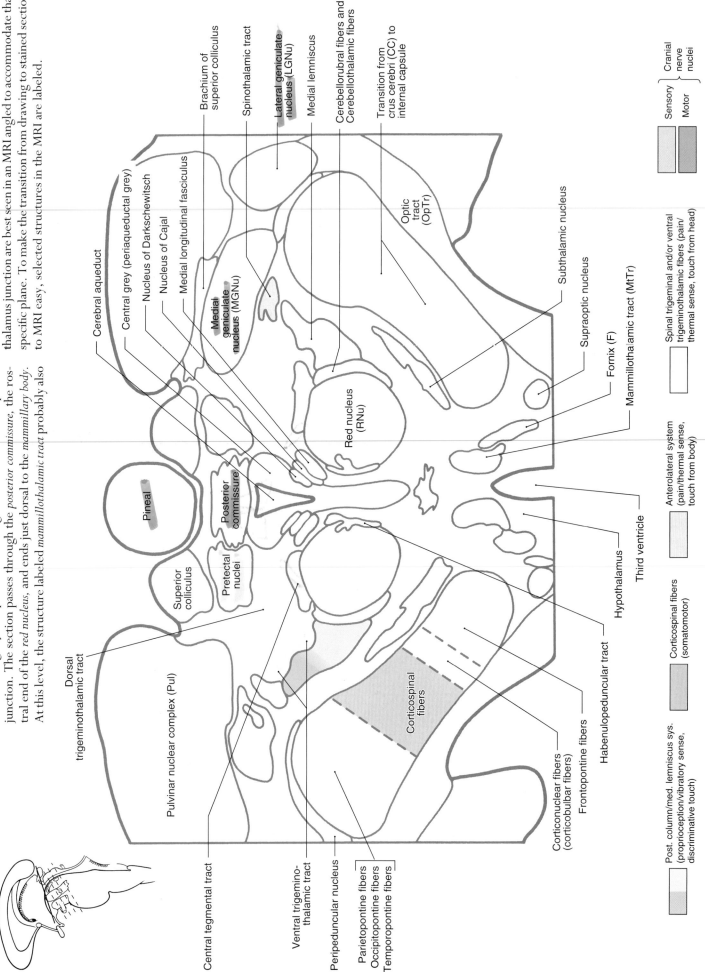

Brachium of superior colliculus

Spinothalamic tract

Lateral geniculate nucleus (LGNu)

Medial lemniscus

Cerebellorubral fibers and Cerebellothalamic fibers

Transition from crus cerebri (CC) to internal capsule

Cerebral aqueduct

Central grey (periaqueductal grey)

Nucleus of Darkschewitsch

Nucleus of Cajal

Medial longitudinal fasciculus

Medial geniculate nucleus (MGNu)

Optic tract (OpTr)

Red nucleus (RNu)

Subthalamic nucleus

Supraoptic nucleus

Fornix (F)

Mammillothalamic tract (MtTr)

Pineal

Posterior commissure

Superior colliculus

Pretectal nuclei

Hypothalamus

Third ventricle

Dorsal trigeminothalamic tract

Pulvinar nuclear complex (Pul)

Corticospinal fibers

Corticonuclear fibers (corticobulbar fibers)

Frontopontine fibers

Habenulopeduncular tract

Central tegmental tract

Ventral trigemino-thalamic tract

Peripeduncular nucleus

Parietopontine fibers
Occipitopontine fibers
Temporopontine fibers

Sensory ⎫ Cranial
         ⎬ nerve
Motor   ⎭ nuclei

Spinal trigeminal and/or ventral trigeminothalamic fibers (pain/thermal sense, touch from head)

Anterolateral system (pain/thermal sense, touch from body)

Corticospinal fibers (somatomotor)

Post. column/med. lemniscus sys. (proprioception/vibratory sense, discriminative touch)

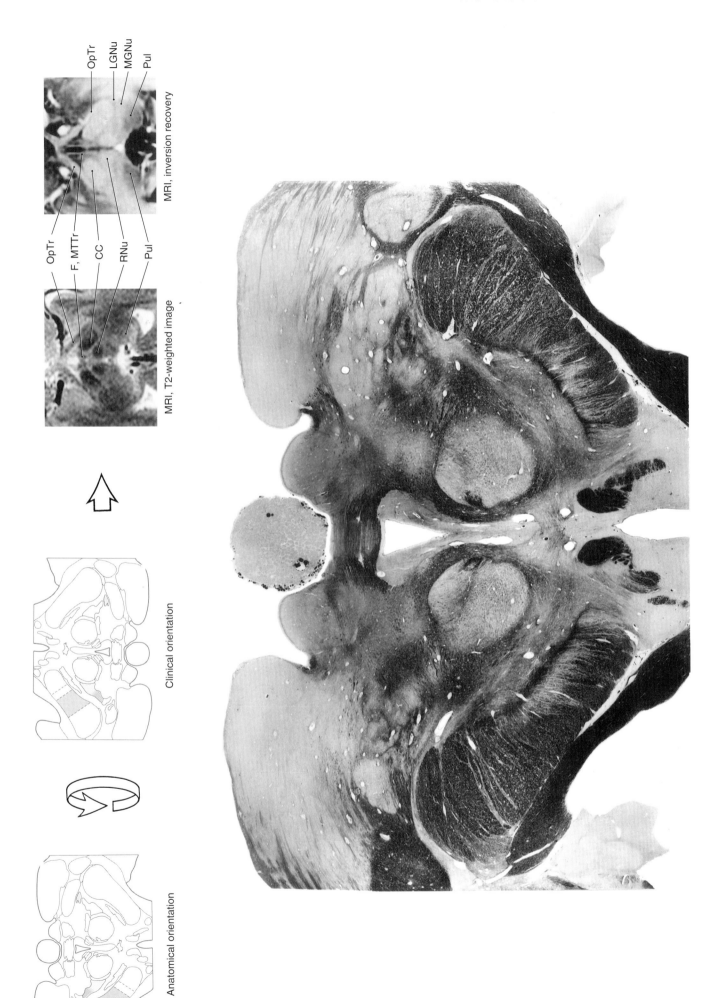

OpTr
LGNu
MGNu
Pul

MRI, inversion recovery

OpTr
F, MTTr
CC
RNu
Pul

MRI, T2-weighted image

Clinical orientation

Anatomical orientation

Vascular Syndromes or Lesions of the Midbrain

Medial Midbrain (Weber) Syndrome: May result from occlusion of paramedian branches of P_1 segment of posterior cerebral artery.

Deficit	Structure Damaged
• Contralateral hemiplegia of arm and leg	• Corticospinal fibers in crus cerebri
• Ipsilateral paralysis of eye movement: eye oriented down and out and pupil dilated and fixed	• Oculomotor nerve

Comment: This combination of motor deficits at this level of the brainstem is called a *superior alternating hemiplegia*. This pattern consists of *ipsilateral paralysis of eye movement* and *contralateral hemiplegia* of the upper and lower extremities. Damage to the corticonuclear (corticobulbar) fibers in the crus cerebri may result in a partial deficit in tongue and facial movement on the contralateral side. These cranial nerve deficits are seen as a *deviation of the tongue to the side opposite the lesion on attempted protrusion* and a *paralysis of the lower half of the facial muscles* on the contralateral side. Although parts of the substantia nigra are frequently involved, *akinesia* or *dyskinesia* are not frequently seen.

Central Midbrain Lesion (Claude syndrome)

Deficit	Structure Damaged
• Ipsilateral paralysis of eye movement: eye oriented down and out and pupil dilated and fixed	• Oculomotor nerve
• Contralateral ataxia and tremor of cerebellar origin	• Red nucleus and cerebellothalamic fibers

Comment: The lesion in this syndrome may extend laterally into the medial lemniscus and the dorsally adjacent ventral trigeminothalamic fibers. If this was the case, there could conceivably be a loss or diminution of position and vibratory sense and of discriminative touch from the contralateral arm and partial loss of pain and thermal sensation from the contralateral face.

Benedikt syndrome: This results from a larger lesion of the midbrain that essentially involves both of the separate areas of Weber and Claude. The main deficits are contralateral hemiplegia of arm and leg (corticospinal fibers), ipsilateral paralysis of eye movement with dilated pupil (oculomotor nerve), and cerebellar tremor and ataxia (red nucleus and cerebellothalamic fibers). Slight variations may be present based on the extent of the lesion.

Parinaud syndrome: This syndrome is usually caused by a tumor in the pineal region, such as germinoma, astrocytoma, pinecytoma/pineoblastoma, or any of a variety of other tumors that impinge on the superior colliculi. The potential for occlusion at the cerebral aqueduct in these cases also indicates that hydrocephalus may be a component of this syndrome. The deficits in these patients consist of a *paralysis of upward gaze* (superior colliculi), *hydrocephalus* (occlusion of the cerebral aqueduct), and eventually a *failure of eye movement* due to pressure on the oculomotor and trochlear nuclei. These patients may also exhibit *nystagmus* due to involvement of the medial longitudinal fasciculus.

Uncal Herniation: Herniation of the uncus occurs in response to large and rapidly expanding lesions in the cerebral hemisphere, this being a supratentorial location. *Uncal herniation* is an extrusion of the uncus through the tentorial notch (tentorial incisura) with resultant pressure on the oculomotor nerve and the crus cerebri of the midbrain. Initially the pupils, unilaterally or bilaterally, may dilate or respond slowly to light, followed by weakness of oculomotor movement. As herniation progresses the pupils will be fully dilated, eye movements regulated by the oculomotor nerve may be slow or absent, and the eyes will deviate slightly laterally due to the unopposed actions of the abducens nerves. There is usually weakness on the contralateral side of the body due to compression of corticospinal fibers in the crus cerebri. However, if pressure is sufficient the entire midbrain may shift so that there can be contralateral as well as ipsilateral weakness due to pressure on the same side and pressure on the opposite side of the crus cerebri. This hemiplegia ipsilateral to the herniation and ipsilateral to the oculomotor deficits is called the *Kernohan phenomenon*. As damage from the pressure on the midbrain extends down and into the upper pons the pupils are dilated and fixed, eye movement is largely absent, respiration is decreased, and the patient will become decerebrate (upper and lower extremities extended, toes pointed inward, fingers flexed, forearm pronated, head and neck extended).

5-27 Semidiagrammatic representation of the internal distribution of arteries in the midbrain. Selected main structures are labeled on the left side of each section; the typical pattern of arterial distribution overlies these structures on the right side. The general distribution patterns of the vessels to the midbrain as shown here may vary somewhat from patient to patient. For example, the adjacent territories served by neighboring vessels may overlap to differing degrees at their margins or the territory of a particular vessel may be larger or smaller than seen in the general pattern.

Abbreviations

BP	Basilar pons
CC	Crus cerebri
DecSCP	Decussation of the superior cerebellar peduncle
IC	Inferior colliculus
LGNu	Lateral geniculate nucleus
MGNu	Medial geniculate nucleus
ML	Medial lemniscus
RNu	Red nucleus
SC	Superior colliculus
SCP	Superior cerebellar peduncle
SN	Substantia nigra

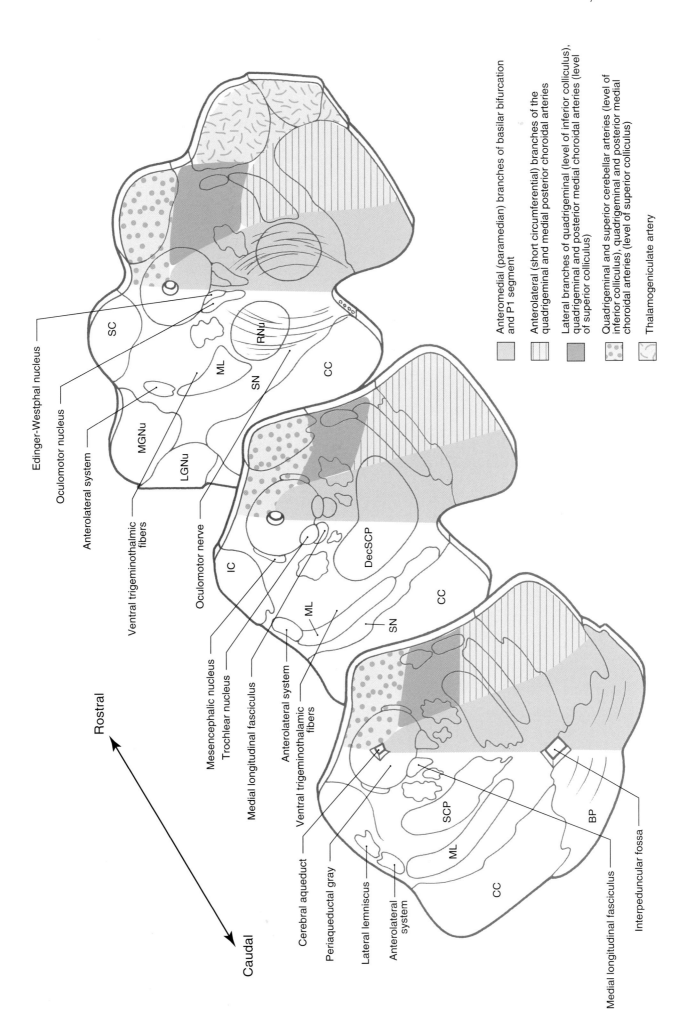

Rostral

Caudal

Edinger-Westphal nucleus

Oculomotor nucleus

Anterolateral system

Ventral trigeminothalmic fibers

Oculomotor nerve

Mesencephalic nucleus

Trochlear nucleus

Medial longitudinal fasciculus

Ventral trigeminothalamic fibers

Anterolateral system

Cerebral aqueduct

Periaqueductal gray

Lateral lemniscus

Anterolateral system

Medial longitudinal fasciculus

Interpeduncular fossa

SC

RNu

ML

SN

CC

MGNu

LGNu

IC

ML

SN

DecSCP

CC

SCP

ML

BP

CC

Anteromedial (paramedian) branches of basilar bifurcation and P1 segment

Anterolateral (short circumferential) branches of the quadrigeminal and medial posterior choroidal arteries

Lateral branches of quadrigeminal (level of inferior colliculus), quadrigeminal and posterior medial choroidal arteries (level of superior colliculus)

Quadrigeminal and superior cerebellar arteries (level of inferior colliculus), quadrigeminal and posterior medial choroidal arteries (level of superior colliculus)

Thalamogeniculate artery

5-28   Coronal section of forebrain through the *splenium of the corpus callosum* and *crus of fornix*, and extending into the *inferior colliculus* and exit of the *trochlear nerve*. Many of the structures labeled in this figure can be easily identified in the T1-weighted MRI adjacent to the photograph.

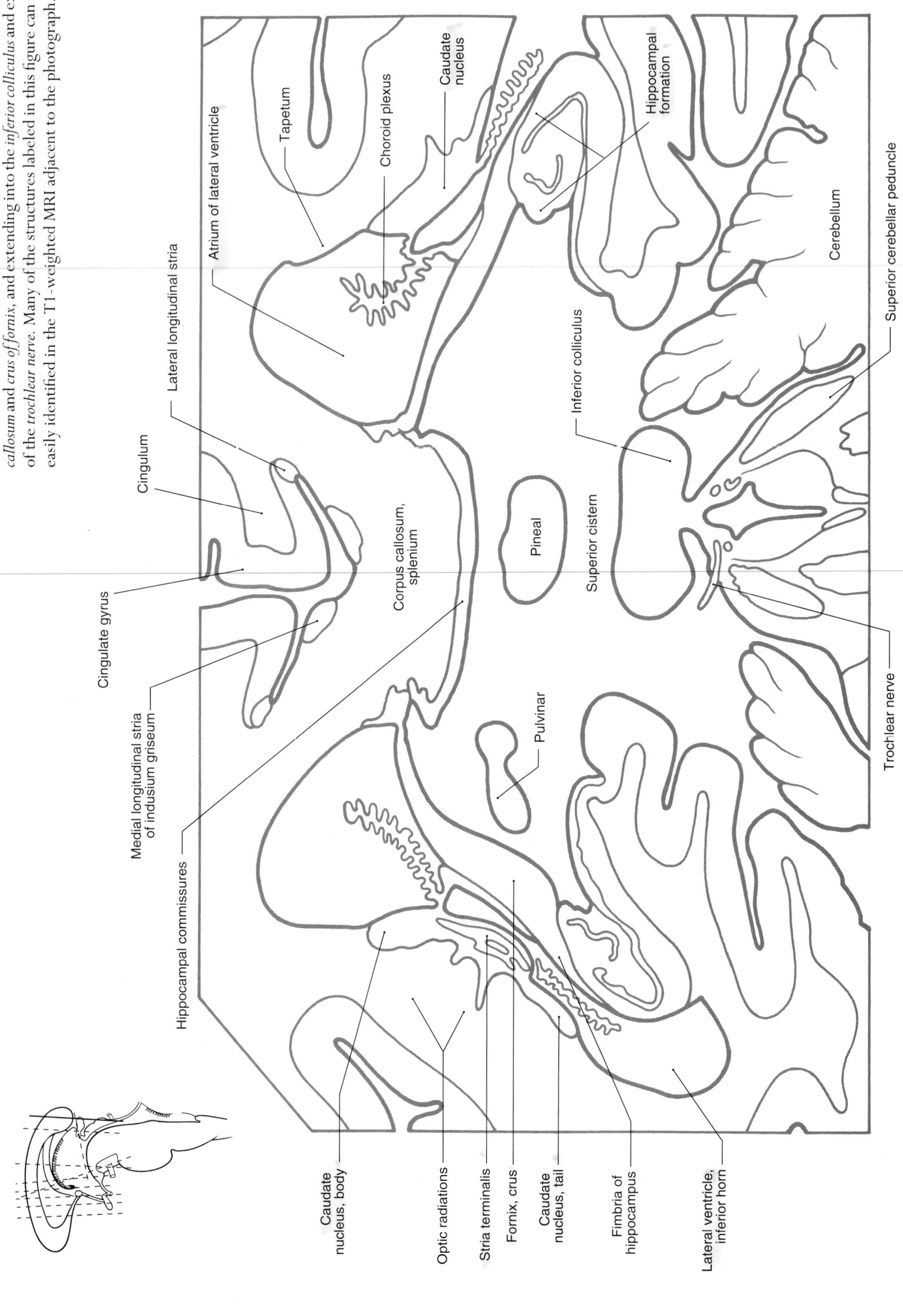

Tapetum

Caudate nucleus

Choroid plexus

Hippocampal formation

Atrium of lateral ventricle

Cingulum

Lateral longitudinal stria

Cerebellum

Inferior colliculus

Superior cerebellar peduncle

Cingulate gyrus

Corpus callosum, splenium

Pineal

Superior cistern

Medial longitudinal stria of indusium griseum

Hippocampal commissures

Pulvinar

Trochlear nerve

Caudate nucleus, body

Optic radiations

Stria terminalis

Fornix, crus

Caudate nucleus, tail

Fimbria of hippocampus

Lateral ventricle, inferior horn

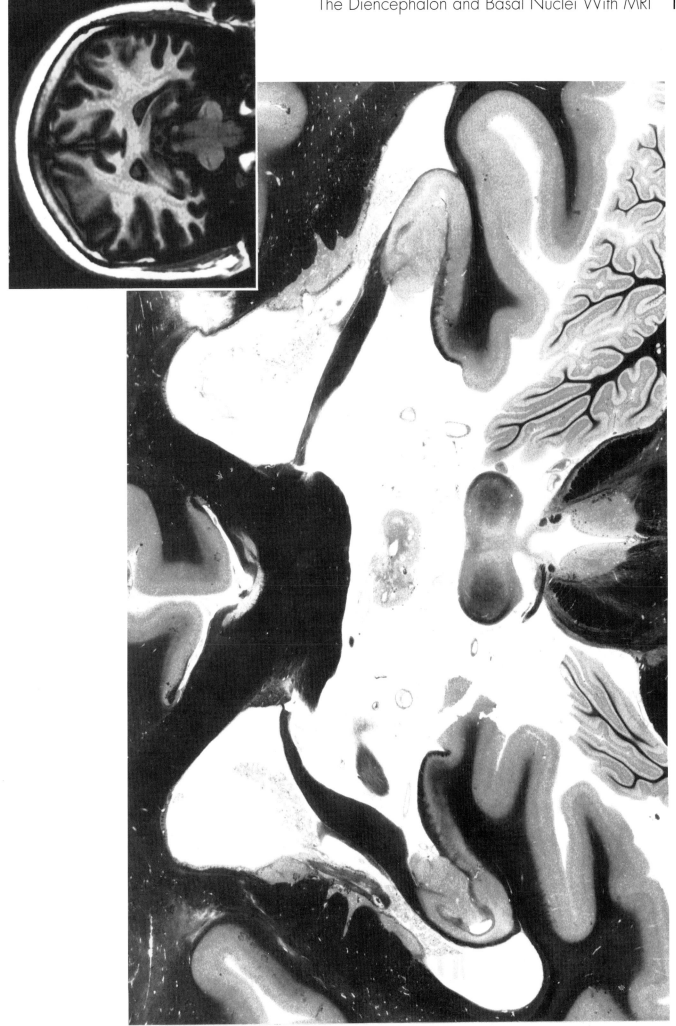

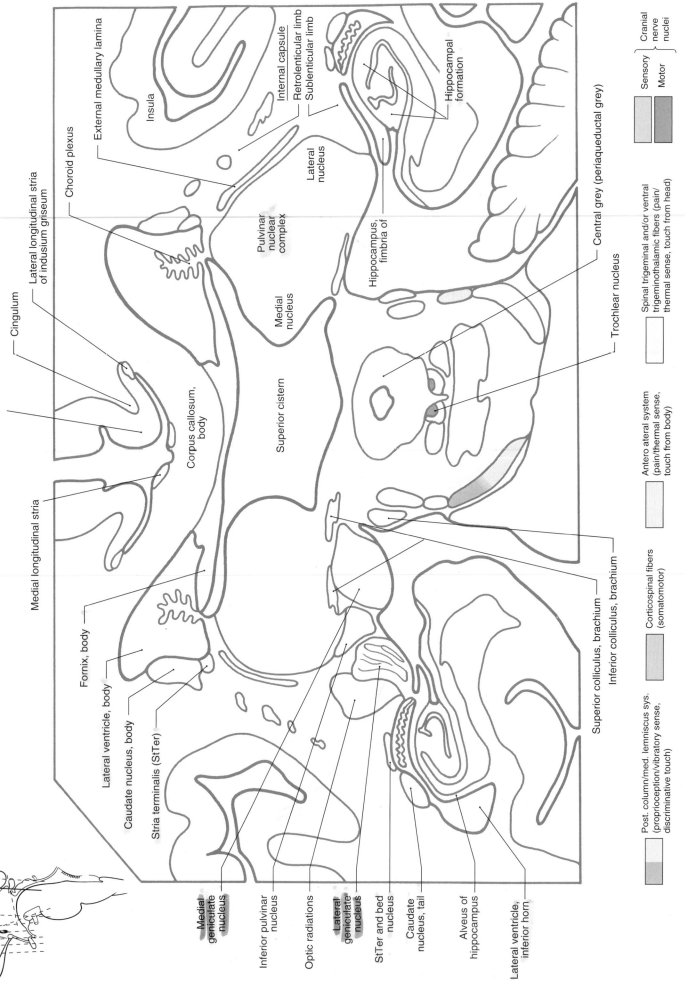

5-29   Coronal section of the forebrain through the *pulvinar* and the *medial* and *lateral geniculate nuclei*. The section extends into upper portions of the *midbrain tegmentum*. Many of the structures la-beled in this figure can be easily identified in the T1-weighted MRI adjacent to the photograph.

Insula

External medullary lamina

Internal capsule
Retrolenticular limb
Sublenticular limb

Lateral nucleus

Hippocampal formation

Choroid plexus

Lateral longitudinal stria of indusium griseum

Cingulum

Pulvinar nuclear complex

Hippocampus, fimbria of

Central grey (periaqueductal grey)

Medial nucleus

Corpus callosum, body

Superior cistern

Trochlear nucleus

Medial longitudinal stria

Fornix, body

Lateral ventricle, body

Caudate nucleus, body

Stria terminalis (StTer)

Medial geniculate nucleus

Inferior pulvinar nucleus

Optic radiations

Lateral geniculate nucleus

StTer and bed nucleus

Caudate nucleus, tail

Alveus of hippocampus

Lateral ventricle, inferior horn

Superior colliculus, brachium

Inferior colliculus, brachium

Post. column/med. lemniscus sys. (proprioception/vibratory sense, discriminative touch)

Corticospinal fibers (somatomotor)

Antero ateral system (pain/thermal sense, touch from body)

Spinal trigeminal and/or ventral trigeminothalamic fibers (pain/thermal sense, touch from head)

Sensory ⎫ Cranial
          ⎬ nerve
Motor   ⎭ nuclei

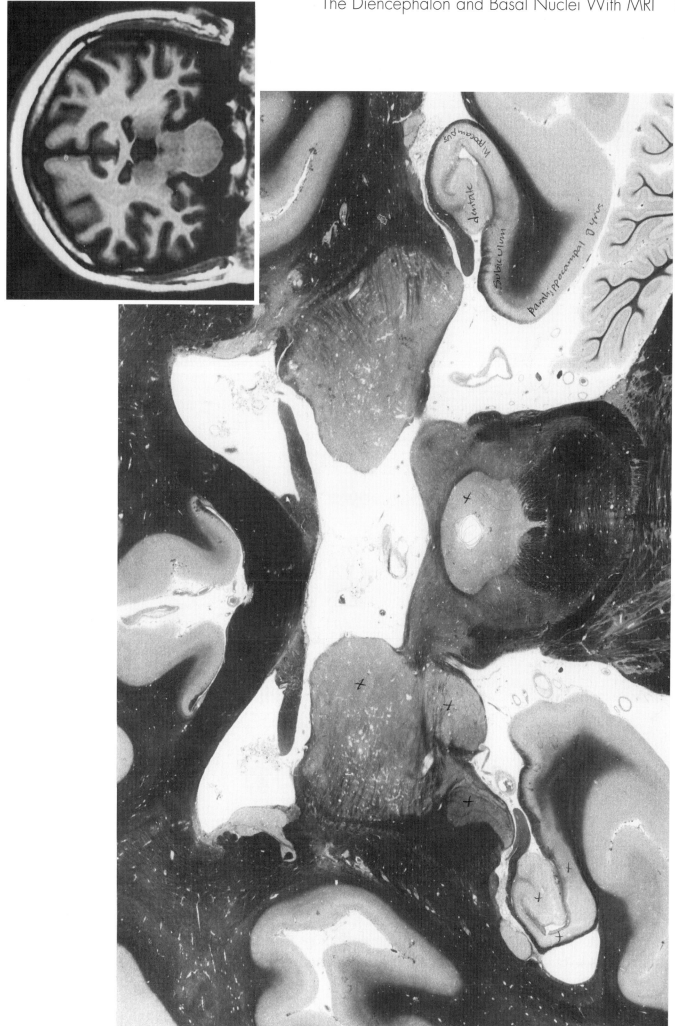

5-30 Slightly oblique section of the forebrain through the *pulvinar, ventral posteromedial,* and *ventral posterolateral* nuclei. The section extends rostrally through the *subthalamic nucleus* and ends in the *caudal hypothalamus* just dorsal to the *mammillary bodies* as seen by the position of the (postcommissural) fornix.

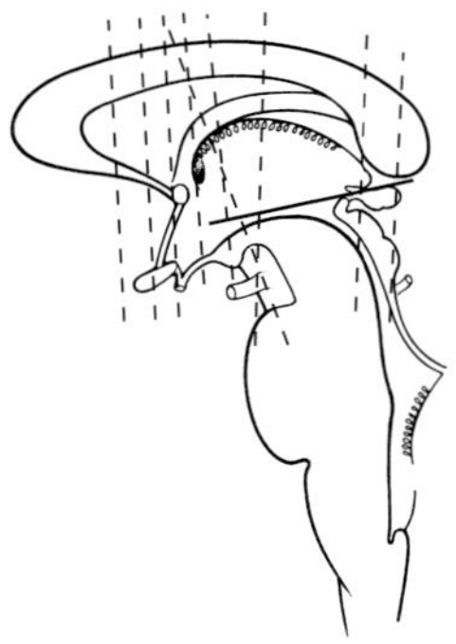

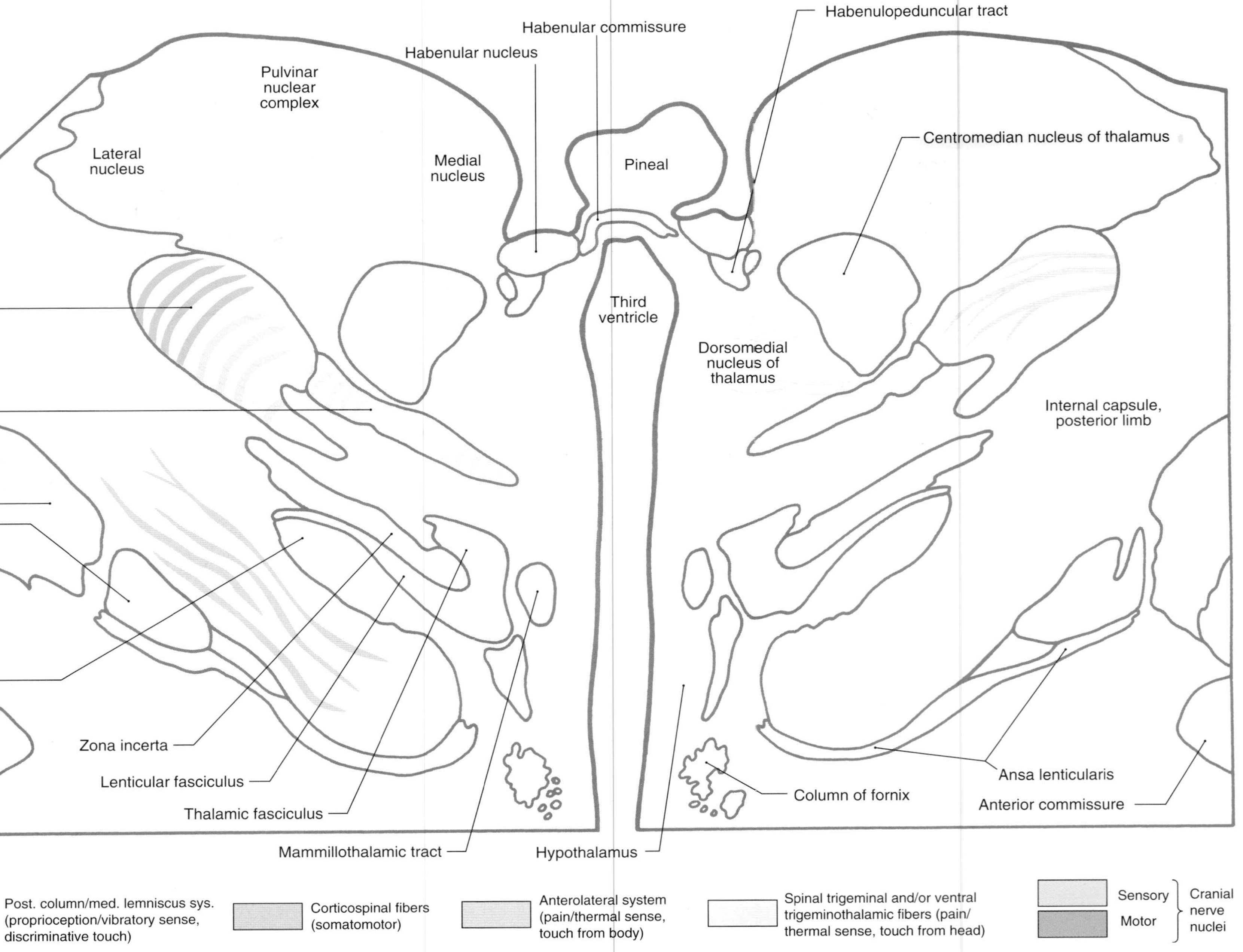

Centromedian nucleus of thalamus

Habenulopeduncular tract

Dorsomedial nucleus of thalamus

Internal capsule, posterior limb

Ansa lenticularis

Anterior commissure

Column of fornix

Habenular commissure

Pineal

Third ventricle

Hypothalamus

Habenular nucleus

Medial nucleus

Pulvinar nuclear complex

Lateral nucleus

Mammillothalamic tract

Zona incerta

Lenticular fasciculus

Thalamic fasciculus

Subthalamic nucleus

Ventral posterolateral nucleus of thalamus

Ventral posteromedial nucleus of thalamus

Globus pallidus:
Lateral segment
Medial segment

Post. column/med. lemniscus sys. (proprioception/vibratory sense, discriminative touch)

Corticospinal fibers (somatomotor)

Anterolateral system (pain/thermal sense, touch from body)

Spinal trigeminal and/or ventral trigeminothalamic fibers (pain/thermal sense, touch from head)

Sensory | Cranial nerve nuclei
Motor |

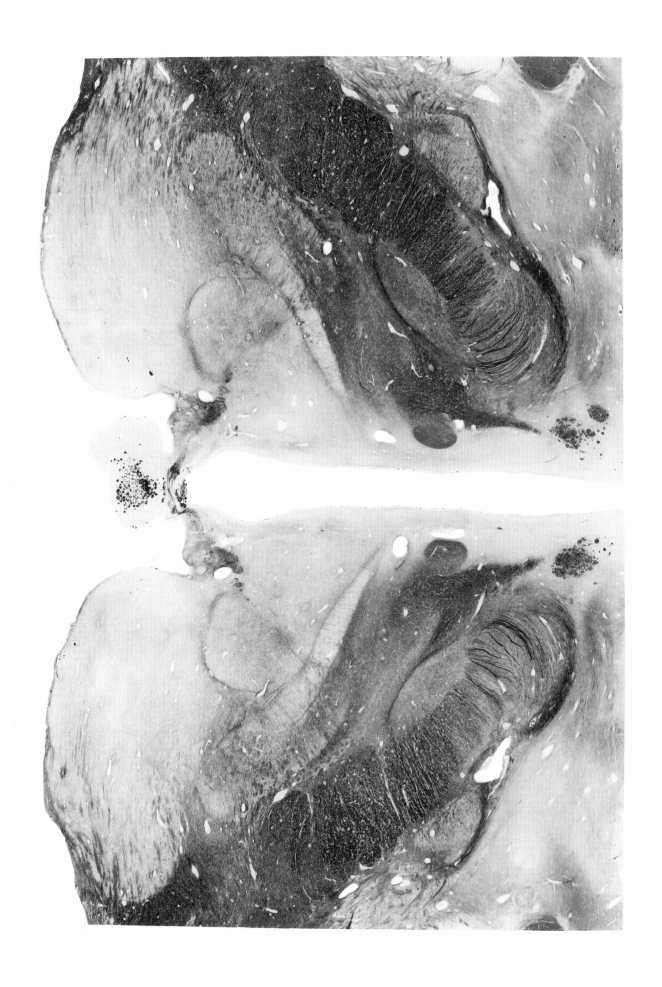

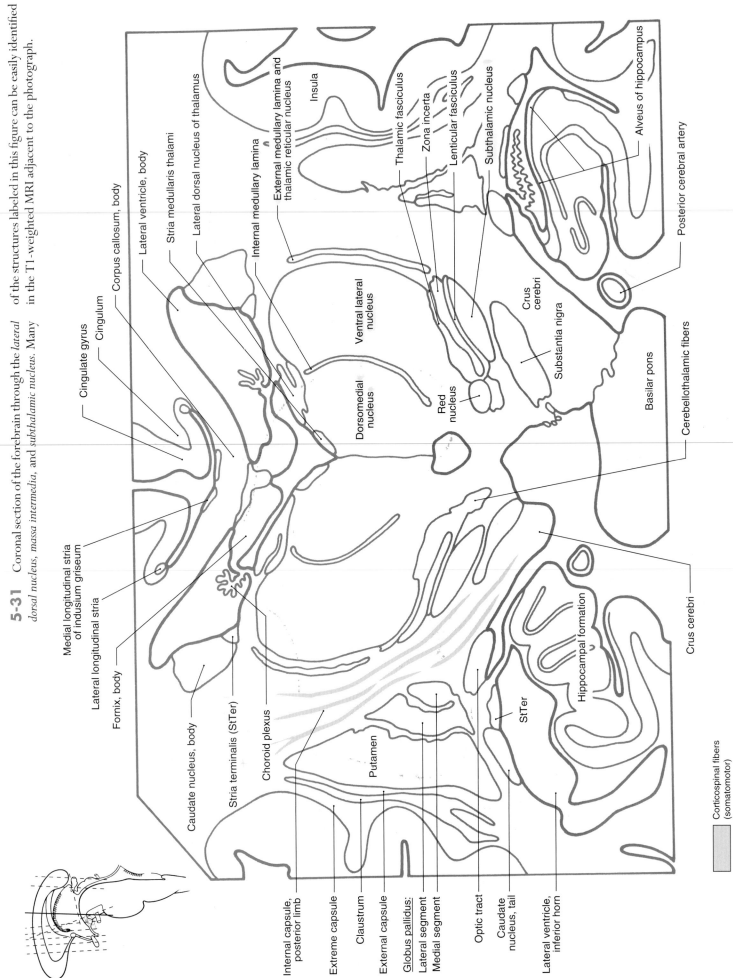

5-31   Coronal section of the forebrain through the *lateral dorsal nucleus, massa intermedia,* and *subthalamic nucleus.* Many of the structures labeled in this figure can be easily identified in the T1-weighted MRI adjacent to the photograph.

Cingulate gyrus

Cingulum

Corpus callosum, body

Lateral ventricle, body

Stria medullaris thalami

Lateral dorsal nucleus of thalamus

Internal medullary lamina

External medullary lamina and thalamic reticular nucleus

Insula

Thalamic fasciculus

Zona incerta

Lenticular fasciculus

Subthalamic nucleus

Alveus of hippocampus

Posterior cerebral artery

Ventral lateral nucleus

Crus cerebri

Substantia nigra

Dorsomedial nucleus

Red nucleus

Basilar pons

Cerebellothalamic fibers

Medial longitudinal stria of indusium griseum

Lateral longitudinal stria

Fornix, body

Caudate nucleus, body

Stria terminalis (StTer)

Choroid plexus

Putamen

StTer

Hippocampal formation

Crus cerebri

Internal capsule, posterior limb

Extreme capsule

Claustrum

External capsule

Globus pallidus:
Lateral segment
Medial segment

Optic tract

Caudate nucleus, tail

Lateral ventricle, inferior horn

Corticospinal fibers (somatomotor)

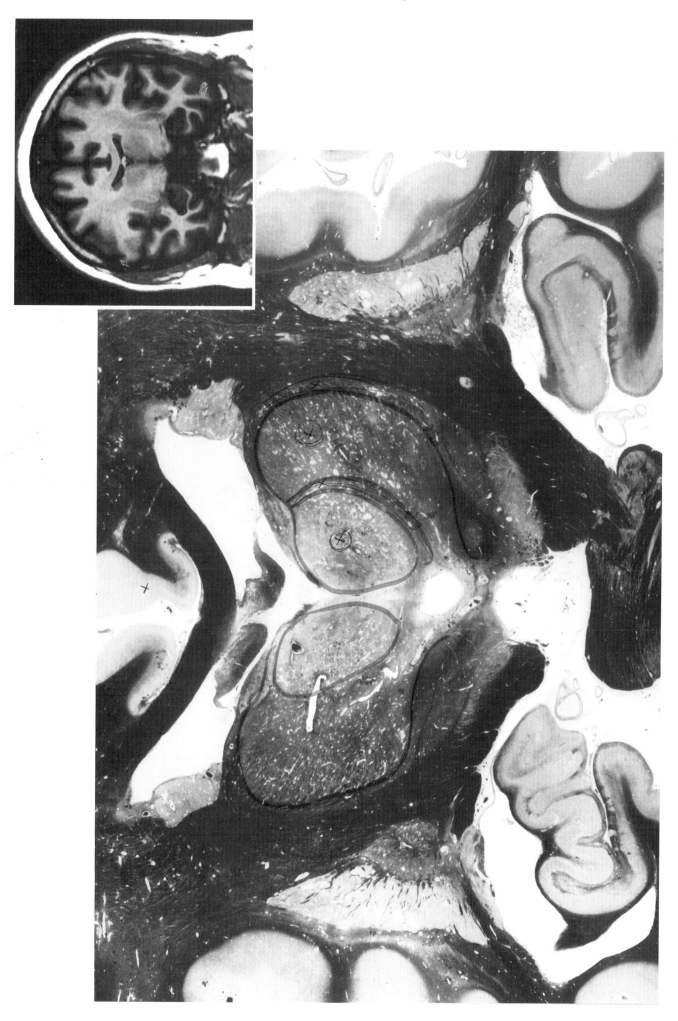

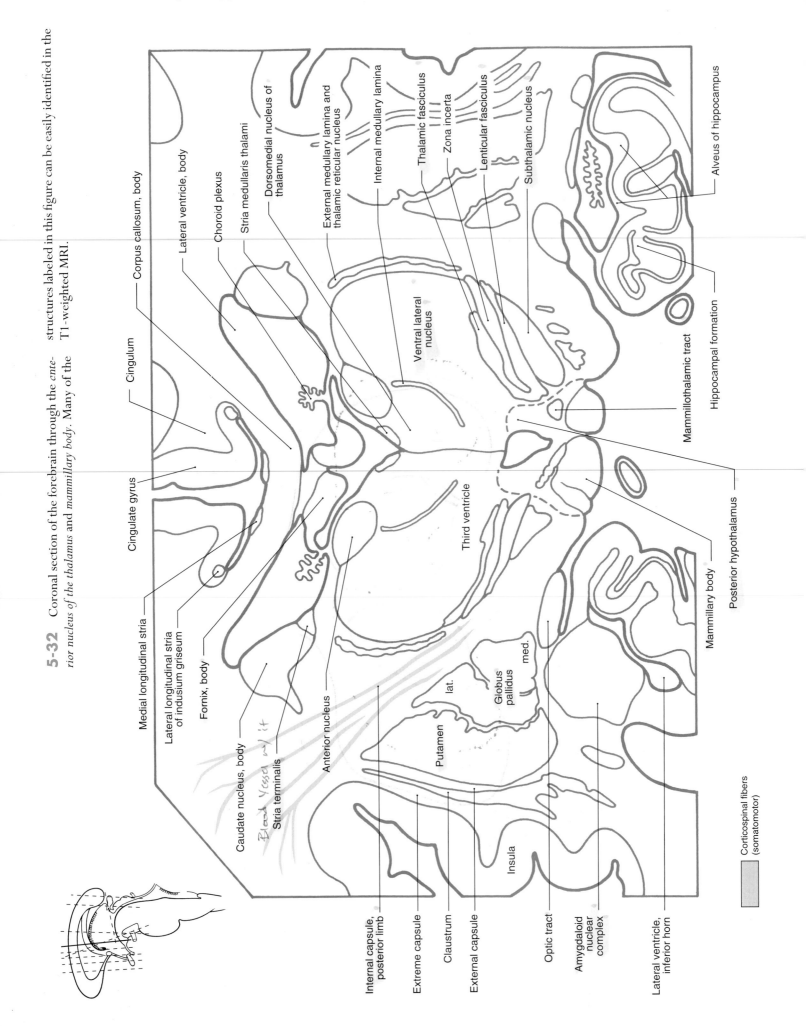

5-32   Coronal section of the forebrain through the *ante-rior nucleus of the thalamus and mammillary body*. Many of the structures labeled in this figure can be easily identified in the T1-weighted MRI.

Cingulum

Corpus callosum, body

Lateral ventricle, body

Choroid plexus

Stria medullaris thalami

Dorsomedial nucleus of thalamus

External medullary lamina and thalamic reticular nucleus

Internal medullary lamina

Thalamic fasciculus

Zona incerta

Lenticular fasciculus

Subthalamic nucleus

Alveus of hippocampus

Cingulate gyrus

Ventral lateral nucleus

Mammillothalamic tract

Hippocampal formation

Medial longitudinal stria

Lateral longitudinal stria of indusium griseum

Fornix, body

Blood Vessel in it

Stria terminalis

Caudate nucleus, body

Anterior nucleus

Third ventricle

Posterior hypothalamus

Mammillary body

Globus pallidus

lat.

med.

Putamen

Insula

Internal capsule, posterior limb

Extreme capsule

Claustrum

External capsule

Optic tract

Amygdaloid nuclear complex

Lateral ventricle, inferior horn

Corticospinal fibers (somatomotor)

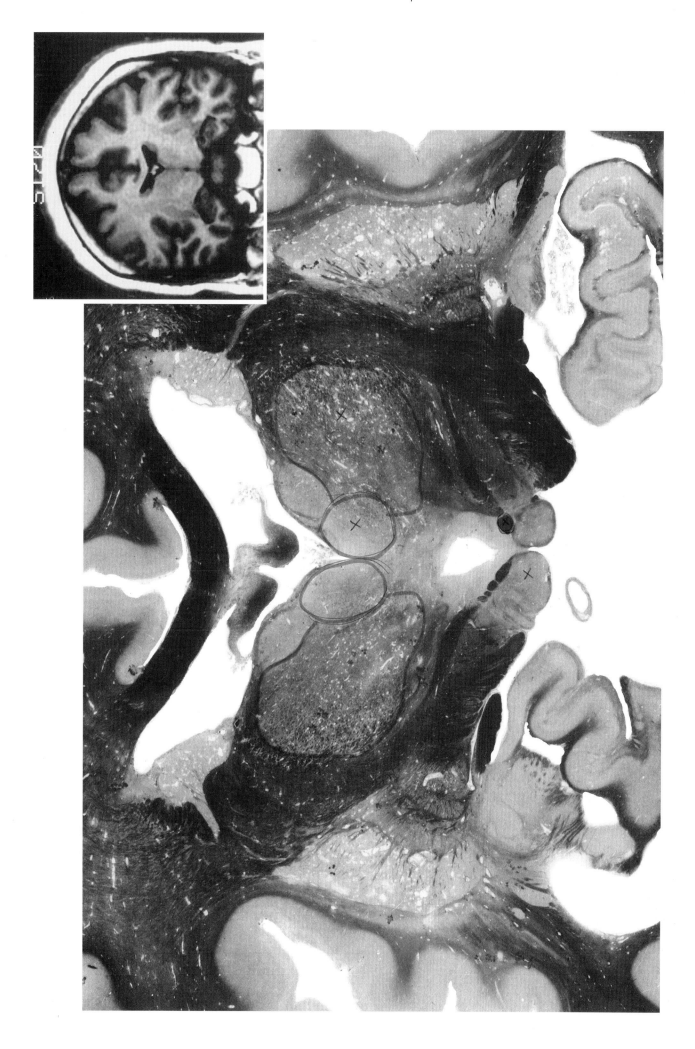

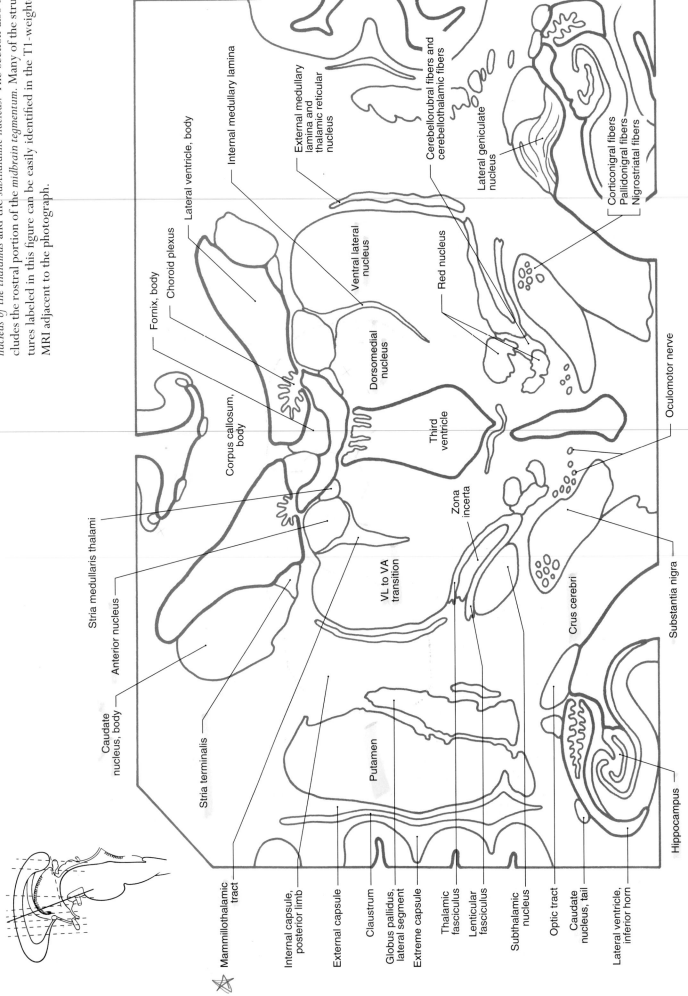

5-33   Slightly oblique section of the forebrain through the *anterior nucleus of the thalamus* and the *subthalamic nucleus*. The section also includes the rostral portion of the *midbrain tegmentum*. Many of the structures labeled in this figure can be easily identified in the T1-weighted MRI adjacent to the photograph.

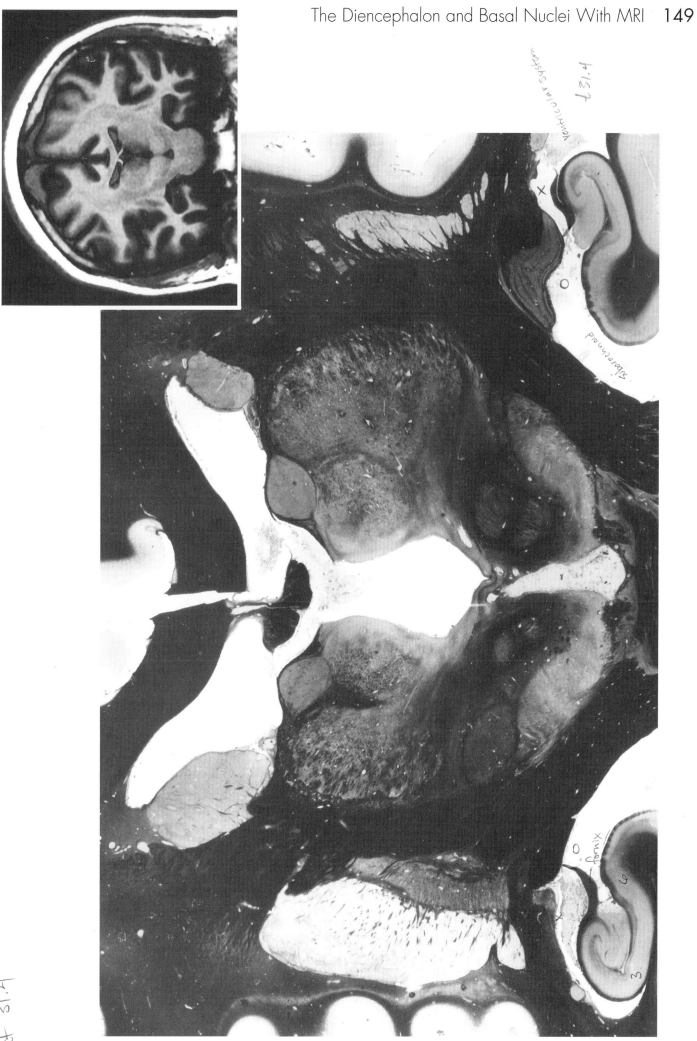

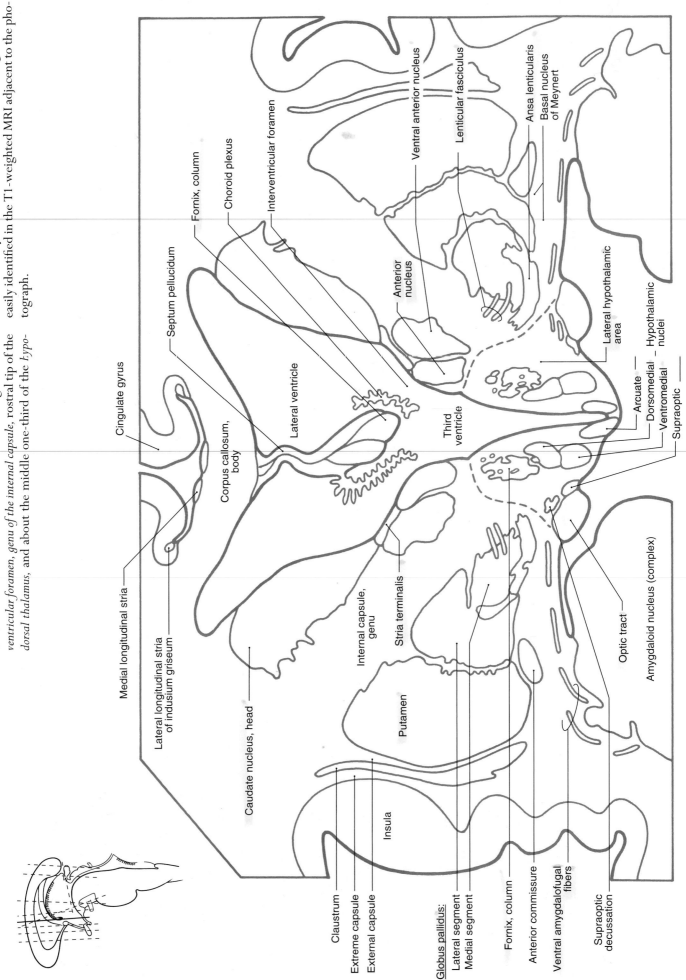

5-34   Coronal section of the forebrain through the *interventricular foramen, genu of the internal capsule, rostral tip of the dorsal thalamus,* and about the middle one-third of the *hypothalamus.* Many of the structures labeled in this figure can be easily identified in the T1-weighted MRI adjacent to the photograph.

Cingulate gyrus

Septum pellucidum

Fornix, column

Choroid plexus

Interventricular foramen

Ventral anterior nucleus

Lenticular fasciculus

Ansa lenticularis

Basal nucleus of Meynert

Anterior nucleus

Lateral ventricle

Lateral hypothalamic area

Third ventricle

Arcuate
Dorsomedial
Ventromedial
Supraoptic

Hypothalamic nuclei

Medial longitudinal stria

Lateral longitudinal stria of indusium griseum

Corpus callosum, body

Internal capsule, genu

Stria terminalis

Optic tract

Amygdaloid nucleus (complex)

Caudate nucleus, head

Putamen

Insula

Claustrum

Extreme capsule

External capsule

Globus pallidus:
Lateral segment
Medial segment

Fornix, column

Anterior commissure

Ventral amygdalofugal fibers

Supraoptic decussation

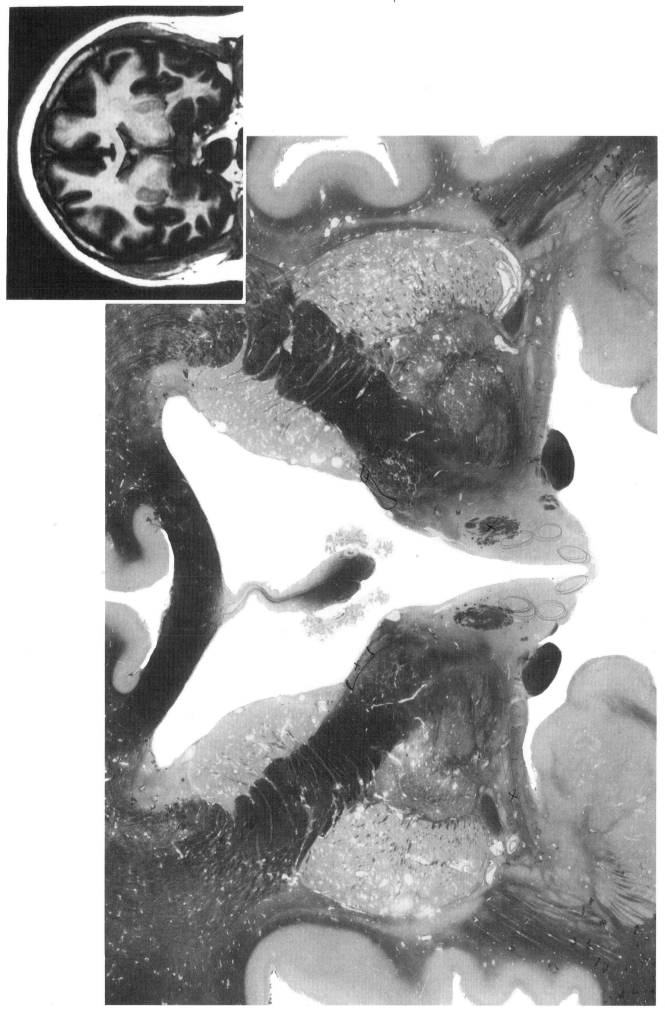

5-35   Coronal section of the forebrain through the *anterior commissure* and rostral aspects of the *hypothalamus.* Many of the structures labeled in this figure can be easily identified in the T1-weighted MRI.

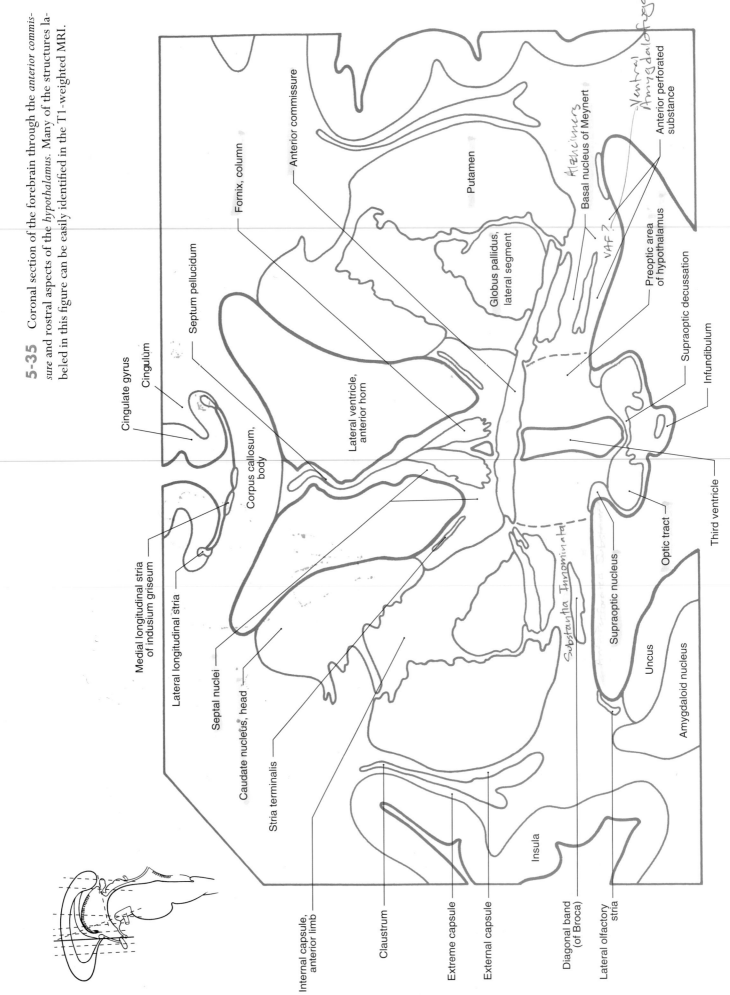

Cingulate gyrus

Cingulum

Septum pellucidum

Medial longitudinal stria of indusium griseum

Lateral longitudinal stria

Septal nuclei

Caudate nucleus, head

Stria terminalis

Corpus callosum, body

Lateral ventricle, anterior horn

Fornix, column

Anterior commissure

Putamen

Globus pallidus, lateral segment

Basal nucleus of Meynert

Alzheimers

VAF?

Preoptic area of hypothalamus

Supraoptic decussation

Infundibulum

Third ventricle

Optic tract

Supraoptic nucleus

Substantia Innominata

Amygdaloid nucleus

Uncus

Lateral olfactory stria

Diagonal band (of Broca)

External capsule

Extreme capsule

Claustrum

Internal capsule, anterior limb

Insula

Ventral Amygdalofrugal

Anterior perforated substance

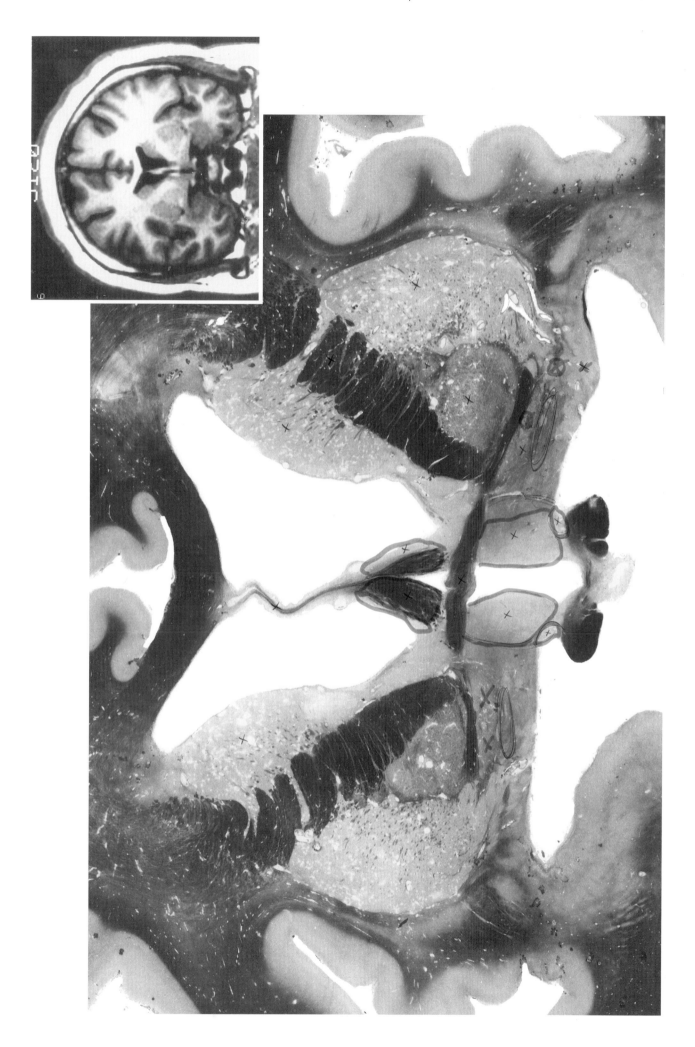

5-36 Coronal section of the forebrain through the *head of the caudate nucleus*, rostral portions of the *optic chiasm*, and the *nucleus accumbens*. Many of the structures labeled in this figure can be easily identified in the T1-weighted MRI adjacent to the photograph.

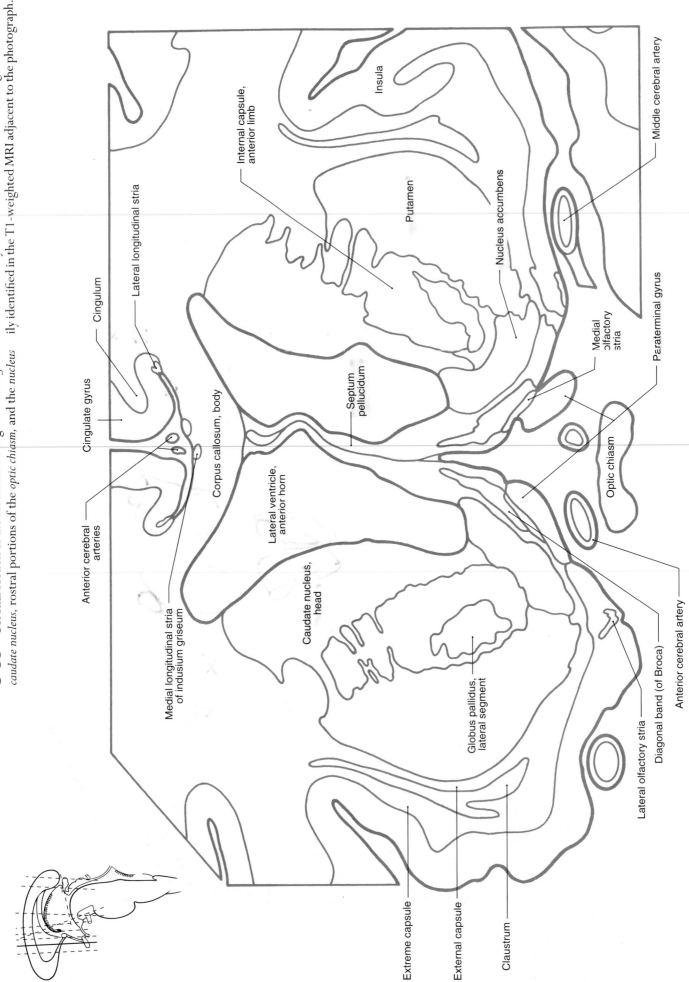

Insula

Internal capsule, anterior limb

Putamen

Lateral longitudinal stria

Cingulum

Cingulate gyrus

Anterior cerebral arteries

Corpus callosum, body

Septum pellucidum

Lateral ventricle, anterior horn

Medial longitudinal stria of indusium griseum

Caudate nucleus, head

Globus pallidus, lateral segment

Extreme capsule

External capsule

Claustrum

Nucleus accumbens

Medial olfactory stria

Paraterminal gyrus

Optic chiasm

Anterior cerebral artery

Lateral olfactory stria

Diagonal band (of Broca)

Middle cerebral artery

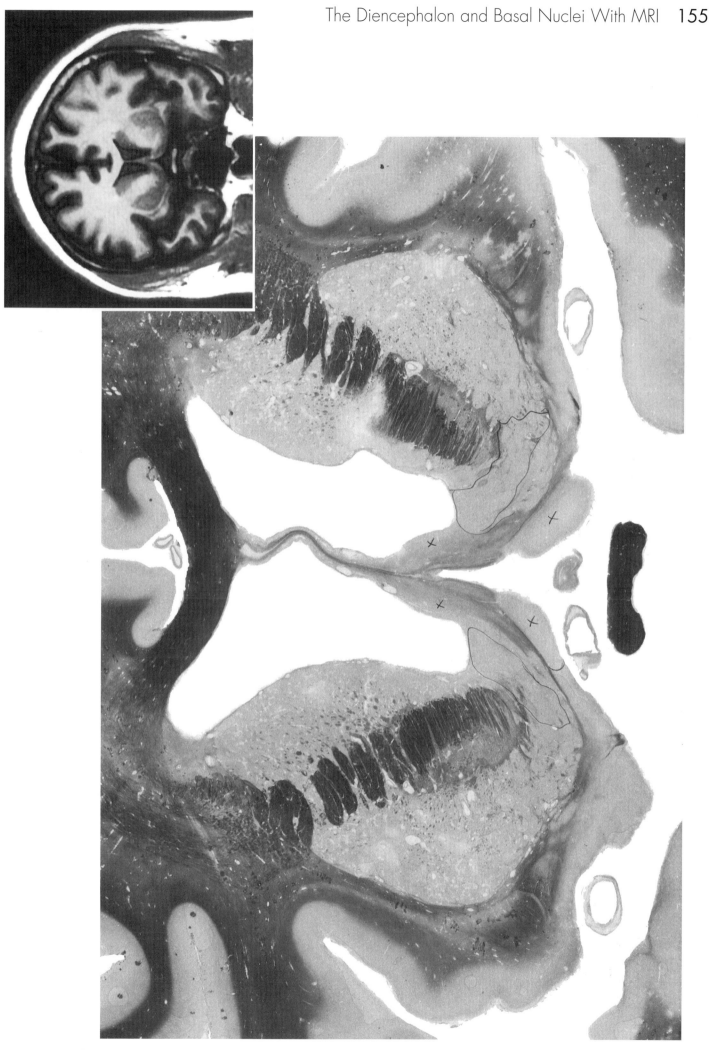

5-37 Coronal section of forebrain through the *head of the caudate nucleus* and the *anterior horn of the lateral ventricle.* Many of the structures labeled in this figure can be easily identified in the T1-weighted MRI adjacent to the photograph.

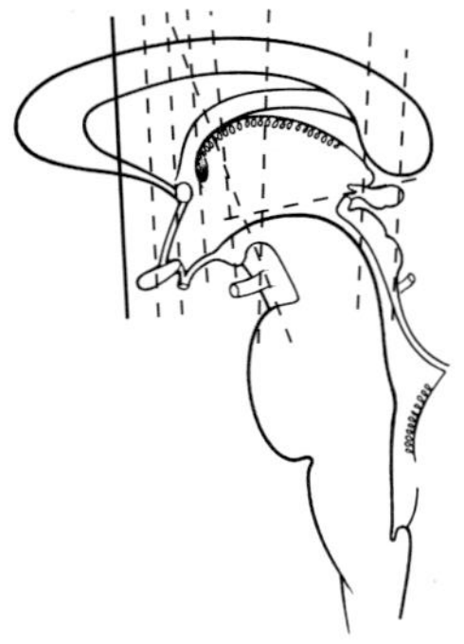

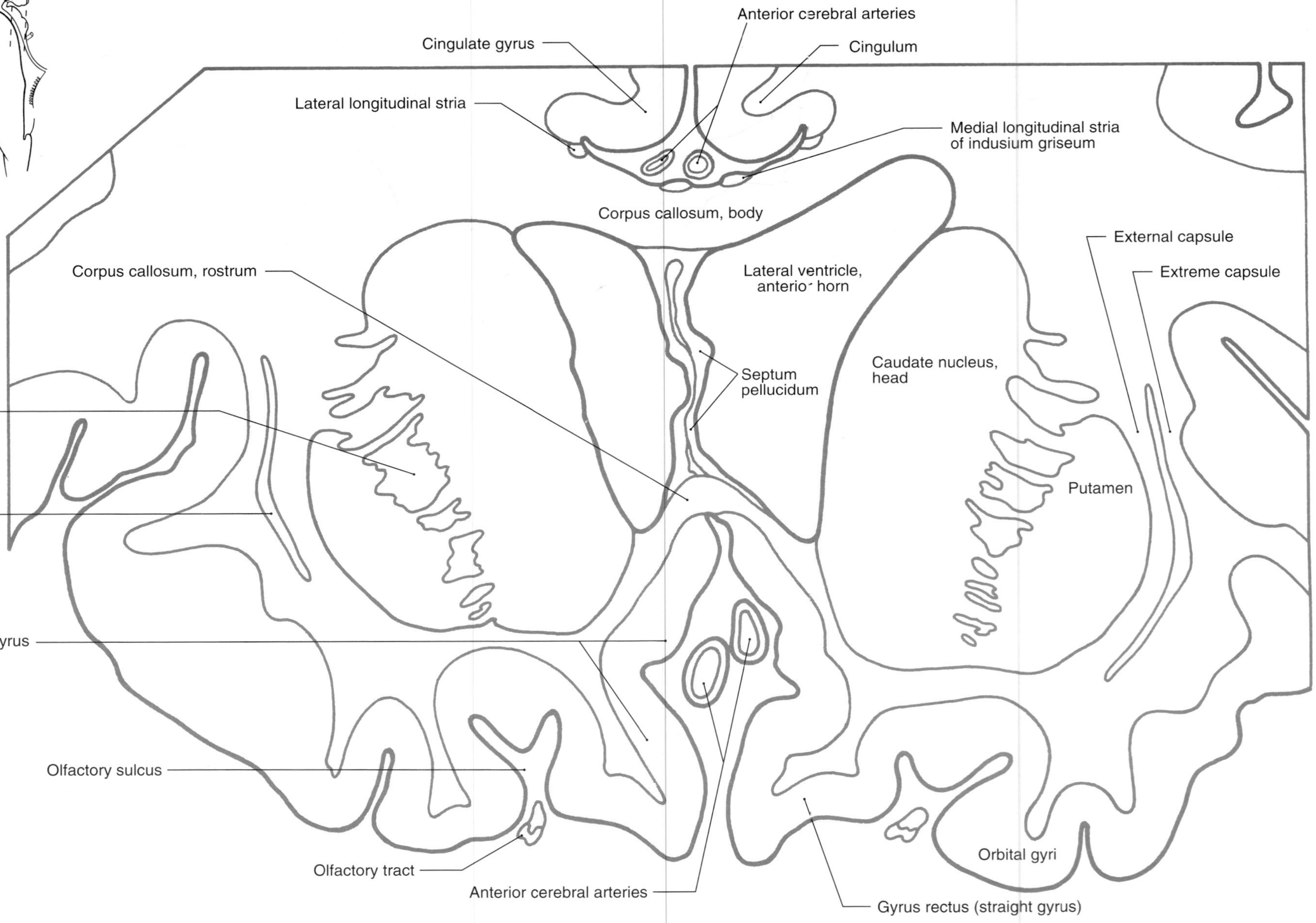

External capsule

Extreme capsule

Putamen

Caudate nucleus, head

Orbital gyri

Gyrus rectus (straight gyrus)

Medial longitudinal stria of indusium griseum

Anterior cerebral arteries

Cingulum

Corpus callosum, body

Lateral ventricle, anterior horn

Septum pellucidum

Cingulate gyrus

Lateral longitudinal stria

Anterior cerebral arteries

Olfactory tract

Corpus callosum, rostrum

Internal capsule, anterior limb

Claustrum

Subcallosal gyrus

Olfactory sulcus

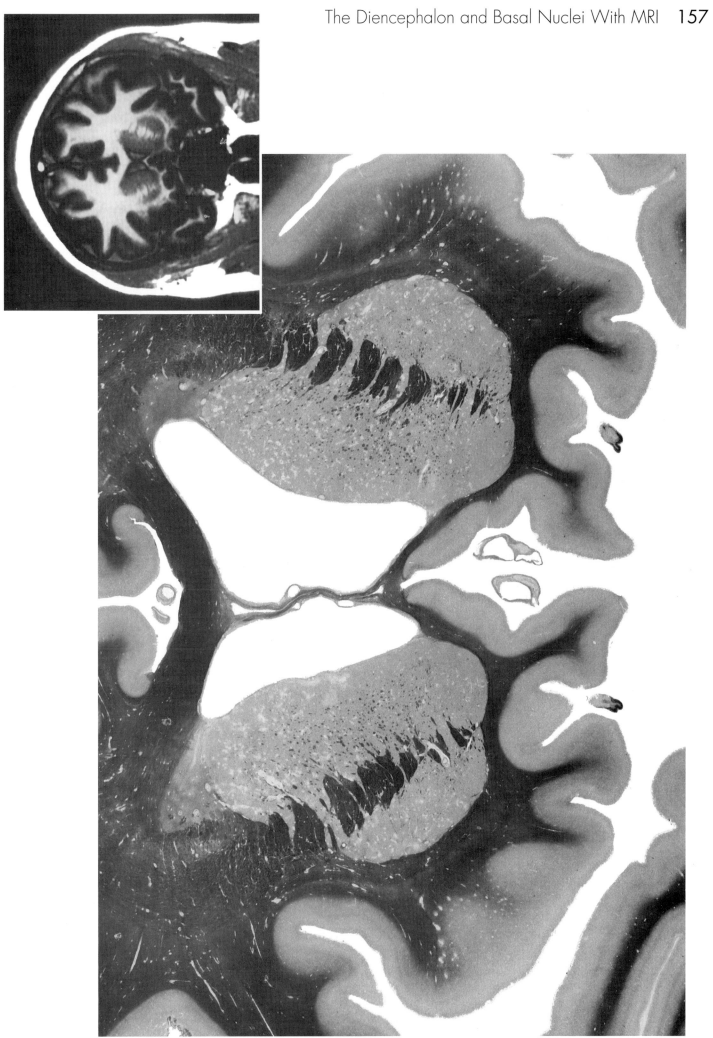

Vascular Syndromes or Lesions of the Forebrain

Forebrain vascular lesions result in a wide range of deficits that include motor and sensory losses and a variety of cognitive disorders. Forebrain vessels may be occluded by a *thrombus*. This is a structure (usually a clot) formed by blood products and frequently attached to the vessel wall. Deficits may appear slowly, or wax and wane, as the blood flow is progressively restricted. Vessels may also be occluded by *embolization*. A foreign body, or *embolus* (fat, air, piece of thrombus, piece of sclerotic plaque, clump of bacteria, etc.), is delivered from some distant site into the cerebral circulation where it lodges in a vessel. Since this is a sudden event deficits usually appear quickly and progress rapidly. Interruption of blood supply to a part of the forebrain will result in an *infarct* of the area served by the occluded vessel.

Lesion in the Subthalamic Nucleus: Small vascular lesions occur in the subthalamic nucleus, resulting in rapid and unpredictable flailing movements of the contralateral extremities (*hemiballismus*). Movements are more obvious in the arm than in the leg. The clinical expression of this lesion is through corticospinal fibers, therefore it is on the contralateral side of the body.

Occlusion of Lenticulostriate Branches to Internal Capsule: Damage to the internal capsule may result in contralateral *hemiplegia* (corticospinal fibers) and a loss, or diminution, of sensory perception (pain, thermal sense, proprioception) caused by damage to thalamocortical fibers traversing the posterior limb to the overlying sensory cortex. If the lesion extends into the genu of the capsule, a partial paralysis of facial muscles and tongue movement may also occur contralaterally.

Infarction of Posterior Thalamic Nuclei: Occlusion of vessels to posterior thalamic regions results in either a *complete sensory loss* (pain/thermal sense, touch, vibratory and position sense) on the contralateral side of the body, or a *dissociated sensory loss*. In the latter case the patient may experience pain/thermal sensory losses but not position/vibratory losses, or vice versa. As the lesion resolves the patient may experience intense persistent pain, *thalamic pain*, or *anesthesia dolorosa*.

Occlusion of Distal Branches of the Anterior (ACA) or Middle (MCA) Cerebral Arteries: Occlusion of distal branches of the ACA results in motor and sensory losses in the contralateral foot, leg, and thigh owing to damage to the anterior and posterior paracentral gyri (primary motor and sensory cortices for lower extremity). Occlusion of distal branches of MCA results in contralateral motor and sensory losses of the upper extremity, trunk, and face with sparing of the leg and foot, and a consensual deviation of the eyes to the ipsilateral side. This represents damage to the precentral and postcentral gyri and to the frontal eye fields.

Watershed Infarct: Sudden systemic hypotension, hypoperfusion, or embolic showers may result in infarcts at border zones between the territories served by the ACA, MCA, and posterior cerebral artery (PCA). *Anterior watershed infarcts* (at the ACA–MCA junction) result in a contralateral hemiparesis (mainly leg) and expressive language or behavioral changes. *Posterior watershed infarcts* (MCA–PCA interface) result in visual deficits and language problems.

Anterior Choroidal Artery Syndrome: Occlusion of this vessel may result from small emboli or small vessel disease. This syndrome may also occur as a complication of temporal lobectomy (removal of the temporal lobe to treat intractable epilepsy). The infarcted area usually includes the optic tract, lower portions of the basal nuclei, and lower aspects of the internal capsule. The patient experiences a contralateral *hemiplegia, hemihypethesia,* and *homonymous hemianopsia.* These deficits are due to, respectively, involvement of corticospinal fibers in the posterior limb of the internal capsule or possibly in the crus cerebri, involvement of thalamocortical fibers in the posterior limb of the internal capsule, and involvement of the fibers of the optic tract.

Parkinson Disease: Parkinson disease (paralysis agitans) results from a loss of the dopamine-containing cells in the substantia nigra. Although this part of the brain is located in the midbrain, the terminals of these nigrostriatal fibers are in the putamen and the caudate nucleus. The classic signs and symptoms of this disease are a *stooped posture, resting tremor, rigidity, shuffling or festinating gait,* and difficulty initiating or maintaining movement (*akinesia, hypokinesia,* or *bradykinesia*). Initially, the tremor and walking difficulty may appear on one side of the body, but these signs usually spread to both sides with time. This is a neurodegenerative disease that has, in its later stages, a dementia component.

Transient Ischemic Attack: A transient ischemic attack, commonly called TIA, is a temporary (and frequently focal) neurologic deficit that usually resolves within 10 to 30 minutes from the onset of symptoms. The cause is temporary occlusion of a vessel or inadequate perfusion of a restricted vascular territory. TIA that last 60+ minutes may result in some permanent deficits. This vascular event may take place anywhere in the central nervous system but is more common in the cerebral hemisphere.

5-38 Semidiagrammatic representation of the internal distribution of arteries to the diencephalon, basal ganglia, and internal capsule. Selected structures are labeled on the left side of each section; the general pattern of arterial distribution overlies these structures on the right side. The general distribution patterns of arteries in the forebrain as shown here may vary from patient to patient. For example, the adjacent territories served by neighboring vessels may overlap to varying degrees at their margins or the territory of a particular vessel may be larger or smaller than seen in the general pattern.

Abbreviations

APS	Anterior perforated substance
BCorCl	Body of corpus callosum
CC	Crus cerebri
CM	Centromedian nucleus of thalamus
DMNu	Dorsomedial nucleus of thalamus
GP	Globus pallidus
HyTh	Hypothalamus
PulNu	Pulvinar nuclear complex
Put	Putamen
SplCorCl	Splenium of the corpus callosum
VA	Ventral anterior nucleus of thalamus
VL	Ventral lateral nucleus of thalamus

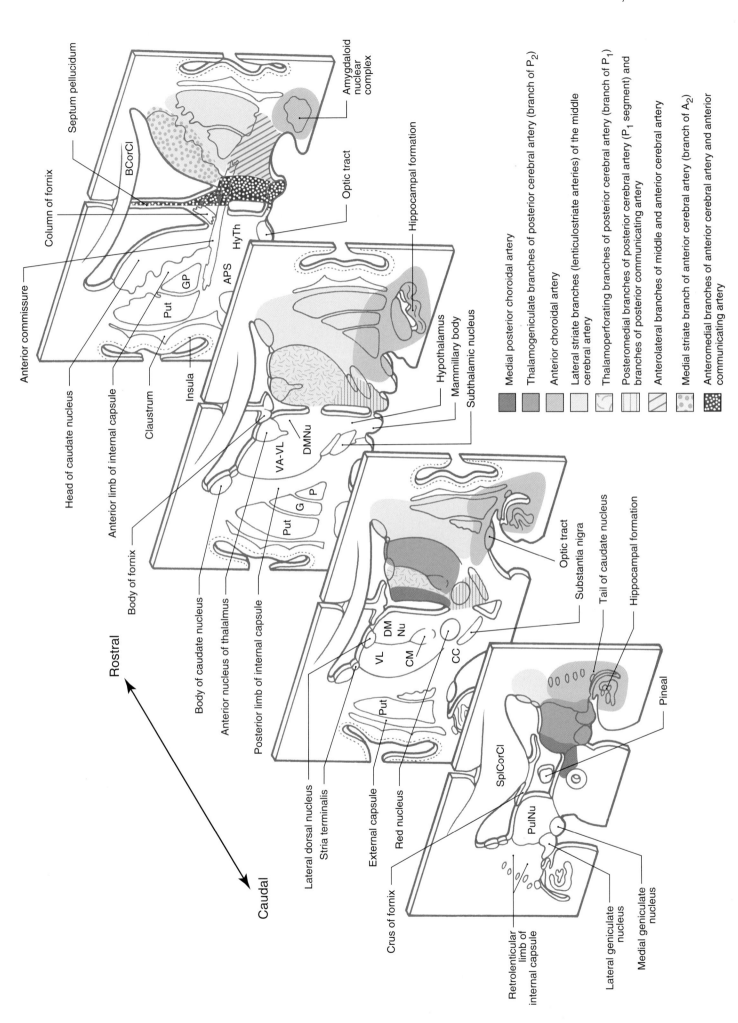

Rostral

Caudal

Septum pellucidum

Amygdaloid nuclear complex

Column of fornix

BCorCl

Optic tract

Hippocampal formation

Anterior commissure

HyTh

APS

GP

Put

Head of caudate nucleus

Insula

Claustrum

Anterior limb of internal capsule

Hypothalamus

Mammillary body

Subthalamic nucleus

Body of fornix

VA-VL

DMNu

Put

G

P

Anterior nucleus of thalamus

Body of caudate nucleus

Posterior limb of internal capsule

Optic tract

Substantia nigra

Tail of caudate nucleus

Hippocampal formation

Lateral dorsal nucleus

Stria terminalis

External capsule

Red nucleus

VL

DM Nu

CM

CC

Put

SplCorCl

Pineal

Crus of fornix

PulNu

Retrolenticular limb of internal capsule

Lateral geniculate nucleus

Medial geniculate nucleus

Medial posterior choroidal artery

Thalamogeniculate branches of posterior cerebral artery (branch of P$_2$)

Anterior choroidal artery

Lateral striate branches (lenticulostriate arteries) of the middle cerebral artery

Thalamoperforating branches of posterior cerebral artery (branch of P$_1$)

Posteromedial branches of posterior cerebral artery (P$_1$ segment) and branches of posterior communicating artery

Anterolateral branches of middle and anterior cerebral artery

Medial striate branch of anterior cerebral artery (branch of A$_2$)

Anteromedial branches of anterior cerebral artery and anterior communicating artery

Internal Morphology of the Brain in Stained Sections: Axial–Sagittal Correlations with MRI

Although the general organization of Chapter 6 has been described in Chapter 1 (the reader may wish to refer back to this section), it is appropriate to reiterate its unique features at this point. Each set of facing pages has photographs of an axial stained section (left-hand page) and a sagittal stained section (right-hand page). In addition to individually labeled structures, a heavy line appears on each photograph. This prominent line on the axial section represents the approximate plane of the sagittal section located on the facing page. On the sagittal section this line signifies the approximate plane of the corresponding axial section. The reader can identify features in each photograph and then, using this line as a reference point, visualize structures that are located either above or below that plane (axial to sagittal comparison) or medial or lateral to that plane (sagittal to axial comparison). This method of presentation provides a format for reconstructing and understanding three-dimensional relationships within the central nervous system.

The magnetic resonance image (MRI) placed on every page

in this chapter gives the reader an opportunity to compare internal brain anatomy, as seen in stained sections, with those structures as visualized in clinical images generated in the same plane. Even a general comparison reveals that many features, as seen in the stained section, can be readily identified in the adjacent MRI.

This chapter is also organized so that one can view structures in either the axial or the sagittal plane only. Axial photographs appear on left-hand pages and are sequenced from dorsal to ventral (odd-numbered Figures 6-1 through 6-9), while sagittal photographs are on the right-hand pages and progress from medial to lateral (even-numbered Figures 6-2 through 6-10). Consequently, the user can identify and follow structures through an axial series by simply flipping through the left-hand pages or through a sagittal series by flipping through the right-hand pages. The inherent flexibility in this chapter should prove useful in a wide variety of instructional/learning situations. The drawings shown in the following illustrate the axial and sagittal planes of the photographs in this chapter.

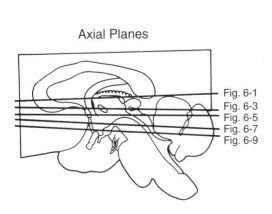

Axial Planes

Fig. 6-1
Fig. 6-3
Fig. 6-5
Fig. 6-7
Fig. 6-9

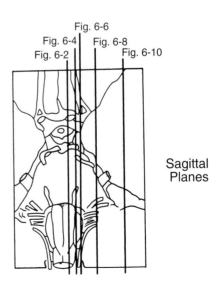

Fig. 6-6
Fig. 6-4   Fig. 6-8
Fig. 6-2   Fig. 6-10

Sagittal Planes

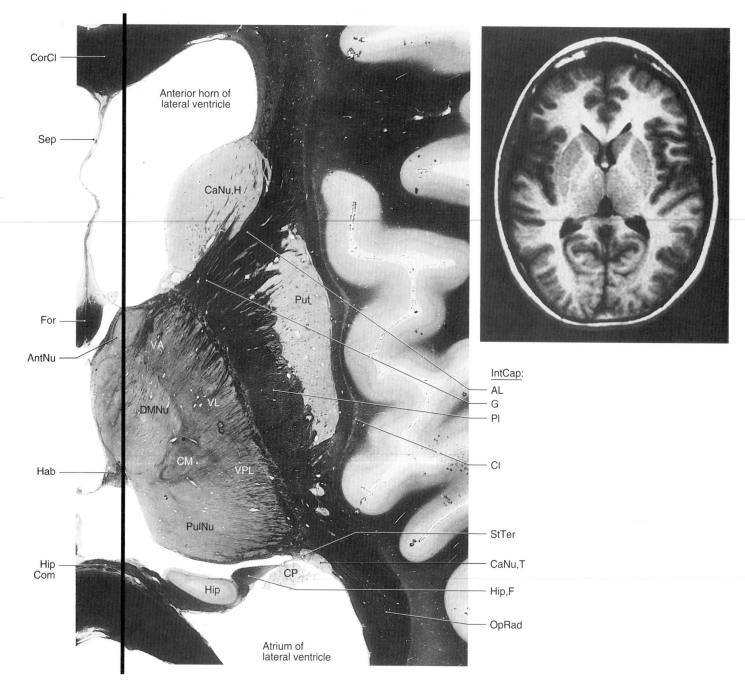

6-1 Axial section through the *head of the caudate nucleus* and several key *thalamic nuclei (anterior, centromedian, pulvinar, habenular)*. The heavy line represents the approximate plane of the sagittal section shown in Figure 6-2 (facing page). Many of the structures labeled in this photograph can be clearly identified in the adjacent T1-weighted MRI.

Abbreviations

AntNu	Anterior nucleus of thalamus	**HipCom**	Hippocampal commissure
CaNu,H	Caudate nucleus, head	**IntCap,AL**	Internal capsule, anterior limb
CaNu,T	Caudate nucleus, tail	**IntCap,G**	Internal capsule, genu
CI	Claustrum	**IntCap,PL**	Internal capsule, posterior limb
CM	Centromedial nucleus of thalamus	**OpRad**	Optic radiations
CorCI	Corpus callosum	**PulNu**	Pulvinar nuclear complex
CP	Choroid plexus	**Put**	Putamen
DMNu	Dorsomedial nucleus of thalamus	**Sep**	Septum pellucidum
For	Fornix, column	**StTer**	Stria terminalis
Hab	Habenular nucleus	**VA**	Ventral anterior nucleus of thalamus
Hip	Hippocampal formation	**VL**	Ventral lateral nucleus of thalamus
Hip,F	Hippocampus, fimbria	**VPL**	Ventral posterolateral nucleus

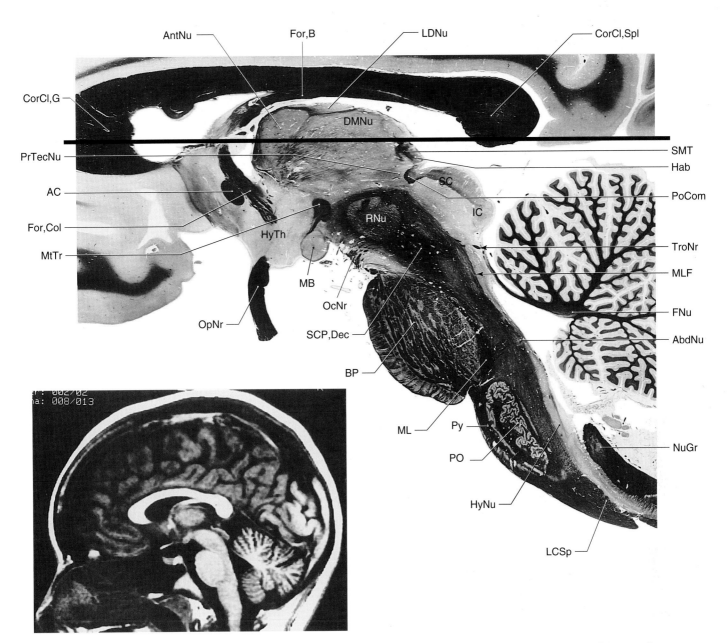

6-2 Sagittal section through the *column of the fornix, anterior thalamic nucleus, red nucleus,* and medial portions of the *pons (abducens nucleus), cerebellum (fastigial nucleus),* and *medulla (nucleus gracilis).* The heavy line represents the approximate plane of the axial section shown in Figure 6-1 (facing page). Many of the structures labeled in this photograph can be clearly identified in the adjacent T1-weighted MRI.

Abbreviations

AbdNu	Abducens nucleus		**MB**	Mammillary body
AC	Anterior commissure		**ML**	Medial lemniscus
AntNu	Anterior nucleus of thalamus		**MLF**	Medial longitudinal fasciculus
BP	Basilar pons		**MtTr**	Mammillothalamic tract
CorCl,G	Corpus callosum, genu		**NuGr**	Nucleus gracilis
CorCl,Spl	Corpus callosum, splenium		**OcNr**	Oculomotor nerve
DMNu	Dorsomedial nucleus of thalamus		**OpNr**	Optic nerve
FNu	Fastigial nucleus (medial cerebellar nucleus)		**PO**	Principal olivary nucleus
For,B	Fornix, body		**PoCom**	Posterior commissure
For,Col	Fornix, column		**PrTecNu**	Pretectal nuclei
Hab	Habenular nuclei		**Py**	Pyramid
HyNu	Hypoglossal nucleus		**RNu**	Red nucleus
HyTh	Hypothalamus		**SC**	Superior colliculus
IC	Inferior colliculus		**SCP,Dec**	Superior cerebellar peduncle, decussation
LCsp	Lateral corticospinal tract		**SMT**	Stria medullaris thalami
LDNu	Lateral dorsal nucleus		**TroNr**	Trochlear nerve

6-3   Axial section through the *head of the caudate nucleus, centromedian nucleus, medial geniculate body,* and *superior colliculus.* The heavy line represents the approximate plane of the sagittal section shown in Figure 6-4 (facing page). Many of the structures labeled in this photograph can be clearly identified in the adjacent T2-weighted MRI.

Abbreviations

CaNu,H	Caudate nucleus, head	**MGNu**	Medial geniculate nucleus
CaNu,T	Caudate nucleus, tail	**MtTr**	Mammillothalamic tract
Cl	Claustrum	**OpRad**	Optic radiations
CM	Centromedian nucleus of thalamus	**PulNu**	Pulvinar nuclear complex
DMNu	Dorsomedial nucleus of thalamus	**Put**	Putamen
ExtCap	External capsule	**SC**	Superior colliculus
For,Col	Fornix, column	**SC,Br**	Superior colliculus, brachium
Sep	Septum pellucidum	**StTer**	Stria terminalis
GPL	Globus pallidus, lateral segment	**VA**	Ventral anterior nucleus of thalamus
Hab,Com	Habenular commissure	**VL**	Ventral lateral nucleus of thalamus
Hip	Hippocampal formation	**VPL**	Ventral posterolateral nucleus of thalamus
Ins	Insula	**VPM**	Ventral posteromedial nucleus of thalamus
IntCap,AL	Internal capsule, anterior limb	**Tap**	Tapetum
IntCap,PL	Internal capsule, posterior limb		

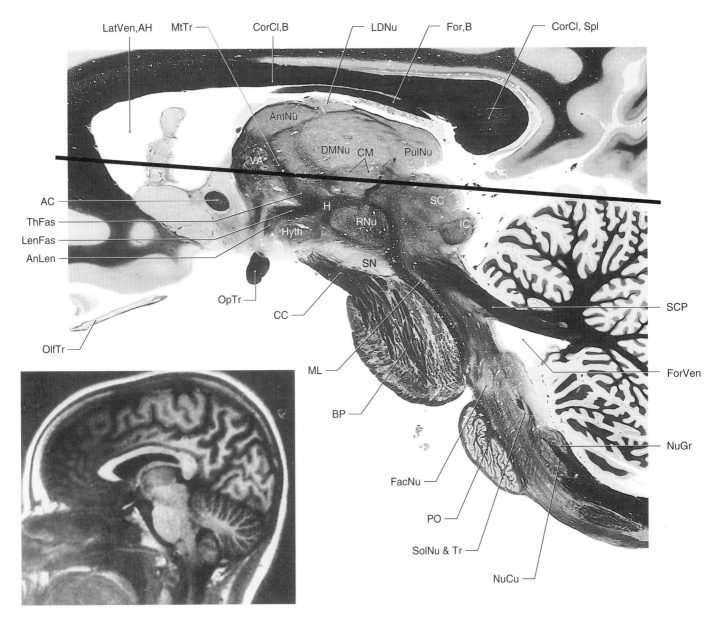

6-4 Sagittal section through *anterior* and *ventral anterior thalamic nuclei, red nucleus* and central areas of the *pons, cerebellum* (*and superior peduncle*), and *medulla* (*solitary nuclei and tract*). Note the position of the *facial motor nucleus* at the pons-medulla junction. The heavy line represents the approximate plane of the axial section shown in Figure 6-3 (facing page). Many of the structures labeled in this photograph can be clearly identified in the adjacent T1-weighted MRI.

Abbreviations

AC	Anterior commissure		**LDNu**	Lateral dorsal nucleus
AnLen	Ansa lenticularis		**ML**	Medial lemniscus
AntNu	Anterior nucleus of thalamus		**MtTr**	Mammillothalamic tract
BP	Basilar pons		**NuCu**	Nucleus cuneatus
CC	Crus cerebri		**NuGr**	Nucleus gracilis
CM	Centromedian nucleus		**OlfTr**	Olfactory tract
CorCl,B	Corpus callosum, body		**OpTr**	Optic tract
CorCl, Spl	Corpus callosum, splenium		**PO**	Principal olivary nucleus
DMNu	Dorsomedial nucleus of thalamus		**PulNu**	Pulvinar nuclear complex
FacNu	Facial nucleus		**RNu**	Red nucleus
For,B	Fornix, body		**SC**	Superior colliculus
ForVen	Fourth ventricle		**SCP**	Superior cerebellar peduncle (brachium conjunctivum)
H	Prerubral field			
HyTh	Hypothalamus		**SN**	Substantia nigra
IC	Inferior colliculus		**SolNu&Tr**	Solitary nuclei and tract
LatVen,AH	Lateral ventricle, anterior horn		**ThFas**	Thalamic fasciculus
LenFas	Lenticular fasciculus		**VA**	Ventral anterior nucleus of thalamus

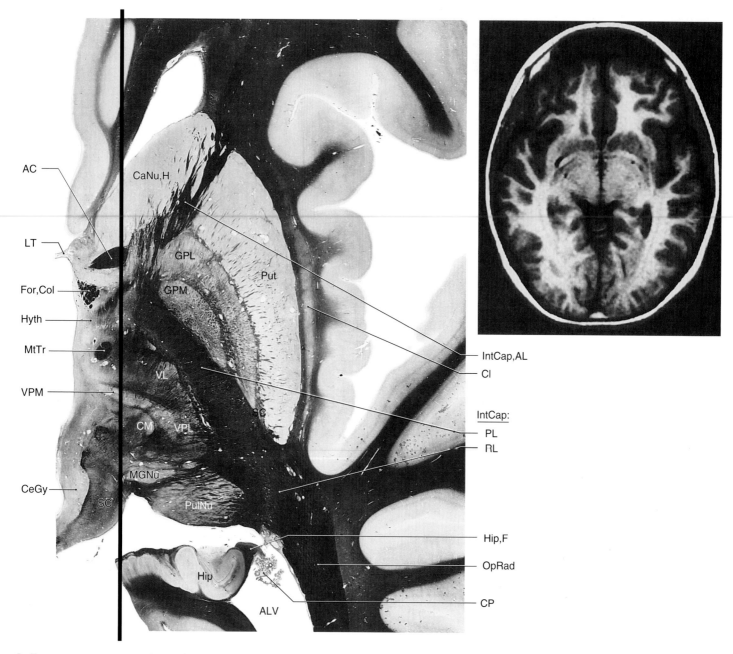

AC
LT
For,Col
Hyth
MtTr
VPM
CeGy

CaNu,H
GPL
GPM
Put
VL
SC
CM VPL
MGNu
SC PulNu
Hip
ALV

IntCap,AL
CI

IntCap:
PL
RL

Hip,F
OpRad

CP

6-5 Axial section through the *head of the caudate nucleus, ventral posteromedial nucleus, medial geniculate body,* and ventral parts of the *pulvinar.* The heavy line represents the approximate plane of the sagittal section shown in Figure 6-6 (facing page). Many of the structures labeled in this photograph can be clearly identified in the adjacent T1-weighted MRI.

Abbreviations

AC	Anterior commissure		**IntCap,AL**	Internal capsule, anterior limb
ALV	Atrium of lateral ventricle		**IntCap,Pl**	Internal capsule, posterior limb
CaNu,H	Caudate nucleus, head		**IntCap,RL**	Internal capsule, retrolenticular limb
CeGy	Central gray (periaqueductal gray)		**LT**	Lamina terminalis
CI	Claustrum		**MGNu**	Medial geniculate nucleus
CM	Centromedian nucleus of thalamus		**MtTr**	Mammillothalamic tract
CP	Choroid plexus		**OpRad**	Optic radiations
For,Col	Fornix, column		**PulNu**	Pulvinar nuclear complex
GPL	Globus pallidus, lateral segment		**Put**	Putamen
GPM	Globus pallidus, medial segment		**SC**	Superior colliculus
Hip	Hippocampal formation		**VL**	Ventral lateral nucleus of thalamus
Hip,F	Hippocampus, fimbria		**VPL**	Ventral posterolateral nucleus of thalamus
HyTh	Hypothalamus		**VPM**	Ventral posteromedial nucleus of thalamus

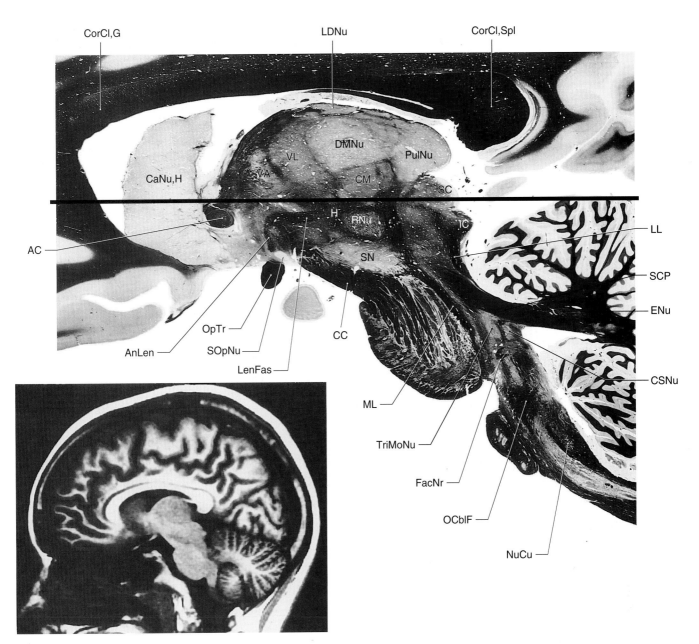

6-6 Sagittal section through central regions of the *diencephalon* (*centromedian nucleus*) and *midbrain* (*red nucleus*), and through lateral areas of the *pons* (*trigeminal motor nucleus*) and *medulla* (*nucleus cuneatus*). The heavy line represents the approximate plane of the axial section shown in Figure 6-5 (facing page). Many of the structures labeled in this photograph can be clearly identified in the adjacent T1-weighted MRI.

Abbreviations

AC	Anterior commissure		**LL**	Lateral lemniscus
AnLen	Ansa lenticularis		**ML**	Medial lemniscus
CaNu,H	Caudate nucleus, head		**NuCu**	Nucleus cuneatus
CC	Crus cerebri		**OCblF**	Olivocerebellar fibers
CM	Centromedian nucleus of thalamus		**OpTr**	Optic tract
CorCl,G	Corpus callosum, genu		**PulNu**	Pulvinar nuclear complex
CorCl,Spl	Corpus callosum, splenium		**RNu**	Red nucleus
CSNu	Chief (prinicipal) sensory nucleus of trigeminal nerve		**SC**	Superior colliculus
DMNU	Dorsomedial nucleus of thalamus		**SCP**	Superior cerebellar peduncle (brachium conjunctivum)
ENu	Emboliform nucleus (anterior interposed cerebellar nucleus)		**SN**	Substantia nigra
FacNr	Facial nerve		**SOpNu**	Supraoptic nucleus
H	Field of Forel (prerubral field)		**TriMoNu**	Trigeminal motor nucleus
IC	Inferior colliculus		**VA**	Ventral anterior nucleus of thalamus
LenFas	Lenticular fasciculus		**VL**	Ventral lateral nucleus of thalamus
LDNu	Lateral dorsal nucleus of thalamus			

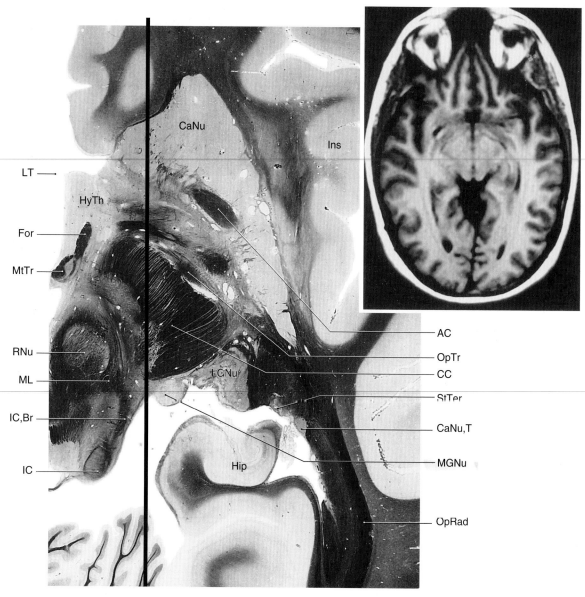

6-7   Axial section through the *hypothalamus, red nucleus, inferior colliculus,* and *lateral geniculate body*. The heavy line represents the approximate plane of the sagittal section shown in Figure 6-8 (facing page). The axial plane through the hemisphere, when continued into the midbrain, represents a slightly oblique section through the mesencephalon. The position of the lamina terminalis is indicated by the double-dashed lines. Many of the structures labeled in this photograph can be clearly identified in the adjacent T1-weighted MRI.

Abbreviations

AC	Anterior commissure	**LGNu**	Lateral geniculate nucleus
CaNu	Caudate nucleus	**LT**	Lamina terminalis
CaNu,T	Caudate nucleus, tail	**MGNu**	Medial geniculate nucleus
CC	Crus cerebri	**ML**	Medial lemniscus
For	Fornix	**MtTr**	Mammillothalamic tract
Hip	Hippocampal formation	**OpRad**	Optic radiation (geniculocalcarine fibers)
HyTh	Hypothalamus	**OpTr**	Optic tract
IC	Inferior colliculus	**RNu**	Red nucleus
IC,Br	Inferior colliculus, brachium	**StTer**	Stria terminalis
Ins	Insula		

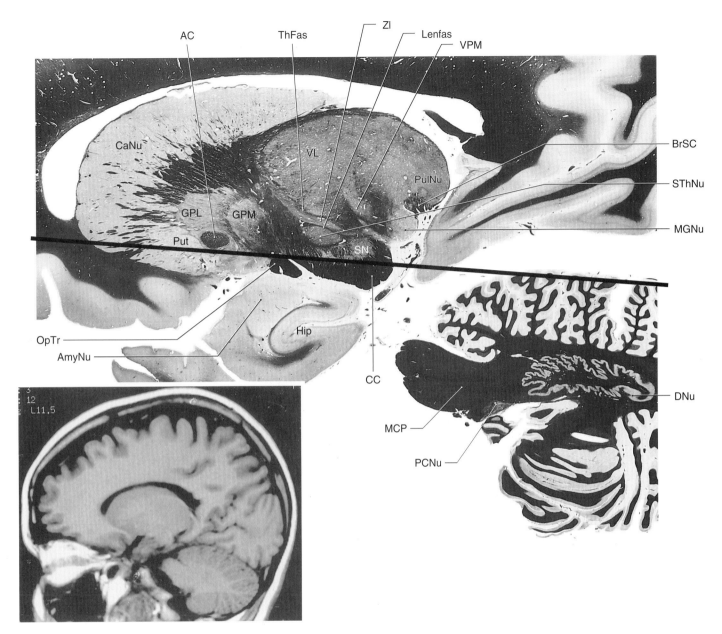

6-8 Sagittal section through the *caudate nucleus,* central parts of the *diencephalon (ventral posteromedial nucleus),* and lateral portions of the *pons* and *cerebellum (dentate nucleus).* The heavy line represents the approximate plane of the axial section shown in Figure 6-7 (facing page). Many of the structures labeled in this photograph can be clearly identified in the adjacent T1-weighted MRI.

Abbreviations

AC	Anterior commissure	**MGNu**	Medial geniculate nucleus
AmyNu	Amygdaloid nucleus (complex)	**OpTr**	Optic tract
BrSC	Brachium of superior colliculus	**PCNu**	Posterior cochlear nucleus
CaNu	Caudate nucleus	**PulNu**	Pulvinar nuclear complex
CC	Crus cerebri	**Put**	Putamen
DNu	Dentate nucleus (lateral cerebellar nucleus)	**SN**	Substantia nigra
GPL	Globus pallidus, lateral segment	**SThNu**	Subthalamic nucleus
GPM	Globus pallidus, medial segment	**ThFas**	Thalamic fasciculus
Hip	Hippocampal formation	**VL**	Ventral lateral nucleus of thalamus
LenFas	Lenticular fasciculus	**VPM**	Ventral posteromedial nucleus of thalamus
MCP	Middle cerebellar peduncle (brachium pontis)	**ZI**	Zona incerta

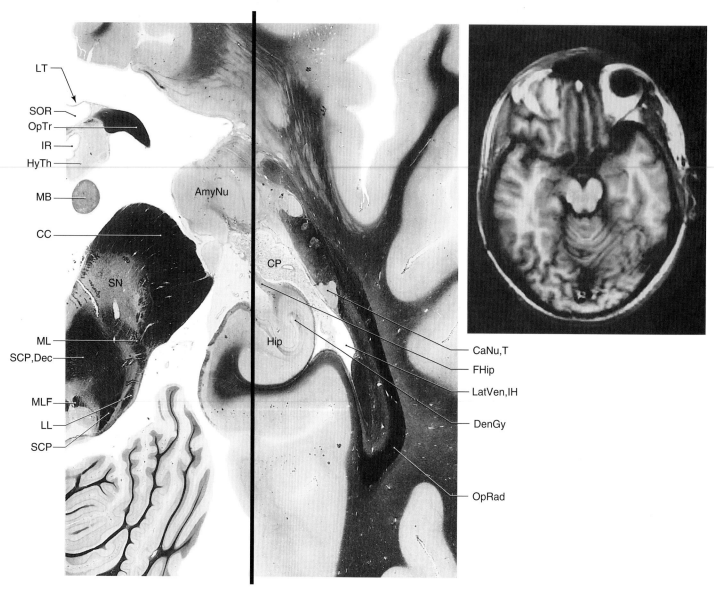

6-9 Axial section through ventral portions of the *hypothalamus* (*supraoptic recess* and *mammillary body*) and forebrain (*amygdaloid nucleus*), and through the *superior cerebellar peduncle decussation* in the midbrain. The heavy line represents the approximate plane of the sagittal section shown in Figure 6-10 (facing page). The axial plane through the hemisphere, when continued into the midbrain, represents a slightly oblique section through the mesencephalon. Many of the structures labeled in this photograph can be clearly identified in the adjacent T1-weighted MRI.

Abbreviations

AmyNu	Amygdaloid nucleus (complex)		**LT**	Lamina terminalis
CaNu,T	Caudate nucleus, tail		**MB**	Mammillary body
CC	Crus cerebri		**ML**	Medial lemniscus
CP	Choroid plexus		**MLF**	Medial longitudinal fasciculus
DenGy	Dentate gyrus		**OpRad**	Optic radiations
FHip	Fimbria of hippocampus		**OpTr**	Optic tract
Hip	Hippocampal formation		**SCP**	Superior cerebellar peduncle (brachium conjunctivum)
HyTh	Hypothalamus			
IR	Infundibular recess of third ventricle		**SCP,Dec**	Superior cerebellar peduncle, decussation
LatVen,lH	Lateral ventricle, inferior (temporal) horn		**SN**	Sustantia nigra
LL	Lateral lemniscus		**SOR**	Supraoptic recess of third ventricle

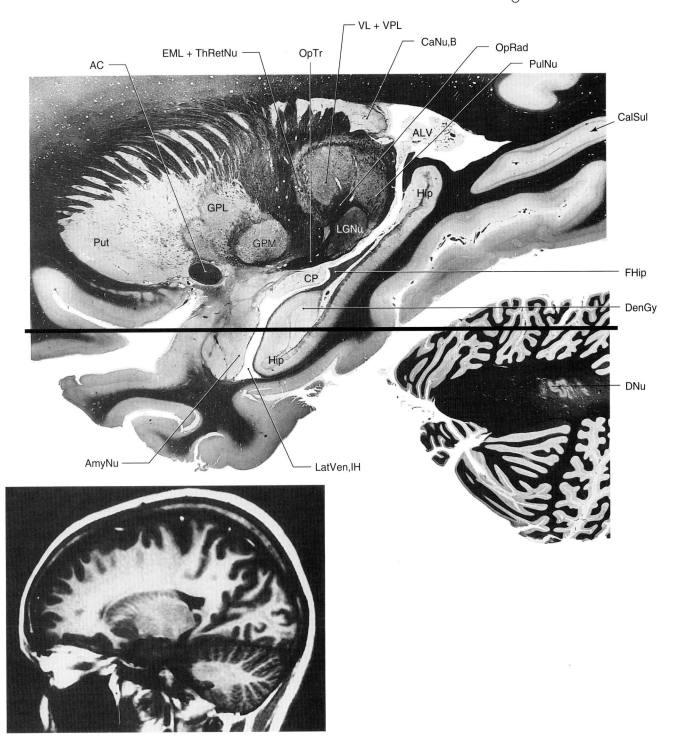

6-10 Sagittal section through the *putamen, amygdaloid nucleus,* and *hippocampus* and through the most lateral portions of the *diencephalon* (*external medullary lamina* and *ventral posterolateral nucleus*). The heavy line represents the approximate plane of the axial section shown in Figure 6-9 (facing page). Many of the structures labeled in this photograph can be clearly identified in the adjacent T1-weighted MRI.

Abbreviations

AC	Anterior commissure		**GPM**	Globus pallidus, medial segment
ALV	Atrium of lateral ventricle		**Hip**	Hippocampal formation
AmyNu	Amygdaloid nucleus (complex)		**LatVen,lH**	Lateral ventricle, inferior (temporal) horn
CalSul	Calcarine sulcus		**LGNu**	Lateral geniculate nucleus
CaNu,B	Caudate nucleus, body		**OpRad**	Optic radiations
CP	Choroid plexus		**OpTr**	Optic tract
DenGy	Dentate gyrus		**PulNu**	Pulvinar nuclear complex
DNu	Dentate nucleus		**Put**	Putamen
EML	External medullary lamina		**ThRetNu**	Thalamic reticular nuclei
FHip	Fimbria of hippocampus		**VL**	Ventral lateral nucleus of thalamus
GPL	Globus pallidus, lateral segment		**VPL**	Ventral posterolateral nucleus of thalamus

Synopsis of Functional Components, Tracts, Pathways, and Systems

The study of *regional neurobiology* (brain structures in gross specimens, in brain slices, in stained sections, and in MRI and CT) is the basis for the study of *systems neurobiology* (tracts, pathways, cranial nerves and their functions), which, in turn, is the basis for understanding and diagnosing the neurologically impaired patient. Building on the concepts learned in earlier chapters on external and internal brain anatomy in specimens and in MRI and CT, on brain vascular patterns, and on the relationships of cranial nerves with long tracts, this chapter explores *systems neurobiology* with a particular emphasis on clinical correlations.

The format of each set of facing pages is designed to summarize, accurately and consisely, the relationships of a given tract or pathway. This includes, but is not limited to, 1) the location of the cells of origin for a given tract/pathway, 2) its entire course throughout the neuraxis and cerebrum, 3) the location of the decussation of these fibers, if applicable, 4) the neurotransmitters associated with the neurons comprising the tract/pathway, 5) a brief review of its blood supply, and 6) a summary of a number of deficits seen as a result of lesions at various points in the tract/pathway. The structure of an atlas does not allow a detailed definition of each clinical term on the printed page. However, the full definition of each clinical term or phrase is available on

the CD that comes with this atlas; these are taken from the current edition of *Stedman's Medical Dictionary*. In this respect, the full definitions are actually available in this book. Researching the full definition of a clinical term or phrase is a powerful and effective learning tool. Also, each clinical term or phrase is available in any standard medical dictionary or comprehensive neurology text.

The layout of the drawings in this chapter clearly shows the laterality of the tract/pathway. That is, the relationship between the location of the cell of origin and the termination of the fibers making up a tract/pathway or the projections of cranial nerve nuclei. *This information is absolutely essential to understanding the position of a lesion and correlating this fact with the deficits seen in the neurologically compromised patient.* For example, is the deficit on the same side as the lesion (ipsilateral), on the opposite side (contralateral), or on both sides (bilateral)? The concept of laterality is usually expressed as "right," "left," or "bilateral" in reference to the side of the deficit(s) when written on the patient's chart.

This chapter is designed to maximize the correlation between structure and function, to provide a range of clinical examples for each tract/pathway, and to help the user develop a knowledge base that can be easily integrated into the clinical setting.

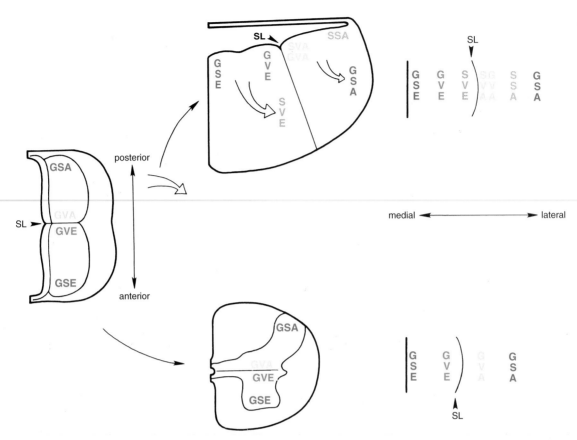

7-1 A semidiagrammatic summary of the positions of functional components as seen in the developing neural tube (left) and in the spinal cord and brainstem of the adult (right). In the neural tube, the alar plate and its associated GSA and GVA components are posterior (dorsal) to the sulcus limitans (SL) while the basal plate and its related GVE and GSE components are anterior (ventral) to the SL. In the adult spinal cord, this general posterior/anterior relationship is maintained, although the neural canal (as central canal) is reduced and/or absent.

Two major changes occur in the transition from spinal cord to brainstem in the adult. First, as the central canal of the cervical cord enlarges into the fourth ventricle and the cerebellum develops, the posterior portion of the neural tube is rotated laterally. Consequently, in the adult, the sulcus limitans is present in the brainstem with motor components (adult derivatives of the basal plate) medial to it, and sensory components (adult derivatives of the alar plate) are located laterally. Second, in the brainstem, special functional components (SVE to muscles of pharyngeal arch origin; SVA taste and olfaction; SSA vestibular, auditory, and visual systems) are intermingled with the rostral continuation of the general functional components as found in the spinal cord.

In the brainstem, however, there is a slight transposition of the SVE and GSA functional components. Embryologically, SVE cell groups appear between those associated with GSE and GVE components. As development progresses, however, SVE cell groups migrate (open arrow) to anterolateral areas of the tegmentum. Cell groups associated with the GSA functional component are displaced from their posterolateral position in the developing brainstem by the newly acquired cell groups having SSA components (as well as other structures). Consequently, structures associated with the GSA component are located (open arrow) in more anterolateral and lateral areas of the brainstem. The approximate border between motor and sensory regions of the brainstem is represented by an oblique line drawn through the brainstem beginning at the SL. The medial (from midline) to lateral positions of the various functional components, as shown on the far right of this figure, are taken from their representative diagrams of brainstem and cord and are directly translatable to Figure 7–2 (facing page). The color-coding of the components on this figure correlate with that in Figure 7–2 on the facing page.

Abbreviations

GSA	General somatic afferent	**SSA**	Special somatic afferent
GSE	General somatic efferent	**SVA**	Special visceral afferent
GVA	General visceral afferent	**SVE**	Special visceral efferent
GVE	General visceral efferent	**SL**	Sulcus limitans

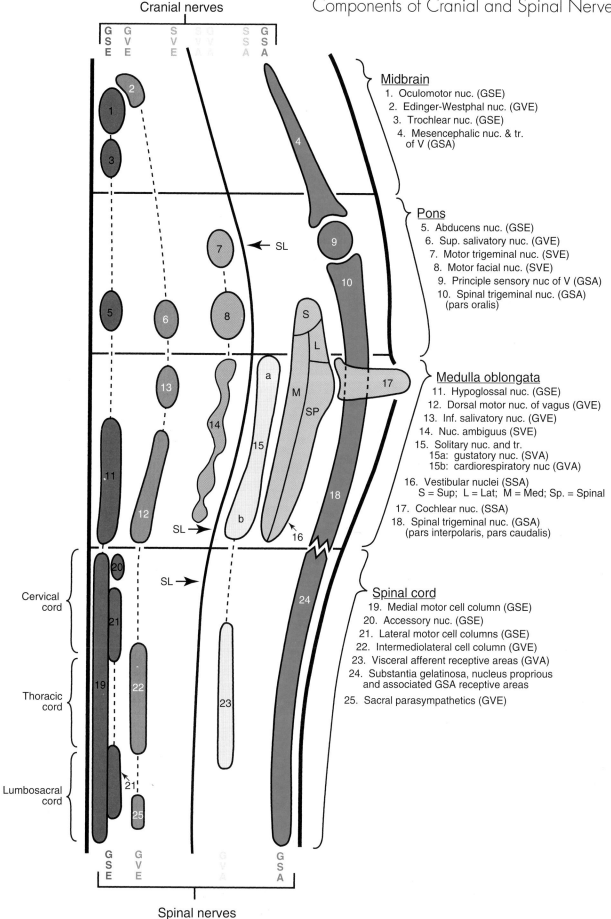

Cranial nerves

Midbrain
1. Oculomotor nuc. (GSE)
2. Edinger-Westphal nuc. (GVE)
3. Trochlear nuc. (GSE)
4. Mesencephalic nuc. & tr. of V (GSA)

Pons
5. Abducens nuc. (GSE)
6. Sup. salivatory nuc. (GVE)
7. Motor trigeminal nuc. (SVE)
8. Motor facial nuc. (SVE)
9. Principle sensory nuc of V (GSA)
10. Spinal trigeminal nuc. (GSA) (pars oralis)

Medulla oblongata
11. Hypoglossal nuc. (GSE)
12. Dorsal motor nuc. of vagus (GVE)
13. Inf. salivatory nuc. (GVE)
14. Nuc. ambiguus (SVE)
15. Solitary nuc. and tr.
    15a: gustatory nuc. (SVA)
    15b: cardiorespiratory nuc (GVA)
16. Vestibular nuclei (SSA)
    S = Sup; L = Lat; M = Med; Sp. = Spinal
17. Cochlear nuc. (SSA)
18. Spinal trigeminal nuc. (GSA) (pars interpolaris, pars caudalis)

Spinal cord
19. Medial motor cell column (GSE)
20. Accessory nuc. (GSE)
21. Lateral motor cell columns (GSE)
22. Intermediolateral cell column (GVE)
23. Visceral afferent receptive areas (GVA)
24. Substantia gelatinosa, nucleus proprious and associated GSA receptive areas
25. Sacral parasympathetics (GVE)

Cervical cord

Thoracic cord

Lumbosacral cord

Spinal nerves

7-2   The medial to lateral positions of brainstem cranial nerve and spinal cord nuclei as shown here are the same as in Figure 7–1. This diagrammatic posterior (dorsal) view shows 1) the relative positions and names of specific cell groups and their associated functional components, 2) the approximate location of particular nuclei in their specific division of brainstem and/or spinal cord, and 3) the rostrocaudal continuity of cell columns (either as continuous or discontinuous cell groups) from one division of the brainstem to the next or from brainstem to spinal cord. The nucleus ambiguus is a column of cells composed of distinct cell clusters interspersed with more diffusely arranged cells, much like a string of beads. Nuclei associated with cranial nerves I (olfaction, SVA) and II (optic, SSA) are not shown. The color-coding used on this figure correlates with that on Figure 7–1 (facing page).

7–3 Orientation drawing for pathways. The trajectory of most pathways illustrated in Chapter 7 appears on individualized versions of this representation of the central nervous system (CNS). Although slight changes are made in each drawing, so as to more clearly diagram a specific pathway, the basic configuration of the CNS is as represented here. This allows the user to move from pathway to pathway without being required to learn a different representation or drawing for each pathway; also, laterality of the pathway, a feature essential to diagnosis (see introduction), is inherently evident in each illustration.

The forebrain (telencephalon and diencephalon) is shown in the coronal plane, and the midbrain, pons, medulla, and spinal cord are represented through their longitudinal axes. The internal capsule is represented in the axial plane in an effort to show the rostrocaudal distribution of fibers located therein.

The reader should become familiar with the structures and regions as shown here because their locations and relationships are easily transferable to subsequent illustrations. It may also be helpful to refer back to this illustration when using subsequent sections of this chapter.

Neurotransmitters: Three important facts are self-evident in the descriptions of neurotransmitters that accompany each pathway drawing. These are illustrated by noting, as an example, that glutamate is found in corticospinal fibers (see Figure 7–10). First, the *location of neuronal cell bodies* containing a specific transmitter is indicated (glutamate-containing cell bodies are found in cortical areas that project to the spinal cord). Second, the *trajectory of fibers* containing a particular neurotransmitter is obvious from the route taken by the tract (glutaminergic corti-

cospinal fibers are found in the internal capsule, crus cerebri, basilar pons, pyramid, and lateral corticospinal tract). Third, the *location of terminals* containing specific neurotransmitters is indicated by the site(s) of termination of each tract (glutaminergic terminals of corticospinal fibers are located in the spinal cord gray matter). In addition, the action of most neuroactive substances is indicated as excitatory (+) or inhibitory (−). This level of neurotransmitter information, as explained here for glutaminergic corticospinal fibers, is repeated for each pathway drawing.

Clinical Correlations: The clinical correlations are designed to give the user an overview of specific deficits (i.e., *hemiplegia, athetosis*) seen in lesions of each pathway and to provide examples of some syndromes or diseases (i.e., *Brown-Sequard syndrome, Wilson disease*) in which these deficits are seen. Although purposefully brief, these correlations highlight examples of deficits for each pathway and provide a built-in mechanism for expanded study. For example, the words in *italics* in each correlation are clinical terms and phrases that are defined on the CD (from Stedman's) included with this atlas or can be found in standard medical dictionaries and clinical neuroscience textbooks. Consulting these sources, especially the CD available in this atlas, will significantly enhance understanding of the deficits seen in the neurologically compromised patient. Expanded information, based on the deficits mentioned in this chapter, is integrated into some of the questions for chapter 7. Referring to such sources will allow the user to glean important clinical points that correlate with the pathway under consideration, and enlarge his or her knowledge and understanding by researching the italicized words and phrases.

Abbreviations

CE	Cervical enlargement of spinal cord	**IntCap,PL**	Internal capsule, posterior limb
Cer	Cervical levels of spinal cord	**LatSul**	Lateral sulcus (Sylvian sulcus)
CinSul	Cingulate sulcus	**LatVen**	Lateral ventricle
CaNu	Caudate nucleus (+ Put = neostriatum)	**LSE**	Lumbosacral enlargement of spinal cord
CM	Centromedian (and intralaminar) nuclei	**LumSac**	Lumbosacral level of spinal cord
CorCl	Corpus callosum	**L-VTh**	Lateral and ventral thalamic nuclei excluding VPM and VPL
Dien	Diencephalon		
DMNu	Dorsomedial nucleus of thalamus	**Mes**	Mesencephalon
For	Fornix	**Met**	Metencephalon
GP	Globus pallidus (paleostriatum)	**Myelen**	Myelencephalon
GPl	Globus pallidus, lateral segment	**Put**	Putamen (+ CaNu = neostriatum)
GPm	Globus pallidus, medial segment	**SThNu**	Subthalamic nucleus
HyTh	Hypothalamic area	**Telen**	Telencephalon
IC	Internal capsule	**Thor**	Thoracic levels of spinal cord
IntCap,AL	Internal capsule, anterior limb	**VPL**	Ventral posterolateral nucleus of thalamus
IntCap,G	Internal capsule, genu	**VPM**	Ventral posteromedial nucleus of thalamus

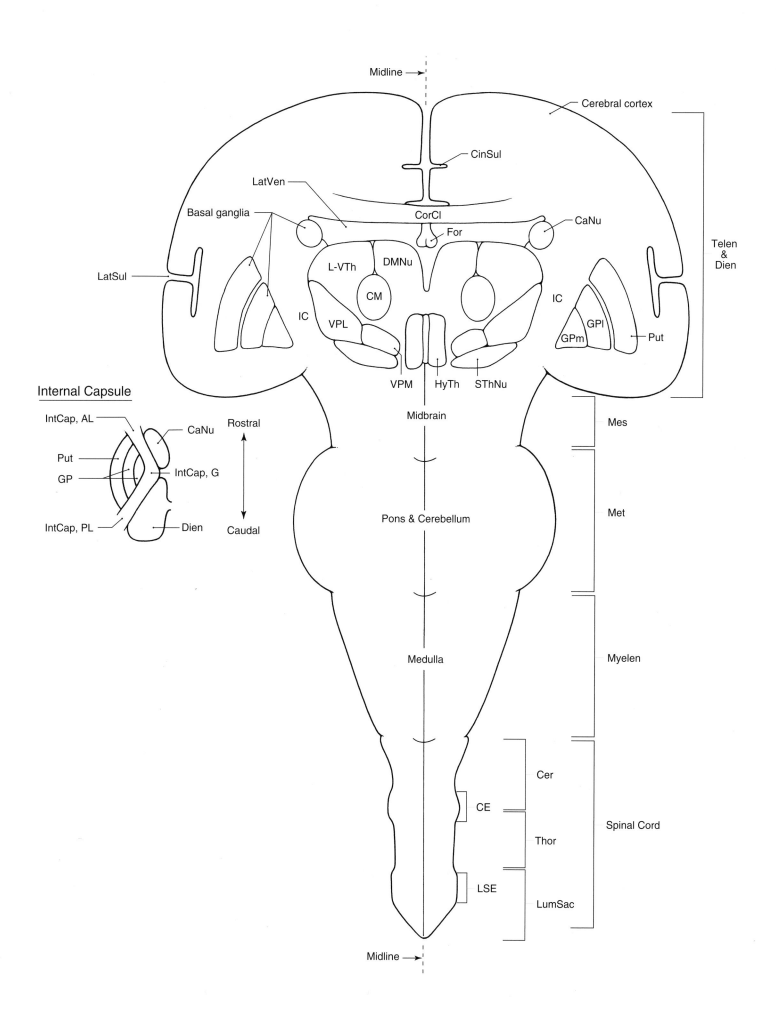

Midline →

Cerebral cortex

CinSul

LatVen

Basal ganglia

CorCl

CaNu

For

L-VTh   DMNu

CM

IC

VPL

GPl

GPm

Put

LatSul

VPM   HyTh   SThNu

Telen & Dien

Internal Capsule

IntCap, AL

Put

GP

IntCap, PL

CaNu

IntCap, G

Dien

Rostral

Caudal

Midbrain

Mes

Pons & Cerebellum

Met

Medulla

Myelen

Cer

CE

Thor

Spinal Cord

LSE

LumSac

Midline →

Posterior (Dorsal) Column-Medial Lemniscus System

7-4 The origin, course, and distribution of fibers composing the posterior (dorsal) column (PC)-medial lemniscus (ML) system. This illustration shows the longitudinal extent, the positions in representative cross-sections of brainstem and spinal cord, and the somatotopy of fibers in the PC and ML. The ML undergoes positional changes as it courses from the myelencephalon (medulla) rostrally toward the mesencephalic-diencephalic junction. In the medulla, ML and ALS fibers are widely separated and receive different blood supplies, whereas in the midbrain, they are served by a common arterial source. As the ML makes positional changes, the somatotopy therein follows accordingly. Fibers of the postsynaptic posterior column system (shown in green) are considered in detail in Figure 7–6 on page 182.

Neurotransmitters: Acetylcholine and the excitatory amino acids glutamate and aspartate are associated with some of the large-diameter, heavily myelinated fibers of the posterior horn and posterior columns.

Clinical Correlations: Damage to posterior column fibers on one side of the spinal cord (as in the *Brown-Sequard syndrome*) results in an ipsilateral loss of vibratory sensation, position sense, and discriminative touch *(asterognosis, stereoagnosis)* below the level of the lesion. The term *stereoanesthesia* is frequently used to specify a lesion of peripheral nerves that results in an inability to perceive proprioceptive and tactile sensations. The term *tactile agnosia* is sometimes considered to be synonymous with these preceding three terms. However, *tactile agnosia* is also used to describe deficits seen in lesions of the parietal cortex. Bilateral damage (as in *tabes dorsalis* or *subacute combined degeneration of the spinal cord*) produces bilateral losses. Although *ataxia* is the most common feature in patients with tabes dorsalis, they also have a loss of *deep tendon reflexes,* severe *lancinating pain* over the body below the head (more common in the lower extremity), and bladder dysfunction. The *ataxia* that may be seen in patients with posterior column lesions (*sensory ataxia*) is due to a lack of proprioceptive input and position sense. These individuals tend to forcibly place their feet to the floor in an attempt to stimulate such sensory input. A patient with mild ataxia due to posterior column disease may compensate for the motor deficit by using visual cues. Patients with subacute combined degeneration (SCD) of the spinal cord first have signs and symptoms of posterior column involvement, followed later by signs of corticospinal tract damage (*spastic weakness of legs, increased deep tendon reflexes, Babinski sign*).

Rostral to the sensory decussation, medial lemniscus lesions result in contralateral losses that include the entire body excluding the head. Brainstem lesions involving medial lemniscus fibers usually include adjacent structures, result in motor and additional sensory losses, and may reflect the distribution patterns of vessels (as in *medial medullary* or *medial pontine syndromes*). Large lesions in the forebrain may result in a complete contralateral loss of modalities carried in the posterior columns and anterolateral systems, or may produce *pain* (as in the *thalamic syndrome*).

Abbreviations

ALS	Anterolateral system		**NuGr**	Gracile nucleus
BP	Basilar pons		**PC**	Posterior column
CC	Crus cerebri		**PO**	Principal olivary nucleus
CTT	Central tegmental tract		**PoCGy**	Postcentral gyrus
FCu	Cuneate fasciculus		**PPGy**	Posterior paracentral gyrus
FGr	Gracile fasciculus		**PRG**	Posterior (dorsal) root ganglia
IAF	Internal arcuate fibers		**Py**	Pyramid
IC	Internal capsule		**RB**	Restiform body
ML	Medial lemniscus		**RNu**	Red nucleus
MLF	Medial longitudinal fasciculus		**SN**	Substantia nigra
NuCu	Cuneate nucleus		**VPL**	Ventral posterolateral nucleus of thalamus

Somatotopy of Body Areas

A	Fibers conveying input from upper extremity		S_5	Fibers from approximately the fifth sacral level
L	Fibers conveying input from lower extremity			
N	Fibers conveying input from neck		T_5	Fibers from approximately the fifth thoracic level
T	Fibers conveying input from trunk			
C_2	Fibers from approximately the second cervical level			

Review of Blood Supply to DC-ML System

STRUCTURES	ARTERIES
PC in Spinal Cord	penetrating branches of arterial vasocorona (see Figure 5–6)
ML in Medulla	anterior spinal (see Figure 5–14)
ML in Pons	overlap of paramedian and long circumferential branches of basilar (see Figure 5–21)
ML in Midbrain	short circumferential branches of posterior cerebral and superior cerebellar (see Figure 5–27)
VPL	thalamogeniculate branches of posterior cerebral (see Figure 5–38)
Posterior Limb of **IC**	lateral striate branches of middle cerebral (see Figure 5–38)

Posterior Column-Medial Lemniscus System

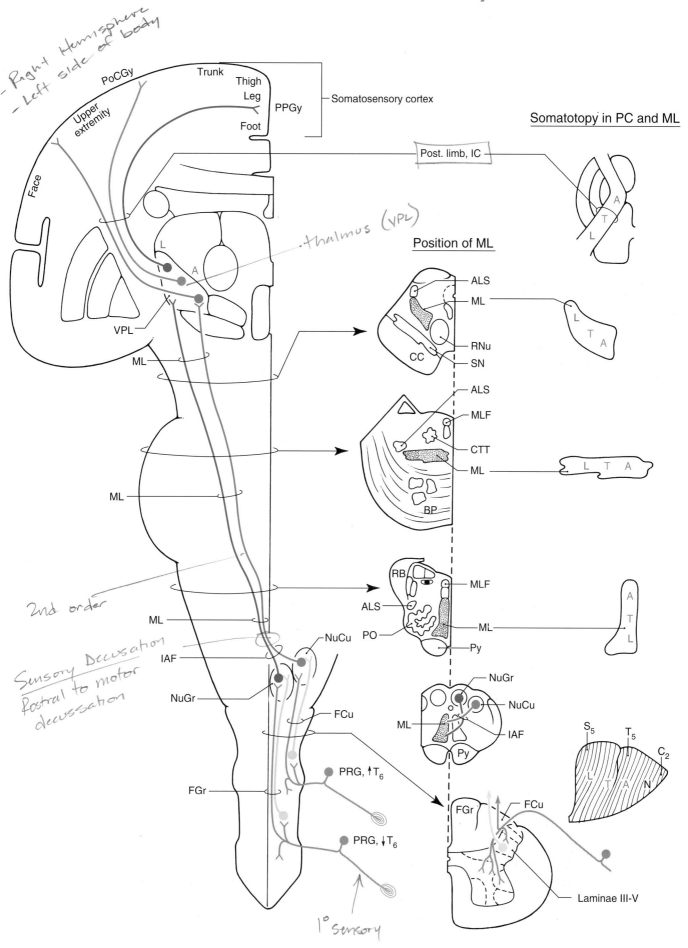

- Right Hemisphere
- Left side of body

PoCGy

Trunk

Thigh

Leg

Foot

Upper extremity

Face

PPGy

Somatosensory cortex

Somatotopy in PC and ML

Post. limb, IC

Position of ML

thalmus (VPL)

VPL

L

A

ML

ALS

ML

RNu

SN

CC

ALS

MLF

CTT

ML

BP

2nd order

RB

MLF

ALS

ML

PO

Py

NuCu

IAF

NuGr

Sensory Decussation
Rostral to motor decussation

ML

FCu

NuGr

NuCu

ML

IAF

Py

PRG, ↑T₆

FGr

PRG, ↓T₆

S₅   T₅   C₂

L   T   A   N

FGr

FCu

Laminae III-V

1° sensory

Anterolateral System

7–5 The longitudinal extent and somatotopy of fibers composing the anterolateral system (ALS). The ALS is a composite bundle containing ascending fibers that terminate in the reticular formation (spinoreticular fibers), the mesencephalon (spinotectal fibers to deep layers of the superior colliculus, spinoperiaqueductal fibers to the periaqueductal grey), the hypothalamus (spinohypothalamic fibers), and the sensory relay nuclei of the dorsal thalamus (spinothalamic fibers). Other fibers in the ALS include spinoolivary projections to the accessory olivary nuclei. Spinothalamic fibers terminate primarily in the VPL and reticulothalamic fibers terminate in some intralaminar nuclei, and in medial areas of the posterior thalamic complex.

Fibers from the PAG and nucleus raphe dorsalis enter the nucleus raphe magnus and adjacent reticular area. These latter sites, in turn, project to laminae I, II, and V of the spinal cord via raphespinal and reticulospinal fibers that participate in the modulation of pain transmission in the spinal cord.

Neurotransmitters: Glutamate (+), calcitonin gene-related peptide, and substance P(+)-containing posterior (dorsal) root ganglion cells project into laminae I, II (heavy), V (moderate), and III, IV (sparse). Some spinoreticular and spinothalamic fibers contain enkephalin (−), somatostatin (−), and cholecystokinin (+). In addition to enkephalin and somatostatin, some spinomesencephalic fibers contain vasoactive intestinal polypeptide (+). Neurons in the PAG and nucleus raphe dorsalis containing serotonin and neurotensin project into the nuclei raphe magnus and adjacent reticular formation. Cells in these latter centers that contain serotonin and enkephalin send processes to spinal cord laminae I, II, and V. Serotonergic raphespinal or enkephalinergic reticulospinal fibers may inhibit primary sensory fibers or projection neurons, conveying nociceptive (pain) information.

Clinical Correlations: Spinal lesions involving the anterolateral system (as in the *Brown-Sequard syndrome*) result in a loss of pain and temperature sensations on the contralateral side of the body beginning one to two levels caudal to the lesion. *Syringomyelia* produces bilateral sensory losses restricted to adjacent dermatomes because of damage to the anterior (ventral) white commissure. Vascular lesions in the spinal cord (such as *acute central cervical cord syndrome*) may result in a bilateral and splotchy loss of pain and thermal sense below the lesion because the ALS has a dual vascular supply.

Vascular lesions in the lateral medulla *(posterior inferior cerebellar artery syndrome)* or lateral pons (anterior inferior cerebellar artery occlusion) result in a loss of pain and thermal sensations over the entire contralateral side of the body (ALS) as well as on the ipsilateral face (spinal trigeminal tract and nucleus), coupled with other motor and/or sensory deficits based on damage to structures these vessels serve. Note that the ALS and PC-ML systems are separated in the medulla (in different vascular territories) but are adjacent to each other in the midbrain (basically in the same vascular territory). Consequently, medullary lesions will not result in deficits related to both pathways, while a lesion in the midbrain may result in a contralateral loss of pain, thermal, vibratory, and discriminative touch sensations on the body, excluding the head.

Profound loss of posterior column and anterolateral system modalities, or *intractable pain* and/or *paresthesias* (as in the *thalamic syndrome*), may result from vascular lesions in the posterolateral thalamus. So-called thalamic pain may also be experienced by patients who have brainstem lesions.

Abbreviations

A	Input from upper extremity regions	**PRG**	Posterior (dorsal) root ganglion
ALS	Anterolateral system	**Py**	Pyramid
AWCom	Anterior (ventral) white commissure	**RaSp**	Raphespinal fibers
CC	Crus cerebri	**RB**	Restiform body
IC	Internal capsule	**RetF**	Reticular formation (of midbrain)
L	Input from lower extremity regions	**RetTh**	Reticulothalamic fibers
MCP	Middle cerebellar peduncle	**RNu**	Red nucleus
ML	Medial lemniscus	**S**	Input from sacral regions
MLF	Medial longitudinal fasciculus	**SC**	Superior colliculus
Nu	Nuclei	**SpRet**	Spinoreticular fibers
NuDark	Nucleus of Darkschewitsch	**SpTec**	Spinotectal fibers
NuRa,d	Nucleus raphe, dorsalis	**SpTh**	Spinothalamic fibers
NuRa,m	Nucleus raphe, magnus	**T**	Input from thoracic regions
PAG	Periaqueductal gray	**VPL**	Ventral posterolateral nucleus of thalamus
PoCGy	Postcentral gyrus	**I-VIII**	Laminae I-VIII of Rexed
PPGy	Posterior paracentral gyrus		

Review of Blood Supply to ALS

STRUCTURES	ARTERIES
ALS in Spinal Cord	penetrating branches of arterial vasocorona and branches of central (see Figures 5–6 and 5–14)
ALS in Medulla	caudal third, vertebral; rostral two-thirds, posterior inferior cerebellar (see Figure 5–14)
ALS in Pons	long circumferential branches of basilar (see Figure 5–21)
ALS in Midbrain	short circumferential branches of posterior cerebral, superior cerebellar (see Figure 5–27)
VPL	thalamogeniculate branches of posterior cerebral (see Figure 5–38)
Posterior Limb of **IC**	lateral striate branches of middle cerebral (see Figure 5–38)

Anterolateral System

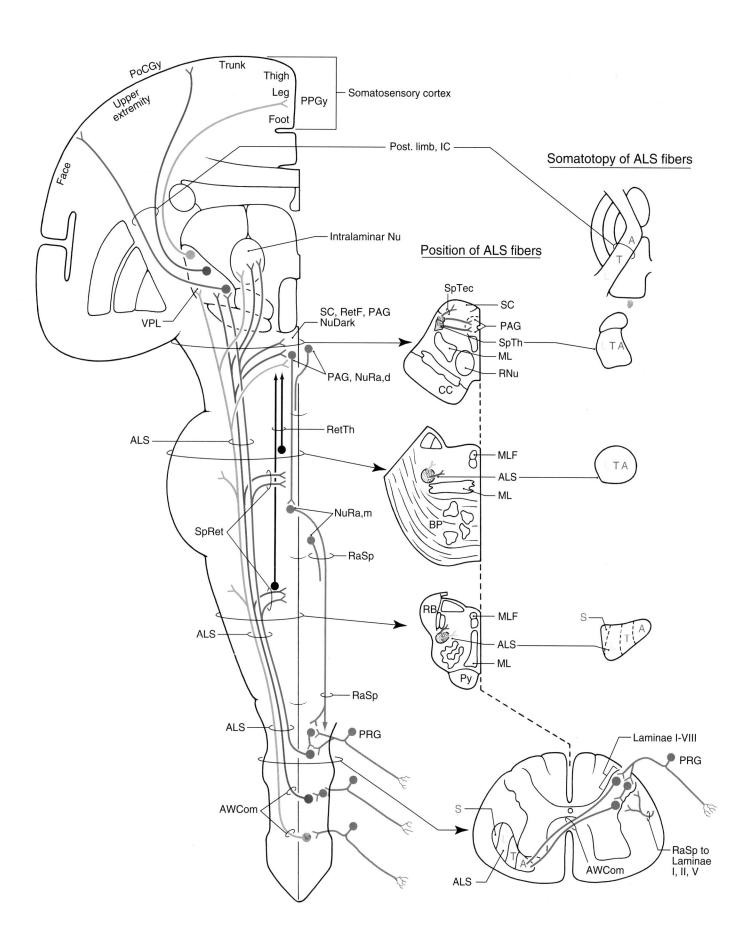

Somatosensory cortex

PoCGy
Trunk
Thigh
Leg
Foot
PPGy
Upper extremity
Face
VPL

Post. limb, IC

Somatotopy of ALS fibers

Intralaminar Nu

Position of ALS fibers

SC, RetF, PAG
NuDark

PAG, NuRa,d

SpTec
SC
PAG
SpTh
ML
RNu
CC

ALS

RetTh

MLF
ALS
ML
BP

SpRet

NuRa,m

RaSp

ALS

RB
MLF
ALS
ML
Py

RaSp

ALS

PRG

Laminae I-VIII
PRG

AWCom

S

RaSp to Laminae I, II, V

AWCom

ALS

Postsynaptic-Posterior (Dorsal) Column System and the Spinocervicothalamic Pathway

7-6 The origin, course, and distribution of fibers composing the postsynaptic-posterior column system (upper) and the spinocervicothalamic pathway (lower). Postsynaptic-posterior column fibers originate primarily from cells in lamina IV (some cells in laminae III and V-II also contribute), ascend in the ipsilateral dorsal fasciculi, and end in their respective nuclei in the caudal medulla. Moderate-to-sparse collaterals project to a few other medullary targets.

Fibers of the spinocervical part of the spinocervicothalamic pathway also originate from cells in lamina IV (less so from III and V). The axons of these cells ascend in the posterior part of the lateral funiculus (this is sometimes called the dorsolateral funiculus) and end in a topographic fashion in the lateral cervical nucleus: lumbosacral projections terminate posterolaterally and cervical projections anteromedially. Cells of the posterior column nuclei and the lateral cervical nucleus convey information to the contralateral thalamus via the medial lemniscus.

Neurotransmitters: Glutamate (+) and possibly substance P (+) are present in some spinocervical projections. Because some cells in laminae III-V have axons that collateralize to both the lateral cervi-cal nucleus *and* the dorsal column nuclei, glutamate (and substance P) may also be present in some postsynaptic dorsal column fibers.

Clinical Correlations: The postsynaptic-posterior column and spinocervicothalamic pathways are not known to be major circuits in the human nervous system. However, the occurrence of these fibers may explain a well known clinical observation. Patients that have received an *anterolateral cordotomy* (this lesion is placed just ventral to the denticulate ligament) for *intractable pain* may experience complete or partial relief, or there may be a recurrence of pain perception within days or weeks. Although the cordotomy transects fibers of the antero-lateral system (the main pain pathway), this lesion spares the posterior horn, posterior columns, and spinocervical fibers. Consequently, the recurrence of pain perception (or even the partial relief of pain) in these patients may be explained by these postsynaptic-dorsal column and spinocervicothalamic projections. Through these connections, some nociceptive (pain) information may be transmitted to the ventral posterolateral nucleus and on to the sensory cortex, via circuits that by-pass the anterolateral system and are spared in a cordotomy.

Abbreviations

ALS	Anterolateral system
AWCom	Anterior (ventral) white commissure
FCu	Cuneate fasciculus
FGr	Gracile fasciculus
IAF	Internal arcuate fibers
LCerNu	Lateral cervical nucleus
ML	Medial lemniscus
NuCu	Cuneate nucleus
NuGr	Gracile nucleus
PRG	Posterior (dorsal) root ganglion

Review of Blood Supply to Dorsal Horn, FGr, FCu, LCerNu

STRUCTURES	ARTERIES
FGr, FCu in Spinal Cord	penetrating branches of arterial vasocorona and some branches from central (sulcal) (see Figure 5–6)
LCerNu	penetrating branches of arterial vasocorona and branches from central (see Figure 5–6)
NuGr NuCu	posterior spinal (see Figure 5–14)

Postsynaptic-Posterior (Dorsal) Column System and the Spinocervicothalamic Pathway

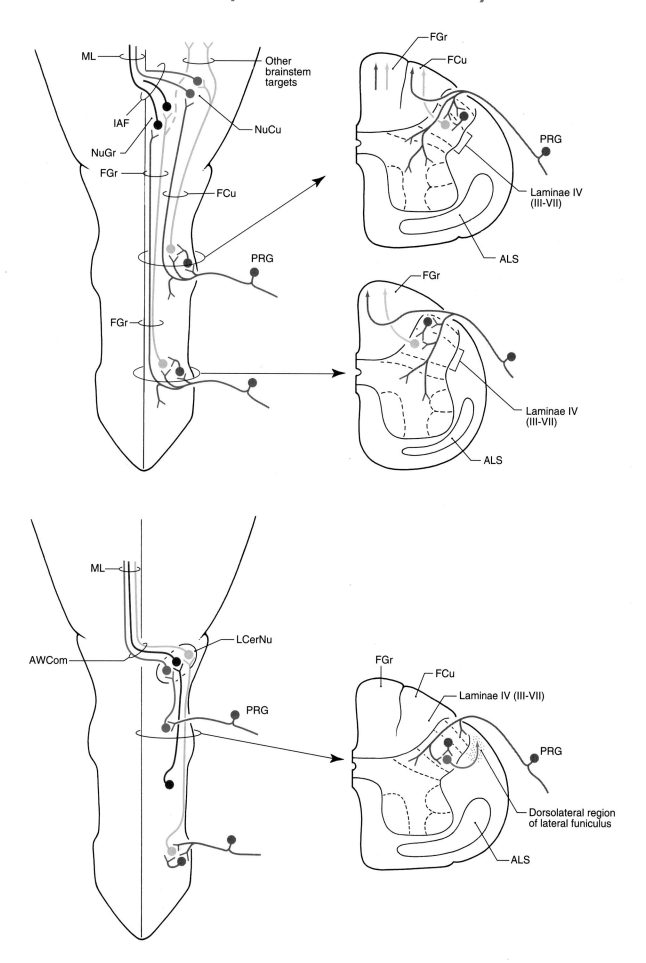

Trigeminal Pathways

7–7 The distribution of general sensory (GSA) information originating on cranial nerves V (trigeminal), VII (facial), IX (glossopharyngeal), and X (vagus). Some of these primary sensory fibers end in the chief sensory nucleus, but most form the spinal trigeminal tract and end in the spinal trigeminal nucleus.

Neurons in the spinal trigeminal nucleus and in ventral parts of the chief sensory nucleus give rise to crossed anterior (ventral) trigeminothalamic fibers. Collaterals of these ascending fibers influence the hypoglossal, facial (*corneal reflex, supraorbital,* or *trigeminofacial reflex*), and trigeminal motor nuclei; mesencephalic collaterals are involved in the *jaw reflex,* also called the *jaw-jerk reflex.* Collaterals also enter the dorsal motor vagal nucleus (*vomiting reflex*), the superior salivatory nucleus (*tearing/lacrimal reflex*), and the nucleus ambiguus and adjacent reticular formation (*sneezing reflex*). Uncrossed posterior (dorsal) trigeminothalamic fibers arise from posterior regions of the chief sensory nucleus.

Neurotransmitters: Substance P (+)-containing and cholecystokinin (+)-containing trigeminal ganglion cells project to the spinal trigeminal nucleus, especially its caudal part (pars caudalis). Glutamate (+) is found in many trigeminothalamic fibers arising from the chief sensory nucleus and the pars interpolaris of the spinal nucleus. It is present in fewer trigeminothalamic fibers from the pars caudalis and in almost none from the pars oralis. The locus ceruleus (noradrenergic fibers) and the raphe nuclei (serotonergic fibers) also project to the spinal nucleus. Enkephalin (−)-containing cells are present in caudal regions of the spinal nucleus, and enkephalinergic fibers are found in the nucleus ambiguus and in the hypoglossal, facial, and trigeminal motor nuclei.

Clinical Correlations: Lesions of the trigeminal ganglion or nerve proximal to the ganglion result in 1) a loss of pain, temperature, and tactile sensation from the ipsilateral face, oral cavity, and teeth; 2) ipsilateral paralysis of masticatory muscles; and 3) ipsilateral loss of the corneal reflex. Damage to peripheral portions of the trigeminal nerve may be traumatic (skull fracture, especially of supraorbital and infraorbital branch), inflammatory (as in *herpes zoster*), or result from tumor growth. The deficit would reflect the peripheral portion of the trigeminal nerve damaged.

Trigeminal neuralgia (tic douloureux) is a severe burning pain restricted to the peripheral distribution of the trigeminal nerve, usually its V_2 (maxillary) division. This pain may be initiated by any contact to areas of the face such as the corner of the mouth, nose, lips, or cheek (e.g., shaving, putting make-up on, chewing, or even smiling). The attacks frequently occur without warning, may happen only a few times a month to many times in a single day, and are usually seen in patients 40 years of age or older. One probable cause of trigeminal neuralgia is compression of the trigeminal root by aberrant vessels, most commonly a loop of the superior cerebellar artery (see page 41). Other causes may include tumor, *multiple sclerosis,* and ephaptic transmission (*ephapse*) in the trigeminal ganglion. This is the most common type of neuralgia.

In the medulla, fibers of the spinal trigeminal tract and ALS are served by the posterior inferior cerebellar artery (PICA). Consequently, an *alternating hemianesthesia* is one characteristic feature of the *PICA syndrome.* This is a loss of pain and thermal sensations on one side of the body and the opposite side of the face. Pontine gliomas may produce a paralysis of masticatory muscles (motor trigeminal damage) and some loss of tactile input (chief sensory nucleus damage), as well as other deficits based on what adjacent structures may be involved.

Abbreviations

ALS	Anterolateral system	**OpthV**	Ophthalmic division of trigeminal nerve	**VPM**	Ventral posteromedial nucleus of thalamus
CC	Crus cerebri				
DTTr	Dorsal trigeminothalamic tract	**PSNu**	Principal (chief) sensory nucleus	**VTTr**	Ventral trigeminothalamic tract
FacNu	Facial nucleus				
GSA	General somatic afferent	**RB**	Restiform body		
HyNu	Hypoglossal nucleus	**RetF**	Reticular formation		**Ganglia**
IC	Internal capsule	**RNu**	Red nucleus	**1**	Trigeminal ganglion
ManV	Mandibular division of trigeminal nerve	**SpTNu**	Spinal trigeminal nucleus	**2**	Geniculate ganglion
		SpTTr	Spinal trigeminal tract	**3**	Superior of glossopharyngeal
MaxV	Maxillary division of trigeminal nerve	**TriMoNu**	Trigeminal motor nucleus	**4**	Superior of vagus
		TMJ	Temporomandibular joint		
MesNu	Mesencephalic nucleus	**VPL**	Ventral posterolateral nucleus of thalamus		
ML	Medial lemniscus				

Review of Blood Supply to SpTT, SpTNu, and Trigeminothalamic Tracts

STRUCTURES	ARTERIES
SpTTr and **SpTNu** in Medulla	caudal third, vertebral; rostral two-thirds, posterior inferior cerebellar (see Figure 5–14)
SpTTr and **SpTNu** in Pons	long circumferential branches of basilar (see Figure 5–21)
Trigeminothalamic Fibers in Midbrain	short circumferential branches of posterior cerebral and superior cerebellar (see Figure 5–27)
VPM	thalamogeniculate branches of posterior cerebral (see Figure 5–38)
Posterior Limb of **IC**	lateral striate branches of middle cerebral (see Figure 5–38)

Trigeminal Pathways

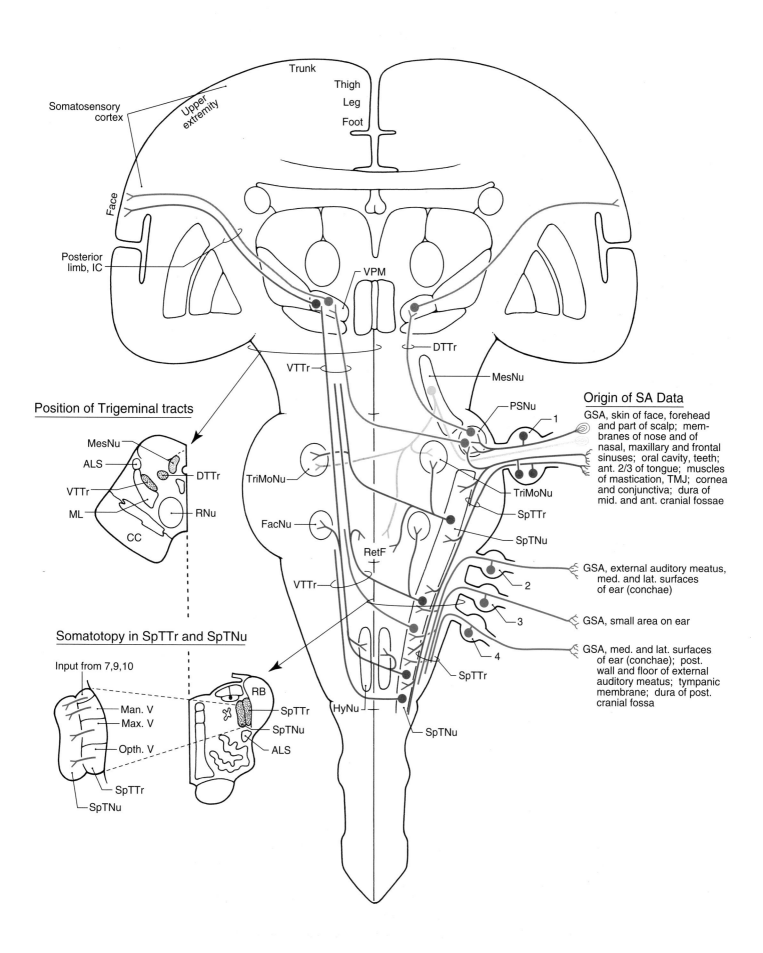

Somatosensory cortex
Face
Trunk
Thigh
Leg
Foot
Upper extremity
Posterior limb, IC
VPM
DTTr
VTTr
MesNu

Position of Trigeminal tracts

MesNu
ALS
VTTr
ML
DTTr
RNu
CC

Somatotopy in SpTTr and SpTNu

Input from 7,9,10
Man. V
Max. V
Opth. V
SpTTr
SpTNu
RB
SpTTr
SpTNu
ALS

TriMoNu
FacNu
RetF
VTTr
HyNu
PSNu
TriMoNu
SpTTr
SpTNu
SpTTr
SpTNu

Origin of SA Data

GSA, skin of face, forehead and part of scalp; membranes of nose and of nasal, maxillary and frontal sinuses; oral cavity, teeth; ant. 2/3 of tongue; muscles of mastication, TMJ; cornea and conjunctiva; dura of mid. and ant. cranial fossae

GSA, external auditory meatus, med. and lat. surfaces of ear (conchae)

GSA, small area on ear

GSA, med. and lat. surfaces of ear (conchae); post. wall and floor of external auditory meatus; tympanic membrane; dura of post. cranial fossa

1
2
3
4

Solitary Pathways

7–8 Visceral afferent input (SVA-taste; GVA general visceral sensation) on cranial nerves VII (facial), IX (glossopharyngeal), and X (vagus) enters the solitary nuclei via the solitary tract. What we commonly call the solitary "nucleus" is actually a series of small nuclei that collectively form this rostrocaudal-oriented cell column.

Solitary cells project to the salivatory, hypoglossal, and dorsal motor vagal nuclei and the nucleus ambiguus. Solitary projections to the nucleus ambiguus are largely bilateral and are the intermediate neurons in the pathway for the *gag reflex*. The afferent limb of the *gag-reflex* is carried on the glossopharyngeal nerve, and the efferent limb originates from the nucleus ambiguus. In this respect, the efferent limb travels on both the glossopharyngeal and vagus nerves. Although not routinely tested, the *gag-reflex* should be evaluated in patients with *dysarthria, dysphagia,* or *hoarseness*. Solitariospinal fibers are bilateral with a contralateral preponderance and project to the phrenic nucleus, the intermediolateral cell column, and the ventral horn. The VPM is the thalamic center through which visceral afferent information is relayed onto the cerebral cortex.

Neurotransmitters: Substance P (+)-containing and cholecystokinin (+)-containing cells in the geniculate ganglion (facial nerve) and in the inferior ganglia of the glossopharyngeal and vagus nerves project to the solitary nucleus. Enkephalin (−), neurotensin, and GABA (+) are present in some solitary neurons that project into the adjacent dorsal motor vagal nucleus. Cholecystokinin (+), somatostatin (−), and enkephalin (−) are present in solitary neurons, in cells of the parabrachial nuclei, and in some thalamic neurons that project to taste, and other visceral areas, of the cortex.

Clinical Correlations: Lesions of the geniculate ganglion, or facial nerve proximal to the ganglion, result in 1) ipsilateral loss of taste *(ageusia)* from the anterior two-thirds of the tongue and 2) an ipsilateral *facial (Bell) palsy*. Although a glossopharyngeal nerve lesion will result in *ageusia* from the posterior third of the tongue on the ipsilateral side, this loss is difficult to test. On the other hand, *glossopharyngeal neuralgia* is an idiopathic pain localized to the peripheral sensory branches of the IXth nerve in the posterior pharynx, posterior tongue, and tonsillar area. Although comparatively rare, glossopharyngeal neuralgia may be aggravated by talking or even swallowing. Occlusion of the posterior inferior cerebellar artery (as in the *posterior inferior cerebellar artery* or *lateral medullary syndrome),* in addition to producing an *alternate hemianesthesia,* will also result in *ageusia* from the ipsilateral side of the tongue because the posterior inferior cerebellar artery serves the solitary tract and nuclei in the medulla.

Interestingly, lesions of the olfactory nerves or tract (*anosmia,* loss of olfactory sensation; *dysosmia,* distorted olfactory sense) may affect how the patient perceives taste. Witness the fact that the nasal congestion accompanying a severe cold will markedly affect the sense of taste.

Abbreviations

AmyNu	Amygdaloid nucleus (complex)	**SalNu**	Salivatory nuclei
CardResp	Cardiorespiratory portion (caudal) of solitary nucleus	**SolTr & Nu**	Solitary tract and nuclei
		SVA	Special visceral afferent
GustNu	Gustatory nucleus (rostral portion of solitary nucleus)	**Tr**	Tract
		VA	Visceral afferent
GVA	General visceral afferent	**VPM**	Ventral posteromedial nucleus of thalamus
HyNu	Hypoglossal nucleus		
HyTh	Hypothalamus		
InfVNu	Inferior (or spinal) vestibular nucleus		

Number Key

MVNu	Medial vestibular nucleus
NuAm	Nucleus ambiguus
PBNu	Parabrachial nuclei
RB	Restiform body

1	Geniculate ganglion of facial
2	Inferior ganglion of glossopharyngeal
3	Inferior ganglion of vagus
4	Dorsal motor vagal nucleus

Review of Blood Supply to SolNu and SolTr

STRUCTURES	ARTERIES
SolNu and **Tr** in inferior cerebellar	caudal medulla, anterior spinal; rostral medulla, posterior inferior cerebellar (See Figure 5–14)
Ascending Fibers in Pons	long circumferential branches of basilar and branches of superior cerebellar (see Figure 5–21)
VPM	thalamogeniculate branches of posterior cerebral (see Figure 5–38)
Posterior Limb of **IC**	lateral striate branches of middle cerebral (see Figure 5–38)

Solitary Pathways

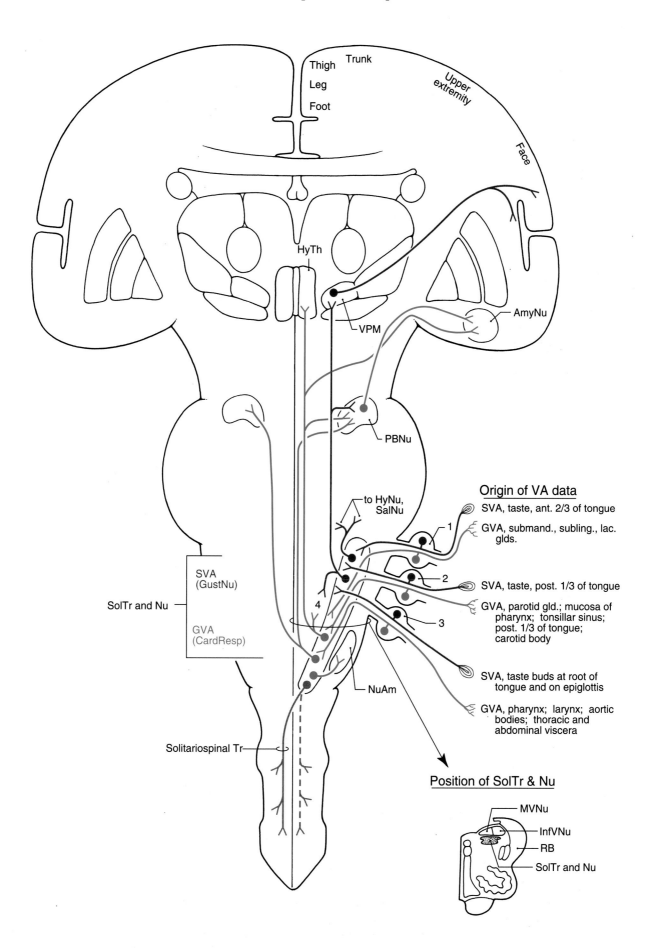

Thigh Trunk

Leg

Foot

Upper extremity

Face

HyTh

VPM

AmyNu

PBNu

to HyNu, SalNu

SVA (GustNu)

SolTr and Nu

GVA (CardResp)

NuAm

Solitariospinal Tr

Origin of VA data

SVA, taste, ant. 2/3 of tongue

GVA, submand., subling., lac. glds.

SVA, taste, post. 1/3 of tongue

GVA, parotid gld.; mucosa of pharynx; tonsillar sinus; post. 1/3 of tongue; carotid body

SVA, taste buds at root of tongue and on epiglottis

GVA, pharynx; larynx; aortic bodies; thoracic and abdominal viscera

1

2

3

4

Position of SolTr & Nu

MVNu

InfVNu

RB

SolTr and Nu

7–9   Blank master drawing for sensory pathways. This illustration is provided for self-evaluation of sensory pathway understanding, for the instructor to expand on sensory pathways not covered in the atlas, or both.

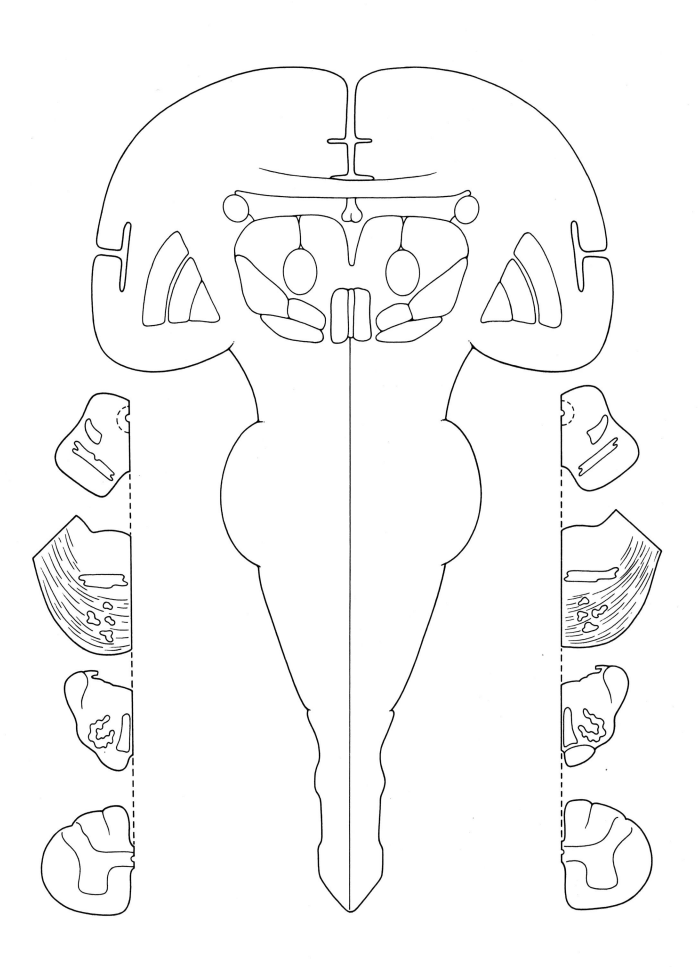

Corticospinal Tracts

7-10　The longitudinal extent of corticospinal fibers and their position and somatotopy at representative levels within the neuraxis. The somatotopy of corticospinal fibers in the basilar pons is less obvious than in the internal capsule, crus cerebri, pyramid, or spinal cord. In the decussation of the pyramids, fibers originating from upper extremity areas of the cerebral cortex cross rostral to those that arise from lower extremity areas. In addition to fibers arising from the somatomotor area of the cerebral cortex (area 4), a significant contingent also originate from the postcentral gyrus (areas 3, 1, 2); the former terminate primarily in laminae VI-IX, while the latter end mainly in laminae IV and V. Prefrontal regions, especially area 6, and parietal areas 5 and 7 also contribute to the corticospinal tract.

Neurotransmitters: Acetylcholine, gamma-aminobutyric acid (−), and substance P (+, plus other peptides) are found in small cortical neurons presumed to function as local circuit cells or in corticocortical connections. Glutamate (+) is present in cortical efferent fibers that project to the spinal cord. Glutaminergic corticospinal fibers and terminals are found in all spinal levels but are especially concentrated in cervical and lumbosacral enlargements. This correlates with the fact that approximately 55% of all corticospinal fibers terminate in cervical levels of the spinal cord, approximately 20% in thoracic levels, and approximately 25% in lumbosacral levels. Some corticospinal fibers may branch and terminate at multiple spinal levels. Lower motor neurons are influenced by corticospinal fibers either directly or indirectly via interneurons. Acetylcholine and calcitonin gene-related peptides are present in these large motor cells and in their endings in skeletal muscle.

Clinical Correlations: *Myasthenia gravis*, a disease characterized by moderate to profound weakness of skeletal muscles, is caused by circulating antibodies that react with postsynaptic nicotinic acetylcholine receptors. Progressive muscle fatigability throughout the day is a hallmark of this disease. Ocular muscles are usually affected first (*diplopia, ptosis*), and in approximately 50% of patients, facial and oropharyngeal muscles are commonly affected (*facial weakness, dysphagia, dysarthria*). Weakness may also be seen in limb muscles but almost always in combination with facial/oral weaknesses.

Injury to corticospinal fibers on one side of the cervical spinal cord (as in the *Brown-Sequard syndrome*) results in weakness (*hemiparesis*) or paralysis (*hemiplegia*) of the ipsilateral upper and lower extremities. In addition, and with time, these patients may exhibit features of an *upper motor neuron lesion (hyperreflexia, spasticity,* loss of superficial abdominal reflexes, and the *Babinski sign*). Bilateral cervical spinal cord damage above C4–C5 may result in paralysis of all four extremities (*quadriplegia*). Unilateral spinal cord lesions in thoracic levels may result in paralysis of the ipsilateral lower extremity (*monoplegia*). If the thoracic spinal cord damage is bilateral both lower extremities may be paralyzed (*paraplegia*). Small lesions within the decussation of the pyramids may result in a bilateral paresis of the upper extremities (lesion in rostral portions) or a bilateral paresis of the lower extremities (lesion in caudal portions) based on the crossing patterns of fibers within the decussation.

Rostral to the pyramidal decussation, vascular lesions in the medulla (the *medial medullary syndrome*), pons (the *Millard-Gubler or Foville syndromes*), or midbrain (the *Weber syndrome*) all produce *alternating (crossed) hemiplegias*. These present as a contralateral hemiplegia of the upper and lower extremities, coupled with an ipsilateral paralysis of the tongue (medulla), facial muscles or lateral rectus muscle (pons), and most eye movements (midbrain). Sensory deficits are frequently seen as part of these syndromes. Lesions in the internal capsule (*lacunar strokes*) produce contralateral hemiparesis sometimes coupled with various cranial nerve signs due to corticonuclear (corticobulbar) fiber involvement. Bilateral weakness, indicative of corticospinal involvement, is also present in *amyotrophic lateral sclerosis*.

Abbreviations

ACSp	Anterior corticospinal tract	**LCSp**	Lateral corticospinal tract	
ALS	Anterolateral system	**ML**	Medial lemniscus	
APGy	Anterior paracentral gyrus	**MLF**	Medial longitudinal fasciculus	
BP	Basilar pons	**PO**	Principal olivary nucleus	
CC	Crus cerebri	**PrCGy**	Precentral gyrus	
CNu	Corticonuclear (corticobulbar) fibers	**Py**	Pyramid	
		RB	Restiform body	
CSp	Corticospinal fibers	**RNu**	Red nucleus	
IC	Internal capsule	**SN**	Substantia nigra	

Somatotopy of CSp Fibers

A　Position of fibers coursing to upper extremity regions of spinal cord

L　Position of fibers coursing to lower extremity regions of spinal cord

T　Position of fibers coursing to thoracic regions of spinal cord

Review of Blood Supply to Corticospinal Fibers

STRUCTURES	ARTERIES
Posterior Limb of **IC**	lateral striate branches of middle cerebral (see Figure 5–38)
Crus Cerebri in Midbrain	paramedian and short circumferential branches of basilar and posterior communicating (see Figure 5–27)
CSp in **BP**	paramedian branches of basilar (see Figure 5–21)
Py in Medulla	anterior spinal (see Figure 5–14)
LCSp in Spinal Cord	penetrating branches of arterial vasocorona (leg fibers), branches of central artery (arm fibers) (See Figure 5–6)

Corticospinal Tracts

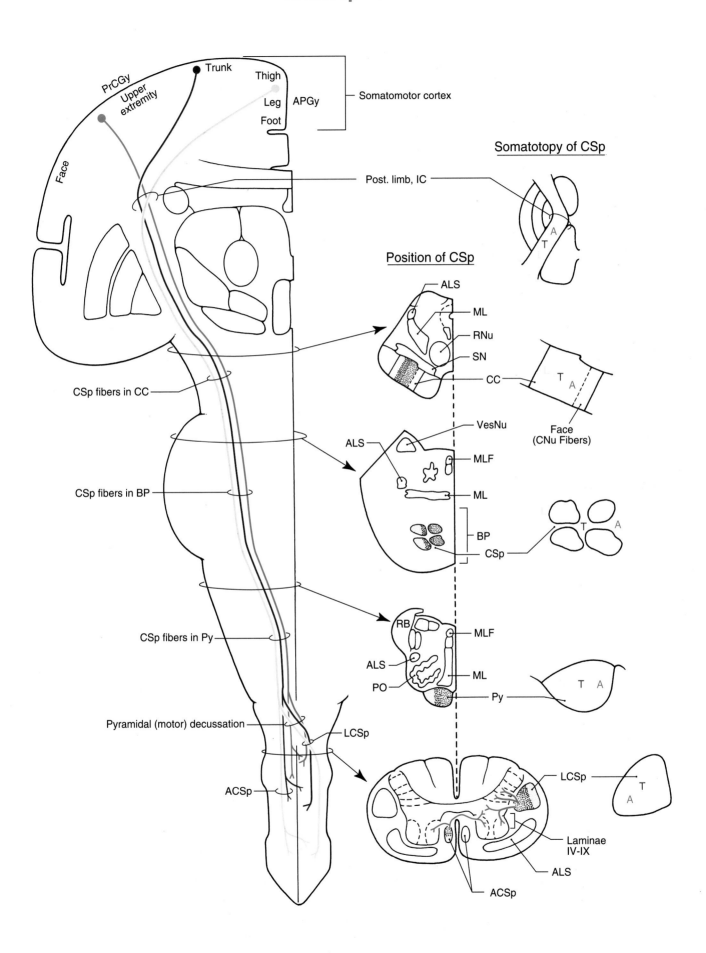

Somatomotor cortex

PrCGy

Upper extremity

Face

Trunk

Thigh

Leg

Foot

APGy

Post. limb, IC

Somatotopy of CSp

Position of CSp

ALS

ML

RNu

SN

CC

Face (CNu Fibers)

CSp fibers in CC

VesNu

ALS

MLF

ML

BP

CSp

CSp fibers in BP

RB

MLF

ALS

ML

PO

Py

CSp fibers in Py

Pyramidal (motor) decussation

LCSp

ACSp

LCSp

Laminae IV-IX

ALS

ACSp

Corticonuclear (Corticobulbar) Fibers

7-11 The origin, course, and distribution of corticonuclear (corticobulbar) fibers to brainstem motor nuclei. These fibers influence—either directly or through neurons in the immediately adjacent reticular formation—the motor nuclei of oculomotor, trochlear, trigeminal, abducens, facial, glossopharyngeal and vagus (both via nucleus ambiguus), spinal accessory, and hypoglossal nerves.

Corticonuclear (corticobulbar) fibers arise in the frontal eye fields (areas 6 and 8 in caudal portions of the middle frontal gyrus), the precentral gyrus (somatomotor cortex, area 4), and some originate from the postcentral gyrus (areas 3,1, 2). Fibers from area 4 occupy the genu of the internal capsule, but those from the frontal eye fields (areas 8,6) may traverse caudal portions of the anterior limb, and some (from areas 3,1,2), may occupy the most rostral portions of the posterior limb. Fibers that arise in areas 8 and 6 terminate in the *rostral interstitial nucleus of the medial longitudinal fasciculus (vertical gaze center)* and in the *paramedian pontine reticular formation (horizontal gaze center)*; these areas, in turn, project respectively to the IIIrd and IVth, and to the VIth nuclei. Fibers from area 4 terminate in, or adjacent to, cranial nerve motor nuclei excluding those of III, IV, and VI.

Although not illustrated here, the superior colliculus receives cortical input from area 8 and from the parietal eye field (area 7) and also projects to the riMLF and PPRF. In addition, it is important to note that descending cortical fibers (many arising in areas 3, 1, 2) project to sensory relay nuclei of some cranial nerves and to other sensory relay nuclei in the brainstem, such as those of the posterior column system.

Neurotransmitters: Glutamate ($+$) is found in many corticofugal axons that directly innervate cranial nerve motor nuclei and in those fibers that terminate near (indirect), but not in, the various motor nuclei.

Clinical Correlations: Lesions involving the motor cortex (as in cerebral artery occlusion) or the internal capsule (as in *lacunar strokes* or occlusion of lenticulostriate branches of M_1) give rise to a contralateral *hemiplegia* of the arm and leg (corticospinal fiber involvement) coupled with certain cranial nerve signs. Strictly cortical lesions may produce a transient *gaze palsy* in which the eyes deviate toward the lesioned side and away from the side of the hemiplegia. In addition to a contralateral *hemiplegia,* common cranial nerve findings in capsular lesions may include 1) deviation of the tongue toward the side of the weakness and away from the side of the lesion when protruded and 2) paralysis of facial muscles on the contralateral lower half of the face *(central facial palsy).* This reflects the fact that corticonuclear (corticobulbar) fibers to genioglossus motor neurons and to facial motor neurons serving the lower face are primarily crossed. Interruption of corticonuclear fibers to the nucleus ambiguus may result in weakness of palatal muscles contralateral to the lesion; the uvula will deviate towards the ipsilateral (lesioned) side on attempted phonation. In addition, a lesion involving corticonuclear fibers to the accessory nucleus may result in drooping of the ipsilateral shoulder (or an inability to elevate the shoulder against resistance) due to trapezius weakness, and difficulty in turning the head (against resistance) to the contralateral side due to weakness of the sternocleidomastoid muscle. In contrast to the *alternating hemiplegia* seen in some brainstem lesions, hemisphere lesions result in spinal and cranial nerve deficits that are generally, but not exclusively, contralateral to the cerebral injury.

Brainstem lesions, especially in the midbrain or pons, may result in the following: 1) *vertical gaze palsies* (midbrain), 2) the *Parinaud syndrome*—paralysis of upward gaze (tumors in area of pineal), 3) *internuclear ophthalmoplegia* (lesion in MLF between motor nuclei of III and VI), 4) *horizontal gaze palsies* (lesion in PPRF), or 5) *the one-and-a-half syndrome.* In the latter case, the lesion is adjacent to the midline and involves the abducens nucleus and adjacent PPRF, internuclear fibers from the ipsilateral abducens that are crossing to enter the contralateral MLF, and internuclear fibers from the contralateral abducens nucleus that cross to enter the MLF on the ipsilateral (lesioned) side. The result is a loss of ipsilateral abduction (lateral rectus) and adduction (medial rectus, the "one") and a contralateral loss of adduction (medial rectus, the "half"); the only remaining horizontal movement is contralateral abduction via the intact abducens motor neurons.

Abbreviations

AbdNu	Abducens nucleus	**OcNu**	Oculomotor nucleus
AccNu	Accessory nucleus (spinal accessory nu.)	**PPRF**	Paramedian pontine reticular formation
FacNu	Facial nucleus	**riMLF**	Rostral interstitial nucleus of the medial longitudinal fasciculus
HyNu	Hypoglossal nucleus		
IC	Internal capsule	**TriMoNu**	Trigeminal motor nucleus
NuAm	Nucleus ambiguus	**TroNu**	Trochlear nucleus

Review of Blood Supply to Cranial Nerve Motor Nuclei

STRUCTURES	ARTERIES
OcNu and **EWNu**	paramedian branches of basilar bifurcation and medial branches of posterior cerebral and posterior communicating (see Figure 5–27)
TriMoNu	long circumferential branches of basilar (see Figure 5–21)
AbdNu and **FacNu**	long circumferential branches of basilar (see Figure 5–21)
NuAm	posterior inferior cerebellar (see Figure 5–14)
HyNu	anterior spinal (see Figure 5–14)

Corticonuclear (Corticobulbar) Fibers

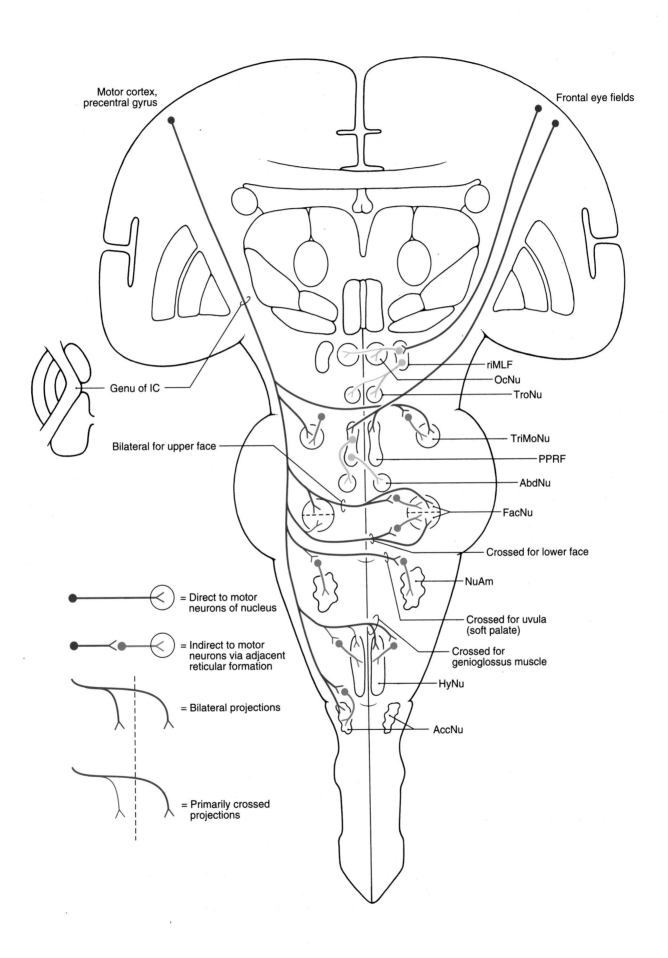

Motor cortex, precentral gyrus

Frontal eye fields

Genu of IC

Bilateral for upper face

riMLF
OcNu
TroNu

TriMoNu
PPRF
AbdNu
FacNu

Crossed for lower face

NuAm

Crossed for uvula (soft palate)

Crossed for genioglossus muscle

HyNu

AccNu

= Direct to motor neurons of nucleus

= Indirect to motor neurons via adjacent reticular formation

= Bilateral projections

= Primarily crossed projections

Tectospinal and Reticulospinal Tracts

7–12　The origin, course, position in representative cross-sections of brainstem and spinal cord, and the general distribution of tectospinal and reticulospinal tracts. Tectospinal fibers originate from deeper layers of the superior colliculus, cross in the posterior (dorsal) tegmental decussation, and distribute to cervical cord levels. Several regions of cerebral cortex (e.g., frontal, parietal, temporal) project to the tectum, but the most highly organized corticotectal projections arise from the visual cortex. Pontoreticulospinal fibers (medial reticulospinal) tend to be uncrossed, while those from the medulla (bulboreticulospinal or lateral reticulospinal) are bilateral but with a pronounced ipsilateral preponderance. Corticoreticular fibers are bilateral with a slight contralateral preponderance and originate from several cortical areas.

Neurotransmitters: Corticotectal projections, especially those from the visual cortex, utilize glutamate (+). This substance is also present in most corticoreticular fibers. Some neurons of the gigantocellular reticular nucleus that send their axons to the spinal cord, as reticulospinal projections, contain enkephalin (−) and substance P (+). Enkephalinergic reticulospinal fibers may be part of the descending system that modulates pain transmission at the spinal level. Many reticulospinal fibers influence the activity of lower motor neurons.

Clinical Correlations: Isolated lesions of only tectospinal and reticulospinal fibers are essentially never seen. Tectospinal fibers project to upper cervical levels where they influence reflex movement of the head and neck. Such movements may be diminished or slowed in patients with damage to these fibers. Pontoreticulospinal (medial reticulospinal) fibers are excitatory to extensor motor neurons and to neurons innervating axial musculature; some of these fibers may also inhibit flexor motor neurons. In contrast, some bulboreticulospinal (lateral reticulospinal) fibers are primarily inhibitory to extensor motor neurons and to neurons innervating muscles of the neck and back; these fibers may also excite flexor motor neurons via interneurons. Reticulospinal (and vestibulospinal) fibers contribute to the *spasticity* that develops in patients having lesions of corticospinal fibers. These reticulospinal and vestibulospinal fibers (see Figure 7-13 on page 196) also contribute to the tonic extension of the arms and legs seen in *decerebrate rigidity* when spinal motor neurons are released from descending cortical control.

Abbreviations

ALS	Anterolateral system	**PO**	Principal olivary nucleus
ATegDec	Anterior tegmental decussation (rubrospinal fibers)	**PTegDec**	Posterior tegmental decussation (tectospinal fibers)
BP	Basilar pons	**Py**	Pyramid
CC	Crus cerebri	**RB**	Restiform body
CRet	Corticoreticular fibers	**RetNu**	Reticular nuclei
CTec	Corticotectal fibers	**RetSp**	Reticulospinal tract(s)
GigRetNu	Gigantocellular reticular nucleus	**RNu**	Red nucleus
LCSp	Lateral corticospinal tract	**RuSp**	Rubrospinal tract
ML	Medial lemniscus	**SC**	Superior colliculus
MLF	Medial longitudinal fasciculus	**SN**	Substantia nigra
MVNu	Medial vestibular nucleus	**SpVNu**	Spinal (or inferior) vestibular nucleus
OcNu	Oculomotor nucleus	**TecSp**	Tectospinal tract

Review of Blood Supply to SC, Reticular Formation of Pons and Medulla, and TecSp and RetSp Tracts in Cord

STRUCTURES	ARTERIES
SC	long circumferential branches (quadrigeminal branch) of posterior cerebral plus some from superior cerebellar and posterior choroidal (see Figure 5–27)
Pontine Reticular Formation	long circumferential branches of basilar plus branches of superior cerebellar in rostral pons (see Figure 5–21)
Medullary Recticular Formation	branches of vertebral plus paramedian branches of basilar at medulla-pons junction (see Figure 5–14)
TecSp and **RetSp**	branches of central artery (TecSp and Medullary RetSp); Tracts penetrating branches of arterial vasocorona (Pontine RetSp) (see Figures 5–14 and 5–6)

Tectospinal and Reticulospinal Tracts

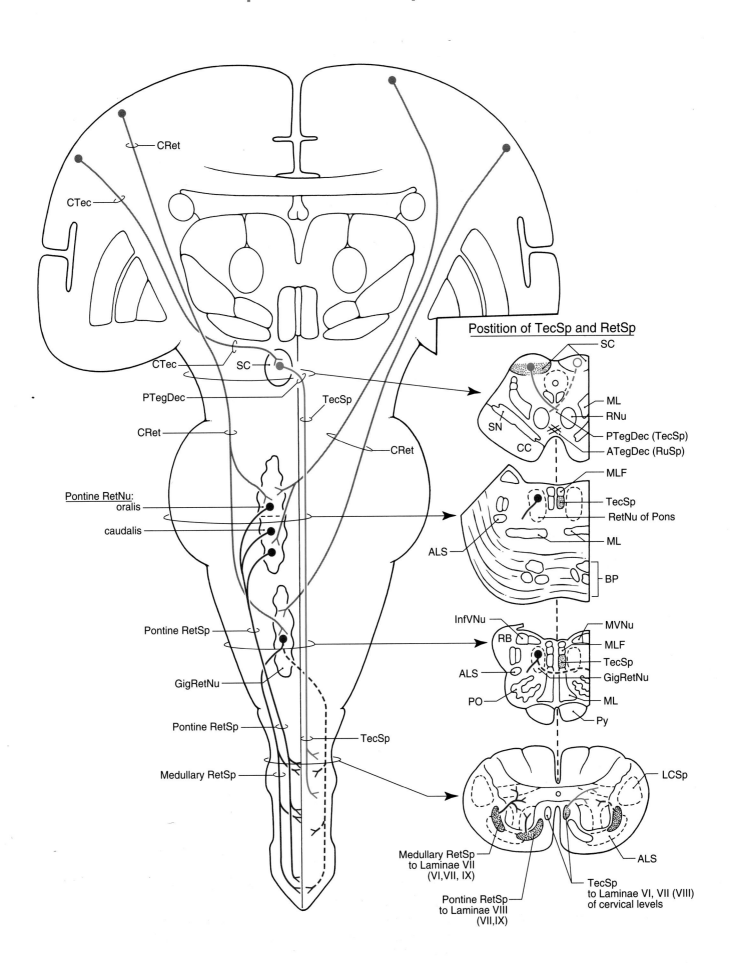

Postition of TecSp and RetSp

Rubrospinal and Vestibulospinal Tracts

7-13   The origin, course, and position in representative cross-sections of brainstem and spinal cord, and the general distribution of rubrospinal and vestibulospinal tracts. Rubrospinal fibers cross in the anterior (ventral) tegmental decussation and distribute to all spinal levels although projections to cervical levels clearly predominate. Cells in dorsomedial regions of the red nucleus receive input from upper extremity areas of the motor cortex and project to cervical cord, but those in ventrolateral areas of the nucleus receive some fibers from lower extremity areas of the motor cortex and may project in sparse numbers to lumbosacral levels. The red nucleus also projects, via the central tegmental tract, to the ipsilateral inferior olivary complex (rubroolivary fibers).

Medial and lateral vestibular nuclei give rise to the medial and lateral vestibulospinal tracts, respectively. The former tract is primarily ipsilateral, projects to upper spinal levels, and is considered a component of the medial longitudinal fasciculus in the spinal cord. The latter tract is ipsilateral and somatotopically organized; fibers to lumbosacral levels originate from dorsal and caudal regions of the lateral nucleus, while those to cervical levels arise from its rostral and more ventral areas.

Neurotransmitters: Glutamate (+) is present in corticorubral fibers. Some lateral vestibulospinal fibers contain aspartate (+), whereas glycine (−) is present in a portion of the medial vestibulospinal projection. There are numerous gamma-aminobutyric acid (−)-containing fibers in the vestibular complex; these represent the endings of cerebellar corticovestibular fibers.

Clinical Correlations: Isolated injury to rubrospinal and vestibulospinal fibers is really not seen in humans. Deficits in fine distal limb movements seen in monkeys following experimental rubrospinal lesions may be present in humans. However, these deficits are overshadowed by the *hemiplegia* associated with injury to the adjacent corticospinal fibers. The contralateral tremor seen in patients with the *Claude syndrome* (a lesion of the medial midbrain) is partially related to damage to the red nucleus as well as to the adjacent cerebellothalamic fibers. These patients may also have a paucity of most eye movement on the ipsilateral side and a dilated pupil (*mydriasis*) due to concurrent damage to exiting rootlets of the oculomotor nerve.

Medial vestibulospinal fibers primarily inhibit motor neurons innervating extensors and neurons serving muscles of the back and neck. Lateral vestibulospinal fibers may inhibit some flexor motor neurons, but they mainly facilitate spinal reflexes via their excitatory influence on spinal motor neurons innervating extensors. Vestibulospinal and reticulospinal (see Figure 7-12 on page 194) fibers contribute to the *spasticity* seen in patients with damage to corticospinal fibers or to the tonic extension of the extremities in patients with *decerebrate rigidity*. In the case of decerebrate rigidity, the descending influences on spinal flexor motor neurons (corticospinal, rubrospinal) is removed; the descending brainstem influence on spinal extensor motor neurons predominates; this is augmented by excitatory spinoreticular input (via ALS) to some of the centers giving rise to reticulospinal fibers (see also Figure 7-12 on page 194).

Abbreviations

ATegDec	Anterior tegmental decussation (rubrospinal fibers)	**MVessp**	Medial vestibulospinal tract
CC	Crus cerebri	**MVNu**	Medial vestibular nucleus
CorRu	Corticorubral fibers	**OcNu**	Oculomotor nucleus
FacNu	Facial nucleus	**PTegDec**	Posterior tegmental decussation (tectospinal fibers)
InfVNu	Inferior (or spinal) vestibular nucleus	**Py**	Pyramid
LCSp	Lateral corticospinal tract	**RNu**	Red nucleus
LRNu	Lateral reticular nucleus	**RuSp**	Rubrospinal tract
LVNu	Lateral vestibular nucleus	**SC**	Superior colliculus
LVesSp	Lateral vestibulospinal tract	**SVNu**	Superior vestibular nucleus
ML	Medial lemniscus	**TecSp**	Tectospinal tract
MLF	Medial longitudinal fasciculus	**VesSp**	Vestibulospinal tracts

Review of Blood Supply to RNu, Vestibular Nuclei, MFL and RuSp, and Vestibulospinal Tracts in Cords

Structures	Arteries
RNu	medial branches of posterior cerebral and posterior communicating plus some from short circumferential branches of posterior cerebral (see Figure 5–27)
Vestibular Nuclei	posterior inferior cerebellar in medulla (see Figure 5–14) and long circumferential branches in pons (see Figure 5–21)
MLF	long circumferential branches of basilar in pons (see Figure 5–21) and anterior spinal in medulla (see Figure 5–14)
MVesSp	branches of central artery (see Figures 5–6 and 5–14)
LVesSp and **RuSp**	penetrating branches of arterial vasocorona plus terminal branches of central artery (see Figure 5–6)

Rubrospinal and Vestibulospinal Tracts

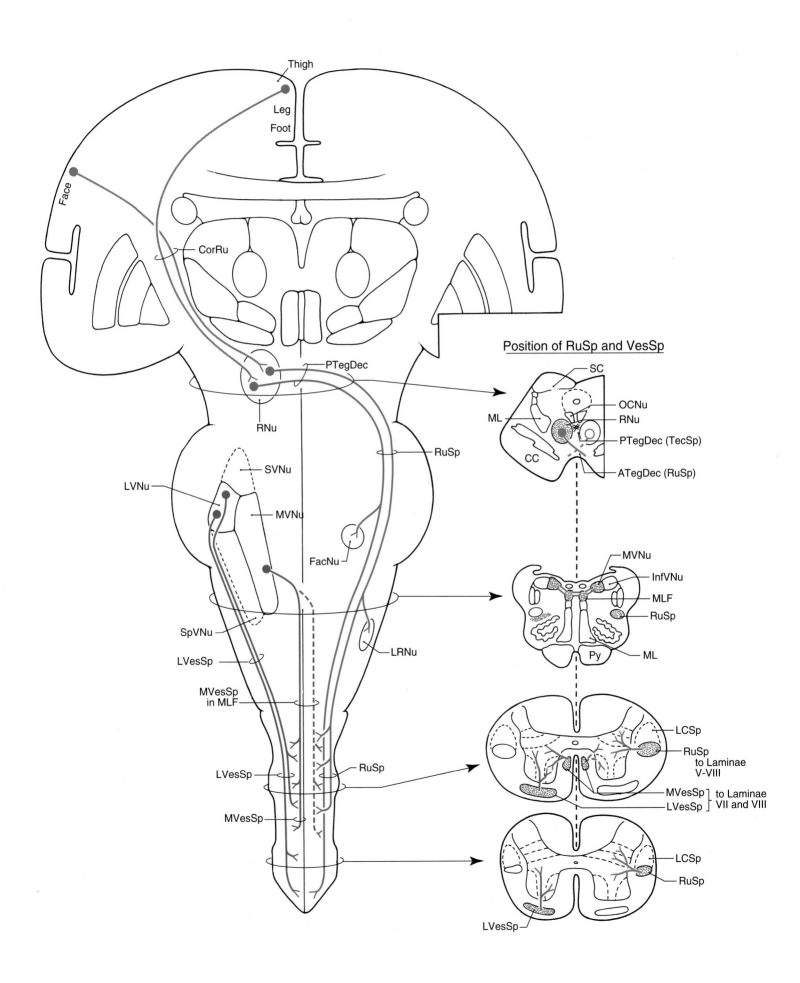

Position of RuSp and VesSp

7-14 Blank master drawing for motor pathways. This illustration is provided for self-evaluation of motor pathways understanding, for the instructor to expand on motor pathways not covered in this atlas, or both.

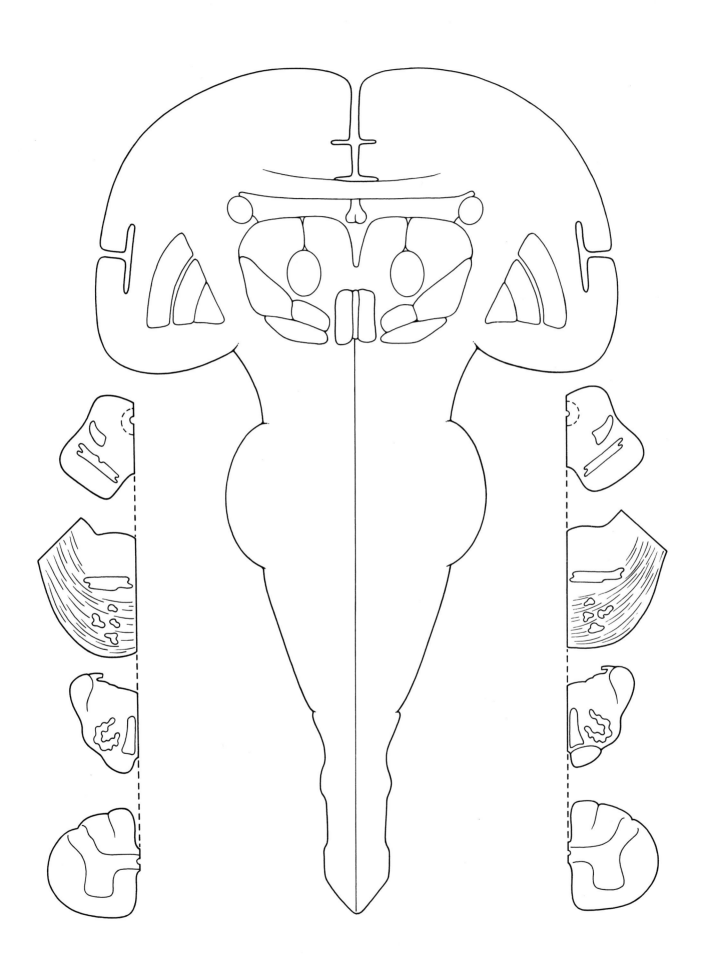

Cranial Nerve Efferents (III, IV, VI, XI-AccNu, XII)

7-15 The origin and peripheral distribution of GSE fibers from the oculomotor, trochlear, abducens, spinal accessory, and hypoglossal nuclei. Also shown are GVE fibers arising from the Edinger-Westphal nucleus and the distribution of postganglionic fibers from the ciliary ganglion. Internuclear abducens neurons project, via the MLF, to contralateral oculomotor neurons that innervate the medial rectus muscle (*internuclear ophthalmoplegia* pathway).

Some authors specify the functional component of neurons in the accessory nucleus as special visceral efferent, some specify it as somatic efferent, and some are noncommittal. Because, in humans, the trapezius and sternocleidomastoid muscles originate from cervical somites located caudal to the last pharyngeal arch, the functional component is designated here as GSE. In addition, experiments in animals reveal that motor neurons innervating the trapezius and sternocleidomastoid muscles are found in cervical cord levels C_1 to approximately C_6.

Neurotransmitters: Acetylcholine (and probably calcitonin gene-related peptide, CGRP) is found in the motor neurons of cranial nerve nuclei and in their peripheral endings. This substance is also found in cells of the Edinger-Westphal nucleus and the ciliary ganglion.

Clinical Correlations: *Myasthenia gravis* (MG) is a disease caused by autoantibodies that may directly block nicotinic acetylcholine receptors or damage the postsynaptic membrane (via complement mediated lysis) thereby reducing the number of viable receptor sites. Ocular movement disorders (*diplopia, ptosis*) are seen first in approximately 50% of patients and are present in approximately 85% of all MG patients. Movements of the neck and tongue may also be impaired, with the latter contributing to *dysphagia* and *dysarthria*.

Lesions of the IIIrd nerve (as in the *Weber syndrome* or in *carotid cavernous aneurysms*) may result in 1) *ptosis*, 2) lateral and downward deviation of the eye, and 3) *diplopia* (except on ipsilateral lateral gaze). In addition, the pupil may be unaffected (pupillary sparing) or dilated and fixed. Lesions in the midbrain that involve the root of the IIIrd nerve and the crus cerebri give rise to a *superior alternating (crossed) hemiplegia*. This is a paralysis of most eye movement and possibly a dilated pupil on the ipsilateral side and a contralateral hemiplegia of the extremities.

Damage to the MLF (as in *multiple sclerosis* or small vessel occlusion) between the VIth and IIIrd nuclei results in *internuclear ophthalmoplegia;* on attempted lateral gaze, the opposite medial rectus muscle will not adduct. A lesion of the IVth nerve (frequently caused by trauma) produces *diplopia* on downward and inward gaze (tilting the head may give some relief), and the eye is slightly elevated when the patient looks straight ahead.

Diabetes mellitus, trauma, or *pontine gliomas* are some causes of VIth nerve dysfunction. In these patients, the affected eye is slightly adducted, and *diplopia* is pronounced on attempted gaze to the lesioned side. Damage in the caudal and medial pons may involve the fibers of the VIth nerve and the adjacent corticospinal fibers in the basilar pons, giving rise to a *middle alternating (crossed) hemiplegia*. The deficits are an ipsilateral paralysis of the lateral rectus muscle and a contralateral hemiplegia of the extremities. The XIth nerve may be damaged centrally (as in *syringobulbia* or *amyotrophic lateral sclerosis*) or at the jugular foramen with resultant paralysis of the ipsilateral sternocleidomastoid and upper parts of the trapezius muscle.

Central injury to the XIIth nucleus or fibers (as in the *medial medullary syndrome* or in *syringobulbia*) or to its peripheral parts (as in *polyneuropathy* or tumors) results in deviation of the tongue toward the lesioned side on attempted protrusion. A lesion in the medial aspects of the medulla will give rise to an *inferior alternating (crossed) hemiplegia*. This is characterized by a paralysis of the ipsilateral side of the tongue (XIIth root damage) and contralateral hemiplegia of the extremities (damage to corticospinal fibers in the pyramid).

Abbreviations

AbdNr	Abducens nerve	**OcNu**	Oculomotor nucleus
AbdNu	Abducens nucleus	**PO**	Principal olivary nucleus
AccNr	Accessory nerve	**Py**	Pyramid
AccNu	Accessory nucleus (spinal accessory nu.)	**RNu**	Red nucleus
BP	Basilar pons	**SC**	Superior colliculus
CC	Crus cerebri	**SCP,Dec**	Superior cerebellar peduncle, decussation
EWNu	Edinger-Westphal nucleus	**TroDec**	Trochlear decussation
FacCol	Facial colliculus	**TroNr**	Trochlear nerve
HyNr	Hypoglossal nerve	**TroNu**	Trochlear nucleus
HyNu	Hypoglossal nucleus		
ML	Medial lemniscus		**Ganglion**
MLF	Medial longitudinal fasciculus	**1**	Ciliary
OcNr	Oculomotor nerve		

Review of Blood Supply to OcNu, TroNu, AbdNu and HyNu, and the Internal Course of their Fibers

STRUCTURES	ARTERIES
OcNu and Fibers	medial branches of posterior cerebral and posterior communicating (see Figure 5–27)
TroNu	paramedian branches of basilar bifurcation (see Figure 5–27)
AbdNu	long circumferential branches of basilar (see Figure 5–21)
Abducens Fibers in **BP**	paramedian branches of basilar (see Figure 5–21)
HyNu and Fibers	anterior spinal (see Figure 5–14)

Cranial Nerve Efferents (III, IV, VI, XI-AccNu, and XII)

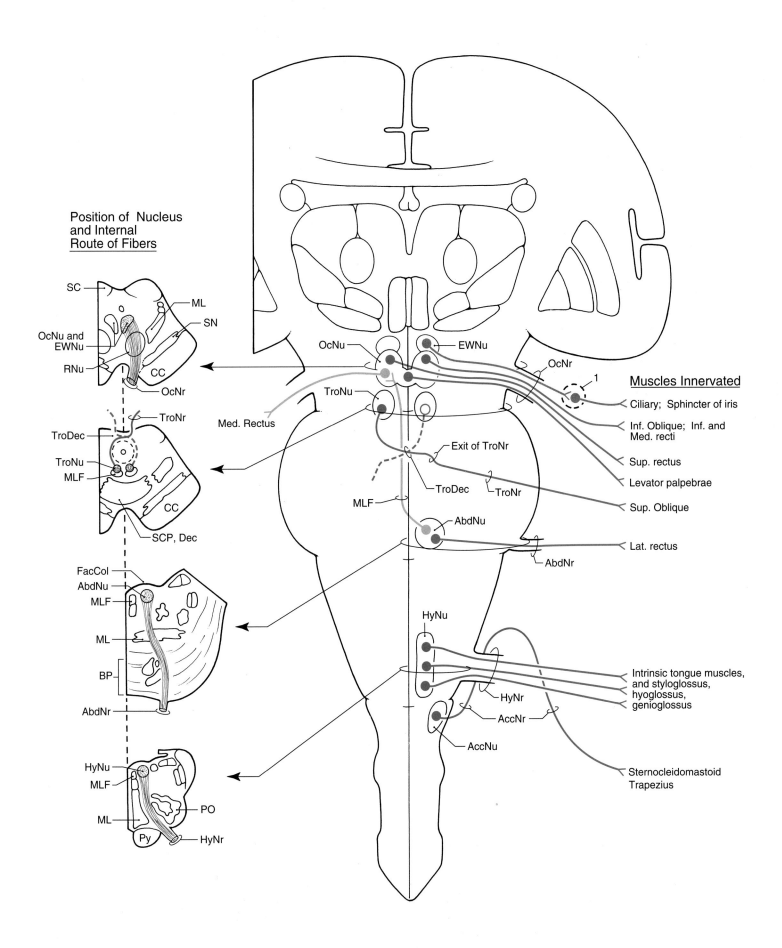

Position of Nucleus
and Internal
Route of Fibers

SC

ML

SN

OcNu and
EWNu

RNu

CC

OcNr

TroDec

TroNr

TroNu

MLF

CC

SCP, Dec

FacCol

AbdNu

MLF

ML

BP

AbdNr

HyNu

MLF

ML

PO

Py

HyNr

OcNu

EWNu

OcNr

TroNu

Med. Rectus

Exit of TroNr

TroDec

TroNr

MLF

AbdNu

AbdNr

HyNu

HyNr

AccNr

AccNu

1

Muscles Innervated

Ciliary; Sphincter of iris

Inf. Oblique; Inf. and
Med. recti

Sup. rectus

Levator palpebrae

Sup. Oblique

Lat. rectus

Intrinsic tongue muscles,
and styloglossus,
hyoglossus,
genioglossus

Sternocleidomastoid
Trapezius

Cranial Nerve Efferents (V, VII, IX, and X)

7–16   The origin and peripheral distribution of fibers arising from the SVE motor nuclei of the trigeminal, facial, and glossopharyngeal and vagus (via the nucleus ambiguus) nerves. Also shown are the origin of GVE preganglionic parasympathetic fibers from the superior (to facial nerve) and inferior (to glossopharyngeal nerve) salivatory nuclei and from the dorsal motor vagal nucleus. Their respective ganglia are indicated as well as the structures innervated by postganglionic fibers arising from each. The SVE functional component specifies cranial nerve motor nuclei that innervate head muscles that arose, embryologically, from pharyngeal arches. Muscles innervated by the trigeminal nerve (V) come from the 1st arch, those served by the facial nerve (VII) from the 2nd arch; the stylopharyngeal muscle originates from the 3rd arch and is innervated by the glossopharyngeal nerve (IX), and the muscles derived from the 4th arch are served by the vagus nerve (X).

Neurotransmitters: The transmitter found in the cells of cranial nerve motor nuclei, and in their peripheral endings, is acetylcholine; CGRP is also colocalized in these motor neurons. This substance is also present in preganglionic and postganglionic parasympathetic neurons.

Clinical Correlations: Patients with *myasthenia gravis* frequently have oropharyngeal symptoms and complications that result in *dysarthria,* and *dysphagia*. These individuals have difficulty chewing and swallowing, their jaw may hang open, and the mobility of facial muscles is decreased. Imparied hearing (weakness of tensor tympani) and *hyperacusis* (weakness of stapedius) may also be present.

Lesions of the Vth nerve (as in *meningiomas* or trauma) result in 1) loss of pain, temperature, and touch on the ipsilateral face and in the oral and nasal cavities; 2) *paralysis* of ipsilateral masticatory muscles (jaw de-

viates to the lesioned side when closed);, and 3) loss of the afferent limb of the *corneal reflex*. If especially large, a vestibular schwannoma may compress the trigeminal nerve root and result in a hemifacial sensory loss that may include the oral cavity. *Trigeminal neuralgia (tic douloureux)* is an intense, sudden, intermittent pain emanating from the area of the cheek, oral cavity, or adjacent parts of the nose (distribution of V_2 or V_3, see also Figure 7-7 on page 184).

Tumors (such as *chordoma* or *vestibular schwannoma*), trauma, or *meningitis* may damage the VIIth nerve, resulting in 1) an ipsilateral *facial palsy* (or Bell palsy); 2) loss of taste from the ipsilateral two-thirds of the tongue; and (3) decreased secretion from the ipsilateral lacrimal, nasal, and sublingual and submandibular glands. Injury distal to the chorda tympani produces only an ipsilateral *facial palsy*. A paralysis of the muscles on one side of the face with no paralysis of the extremities is a *facial hemiplegia*. On the other hand, intermittent and involuntary contraction of the facial muscles is called *hemifacial spasm*. One cause is compression of the facial root by an artery, most commonly a loop of the anterior inferior cerebellar artery or its branches. These patients may also have deficits (*vertigo, tinnitus, hearing loss*) suggesting involvement of the adjacent vestibulocochlear nerve.

Because of their common origin from NuAm, adjacent exit from the medulla, and passage through the jugular foramen, the IXth and Xth nerves may be damaged together (as in *amyotrophic lateral sclerosis* or in *syringobulbia*). The results are *dysarthria, dysphagia, dyspnea,* loss of taste from the ipsilateral caudal tongue, and loss of the *gag reflex,* but no significant autonomic deficits. Bilateral lesions of the Xth nerve are life-threatening because of the resultant total paralysis (and closure) of the muscles in the vocal folds (vocalis muscle).

Abbreviations

AbdNu	Abducens nucleus	**SpTNu**	Spinal trigeminal nucleus
ALS	Anterolateral system	**SpTTr**	Spinal trigeminal tract
BP	Basilar pons	**SSNu**	Superior salivatory nucleus
DVagNu	Dorsal motor nucleus of vagus	**TecSp**	Tectospinal tract
FacNr	Facial nerve	**TriMoNu**	Trigeminal motor nucleus
FacNu	Facial nucleus	**TriNr**	Trigeminal nerve
GINr	Glossopharyngeal nerve	**VagNr**	Vagus nerve
HyNu	Hypoglossal nucleus		
ISNu	Inferior salivatory nucleus		**Ganglia**
MesNu	Mesencephalic nucleus	**1**	Pterygopalatine
ML	Medial lemniscus	**2**	Submandibular
MLF	Medial longitudinal fasciculus	**3**	Otic
NuAm	Nucleus ambiguus	**4**	Terminal and/or intramural
PSNu	Principal (chief) sensory nucleus		

Review of Blood Supply to TriMoNu, FacNu, DMNu and NuAm, and the Internal Course of Their Fibers

STRUCTURES	ARTERIES
TriMoNu and Trigeminal Root	long circumferential branches of basilar (see Figure 5–21)
FacNu and Internal Genu	long circumferential branches of basilar (see Figure 5–21)
DMNu and **NuAm**	branches of vertebral and posterior inferior cerebellar (see Figure 5–14)

Cranial Nerve Efferents (V, VII, IX, and X)

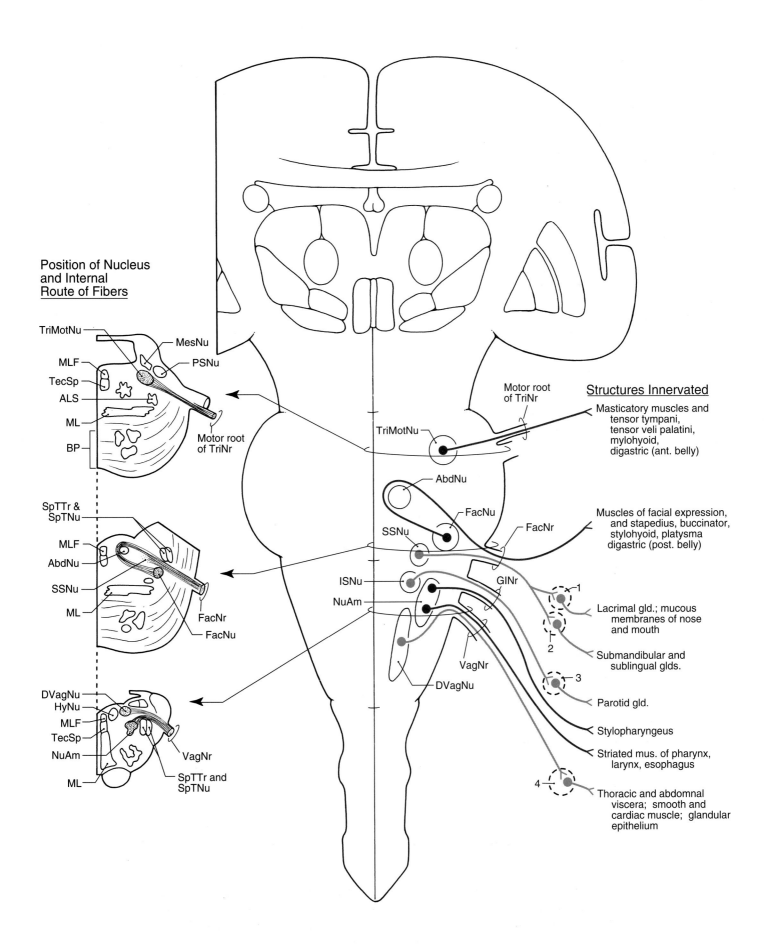

Position of Nucleus and Internal Route of Fibers

TriMotNu
MesNu
MLF
PSNu
TecSp
ALS
ML
BP
Motor root of TriNr

SpTTr & SpTNu
MLF
AbdNu
SSNu
ML
FacNr
FacNu

DVagNu
HyNu
MLF
TecSp
NuAm
ML
VagNr
SpTTr and SpTNu

Motor root of TriNr
TriMotNu
AbdNu
FacNu
SSNu
FacNr
ISNu
GlNr
NuAm
VagNr
DVagNu

Structures Innervated

Masticatory muscles and tensor tympani, tensor veli palatini, mylohyoid, digastric (ant. belly)

Muscles of facial expression, and stapedius, buccinator, stylohyoid, platysma digastric (post. belly)

1

Lacrimal gld.; mucous membranes of nose and mouth

2

Submandibular and sublingual glds.

3

Parotid gld.

Stylopharyngeus

Striated mus. of pharynx, larynx, esophagus

4

Thoracic and abdomnal viscera; smooth and cardiac muscle; glandular epithelium

Spinocerebellar Tracts

7-17 The origin, course, and distribution pattern of fibers to the cerebellar cortex and nuclei from the spinal cord (posterior [dorsal] and anterior [ventral] spinocerebellar tracts, rostral spinocerebellar fibers) and from the external cuneate nucleus (cuneocerebellar fibers). Also illustrated is the somatotopy of those fibers originating from the spinal cord. These fibers enter the cerebellum via the restiform body, the larger portion of the inferior cerebellar peduncle, or in relationship to the superior cerebellar peduncle. After these fibers enter the cerebellum, collaterals are given off to the cerebellar nuclei while the parent axons of spinocerebellar and cuneocerebellar fibers pass on to the cortex, where they end as mossy fibers in the graunular layer. Although not shown here, there are important ascending spinal projections to the medial and dorsal accessory nuclei of the inferior olivary complex (spino-olivary fibers). The accessory olivary nuclei (as well as the principal olivary nucleus) project to the cerebellar cortex and send collaterals into the nuclei (see Figure 7-18 on page 206).

Neurotransmitters: Glutamate (+) is found in some spinocerebellar fibers, in their mossy fiber terminals in the cerebellar cortex, and in their collateral branches that innervate the cerebellar nuclei.

Clinical Correlations: Lesions, or tumors, that selectively damage only spinocerebellar fibers are rarely, if ever, seen in humans. The *ataxia* one might expect to see in patients with a spinal cord hemisection (as in the *Brown-Sequard syndrome*) is masked by the *hemiplegia* resulting from the concomitant damage to lateral corticospinal (and other) fibers.

Friedreich ataxia (hereditary spinal ataxia) is an autosomal recessive disorder the symptoms of which usually appear between 8 and 15 years of age. There is degeneration of anterior and posterior spinocerebellar tracts plus the posterior columns and corticospinal tracts. Degenerative changes are also seen in Purkinje cells in the cerebellum, in posterior root ganglion cells, in neurons of the Clarke column, and in some nuclei of the pons and medulla. The axial and appendicular *ataxia* seen in these patients correlates partially with the spinocerebellar degeneration and also partially with proprioceptive losses via the degeneration of posterior column fibers.

Abbreviations

ACNu	Accessory (external or lateral) cuneate nucleus	**PSCT**	Posterior (dorsal) spinocerebellar tract
ALS	Anterolateral system	**PSNu**	Principal (chief) sensory nucleus of trigeminal nerve
AMV	Anterior medullary velum	**Py**	Pyramid
ASCT	Anterior (ventral) spinocerebellar tract	**RB**	Restiform body
Cbl	Cerebellum	**RSCF**	Rostral spinocerebellar fibers
CblNu	Cerebellar nuclei	**RuSp**	Rubrospinal tract
CCblF	Cuneocerebellar fibers	**S**	Sacral representation
DNuC	Dorsal nucleus of Clarke	**SBC**	Spinal border cells
FNL	Flocculonodular lobe	**SCP**	Superior cerebellar peduncle
IZ	Intermediate zone	**SpTNu**	Spinal trigeminal nucleus
L	Lumbar representation	**SpTTr**	Spinal trigeminal tract
MesNu	Mesencephalic nucleus	**T**	Thoracic representation
ML	Medial lemniscus	**TriMoNu**	Trigeminal motor nucleus
PRG	Posterior (dorsal) root ganglion	**VesNu**	Vestibular nuclei

Review of Blood Supply to Spinal Cord Grey Matter, Spinocerebellar Tracts, RB, and SCP

STRUCTURES	ARTERIES
Spinal Cord Grey	branches of central artery (see Figure 5–6)
PSCT and **ASCT** in Cord	penetrating branches of arterial vasocorona (see Figure 5–6)
RB	posterior inferior cerebellar (See Figure 5–14)
SCP	long circumferential branches of basilar and superior cerebellar (see Figure 5–21)
Cerebellum	posterior and anterior inferior cerebellar and superior cerebellar

Spinocerebellar Tracts

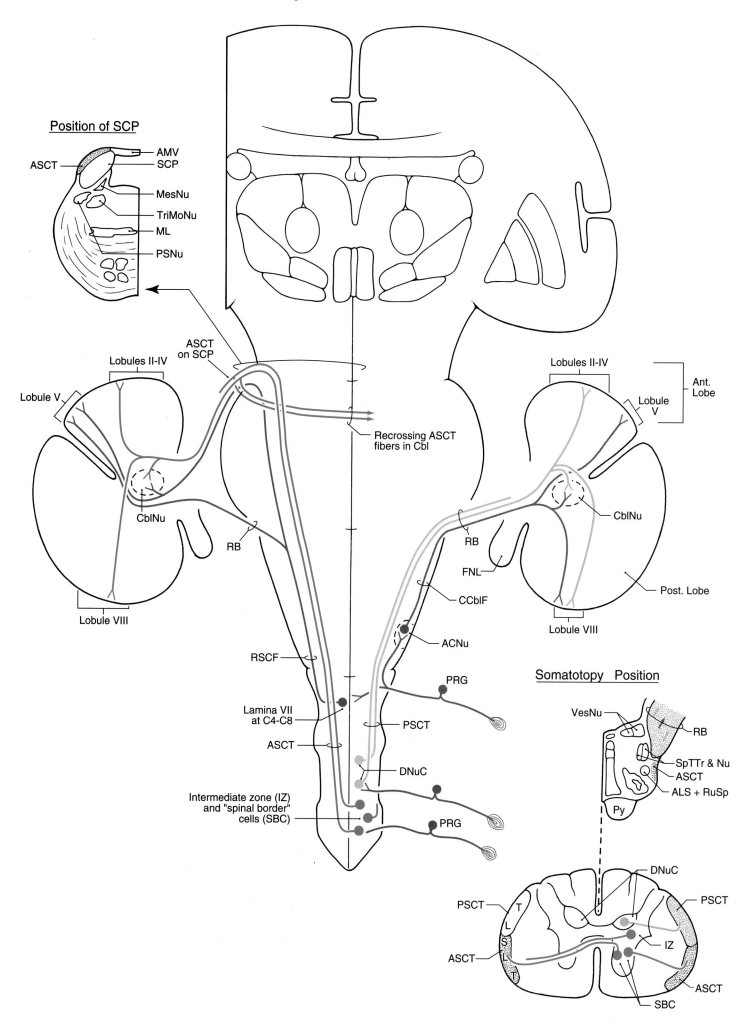

Position of SCP

ASCT

AMV
SCP
MesNu
TriMoNu
ML
PSNu

ASCT
on SCP

Lobules II-IV
Lobule V
Lobule VIII
CblNu
RB
RSCF
Lamina VII
at C4-C8
ASCT
Intermediate zone (IZ)
and "spinal border"
cells (SBC)

Recrossing ASCT
fibers in Cbl

Lobules II-IV
Lobule V
Ant.
Lobe
CblNu
RB
FNL
CCblF
Post. Lobe
Lobule VIII
ACNu
PRG
PSCT
DNuC
PRG

Somatotopy Position

VesNu
RB
SpTTr & Nu
ASCT
ALS + RuSp
Py

PSCT
T
L
S
L
T
ASCT

DNuC
PSCT
IZ
ASCT
SBC

Pontocerebellar, Reticulocerebellar, Olivocerebellar, Ceruleocerebellar, Hypothalamocerebellar, and Raphecerebellar Fibers

7–18 Afferent fibers to the cerebellum from selected brainstem areas and the organization of corticopontine fibers in the internal capsule and crus cerebri as shown here. The cerebellar peduncles are also indicated. Pontocerebellar axons are mainly crossed, reticulocerebellar fibers may be bilateral (from RetTegNu) or mainly uncrossed (from LRNu and PRNu), and olivocerebellar fibers (OCblF) are exclusively crossed. Raphecerebellar, hypothalamocerebellar, and ceruleocerebellar fibers are, to varying degrees, bilateral projections. Although all afferent fibers to the cerebellum give rise to collaterals to the cerebellar nuclei, those from pontocerebellar axons are relatively small, having comparatively small diameters. Olivocerebellar axons end as climbing fibers, reticulocerebellar and pontocerebellar fibers as mossy fibers, and hypothalamocerebellar and ceruleocerebellar axons end in all cortical layers. These latter fibers have been called multilayered fibers in the literature because they branch in all layers of the cerebellar cortex.

Neurotransmitters: Glutamate (+) is found in corticopontine projections and in most pontocerebellar fibers. Aspartate (+) and cor-ticotropin (+)-releasing factor are present in many olivocerebellar fibers. Ceruleocerebellar fibers contain noradrenalin, histamine is found in hypothalamocerebellar fibers, and some reticulocerebellar fibers contain enkephalin. Serotonergic fibers to the cerebellum arise from neurons found in medial areas of the reticular formation (open cell in Figure 7–18) and, most likely, from some cells in the adjacent raphe nuclei.

Clinical Correlations: Common symptoms seen in patients with lesions involving nuclei and tracts that project to the cerebellum are *ataxia* (of trunk or limbs), an *ataxic gait, dysarthria, dysphagia,* and disorders of eye movement such as *nystagmus.* These deficits are seen in some hereditary diseases (such as *olivopontocerebellar degeneration, ataxia telangiectasia,* or *hereditary cerebellar ataxia*), in tumors (brainstem gliomas), in vascular diseases *(lateral pontine syndrome),* or in other conditions such as *alcoholic cerebellar degeneration* or pontine hemorrhages (see Figure 7-19 on page 208 for more information on cerebellar lesions).

Abbreviations

AntLb	Anterior limb of internal capsule	**PonNu**	Pontine nuclei
CblNu	Cerebellar nuclei	**PO**	Principal olivary nucleus
CerCblF	Ceruleocerebellar fibers	**PPon**	Parietopontine fibers
CPonF	Cerebropontine fibers	**PRNu**	Paramedian reticular nuclei
CSp	Corticospinal fibers	**Py**	Pyramid
DAO	Dorsal accessory olivary nucleus	**RB**	Restiform body
FPon	Frontopontine fibers	**RCblF**	Reticulocerebellar fibers
Hyth	Hypothalamus	**RetLenLb**	Retrolenticular limb of internal capsule
HythCblF	Hypothalamocerebellar fibers	**RNu**	Red nucleus
IC	Internal capsule	**RetTegNu**	Reticulotegmental nucleus
LoCer	Nucleus (locus) ceruleus	**SCP**	Superior cerebellar peduncle
LRNu	Lateral reticular nucleus	**SubLenLb**	Sublenticular limb of internal capsule
MAO	Medial accessory olivary nucleus	**SN**	Substantia nigra
MCP	Middle cerebellar peduncle	**TPon**	Temporopontine fibers
ML	Medial lemniscus		
NuRa	Raphe nuclei		

Number Key

1	Nucleus raphe, pontis
2	Nucleus raphe, magnus
3	Raphecerebellar fibers

Other abbreviations:

OCblF	Olivocerebellar fibers
OPon	Occipitopontine fibers
PCbIF	Pontocerebellar fibers
PostLb	Posterior limb of internal capsule

Review of Blood Supply to Precerebellar Relay Nuclei in Pons and Medulla, MCP, and RB

STRUCTURES	ARTERIES
Pontine Tegmemtum	long circumferential branches of basilar plus some from superior cerebellar (see Figure 5–21)
Basilar Pons	paramedian and short circumferential branches of basilar (See Figure 5–21)
Medulla **RetF** and **IO**	branches of vertebral and posterior inferior cerebellar (see Figure 5–14)
MCP	long circumferential branches of basilar and branches of anterior inferior and superior cerebellar (see Figure 5–21)
RB	posterior inferior cerebellar (see Figure 5–14)

Pontocerebellar, Reticulocerebellar, Olivocerebellar, Ceruleocerebellar, Hypothalamocerebellar, and Raphecerebellar Fibers

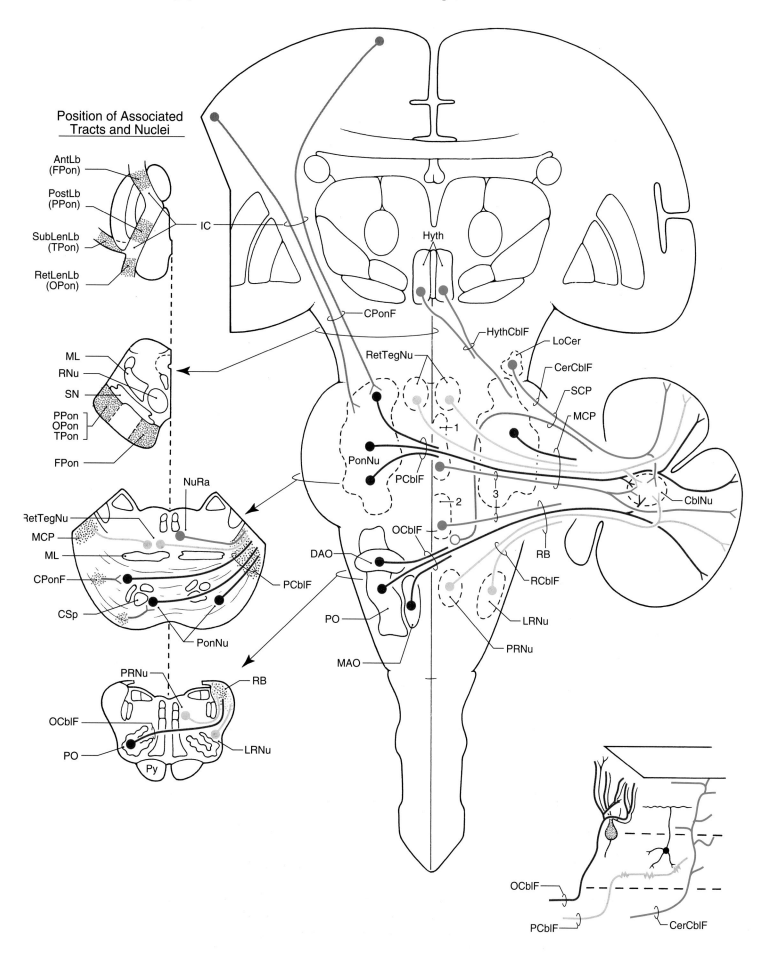

Position of Associated Tracts and Nuclei

Cerebellar Cortioconuclear, Nucleocortical, and Corticovestibular Fibers

7–19 Cerebellar corticonuclear fibers arise from all regions of the cortex and terminate in an orderly (mediolateral and rostrocaudal) sequence in the ipsilateral cerebellar nuclei. For example, corticonuclear fibers from the vermal cortex terminate in the fastigial nucleus, those from the intermediate cortex terminate in the emboliform and globosus nuclei, and those from the lateral cortex terminate in the dentate nucleus. Also, cerebellar corticonuclear fibers from the anterior lobe typically terminate in more rostral regions of these nuclei while those from the posterior lobe terminate more caudally. Cerebellar corticovestibular fibers originate primarily from the vermis and flocculonodular lobe, exit the cerebellum via the juxtarestiform body, and end in the ipsilateral vestibular nuclei. These projections arise from Purkinje cells.

Nucleocortical processes originate from cerebellar nuclear neurons and pass to the overlying cortex in a pattern that basically reciprocates that of the corticonuclear projection; they end as mossy fibers. Some nucleocortical fibers are collaterals of cerebellar efferent axons. The cerebellar cortex may influence the activity of lower motor neurons through, for example, the cerebellovestibular-vestibulospinal route.

Neurotransmitters: Gamma-aminobutyric acid (GABA) (−) is found in Purkinje cells and is the principal transmitter substance present in cerebellar corticonuclear and corticovestibular projections. However, taurine (−) and motilin (−) are also found in some Purkinje cells. GABA-ergic terminals are numerous in the cerebellar nuclei and vestibular complex. Some of the glutamate-containing mossy fibers in the cerebellar cortex represent the endings of nucleocortical fibers that originate from cells in the cerebellar nuclei.

Clinical Correlations: Numerous disease entities can result in cerebellar dysfunction including viral infections *(echovirus)*, hereditary diseases (see Figure 7–18), trauma, tumors *(glioma, medulloblastoma)*, occlusion of cerebellar arteries (cerebellar stroke), *arteriovenous malformation* of cerebellar vessels, developmental errors (such as the *Dandy-Walker syndrome* or the *Arnold-Chiari deformity*), or the intake of toxins. Usually, damage to only the cortex results in little or no dysfunction unless the lesion is quite large or causes an increase in intracranial pressure. However, lesions involving both the cortex and nuclei, or only the nuclei, will produce obvious cerebellar signs.

Lesions involving midline structures (vermal cortex, fastigial nuclei) and/or the flocculonodular lobe result in *truncal ataxia (titubation or tremor), nystagmus,* and head tilting. These patients may also have a wide-based *(cerebellar) gait,* are unable to walk in tandem (heel to toe), and may be unable to walk on their heels or on their toes. Generally, midline lesions result in bilateral motor deficits affecting axial and proximal limb musculature.

Damage to the intermediate and lateral cortices and the globose, emboliform, and dentate nuclei results in various combinations of the following deficits: *dysarthria, dysmetria (hypometria, hypermetria), dysdiadochokinesia, tremor (static, kinetic, intention), rebound phenomenon,* unsteady and wide-based *(cerebellar) gait,* and *nystagmus.* One of the more commonly observed deficits in patients with cerebellar lesions is an *intention tremor,* which is best seen in the *finger-nose test.* The *finger-to-finger test* is also used to demonstrate an intention tremor and to assess cerebellar function. The *heel-to-shin test* will show *dysmetria* in the lower extremity. If the heel-to-shin test is normal in a patient with his/her eyes open, the cerebellum is intact. If this test is repeated in the same patient with eyes closed and is abnormal, this would suggest a lesion in the posterior column-medial lemniscus system.

Cerebellar damage in intermittent and lateral areas (nuclei or cortex plus nuclei) causes movement disorders on the side of the lesion with ataxia and gait problems on that side; the patient may tend to fall toward the side of the lesion. This is because the cerebellar nuclei project to the contralateral thalamus, which projects to the motor cortex on the same side, which projects to the contralateral side of the spinal cord via the corticospinal tract. Other circuits (cerebellorubal-rubospinal) and feedback loops (cerebelloolivary-olivocerebellar) follow similar routes. Consequently, the motor expression of unilateral cerebellar damage is toward the lesioned side because of these doubly crossed pathways.

Lesions of cerebellar efferent fibers, after they cross the midline in the decussation of the superior cerebellar peduncle, will give rise to motor deficits on the side of the body (excluding the head) contralateral to the lesion. This is seen in midbrain lesions such as the *Claude syndrome.*

Abbreviations

CorNu	Corticonuclear fibers	**MVesSp**	Medial vestibulospinal tract
CorVes	Corticovestibular fibers	**MVNU**	Medial vestibular nucleus
Flo	Flocculus	**NL, par**	Lateral cerebellar nucleus, parvocellular region
IC	Intermediate cortex		
InfVesNu	Inferior (spinal) vestibular nucleus	**NM, par**	Medial cerebellar nucleus, parvocellular region
JRB	Juxtarestiform body		
LC	Lateral cortex	**NuCor**	Nucleocortical fibers
LVesSp	Lateral vestibulospinal tract	**SVNu**	Superior vestibular nucleus
LVNu	Lateral vestibular nucleus	**VC**	Vermal cortex
MLF	Medial longitudinal fasciculus		

Review of Blood Supply to Cerebellum and Vestibular Nuclei

STRUCTURES	ARTERIES
Cerebellar Cortex	branches of posterior and anterior inferior cerebellar and superior cerebellar
Cerebellar Nuclei	anterior inferior cerebellar and superior cerebellar
Vestibular Nuclei	posterior inferior cerebellar in medulla, long circumferential branches of basilar in pons

Cerebellar Corticonuclear, Nucleocortical, and Corticovestibular Fibers

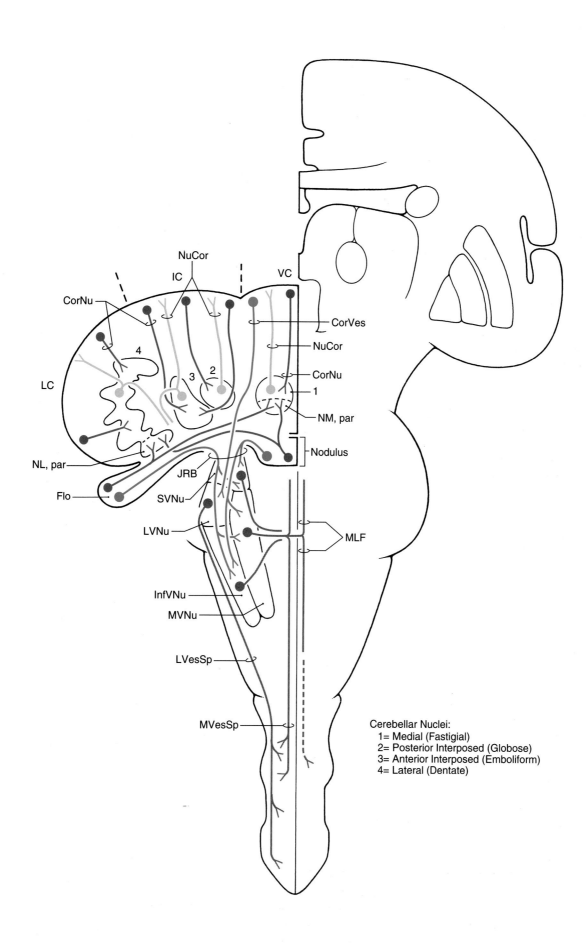

CorNu

NuCor

IC

VC

CorVes

NuCor

CorNu

1

NM, par

Nodulus

LC

4

3

2

NL, par

JRB

Flo

SVNu

LVNu

MLF

InfVNu

MVNu

LVesSp

MVesSp

Cerebellar Nuclei:
1= Medial (Fastigial)
2= Posterior Interposed (Globose)
3= Anterior Interposed (Emboliform)
4= Lateral (Dentate)

Cerebellar Efferent Fibers

7–20 The origin, course, topography, and general distribution of fibers arising in the cerebellar nuclei. Cerebellofugal fibers project to several thalamic areas (VL and VA), to intralaminar relay nuclei in addition to the centromedian, and to a number of midbrain, pontine, and medullary targets. Most of the latter nuclei project back to the cerebellum (e.g., reticulocerebellar, pontocerebellar), some in a highly organized manner. For example, cerebello-olivary fibers from the dentate nucleus (DNu) project to the principal olivary nucleus (PO), and neurons of the PO send their axons back to the lateral cerebellar cortex, with collaterals going to the DNu.

The cerebellar nuclei can influence motor activity through, as examples, the following routes: 1) cerebellorubral-rubrospinal, 2) cerebelloreticular-reticulospinal, 3) cerebellothalamic-thalamocortical-corticospinal, and others. In addition, some direct cerebellospinal fibers arise in the fastigial nucleus as well as in the interposed nuclei.

Neurotransmitters: Many cells in the cerebellar nuclei contain glutamate (+), aspartate (+), or gamma-aminobutyric acid (−). Glutamate and aspartate are found in cerebellorubral and cerebellothalamic fibers, whereas some GABA-containing cells give rise to cerebellopontine and cerebello-olivary fibers. Some cerebelloreticular projections may also contain GABA.

Clinical Correlations: Lesions of the cerebellar nuclei result in a range of motor deficits depending on the location of the injury. Many of these are described in Figure 7–19 on page 208.

Abbreviations

ALS	Anterolateral system		**OcNu**	Oculomotor nucleus
AMV	Anterior medullary velum		**PO**	Principal olivary nucleus
BP	Basilar pons		**PonNu**	Pontine nuclei
CblOl	Cerebello-olivary fibers		**RetForm**	Reticular formation
CblTh	Cerebellothalamic fibers		**RNu**	Red nucleus
CblRu	Cerebellorubral fibers		**RuSp**	Rubrospinal tract
CC	Crus cerebri		**SC**	Superior colliculus
CeGy	Central grey (periaqueductal grey)		**SCP**	Superior cerebellar peduncle
CM	Centromedian nucleus of thalamus		**SCP, Dec**	Superior cerebellar peduncle, decussation
CSp	Corticospinal fibers		**SN**	Substantia nigra
DAO	Dorsal accessory olivary nucleus		**SVNu**	Superior vestibular nucleus
DNu	Dentate nucleus (lateral cerebellar nucleus)		**ThCor**	Thalamocortical fibers
ENu	Emboliform nucleus (anterior interposed cerebellar nucleus)		**ThFas**	Thalamic fasciculus
			TriMoNu	Trigeminal motor nucleus
EWNu	Edinger-Westphal nucleus		**VL**	Ventral lateral nucleus of thalamus
FNu	Fastigial nucleus (medial cerebellar nucleus)		**VPL**	Ventral posterolateral nucleus of thalamus
GNu	Globose nucleus (posterior interposed cerebellar nucleus)		**VSCT**	Ventral spinocerebellar tract
			ZI	Zona incerta
IC	Inferior colliculus			
InfVNu	Inferior (spinal) vestibular nucleus			**Number Key**
INu	Interstitial nucleus		**1**	Ascending projections to superior colliculus, and possibly ventral lateral and ventromedial thalamic nuclei
LRNu	Lateral reticular nucleus			
LVNu	Lateral vestibular nucleus			
MAO	Medial accessory olivary nucleus		**2**	Descending crossed fibers from superior cerebellar peduncle
ML	Medial lemniscus			
MLF	Medial longitudinal fasciculus		**3**	Uncinate fasciculus (of Russell)
MVNu	Medial vestibular nucleus		**4**	Juxtarestiform body to vestibular nuclei
NuDark	Nucleus of Darkschewitsch		**5**	Reticular formation

Review of Blood Supply to Cerebellar Nuclei and Their Principal Efferent Pathways

STRUCTURES	ARTERIES
Cerebellar Nuclei	anterior inferior cerebellar and superior cerebellar
SCP	long circumferential branches of basilar and superior cerebellar (see Figure 5–21)
Midbrain Tegmemtum **(RNu, CblTh, CblRu, OcNu)**	paramedian branches of basilar bifurcation, short circumferential branches of posterior cerebral, branches of superior cerebellar (see Figure 5–27)
VPL, CM, VL, VA	thalamogeniculate branches of posterior cerebral, thalamoperforating branches of the posteromedial group of posterior cerebral (see Figure 5–38)
IC	lateral striate branches of middle cerebral (see Figure 5–38)

Cerebellar Efferent Fibers

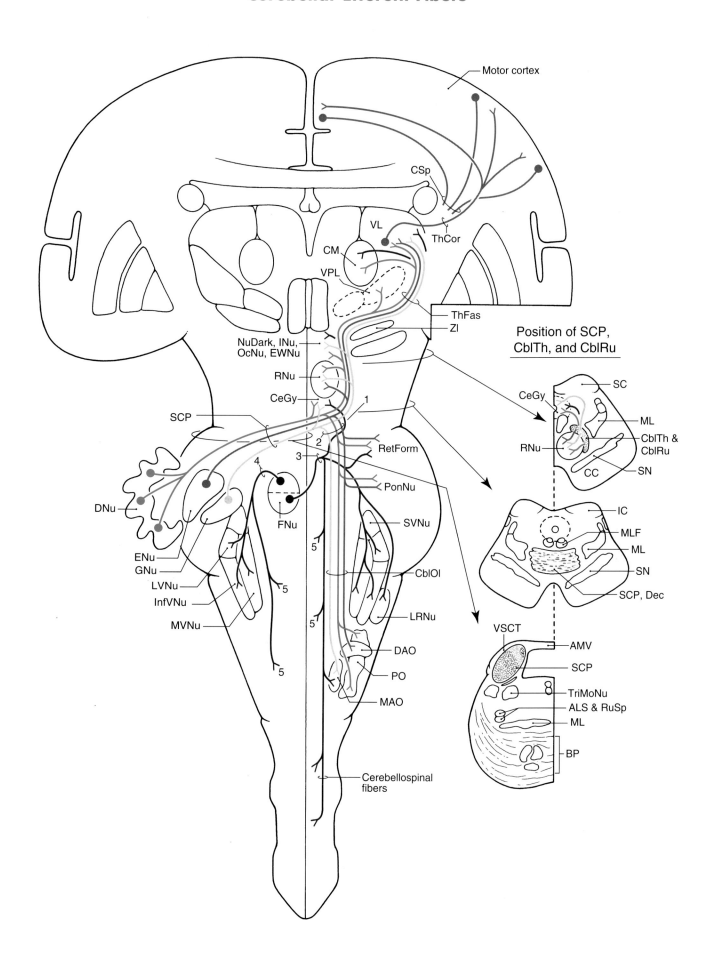

7-28   Blank master drawing of visual pathways. This illustration is provided for self-evaluation of visual pathway understanding, for the instructor to expand on aspects of the visual pathways not covered in the atlas, or both.

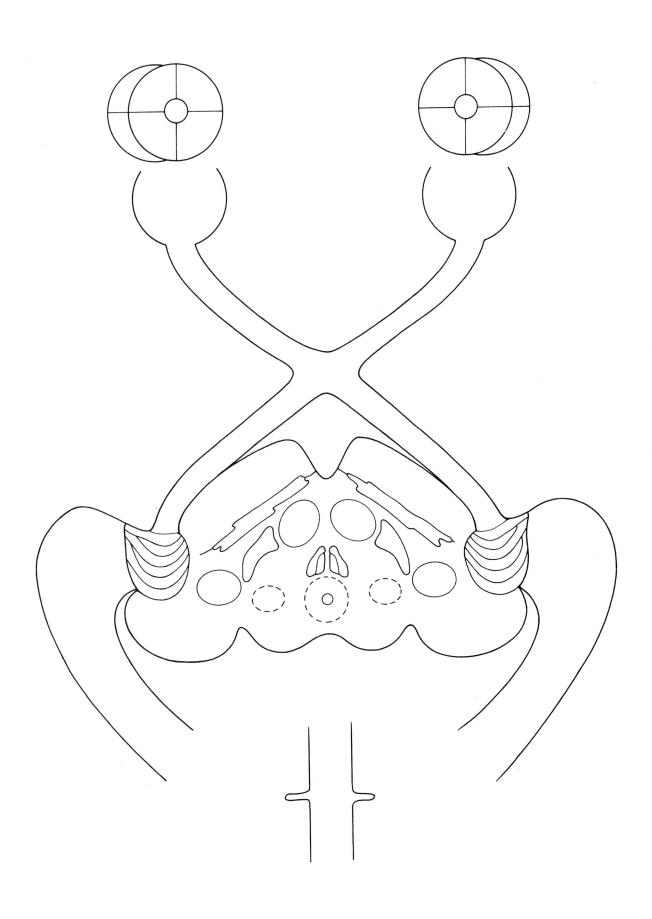

Auditory Pathways

7-29 The origin, course, and distribution of the fibers collectively composing the auditory pathway. Central to the cochlear nerve and dorsal and ventral cochlear nuclei this system is, in a general sense, bilateral and multisynaptic, as input is relayed through brainstem nuclei en route to the auditory cortex. Synapse and crossing (or re-crossing) of information can occur at several levels in the neuraxis. Consequently, central lesions rarely result in a total unilateral hearing loss. The medial geniculate body is the thalamic station for the relay of auditory information to the temporal cortex.

Neurotransmitters: Glutamate (+) and aspartate (+) are found in some spiral ganglion cells and in their central terminations in the cochlear nuclei. Dynorphin-containing and histamine-containing fibers are also present in the cochlear nuclei; the latter arises from the hypothalamus. A noradrenergic projection to the cochlear nuclei and to the inferior colliculus originates from the nucleus locus ceruleus. Cells in the superior olive that contain cholecystokinin and cells in the nuclei of the lateral lemniscus that contain dynorphin project to the inferior colliculus. Although the olivocochlear bundle is not shown, it is noteworthy that enkephalin is found in some of the cells that contribute to this projection.

Clinical Correlations: There are three categories of deafness. *Conductive deafness* is due to problems of the external ear (obstruction of the canal, wax build-up) or disorders of the middle ear (*otitis media, otosclerosis*). *Nerve deafness* (*sensorineural hearing loss*) results from diseases involving the cochlea or the cochlear portion of the vestibulocochlear nerve. *Central deafness* results from damage to the cochlear nuclei or possibly their central connections.

Hearing loss may result from trauma (such as fracture of the petrous bone), demyelinating diseases, tumors, certain medications (*streptomycin*), or occlusion of the labyrinthine artery. Damage to the cochlear part of the VIIIth nerve (as in *vestibular schwannoma*) results in *tinnitus* and/or *deafness* (partial or total) in the ipsilateral ear. High-frequency hearing losses are most common.

The *Weber test* and *Rinne test* are used to differentiate between neural hearing loss and conduction hearing loss, and to lateralize the deficit. In the *Weber test*, a tuning fork (512 Hz) is applied to the midline of the forehead or apex of the skull. In the normal patient, the sound (conducted through the bones of the skull) is heard the same in each year. In the case of *nerve deafness* (lesions of the cochlea or cochlear nerve), the sound is best heard in the normal ear, while in *conductive deafness,* the sound is best heard in the abnormal ear. In the *Rinne test,* a tuning fork (512 Hz) is placed against the mastoid process. When the sound is no longer perceived, the prongs are moved close to the external acoustic meatus, where the sound is again heard; this is the situation in a normal individual (positive Rinne test). In middle ear disease, the sound is not heard at the external meatus after it has disappeared from touching the mastoid bone (abnormal or negative Rinne test). Therefore, a negative Rinne test signifies conductive hearing loss in the ear tested. In mild nerve deafness (cochlea or cochlear nerve lesions), the sound is heard by application of the tuning fork to the mastoid and movement to the ear (the Rinne test is positive). In severe nerve deafness, the sound may not be heard at either position.

In addition to hearing loss and tinnitus, large vestibular schwannomas may result in other signs and symptoms. These include nausea, vomiting and ataxia/unsteady gait (vestibular root involvement), weakness of facial muscles (facial root involvement), and altered sensation from the face and a diminished corneal reflex (trigeminal root involvement). There may also be general signs associated with increased intracranial pressure (lethargy, headache, and vomiting).

Central lesions (as in gliomas or vascular occlusions) rarely produce unilateral or bilateral hearing losses that can be detected, the possible exception being pontine lesions that damage the trapezoid body and nuclei. Injury to central auditory pathways and/or primary auditory cortex may diminish auditory acuity, decrease the ability to hear certain tones, or make it difficult to precisely localize sounds in space. Patients with damage to secondary auditory cortex in the temporal lobe experience difficulty in understanding and/or interpreting sounds (*auditory agnosia*).

Abbreviations

AbdNu	Abducens nucleus	**MLF**	Medial longitudinal fasciculus
ACNu	Anterior (ventral) cochlear nucleus	**PCNu**	Posterior (dorsal) cochlear nucleus
ALS	Anterolateral system	**PulNu**	Pulvinar nuclear complex
CC	Crus cerebri	**RB**	Restiform body
FacNu	Facial nucleus	**RetF**	Reticular formation
IC	Inferior colliculus	**SC**	Superior colliculus
IC,Br	Inferior colliculus, brachium	**SCP,Dec**	Superior cerebellar peduncle, decussation
IC,Com	Inferior colliculus, commissure	**SO**	Superior olive
IC,SL	Internal capsule, sublenticular limb	**SpGang**	Spiral ganglion
LGNu	Lateral geniculate nucleus	**SpTTr**	Spinal trigeminal tract
LL	Lateral lemniscus	**TrapB**	Trapezoid body
LL,Nu	Lateral lemniscus, nucleus	**TrapNu**	Trapezoid nucleus
MGNu	Medial geniculate nucleus	**TTGy**	Transverse temporal gyrus
ML	Medial lemniscus		

Review of Blood Supply to Cochlear Nuclei, LL (and associated structures), Pontine Tegmentum, IC, and MGB

STRUCTURES	ARTERIES
Cochlear Nuclei	anterior inferior cerebellar (see Figure 5–14)
LL, SO in Pons	long circumferential branches of basilar (see Figure 5–21)
IC	long circumferential branches (quadrigeminal branches) of basilar, superior cerebellar (see Figure 5–27)
MGB	thalamogeniculate branches of posterior cerebral (see Figure 5–38)

Auditory Pathways

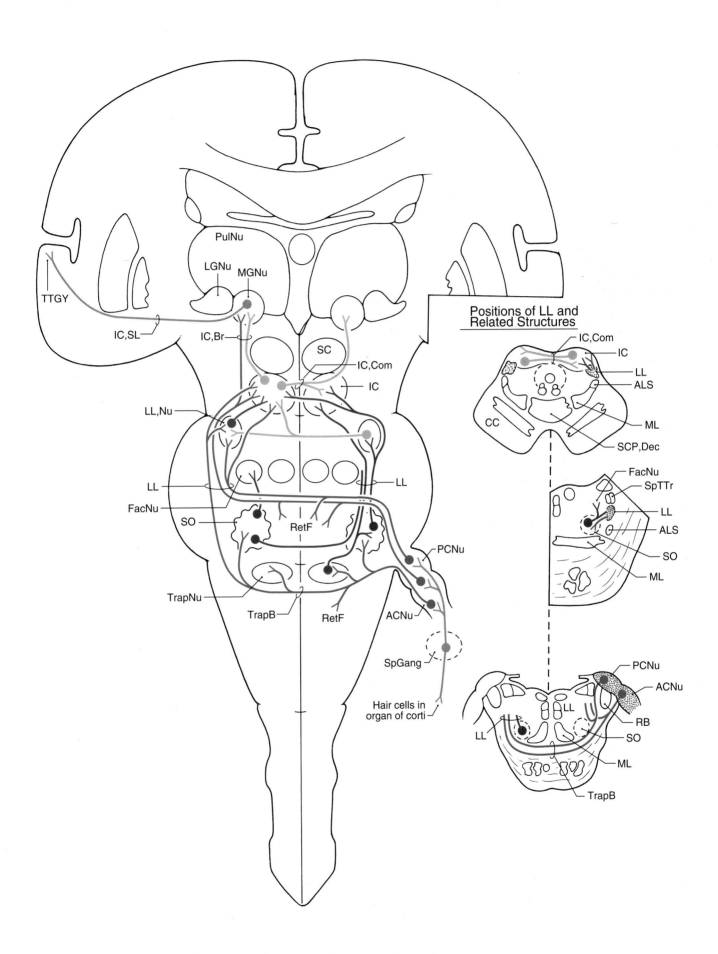

Positions of LL and
Related Structures

Vestibular Pathways

7–30 The origin, course, and distribution of the main afferent and efferent connections of the vestibular nuclei (see also Figures 7–13, 7–19, and 7–20). Primary vestibular afferent fibers may end in the vestibular nuclei or pass to cerebellar structures via the juxtarestiform body. Secondary vestibulocerebellar axons originate from the vestibular nuclei and follow a similar path to the cerebellum. Efferent projections from the vestibular nuclei also course to the spinal cord through vestibulospinal tracts (see Figure 7–13), as well as to the motor nuclei of the oculomotor, trochlear, and abducens nerves via the MLF. Cerebellar structures most extensively interconnected with the vestibular nuclei include the lateral regions of the vermal cortex of anterior and posterior lobes, the flocculonodular lobe, and the fastigial (medial) cerebellar nucleus.

Neurotransmitters: Gamma-aminobutyric (−) is the transmitter associated with many cerebellar corticovestibular fibers and their terminals in the vestibular complex; this substance is also seen in cerebellar corticonuclear axons. The medial vestibular nucleus also has fibers that are dynorphin-positive and histamine-positive; the latter arise from cells in the hypothalamus.

Clinical Correlations: The vestibular part of the VIIIth nerve can be damaged by many of the same insults that affect the cochlear nerve (see Figure 7–29). Damage to vestibular receptors of the vestibular nerve commonly results in *vertigo*. The patient may feel that his or her body is moving *(subjective vertigo)* or that objects in the environment are moving *(objective vertigo)*. They have equilibrium problems, an *unsteady (ataxic) gait,* and a tendency to fall to the lesioned side. Deficits seen in nerve lesions—or in brainstem lesions involving the vestibular nuclei, include *nystagmus, nausea,* and vomiting, along with *vertigo* and gait problems. A *facial palsy* may also appear in concert with VIIIth nerve damage in patients who have a vestibular schwannoma. These vestibular deficits, along with partial or complete deafness, are seen in Ménière disease.

Lesions of those parts of the cerebellum with which the vestibular nerve and nuclei are most intimately connected (flocculonodular lobe and fastigial nucleus) result in *nystagmus, truncal ataxia, ataxic gait,* and a propensity to fall to the injured side. The nystagmus seen in patients with vestibular lesions and the *internuclear ophthalmoplegia* seen in some patients with *multiple sclerosis* are signs that correlate with the interruption of vestibular projections to the motor nuclei of III, IV, and VI via the MLF.

Abbreviations

AbdNu	Abducens nucleus	**PAG**	Periaqueductal gray
ALS	Anterolateral system	**Py**	Pyramid
Cbl	Cerebellar	**RB**	Restiform body
Cbl-CoVes	Cerebellar corticovestibular fibers	**RNu**	Red nucleus
CblNu	Cerebellar nuclei	**SC**	Superior colliculus
HyNu	Hypoglossal nucleus	**SCP,Dec**	Superior cerebellar peduncle, decussation
IC	Inferior colliculus		
InfVNu	Inferior (spinal) vestibular nucleus	**SN**	Substantia nigra
JRB	Juxtarestiform body	**SolNu**	Solitary nucleus
LVesSp	Lateral vestibulospinal tract	**SolTr**	Solitary tract
LVNu	Lateral vestibular nucleus	**SpTTr**	Spinal trigeminal tract
MesNu	Mesencephalic nucleus	**SVNu**	Superior vestibular nucleus
ML	Medial lemniscus	**TroNu**	Trochlear nucleus
MLF	Medial longitudinal fasciculus	**VesGang**	Vestibular ganglion
MVesSp	Medial vestibulospinal tract	**VesCbl,Prim**	Vestibulocerebellar fibers, primary
MVNu	Medial vestibular nucleus	**VesCbl,Sec**	Vestibulocerebellar fibers, secondary
OcNu	Oculomotor nucleus		

Review of Blood Supply to Vestibular Nuclei, TroNu, and OcNu

STRUCTURES	ARTERIES
Vestibular Nuclei	posterior inferior cerebellar in medulla (see Figure 5–14), long circumferential branches of basilar in pons (see Figure 5–21)
TroNu and **OcNu**	paramedian branches of basilar bifurcation, medial branches of posterior cerebral and posterior communicating, short circumferential branches of posterior cerebral (see Figure 5–27)

Vestibular Pathways

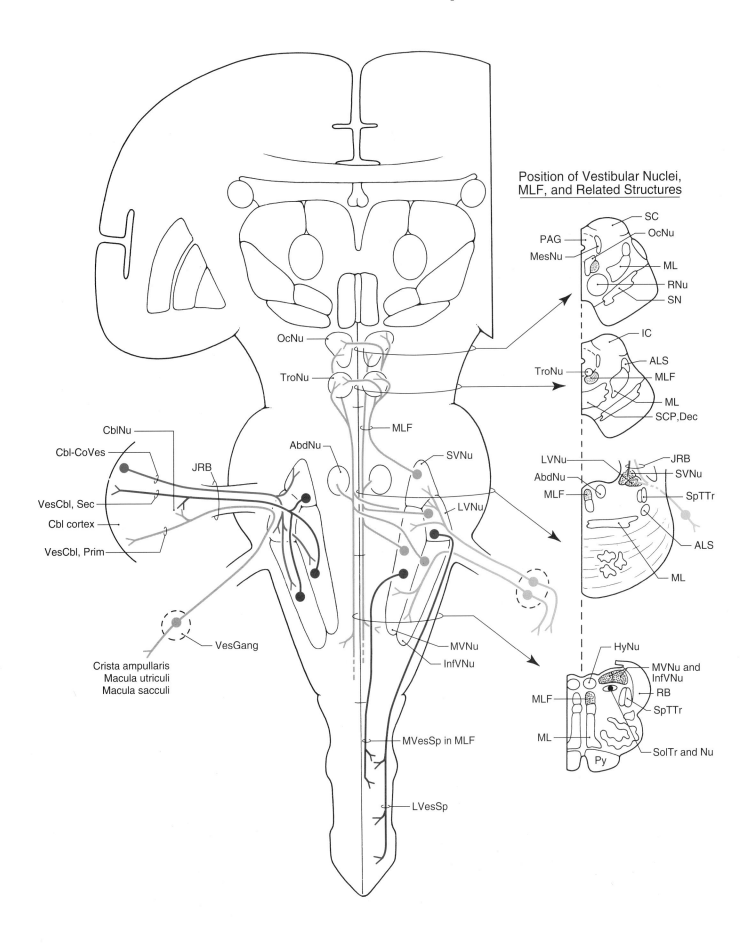

Position of Vestibular Nuclei, MLF, and Related Structures

7-31   Blank master drawing for auditory or vestibular pathway. This illustration is provided for self-evaluation of auditory or vestibular pathway understanding, for the instructor to expand on aspects of these pathways not covered in the atlas, or both.

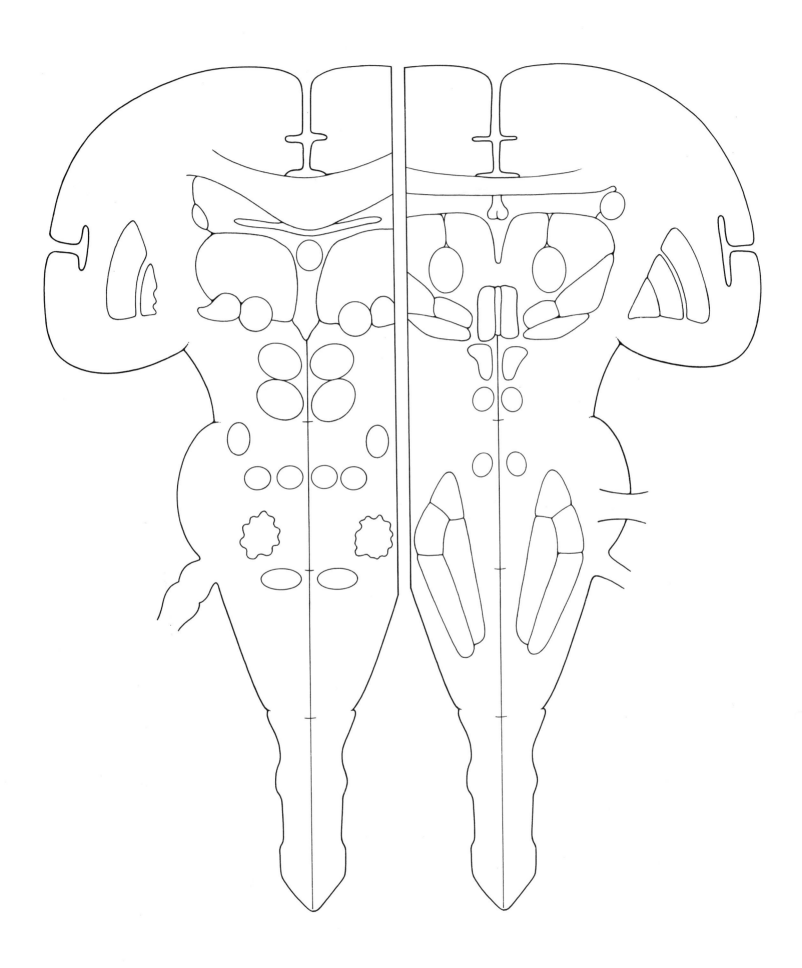

Hippocampal Connections

7–32   Selected afferent and efferent connections of the hippocampus (upper) and the mammillary body (lower) with emphasis on the circuit of Papez. The hippocampus receives input from, and projects to, diencephalic nuclei (especially the mammillary body via the postcommissural fornix), the septal region, and amygdala. The hippocampus receives cortical input from the superior and middle frontal gyri, superior temporal and cingulate gyri, precuneus, lateral occipital cortex, occipitotemporal gyri, and subcallosal cortical areas. The mammillary body is connected with the dorsal and ventral tegmental nuclei, anterior thalamic nucleus (via the mammillothalamic tract), septal nuclei, and through the mammillotegmental tract, to the tegmental pontine and reticulotegmental nuclei.

Neurotransmitters: Glutamate (+)-containing cells in the subiculum and Ammon's horn project to the mammillary body, other hypothalamic centers, and the lateral septal nucleus through the fornix. Cholecystokinin (+) and somatostatin (−) are also found in hippocampal cells that project to septal nuclei and hypothalamic structures. The septal nuclei and the nucleus of the diagonal band give rise to cholinergic afferents to the hippocampus that travel in the fornix. In addition, a gamma-aminobutyric acid (−) septohippocampal projection originates from the medial septal nucleus. Enkephalin and glutamate containing hippocampal afferent fibers arise from the adjacent entorhinal cortex; the locus ceruleus gives origin to noradrenergic fibers to the dentate gyrus, Ammon's horn, and subiculum; and serotoninergic fibers arise from the rostral raphe nuclei.

Clinical Correlations: Dysfunction associated with damage to the hippocampus is seen in patients with trauma to the temporal lobe, as a sequel to alcoholism, and as a result of neurodegenerative changes seen in the dementing diseases (such as *Alzheimer disease* and *Pick disease*). Bilateral injury to the hippocampus results in loss of recent memory (remote memory is unaffected), impaired ability to remember recent (new) events, and difficulty in turning a new experience (something just done or experienced) into a longer-term memory that can be retrieved at a later time. Also, memory that depends on visual, tactile, or auditory discrimination is noticeably affected. These represent *visual agnosia, tactile agnosia,* and *auditory agnosia,* respectively.

In the *Korsakoff syndrome (amnestic confabulatory syndrome)* there is memory loss, dementia, amnesia, and a tendency to give confabulated responses. This type of response is fluent but consists of a string of unrelated, or even made up, "memories" that never actually occurred or make no sense. This may lead to an incorrect conclusion that the patient is suffering from *dementia.* In addition to lesions in the hippocampus in these patients, the mammillary bodies and dorsomedial nucleus of the thalamus are noticeably affected. The Korsakoff syndrome (see also the *Wernicke-Korsakoff* syndrome) as seen in chronic alcoholics is largely owing to thiamine deficiency and can be treated with therapeutic doses of this vitamin.

Abbreviations

AC	Anterior commissure	**LT**	Lamina terminalis
AmHrn	Ammon's horn	**MB**	Mammillary body
Amy	Amygdaloid nucleus (complex)	**MedFCtx**	Medial frontal cortex
AntNu	Anterior nucleus of thalamus	**MedTh**	Medial thalamus
CC, G	Corpus callosum, genu	**MTegTr**	Mammillotegmental tract
CC,Spl	Corpus callosum, splenium	**MtTr**	Mammillothalamic tract
Cing	Cingulum	**NuAcc**	Nucleus accumbens
CingGy	Cingulate gyrus	**OpCh**	Optic chiasm
CorHip	Corticohippocampal fibers	**Pi**	Pineal
DenGy	Dentate gyrus	**RSplCtx**	Retrosplenial cortex
EnCtx	Entorhinal cortex	**SepNu**	Septal nuclei
For	Fornix	**SMNu**	Supramammillary nucleus
GyRec	Gyrus rectus	**Sub**	Subiculum
Hip	Hippocampus	**TegNu**	Tegmental nuclei
Hyth	Hypothalamus	**VmNu**	Ventromedial hypothalamic nucleus
IC,G	Internal capsule, genu		

Review of Blood Supply to Hip, MB, Hyth, and CingGy

STRUCTURES	ARTERIES
Hip	anterior choroidal (see Figure 5–38)
MB, Hyth	branches of circle of Willis (see Figure 2–21)
AntNu	thalamoperforating (see Figure 5–38)
CingGy	branches of anterior cerebral

Hippocampal Connections

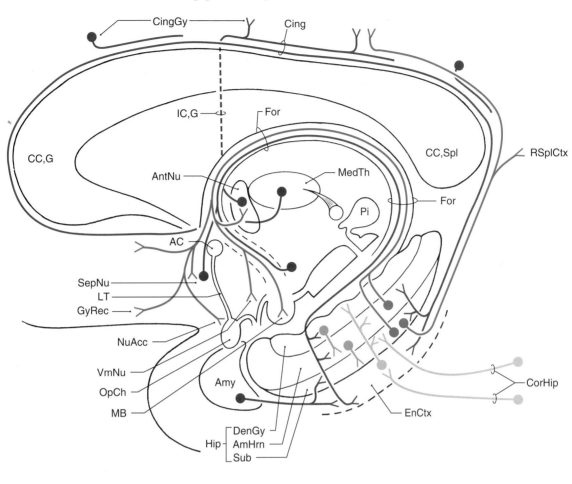

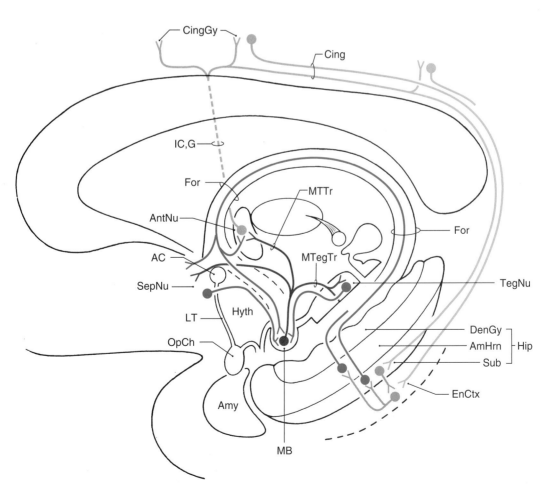

Amygdaloid Connections

7-33 The origin, course, and distribution of selected afferent and efferent connections of the amygdaloid nuclear complex in sagittal (upper) and coronal (lower) planes. The amygdala receives input from, and projects to, brainstem and forebrain centers via the stria terminalis and the ventral amygdalofugal pathway. Corticoamygdaloid and amygdalocortical fibers interconnect the basal and lateral amygdaloid nuclei with select cortical areas.

Neurotransmitters: Cells in the amygdaloid complex contain vasoactive intestinal polypeptide (VIP, +), neurotensin (NT), somatostatin (SOM, −), enkephalin (ENK, −), and substance P (SP, +). These neurons project, via the stria terminalis or the ventral amygdalofugal path, to the septal nuclei (VIP, NT), the bed nucleus of the stria terminalis (NT, ENK, SP), the hypothalamus (VIP, SOM, SP), the nucleus accumbens septi, and the caudate and putamen (NT). Serotonergic amygdaloid fibers originate from the nucleus raphe dorsalis and the superior central nucleus, dopaminergic axons from the ventral tegmental area and the substantia nigra-pars compacta, and noradrenalin-containing fibers from the locus ceruleus. Glutamate (+) is found in olfactory projections to the prepiriform cortex and the amygdaloid complex. Acetylcholine is present in afferents to the amygdala from the substantia innominata, as well as from the septal area. In patients with Alzheimer disease and the associated dementia, there is a marked loss of acetylcholine-containing neurons in the basal nucleus of the substantia innominata, in the cortex, and in the hippocampus.

Clinical Correlations: Dysfunctions related to damage to the amygdaloid complex are seen in patients with trauma to the temporal lobes, *herpes simplex encephalitis*, bilateral temporal lobe surgery to treat intractable epileptic activity, and in some CNS degenerative disorders (such as *Alzheimer disease* and *Pick disease*). The behavioral changes seen in individuals with amygdala lesions collectively form the *Klüver-Bucy syndrome*. In humans these changes/deficits are 1) *hyperorality;* 2) *visual, tactile,* and *auditory agnosia;* 3) *placidity;* 4) *hyperphagia* or other dietary manifestations; 5) an intense desire to explore the immediate environment *(hypermetamorphosis),* and 6) what is commonly called *hypersexuality.* These changes in sexual attitudes are usually in the form of comments, suggestions, and attempts to make a sexual contact (such as touching) rather than in actual intercourse or masturbation. These patients may also show *aphasia, dementia,* and *amnesia.*

Abbreviations

AC	Anterior commissure	**NuRa,d**	Nucleus raphe, dorsalis
Amy	Amygdaloid nuclear complex	**NuRa,m**	Nucleus raphe, magnus
AmyCor	Amygdalocortical fibers	**NuRa,o**	Nucleus raphe, obscurus
AmyFugPath	Amygdalofugal pathway	**NuRa,p**	Nucleus raphe, pallidus
AntHyth	Anterior hypothalamus	**NuStTer**	Nucleus of the stria terminalis
Ba-LatNu	Basal and lateral nuclei	**OlfB**	Olfactory bulb
CaNu	Caudate nucleus	**OpCh**	Optic chiasm
Cen-MedNu	Central, cortical and medial nuclei	**PAG**	Periaqueductal (central) gray
CorAmy	Corticoamygdaloid fibers	**PBrNu**	Parabrachial nuclei
DVagNu	Dorsal motor vagal nucleus	**PfNu**	Parafascicular nucleus
EnCtx	Entorhinal cortex	**Pi**	Pineal
For	Fornix	**POpNu**	Preoptic nucleus
GP	Globus pallidus	**PPriCtx**	Prepiriform cortex
Hyth	Hypothalamus	**Put**	Putamen
LT	Lamina terminalis	**SepNu**	Septal nuclei
LHAr	Lateral hypothalamic area	**SNpc**	Substantia nigra, pars compacta
MedThNu	Medial thalamic nuclei	**SolNu**	Solitary nucleus
MGNu	Medial geniculate nucleus	**StTer**	Stria terminalis
MidTh	Midline thalamic nuclei	**Sub**	Subiculum
NuAcc	Nucleus accumbens	**SubIn**	Substantia innominata
NuCen,s	Nucleus centralis, superior	**VenTegAr**	Ventral tegmental area
NuCer	Nucleus ceruleus	**VmNu**	Ventromedial hypothalamic nucleus

Review of Blood Supply to Amy and Related Centers

STRUCTURES	ARTERIES
Amy	anterior choroidal (see Figure 5–38)
Hyth	branches of circle of Willis (see Figure 5–38)
Brainstem	(see Figures 5–14, 5–21, and 5–27)
Thalamus	thalamoperforating, thalamogeniculate (see Figure 5–38)

Amygdaloid Connections

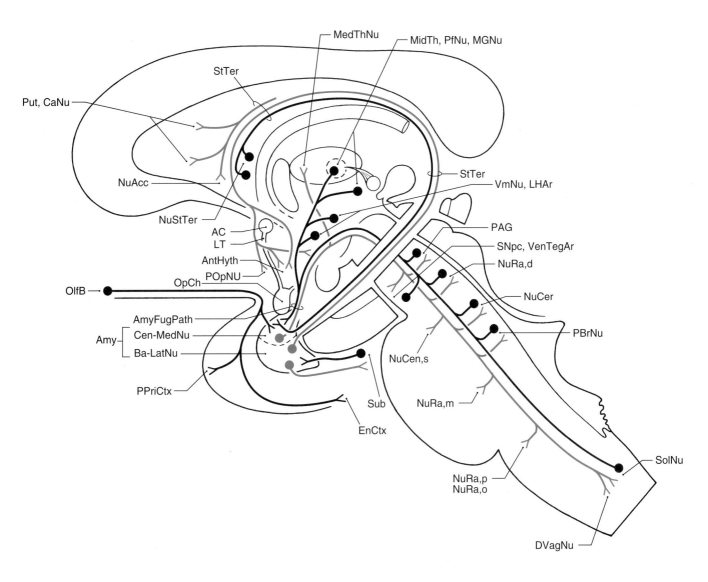

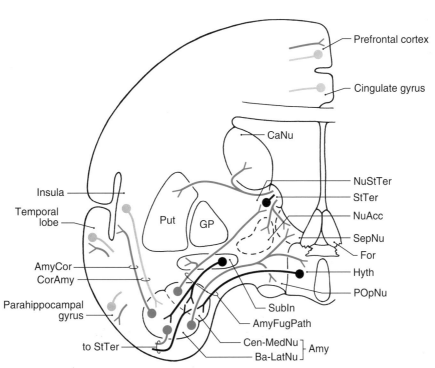

7–34   Blank master drawing for limbic pathways. This illustration is provided for self-evaluation of limbic pathways or connections, for the instructor to expand on aspects of these pathways not covered in the atlas, or both.

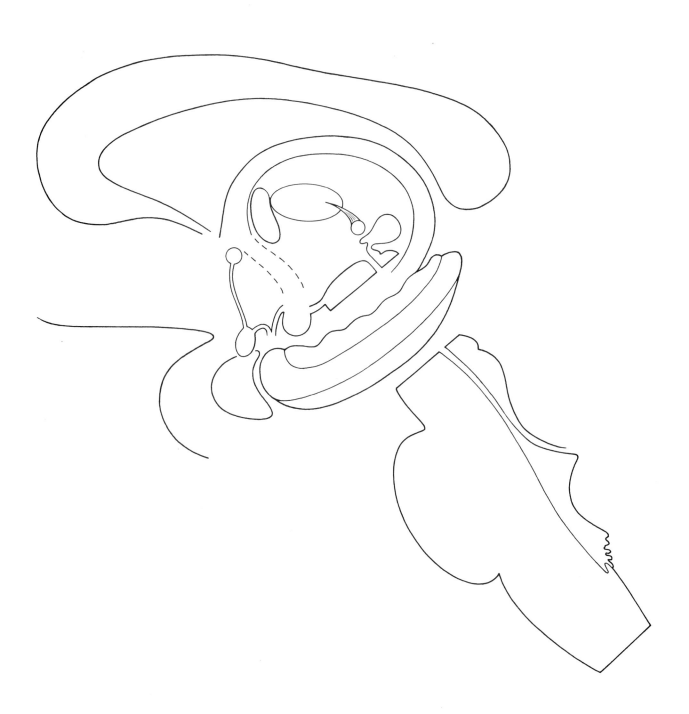

Anatomical–Clinical Correlations: Cerebral Angiogram, MRA, and MRV

A

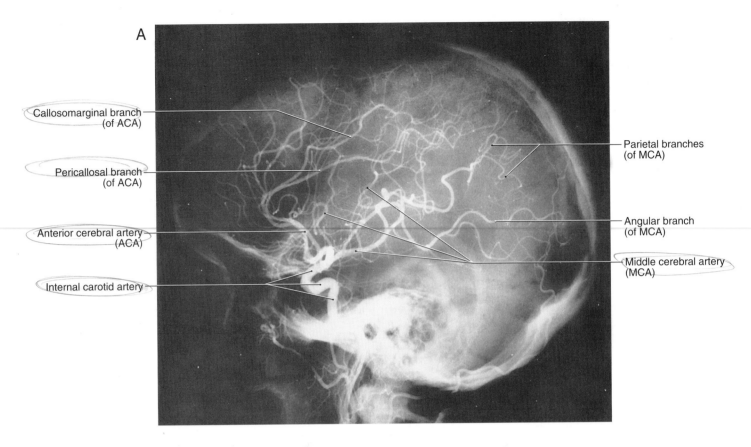

Callosomarginal branch
(of ACA)

Pericallosal branch
(of ACA)

Anterior cerebral artery
(ACA)

Internal carotid artery

Parietal branches
(of MCA)

Angular branch
(of MCA)

Middle cerebral artery
(MCA)

B

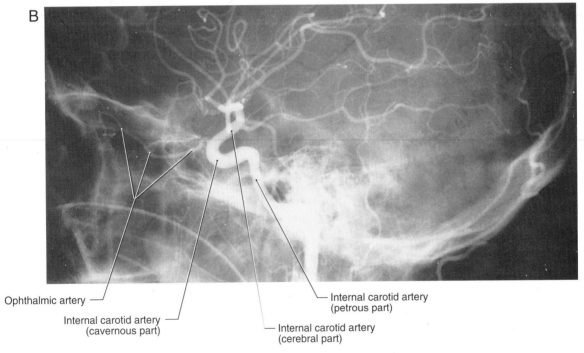

Ophthalmic artery

Internal carotid artery
(cavernous part)

Internal carotid artery
(cerebral part)

Internal carotid artery
(petrous part)

8-1 Internal carotid angiogram (left lateral projection, arterial phase) showing the general patterns of the internal carotid, middle, and anterior cerebral arteries **(A, B)** and an image with especially good filling of the ophthalmic artery **(B).** The ophthalmic artery leaves the cerebral part of the internal carotid and enters the orbit via the optic canal. This vessel gives rise to the central artery of the retina, which is an important source of blood supply to the retina. Occlusion of the ophthalamic artery may result in blindness in the eye on that side. The terminal branches of the ophthalmic artery will anastomose with superficial vessels around the orbit. Compare with Figures 2-12 (page 19) and 2-25 (page 27).

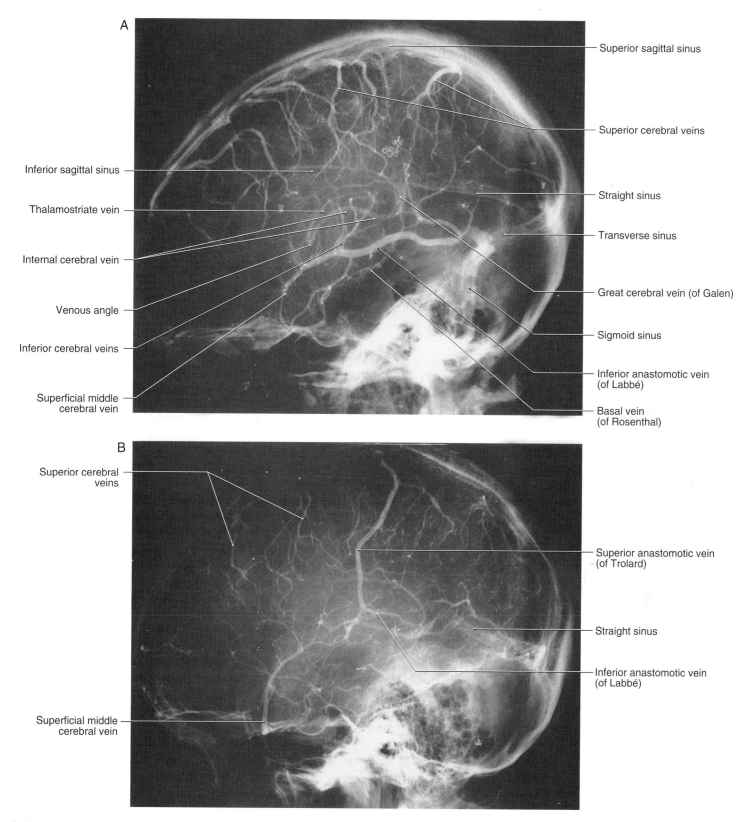

A

Superior sagittal sinus

Superior cerebral veins

Inferior sagittal sinus

Thalamostriate vein

Internal cerebral vein

Venous angle

Inferior cerebral veins

Superficial middle cerebral vein

Straight sinus

Transverse sinus

Great cerebral vein (of Galen)

Sigmoid sinus

Inferior anastomotic vein (of Labbé)

Basal vein (of Rosenthal)

B

Superior cerebral veins

Superficial middle cerebral vein

Superior anastomotic vein (of Trolard)

Straight sinus

Inferior anastomotic vein (of Labbé)

8-2 Two internal carotid angiograms (left lateral projection, venous phase). Superficial and deep venous structures are clear in **A,** but **B** shows a particularly obvious vein of Trolard. The thalamostriate vein **(A)** at this location can also be called the superior thalamostriate vein. The junction of the superior thalamostriate vein with the internal cerebral vein is called the venous angle **(A)**. The interventricular foramen is located immediately rostral to this point. Compare these images with the drawings of veins and sinuses in Figures 2-13 (page 19) and 2-28 (page 29).

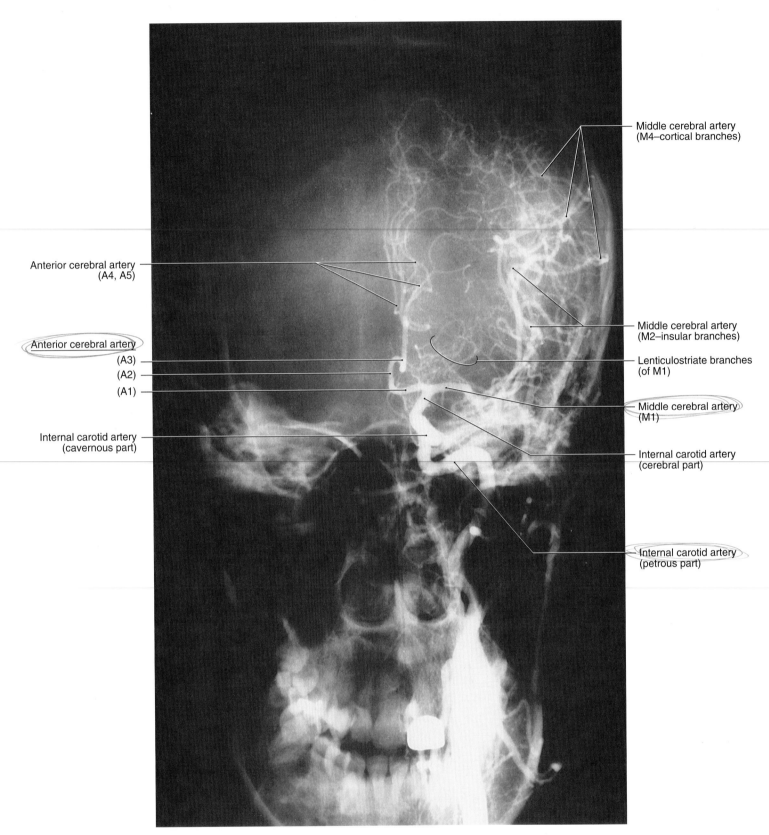

Middle cerebral artery
(M4–cortical branches)

Anterior cerebral artery
(A4, A5)

Anterior cerebral artery
(A3)
(A2)
(A1)

Internal carotid artery
(cavernous part)

Middle cerebral artery
(M2–insular branches)

Lenticulostriate branches
(of M1)

Middle cerebral artery
(M1)

Internal carotid artery
(cerebral part)

Internal carotid artery
(petrous part)

8-3 Internal carotid angiogram (anterior–posterior projection, arterial phase). Note general distribution patterns of anterior and middle cerebral arteries and the location of lenticulostriate branches. The A_1 segment of the anterior cerebral artery is located between the internal carotid bifurcation and the anterior communicating artery. The distal portion of the anterior cerebral artery (ACA) immediately rostral to the anterior communicating artery and inferior to the rostrum of the corpus callosum is the A2 segment (infracallosal). The portion of the ACA arching around the genu of the corpus callosum is the A3 segment (precallosal) and the A4 (supracallosal) and A5 (postcallosal) segments are located superior (above) the corpus callosum.

The M_1 segment of the middle cerebral artery is located between the internal carotid bifurcation and the point at which this vessel branches into superior and inferior trunks on the insular cortex. As branches of the middle cerebral artery pass over the insular cortex they are designated as M_2, as M_3 when these branches are located on the inner surface of the frontal, parietal, and temporal opercula, and as M_4 where they exit the lateral sulcus and fan out over the lateral aspect of the cerebral hemisphere. Compare with Figure 2-21 on page 25.

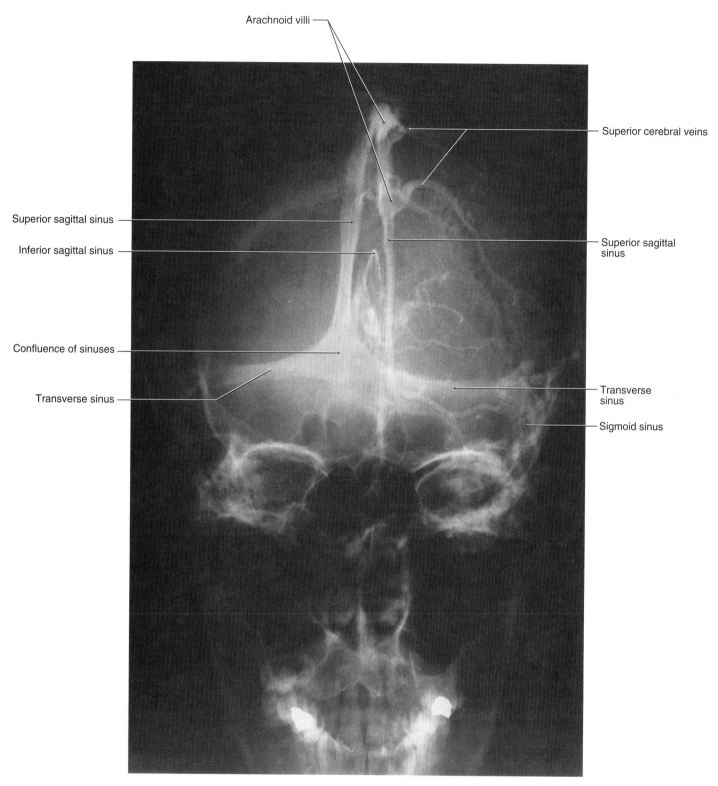

Arachnoid villi

Superior cerebral veins

Superior sagittal sinus

Inferior sagittal sinus

Superior sagittal sinus

Confluence of sinuses

Transverse sinus

Transverse sinus

Sigmoid sinus

8-4 Internal carotid angiogram (anterior–posterior projection, venous phase). The patient's head is tilted slightly; this shows the arching shapes of the superior and inferior sagittal sinuses to full advantage. Note the other venous structures in this image and compare with the arterial phase shown in Figure 8-3 on page 242 and the images in Figures 8-5 and 8-6 on pages 244 and 245. Also compare with Figure 2-28 on page 29.

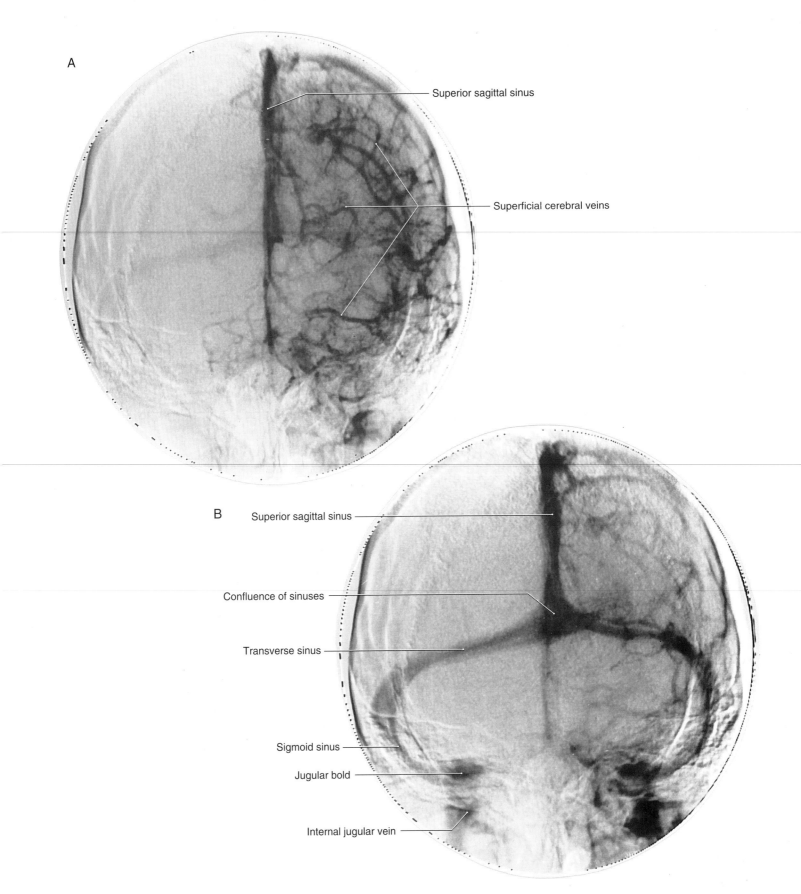

A

Superior sagittal sinus

Superficial cerebral veins

B

Superior sagittal sinus

Confluence of sinuses

Transverse sinus

Sigmoid sinus

Jugular bold

Internal jugular vein

8-5 Digital subtraction image of an internal carotid angiogram (anterior–posterior projection, venous phase). Image **A** is early in the venous phase (greater filling of cortical veins), whereas image **B** is later in the venous phase (greater filling of the sinuses and jugular vein). Both images are of the same patient.

The jugular bulb is a dilated portion of internal jugular vein (IJV) in the jugular fossa at the point where the sigmoid sinus is continuous with the IJV; this continuity is through the jugular foramen. The jugular foramen also contains the roots of cranial nerves IX, X, and XI, the continuation of inferior petrosal sinus with the IJV and several small arteries. Compare with Figures 2-16 (page 21) and 2-19 (page 23).

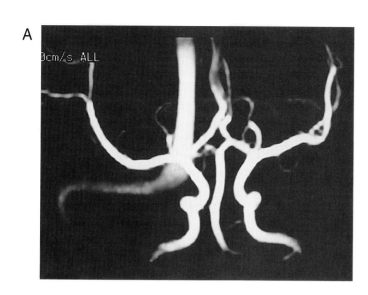

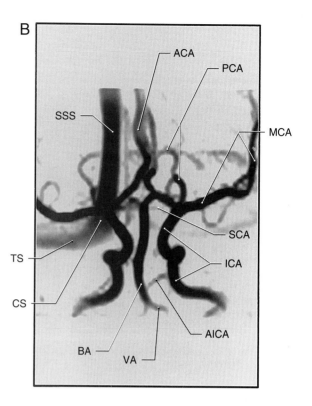

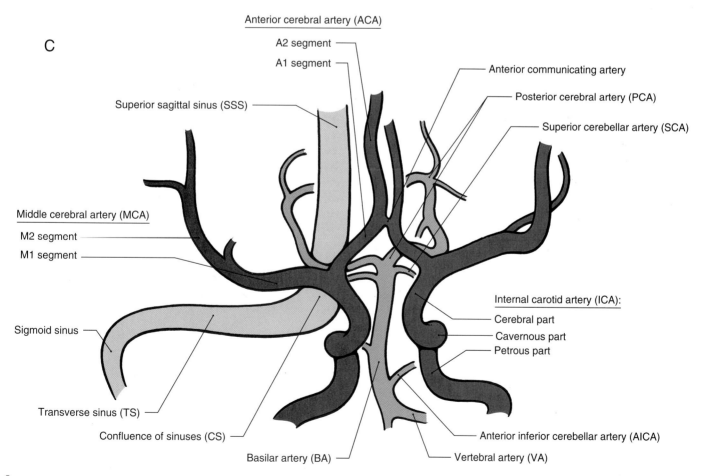

C

Anterior cerebral artery (ACA)

A2 segment

A1 segment

Anterior communicating artery

Posterior cerebral artery (PCA)

Superior sagittal sinus (SSS)

Superior cerebellar artery (SCA)

Middle cerebral artery (MCA)

M2 segment

M1 segment

Internal carotid artery (ICA):

Cerebral part

Cavernous part

Petrous part

Sigmoid sinus

Transverse sinus (TS)

Confluence of sinuses (CS)

Basilar artery (BA)

Anterior inferior cerebellar artery (AICA)

Vertebral artery (VA)

8-6   Magnetic resonance angiography (MRA) is a noninvasive method for imaging cerebral arteries, veins, and sinuses simultaneously. A 3-D phase contrast MRA **(A)** and an inverted video image window **(B)** of the same view show major vessels and sinuses from anterior to posterior. **C** shows the relative position of the major vessels and dural sinuses as imaged in **A** and **B.** The superior sagittal sinus, as seen in A and B, is usually continuous with the right transverse sinus at the confluence of sinuses.

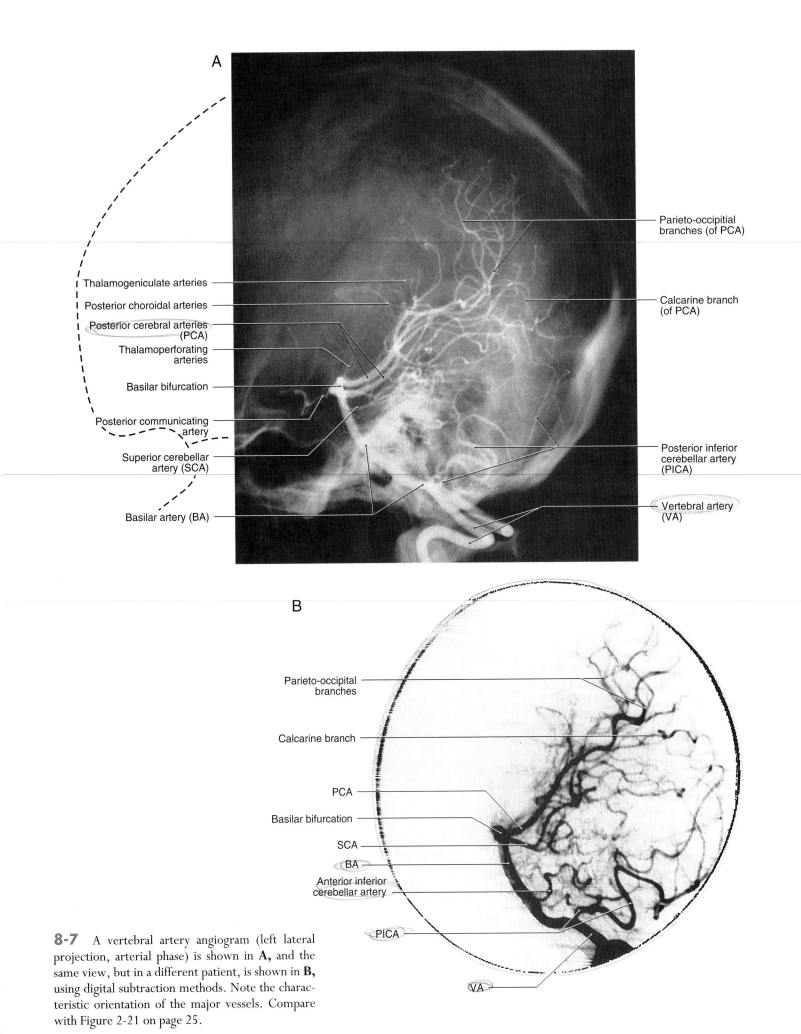

A

Parieto-occipitial
branches (of PCA)

Thalamogeniculate arteries

Posterior choroidal arteries

Posterior cerebral arteries
(PCA)

Thalamoperforating
arteries

Basilar bifurcation

Posterior communicating
artery

Superior cerebellar
artery (SCA)

Basilar artery (BA)

Calcarine branch
(of PCA)

Posterior inferior
cerebellar artery
(PICA)

Vertebral artery
(VA)

B

Parieto-occipital
branches

Calcarine branch

PCA

Basilar bifurcation

SCA

BA

Anterior inferior
cerebellar artery

PICA

VA

8-7 A vertebral artery angiogram (left lateral projection, arterial phase) is shown in **A,** and the same view, but in a different patient, is shown in **B,** using digital subtraction methods. Note the characteristic orientation of the major vessels. Compare with Figure 2-21 on page 25.

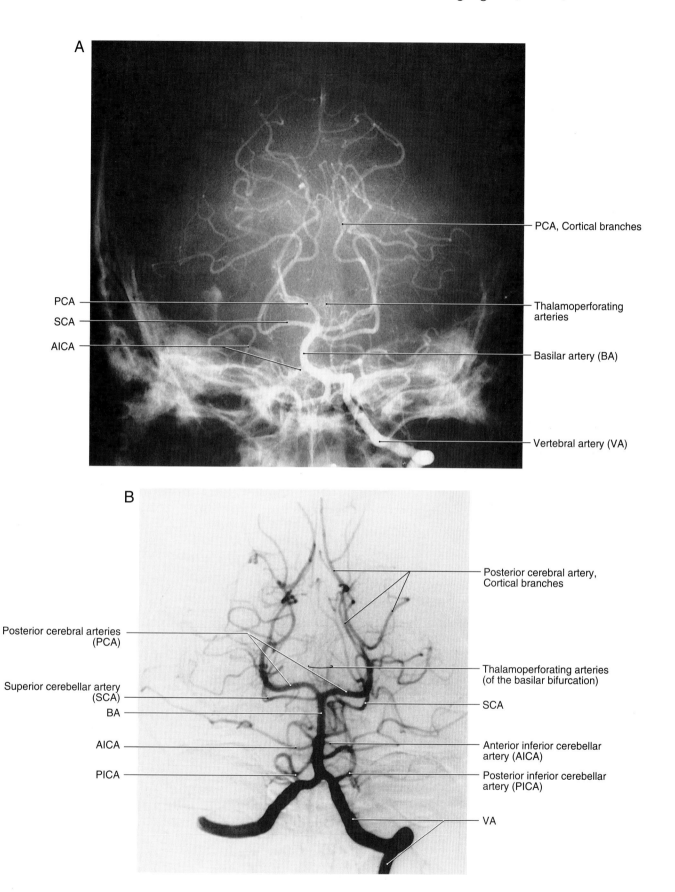

A

PCA, Cortical branches

PCA

SCA

AICA

Thalamoperforating
arteries

Basilar artery (BA)

Vertebral artery (VA)

B

Posterior cerebral arteries
(PCA)

Superior cerebellar artery
(SCA)

BA

AICA

PICA

Posterior cerebral artery,
Cortical branches

Thalamoperforating arteries
(of the basilar bifurcation)

SCA

Anterior inferior cerebellar
artery (AICA)

Posterior inferior cerebellar
artery (PICA)

VA

8-8 A vertebral artery angiogram (anterior–posterior projection, arterial phase) is shown in **A;** the same view, but in a different patient, is shown in **B,** using digital subtraction methods. Even though the injection is into the left vertebral, there is bilateral filling of the vertebral arteries and of branches of the basilar artery. The thalamoperforating arteries are important branches of P1 that generally serve rostral portions of the diencephalon.

The root of the oculomotor (IIIrd) nerve, after exiting the inferior aspect of the midbrain, characteristically passes through the interpeduncular cistern and between the superior cerebellar and posterior cerebral arteries en route to its exit from the skull through the superior orbital fissure. In this position the IIIrd nerve may be damaged by large aneurysms that impinge on the nerve root. Compare with Figures 2-40 (page 39) and 2-41 (page 40).

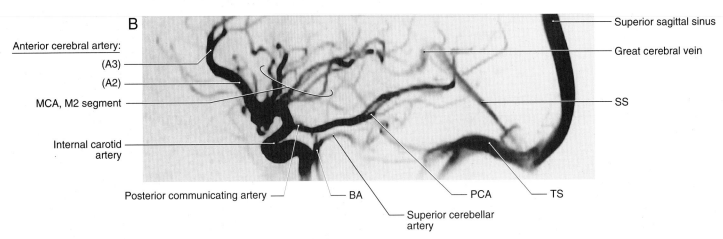

A

Anterior cerebral artery:

A3 segment

A2 segment

A1 segment

Basilar artery (BA)

PCA, Temporal branch

Lateral ventricular vein

Transverse sinus (TS)

Middle cerebral artery (MCA):

M1 segment

M2 segment

MCA, Insular branches

Posterior cerebral artery (PCA)

MCA, Cortical branches (M4 segment)

Internal cerebral vein

Superior petrosal sinus

Great cerebral vein (of Galen)

Straight sinus (SS)

TS

B

Anterior cerebral artery:

(A3)

(A2)

MCA, M2 segment

Internal carotid artery

Posterior communicating artery

BA

Superior cerebellar artery

PCA

TS

Superior sagittal sinus

Great cerebral vein

SS

8-9 MRA images arteries, veins, and sinuses simultaneously, based on the movement of fluid in these structures. These are inverted video images of 3-D phase contrast MRA images as viewed from the dorsal to ventral **(A)** and from the lateral aspect **(B)**. The distal portion of the anterior cerebral artery (ACA) immediately rostral to the anterior communicating artery and inferior to the rostrum of the corpus callo- sum is the A2 segment (infracallosal). The portion of the ACA arching around the genu of the corpus callosum is the A3 segment (precallosal) and the A4 (supracallosal) and A5 (postcallosal) segments are located superior to (above) the corpus callosum. Compare these images with arteries and veins as depicted in Figures 2-18 and 2-19 (page 23), 2-21 (page 25), and 2-23 (page 27).

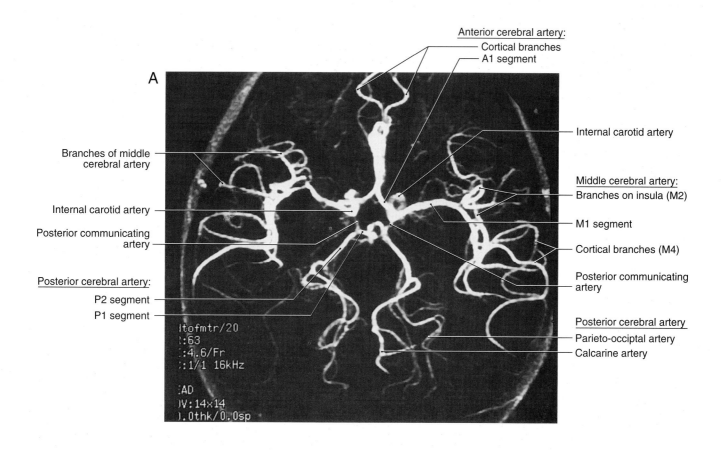

Anterior cerebral artery:
— Cortical branches
— A1 segment

— Internal carotid artery

Middle cerebral artery:
— Branches on insula (M2)

— M1 segment

— Cortical branches (M4)

Posterior communicating artery

Posterior cerebral artery
— Parieto-occiptal artery
— Calcarine artery

Branches of middle cerebral artery

Internal carotid artery

Posterior communicating artery

Posterior cerebral artery:
P2 segment
P1 segment

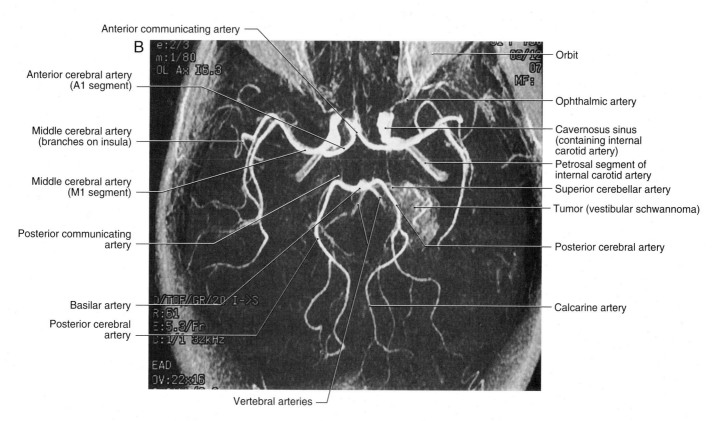

Anterior communicating artery

Anterior cerebral artery (A1 segment)

Middle cerebral artery (branches on insula)

Middle cerebral artery (M1 segment)

Posterior communicating artery

Basilar artery
Posterior cerebral artery

Vertebral arteries

Orbit

Ophthalmic artery

Cavernosus sinus (containing internal carotid artery)

Petrosal segment of internal carotid artery

Superior cerebellar artery

Tumor (vestibular schwannoma)

Posterior cerebral artery

Calcarine artery

8-10   MRA images of the vessels at the base of the brain forming much of the cerebral arterial circle (of Willis) **(A, B).** Note the anterior, middle, and posterior cerebral arteries as they extend outward from the circle. The upper image is from a normal individual, and the lower image is from a patient with a vestibular schwannoma. Descriptions of the segments of the anterior, middle, and posterior cerebral arteries are found on pages 25 and 242.

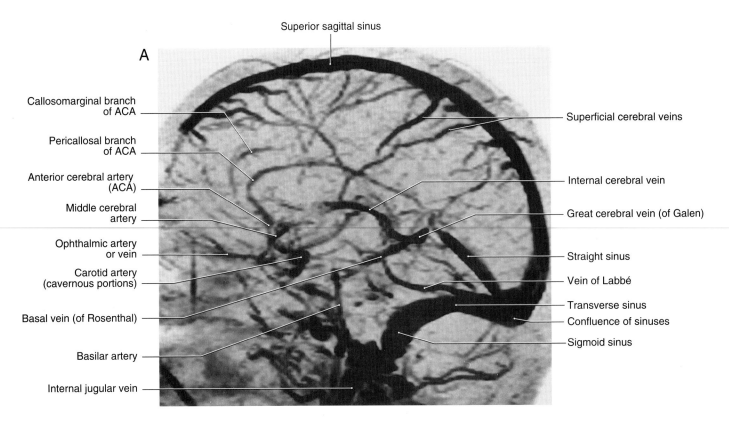

A

Superior sagittal sinus

Callosomarginal branch of ACA

Pericallosal branch of ACA

Anterior cerebral artery (ACA)

Middle cerebral artery

Ophthalmic artery or vein

Carotid artery (cavernous portions)

Basal vein (of Rosenthal)

Basilar artery

Internal jugular vein

Superficial cerebral veins

Internal cerebral vein

Great cerebral vein (of Galen)

Straight sinus

Vein of Labbé

Transverse sinus

Confluence of sinuses

Sigmoid sinus

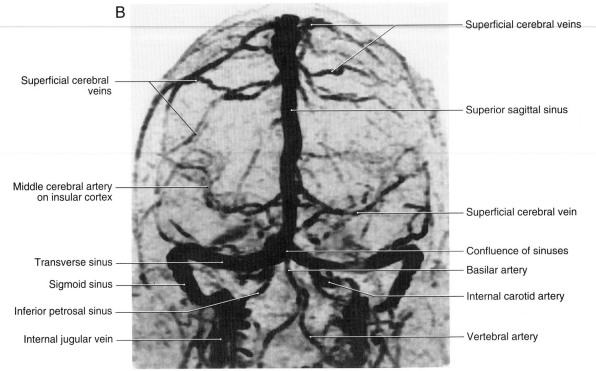

B

Superficial cerebral veins

Superficial cerebral veins

Superior sagittal sinus

Middle cerebral artery on insular cortex

Superficial cerebral vein

Confluence of sinuses

Transverse sinus

Basilar artery

Sigmoid sinus

Internal carotid artery

Inferior petrosal sinus

Internal jugular vein

Vertebral artery

8-11   Magnetic resonance venography (MRV) primarily demonstrates veins and venous sinuses although arteries (seen in **A** and **B**) will also sometimes be visualized. Many veins and venous sinuses can be seen in this lateral view **(A)** and in the anterior-posterior view **(B).** Note that the continuation of the superior sagittal sinus is most prominent into the right transverse sinus (**B,** compare with Figure 8-6 on page 245). Compare with Figures 2-13 (page 19), 2-16 (page 21), 2-19 (page 27), and 2-28 (page 29).

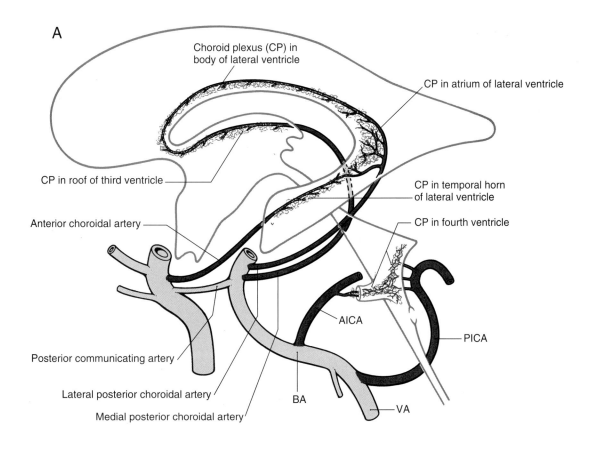

A

Choroid plexus (CP) in body of lateral ventricle

CP in atrium of lateral ventricle

CP in roof of third ventricle

CP in temporal horn of lateral ventricle

Anterior choroidal artery

CP in fourth ventricle

AICA

PICA

Posterior communicating artery

Lateral posterior choroidal artery

Medial posterior choroidal artery

BA

VA

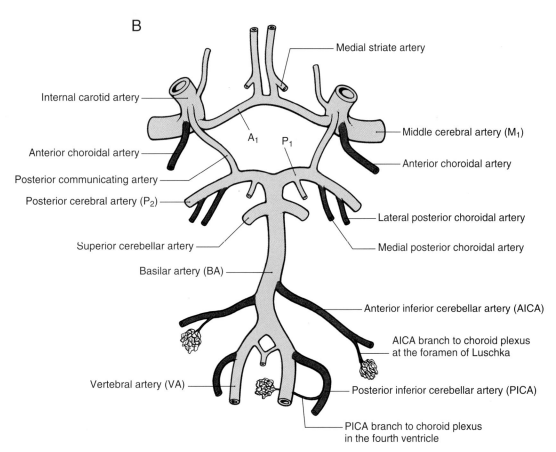

B

Medial striate artery

Internal carotid artery

A_1 P_1

Middle cerebral artery (M_1)

Anterior choroidal artery

Anterior choroidal artery

Posterior communicating artery

Posterior cerebral artery (P_2)

Lateral posterior choroidal artery

Superior cerebellar artery

Medial posterior choroidal artery

Basilar artery (BA)

Anterior inferior cerebellar artery (AICA)

AICA branch to choroid plexus at the foramen of Luschka

Vertebral artery (VA)

Posterior inferior cerebellar artery (PICA)

PICA branch to choroid plexus in the fourth ventricle

8-12   Blood supply to the choroid plexus of the lateral, third, and fourth ventricles. Those branches of the vertebrobasilar system and of the internal carotid artery and P2 segment of the posterior cerebral artery that supply the choroid plexus are accentuated by appearing in a darker red shade. In **A,** a representation of these vessels (origin, course, termination) is shown from the lateral aspect. Anterior, posterior medial, and poste- rior lateral choroidal arteries serve the plexuses of the lateral and third ventricles. The choroid plexus in the fourth ventricle and the clump of choroid plexus protruding out of the foramen of Luschka are served by posterior inferior and anterior inferior cerebellar arteries, respectively. In **B,** the origins of these branches from their main arterial trunks are shown. See also Figures 2-21 (page 25), 2-24 (page 27), and 2-35 (page 35).

A

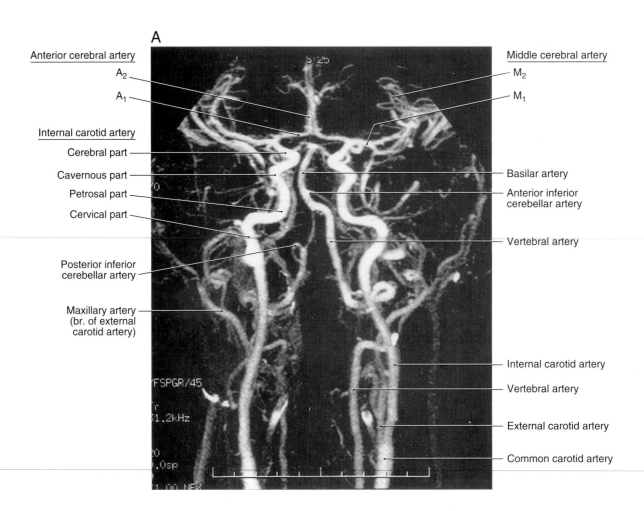

Anterior cerebral artery
- A₂
- A₁

Internal carotid artery
- Cerebral part
- Cavernous part
- Petrosal part
- Cervical part

Posterior inferior cerebellar artery

Maxillary artery (br. of external carotid artery)

Middle cerebral artery
- M₂
- M₁

Basilar artery

Anterior inferior cerebellar artery

Vertebral artery

Internal carotid artery

Vertebral artery

External carotid artery

Common carotid artery

B

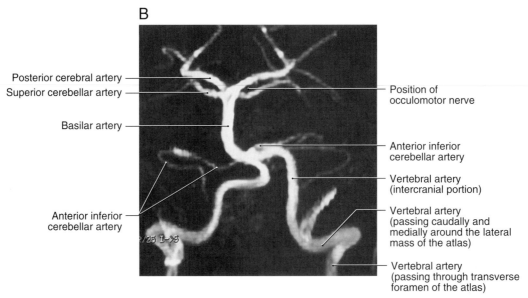

Posterior cerebral artery

Superior cerebellar artery

Basilar artery

Anterior inferior cerebellar artery

Position of occulomotor nerve

Anterior inferior cerebellar artery

Vertebral artery (intercranial portion)

Vertebral artery (passing caudally and medially around the lateral mass of the atlas)

Vertebral artery (passing through transverse foramen of the atlas)

8-13　Overview (**A**) of the arteries in the neck that serve the brain (internal carotid and vertebral) and of their main terminal branches (anterior cerebral artery and middle cerebral artery, vertebrobasilar system) as seen in an MRA (anterior-posterior view). In approximately 40–45% of individuals the left vertebral artery is larger, as seen here, and in about 5–10% of individuals one or the other of the vertebral arteries may be hypoplastic as seen here on the patient's right. The MRI in **B** is a detailed view of the vertebrobasilar system from the point where the vertebral arteries exit the transverse foramen to where the basilar artery bifurcates into the posterior cerebral arteries. Compare this image with Figure 2-21 on page 25.

The vertebral artery (VA) is generally described as being composed of 4 segments sometimes designated as V_1 to V_4. The first segment (V_1) is between the VA origin from the subclavian artery and the entrance of VA into the first transverse foramen (usually C6); the second segment V_2 is that part of VA ascending through the transverse foramen of C6 to C2; the third segment (V_3) is between the exit of VA from the transverse foramen of the axis and the dura at the foramen magnum (this includes the loop of the VA that passes through the transverse foramen of C1/the atlas); the fourth segment (V_4) pierces the dura and joins its counterpart to form the basilar artery.

9

Q & A's: A Sampling of Study and Review Questions, Many in the USMLE Style, All With Explained Answers

D. E. Haines and J. A. Lancon

There are two essential goals of a student studying human neurobiology, or, for that matter, the student of any of the medical sciences. The first is to gain the knowledge base and diagnostic skills to become a competent health care professional. Addressing the medical needs of the patient with insight, skill, and compassion is paramount. The second is to successfully negotiate whatever examination procedures are used in a given setting. These may be standard class examinations, Subject National Board Examination (now used/required in many courses), the USMLE Step 1 Examination (required of all U.S. medical students), or simply the desire, on the part of the student, for self-assessment.

The questions in this chapter are prepared in two general styles. First, there are *study* or *review* questions that test general knowledge concerning the structure of the central nervous system. Many of these have a functional flavor. Second, there are single one best answer questions in the *USMLE style* that use a patient vignette approach in the stem. These questions have been carefully reviewed for clinical accuracy and relevance as used in these examples. At the end of each explained answer, page numbers appear in parentheses that specify where the *correct answer,* be it in a figure or in the text, may be found. In order to make this a fruitful learning exercise, some answers may contain additional relevant information to extend the educational process.

In general, the questions are organized by individual chapters, although chapters 1 and 2 and chapters 3 and 4 are combined. Reference to the page (or pages) containing the correct answer are usually to the chapter(s) from which the question originated. However, recognizing that neuroscience is dynamic and three-dimensional, some answers contain references to chapters other than that from which the question originated. This provides a greater level of integration by bringing a wider range of information to bear on a single question.

Correct diagnosis of the neurologically compromised patient not only requires integration of information contained in different chapters but may also require inclusion of concepts gained in other basic science courses. In this regard a few questions, and their answers, may include such additional basic concepts.

This is not an all-inclusive list of questions, but rather a sampling that covers a wide variety of neuroanatomical and clinically relevant points. There is certainly a much larger variety of questions that could be developed from the topics covered in this atlas. It is hoped that this sample will give the user a good idea of how basic neuroscience information correlates with a range of clinically relevant topics.

Review and Study Questions for Chapters 1 and 2

1. A 71-year-old man complains to his family physician that his face "feels funny." The examination reveals numbness on his face and on the same side of his tongue. MRI shows a lesion in the cerebral cortex. This man's lesion is most likely located in which of the following cortical regions?

- ○ (A) Anterior paracentral
- ○ (B) Lateral one-third of the postcentral
- ○ (C) Lateral one-third of the precentral
- ○ (D) Middle one-third of the postcentral
- ○ (E) Posterior paracentral

2. A 41-year-old woman complains to her family physician about recurring episodes of sharp pain that seem to originate from around her mouth and cheek. The pain is so intense that she is unable to eat, brush her teeth, or apply make-up. Which of the following cranial nerves is the most likely source of this pain?

- ○ (A) Facial (VII)
- ○ (B) Glossopharyngeal (IX)
- ○ (C) Hypoglossal (XII)
- ○ (D) Trigeminal (V)
- ○ (E) Vagus (X)

3. The labyrinthine artery is an important source of blood supply to the inner ear. Which of the following arteries represents the major vessel from which this branch usually arises?

- ○ (A) Anterior inferior cerebellar
- ○ (B) Basilar
- ○ (C) Posterior inferior cerebellar
- ○ (D) Superior cerebellar
- ○ (E) Vertebral

4. The quadrigeminal artery in a 20-year-old man is occluded by a fat embolus originating from a compound fracture of the humerus. Which of the following structures does this occluded vessel most directly affect?

- ○ (A) Superior cerebellar peduncle
- ○ (B) Mammillary bodies
- ○ (C) Medial and lateral geniculate bodies
- ○ (D) Pineal and habenula
- ○ (E) Superior and inferior colliculi

Questions 5 and 6 are based on the following patient.

A 63-year-old man has hearing loss, tinnitus (ringing or buzzing sounds in the ear), vertigo, and unsteady gait; all of these have developed over several years. MRI reveals a large tumor (3 cm in diameter) at the cerebellopontine angle, most likely a vestibular schwannoma (sometimes incorrectly called an acoustic neuroma).

5. What additional deficit could this patient also have?

- ○ (A) Anosmia
- ○ (B) Hemianopsia
- ○ (C) Numbness on the face
- ○ (D) Visual field deficits
- ○ (E) Weakness of the tongue

6. In addition to the vestibulocochlear nerve, which of the following structures would most likely also be affected by the tumor in this man?

- ○ (A) Anterior inferior cerebellar artery
- ○ (B) Facial nerve
- ○ (C) Glossopharyngeal nerve
- ○ (D) Posterior inferior cerebellar artery
- ○ (E) Vagus nerve

7. A 67-year-old man complains to his family physician of severe headaches. The examination reveals visual deficits in both eyes, and MRI shows a lesion in the cerebral cortex. Which of the following cortical structures represents the most likely location of this lesion?

- ○ (A) Angular gyrus
- ○ (B) Cingulate gyrus
- ○ (C) Lingual gyrus
- ○ (D) Parahippocampal gyrus
- ○ (E) Precuneus

8. A sagittal MRI of a 23-year-old woman is located at, or immediately adjacent to, the midline. Which of the following spaces or structures would be in the image and would indicate a midline plane?

- ○ (A) Cerebral aqueduct
- ○ (B) Corpus callosum
- ○ (C) Interpeduncular fossa
- ○ (D) Interventricular foramen
- ○ (E) Superior colliculus

9. A 20-year-old man is brought to the emergency department from the site of a motorcycle accident. He is unconscious and has a broken femur, humerus, and extensive facial injuries. Axial CT shows a white layer on the lateral aspect of the left hemisphere that is approximately 5 mm thick and extends for 12 cm. This observation most likely represents:

- ○ (A) Epidural hemorrhage/hematoma
- ○ (B) Parenchymatous hemorrhage in the cortex
- ○ (C) Subarachnoid hemorrhage
- ○ (D) Subdural hemorrhage/hematoma
- ○ (E) Ventricular hemorrhage

10. Which of the following portions of the ventricular system does not contain choroid plexus?

- ○ (A) Cerebral aqueduct
- ○ (B) Fourth ventricle
- ○ (C) Lateral ventricle
- ○ (D) Interventricular foramen
- ○ (E) Third ventricle

11. A 47-year-old man presents with an intense pain on his face arising from stimulation at the corner of his mouth. This is characteristic of trigeminal neuralgia (tic douloureux). MRI shows a vessel compressing the root of the trigeminal nerve. Which of the following vessels would most likely be involved?

- ○ (A) Anterior inferior cerebellar artery
- ○ (B) Basal vein (of Rosenthal)
- ○ (C) Basilar artery
- ○ (D) Posterior cerebral artery
- ○ (E) Superior cerebellar artery

12. Which of the following cranial nerves contain the afferent and efferent limbs of the corneal reflex?

   ○ (A) II and III (optic and oculomotor)
   ○ (B) III, IV, VI (oculomotor, trochlear, abducens)
   ○ (C) V and VII (trigeminal, facial)
   ○ (D) VIII and IX (vestibulocochlear, glossopharyngeal)
   ○ (E) IX and X (glossopharyngeal, vagus)

13. A 73-year-old man is brought to the emergency department after being found in his garage in a state of confusion. CT shows an infarct involving much of the superior frontal gyrus. Which of the following vessels is most likely occluded in this patient?

   ○ (A) Angular artery
   ○ (B) Callosomarginal artery
   ○ (C) Lenticulostriate arteries
   ○ (D) Middle cerebral artery, M_4 segments
   ○ (E) Posterior cerebral artery, P_4 segments

14. The MRI of a 49-year-old woman shows a tumor located immediately superior to the corpus callosum. This lesion is most likely located in which of the following lobes?

   ○ (A) Frontal
   ○ (B) Limbic
   ○ (C) Occipital
   ○ (D) Parietal
   ○ (E) Temporal

15. A 69-year-old woman is brought to the emergency department. The daughter reports that her mother suddenly seemed to be unable to speak. The examination reveals that the woman has a nonfluent (Broca) aphasia. A sagittal MRI shows a lesion in which of the following gyri?

   ○ (A) Angular
   ○ (B) Inferior frontal
   ○ (C) Lateral one-third of the precentral
   ○ (D) Middle frontal
   ○ (E) Supramarginal

16. Which of the following Brodmann areas represents the primary somatosensory cortex?

   ○ (A) Areas 3, 1, 2
   ○ (B) Area 4
   ○ (C) Area 17
   ○ (D) Area 22
   ○ (E) Area 40

17. A 64-year-old man awakens with a profound weakness of his right hand. The man is transported by ambulance to a major medical center, a distance of 240 miles and taking several hours. About 2.5 hours after his arrival, an MRI shows a small lesion in the cerebral cortex. Which of the following gyri represents the most likely location of this lesion?

   ○ (A) Anterior paracentral
   ○ (B) Medial one-third of precentral
   ○ (C) Middle frontal
   ○ (D) Middle one-third of precentral
   ○ (E) Lateral one-third of precentral

18. A lumbar puncture, commonly called a "lumbar tap," consists of a needle being inserted through an intervertebral space into the lumbar cistern to retrieve a sample of cerebrospinal fluid. Which of the following is the most likely level for the insertion of the needle?

   ○ (A) L1–L2
   ○ (B) L2–L3
   ○ (C) L4–L5
   ○ (D) S1–S2
   ○ (E) T12–L1

19. A 59-year-old man complains of persistent headache. An MRA (Magnetic Resonance Angiography) shows an aneurysm in the interpeduncular fossa (and cistern) arising from the basilar tip. Which of the following cranial nerves would be most directly affected by this aneurysm?

   ○ (A) Abducens (VI)
   ○ (B) Oculomotor (III)
   ○ (C) Optic (II)
   ○ (D) Trigeminal, V1 (V)
   ○ (E) Trochlear (IV)

20. A 71-year-old man presents with a Broca (nonfluent) aphasia. MRI reveals a lesion in Brodmann area 44. As this lesion expands, due to edema, and impinges on the immediately adjacent cortical areas, which of the following deficits would most likely be seen?

   ○ (A) Loss of hearing in one ear
   ○ (B) Numbness and prickly sensation on the hand
   ○ (C) Visual field deficits in both eyes
   ○ (D) Weakness of facial muscles
   ○ (E) Weakness of the upper extremity

21. A 47-year-old woman presents with seizures and ill-defined neurologic complaints. The examination reveals a bruit on the lateral aspect of the head immediately rostral and superior to the ear. A CT shows a large arteriovenous malformation in the area of the lateral sulcus. The feeding artery(ies) is M_4 branches. Which of the following most likely represents the major draining vein?

   ○ (A) Inferior sagittal sinus
   ○ (B) Internal cerebral vein
   ○ (C) Ophthalmic vein
   ○ (D) Superficial middle cerebral vein
   ○ (E) Superior petrosal sinus

22. The collection of posterior and anterior roots that occupy the lumbar cistern are collectively known as which of the following?

   ○ (A) Cauda equina
   ○ (B) Conus medullaris
   ○ (C) Denticulate ligament
   ○ (D) Filum terminale externum
   ○ (E) Filum terminale internum

23. Which of the following Brodmann areas represents the primary somatomotor cortex?

   ○ (A) Areas 3,1,2
   ○ (B) Area 4
   ○ (C) Area 5
   ○ (D) Area 6
   ○ (E) Area 7

24. A 39-year-old woman complains of weakness in her right lower extremity. The history suggests that this deficit has developed slowly, perhaps over several years. MRI shows a meningioma imposing on the cerebral cortex. Which of the following gyri is most likely involved in this patient?

    ○ (A)   Anterior paracentral
    ○ (B)   Lateral part of precentral
    ○ (C)   Medial part of precentral
    ○ (D)   Medial part of postcentral
    ○ (E)   Posterior paracentral

25. A 71-year-old woman presents with motor and sensory deficits affecting her face and upper extremity. CT shows a hemorrhage that is confined largely to the cortex and adjacent subcortical areas. Which of the following vessels/segments are most likely involved?

    ○ (A) A_1
    ○ (B) M_2
    ○ (C) M_3
    ○ (D) M_4
    ○ (E) P_4

26. A 22-year-old man is brought to the emergency department with a gunshot wound to the head. He is decorticate but soon becomes decerebrate. This change in status is due to uncal herniation. Which of the following most specifically describes the position of the uncus prior to herniation?

    ○ (A)   At the temporal lobe
    ○ (B)   Caudal aspect of the cingulate gyrus
    ○ (C)   Caudal aspect of the gyrus rectus
    ○ (D)   Medial edge of occipitotemporal gyri
    ○ (E)   Rostromedial aspect of the parahippocampal gyrus

27. A 73-year-old woman presents with visual deficits in both eyes. No other cranial nerve deficits or motor or sensory deficits are seen. CT shows a hemorrhage in the cerebral cortex. Which of the following vessels/segments is most likely involved in this hemorrhage?

    ○ (A) A_1
    ○ (B) M_3
    ○ (C) M_4
    ○ (D) P_2
    ○ (E) P_4

28. The CT of a 77-year-old man shows a calcified tuft of choroid plexus, the glomus choroideum. Which of the following represents the location of this part of the choroid plexus?

    ○ (A)   Anterior horn of the lateral ventricle
    ○ (B)   Atrium of the lateral ventricle
    ○ (C)   Body of the lateral ventricle
    ○ (D)   Caudal roof of the third ventricle
    ○ (E)   Temporal horn of the lateral ventricle

29. Which of the following represents the most common cause of blood in the subarachnoid space (subarachnoid hemorrhage)?

    ○ (A)   Bleeding from an arteriovenous malformation
    ○ (B)   Bleeding from a meningioma
    ○ (C)   Bleeding from a tumor
    ○ (D)   Rupture of an aneurysm
    ○ (E)   Trauma to the brain

30. The abducens nerve exits the brainstem at the pons-medulla junction generally in line with the preolivary sulcus and passes rostrally just lateral to, and in the same cistern as, the basilar artery. Which of the following cisterns contains the abducens nerve and basilar artery?

    ○ (A)   Ambient
    ○ (B)   Inferior cerebellopontine
    ○ (C)   Premedullary
    ○ (D)   Prepontine
    ○ (E)   Superior cerebellopontine

31. An 81-year-old woman is brought to the emergency department by her son with a complaint of weakness on the same side of her body and face. CT shows a hemorrhage in the territory of the lenticulostriate arteries. Which of the following represents the most likely origin of these vessels?

    ○ (A) A_1
    ○ (B) M_1
    ○ (C) M_2
    ○ (D) P_1
    ○ (E) P_2

32. The MRI of a 27-year-old woman shows a meningioma impinging on the gyrus rectus in axial and coronal MRI. This lesion is located on which of the following lobes of the cerebral hemisphere?

    ○ (A)   Frontal
    ○ (B)   Insular
    ○ (C)   Occipital
    ○ (D)   Parietal
    ○ (E)   Temporal

33. A 51-year-old man presents with visual field deficits in both eyes and a right-sided weakness of the upper and lower extremities. MRI shows a lesion in the optic tract that has spread into a structure located immediately adjacent to this tract. Based on its anatomical relationship, which of the following structures is most likely involved in a lesion spreading from the optic tract?

    ○ (A)   Left basilar pons
    ○ (B)   Left crus cerebri
    ○ (C)   Left pyramid
    ○ (D)   Right crus cerebri
    ○ (E)   Right optic nerve

34. A 19-year-old man presents with significant paralysis of movement in his left eye and a dilated pupil. No other deficits are seen. Suspecting some type of lesion on the root or along the intracranial course of the oculomotor (III) nerve, the neurologist orders an MRI. Which of the following describes the appearance of the subarachnoid and ventricular spaces in a T2-weighted image?

    ○ (A)   Black (hypointense)
    ○ (B)   Dark grey
    ○ (C)   Light grey
    ○ (D)   Medium grey
    ○ (E)   White (hyperintense)

35. A 49-year-old woman presents with ill-defined neurologic deficits that have persisted over several months. As part of the evaluation, the neurologist orders an MRI. Which of the following describes the appearance of CSF in the ventricular spaces, and consequently the outline and shape of the ventricles, in a T1-weighted image?

   ○ (A) Black (hypointense)
   ○ (B) Dark grey
   ○ (C) Light grey
   ○ (D) Medium grey
   ○ (E) White (hyperintense)

36. A 71-year-old morbidly obese man is brought to the emergency department by his son. The son reports that the man complained of a sudden excruciating headache and then became stuporous. Suspecting a ruptured aneurysm the physician orders a CT. Which of the following describes the appearance of acute blood in the subarachnoid space in CT?

   ○ (A) Black (hypodense)
   ○ (B) Black to grey
   ○ (C) Light grey
   ○ (D) Medium grey
   ○ (E) White (hyperdense)

37. Which of the following cranial nerves exits the brainstem via the preolivary sulcus?

   ○ (A) Abducens (VI)
   ○ (B) Facial (VII)
   ○ (C) Hypoglossal (XII)
   ○ (D) Vagus (X)
   ○ (E) Trigeminal (V)

38. A 29-year-old woman becomes acutely ill with high fever, a stiff neck, and stupor. A lumbar puncture reveals cloudy cerebrospinal fluid from which organisms are cultured. Which of the following represents the most frequently seen organisms in cases of adult bacterial meningitis?

   ○ (A) *Escherichia coli*
   ○ (B) *Haemophilus influenzae*
   ○ (C) *Herpes simplex*
   ○ (D) *Listeria monocytogenes*
   ○ (E) *Streptococcus pneumoniae*

39. Which of the following cranial nerves exits the posterior (dorsal) aspect of the brainstem?

   ○ (A) Abducens (VI)
   ○ (B) Hypoglossal (XII)
   ○ (C) Trigeminal (V)
   ○ (D) Trochlear (IV)
   ○ (E) Vestibulocochlear (VIII)

40. Which of the following cranial nerves passes between the posterior cerebral artery and the superior cerebellar artery as it exits the brainstem?

   ○ (A) Abducens
   ○ (B) Oculomotor
   ○ (C) Optic
   ○ (D) Trigeminal
   ○ (E) Vestibulocochlear

41. The MRI of an 11-year-old boy shows a tumor in the pontine portion of the fourth ventricle. The rostral edge of which of the following structures represents the border between the medullary and pontine parts of the fourth ventricle?

   ○ (A) Facial colliculus
   ○ (B) Hypoglossal trigone
   ○ (C) Medial eminence
   ○ (D) Stria medullares
   ○ (E) Vagal trigone

42. A 61-year-old man presents with a tremor and unsteady gait; these problems are on the same side of his body. Sagittal MRI shows a lesion in the anterior lobe of the cerebellum. Which of the following represents the fissure separating the anterior and posterior lobes of the cerebellum?

   ○ (A) Horizontal fissure
   ○ (B) Posterior superior fissure
   ○ (C) Posterolateral fissure
   ○ (D) Primary fissure
   ○ (E) Secondary fissure

43. The MRI of a 49-year-old woman with a brain tumor shows tonsillar herniation. Based on its anatomical position, which of the following portions of the brainstem would be most adversely affected by tonsillar herniation?

   ○ (A) Caudal midbrain
   ○ (B) Caudal pons
   ○ (C) Medulla
   ○ (D) Rostral midbrain
   ○ (E) Rostral pons

44. A 4-year-old boy is brought to the emergency department by his mother who explains that the boy fell off a porch onto a concrete sidewalk. The examination reveals that the boy has a parietal scalp laceration, is stuporous, and has reactive pupils. Suspecting that this boy may have a possible skull fracture with some type of intracranial bleeding, which of the following imaging tests would be most immediately (and appropriately) useful?

   ○ (A) CT
   ○ (B) MRI, gadolinium enhanced
   ○ (C) MRI, T1-weighted
   ○ (D) MRI, T2-weighted
   ○ (E) PET (Positron Emission Tomography)

45. A sagittal MRI of a 52-year-old man clearly shows a small tumor in the area of the long and short gyri. These gyri are characteristically found in which of the following lobes?

   ○ (A) Frontal
   ○ (B) Insular
   ○ (C) Limbic
   ○ (D) Occipital
   ○ (E) Parietal

46. A lesion involving the root of which of the following nerves would most likely have an effect on the gag reflex?

   ○ (A) Accessory
   ○ (B) Facial
   ○ (C) Glossopharyngeal
   ○ (D) Hypoglossal
   ○ (E) Trigeminal

Answers for Chapters 1 and 2

1. Answer **B**:   Numbness on the face, resulting from a lesion in the cerebral cortex, indicates a lesion in the lateral one-third of the postcentral gyrus (face area of the somatosensory cortex). The anterior paracentral gyrus and the precentral gyrus are somatomotor areas of the cerebral cortex. The upper extremity is represented in the middle one-third of the postcentral gyrus and the lower extremity is represented in the posterior paracentral gyrus. (p. 15)

2. Answer **D**:   Tic douloureux (trigeminal neuralgia) is a lancinating pain that originates from the territories of the trigeminal nerve, primarily its V2 or V3 territories. The trigger zone is frequently around the corner of the mouth. There is a geniculate neuralgia (related to the ear) and a glossopharyngeal neuralgia (related to the throat or palate), but neither of these originates from the surface of the face near the oral cavity. The hypoglossal nerve is the motor for the tongue and the vagus is the motor for most of the pharynx and larynx, visceromotor for much of the gut, and contains viscerosensory fibers from the gut. (p. 41)

3. Answer **A**:   In most cases (85–100%), the labyrinthine artery, also called the internal auditory artery, originates from the anterior inferior cerebellar artery. It enters the internal acoustic meatus, serves bone and dura of the canal, the nerves of the canal, and vestibular and cochlear structures. In a few cases (15% or less), this artery originates from the basilar artery. None of the other choices gives rise to vessels that serve the inner ear. (p. 25, 27)

4. Answer **E**:   The quadrigeminal artery is the primary blood supply to the superior and inferior colliculi: this vessel originates from P_1. The geniculate bodies receive their blood supply from the thalamogeniculate arteries, and the pineal and habenula from the posterior medial choroidal artery. The superior cerebellar peduncle receives its blood supply via the medial branch of the superior cerebellar artery, and branches of the cerebral circle (of Willis) serve the mammillary bodies. (p. 25, 35)

5. Answer **C**:   Vestibular schwannomas larger than 2.0 cm in diameter may impinge on the root of the trigeminal nerve and cause numbness on the same side of the face. Although the other deficits listed are not seen in these patients, diplopia (involvement of oculomotor, abducens or trochlear nerves, singularly or in combination) may be present, but in fewer than 10% of these individuals. (p. 42)

6. Answer **B**:   The internal acoustic meatus contains the vestibulocochlear nerve, the facial nerve, and the labyrinthine artery, a branch of the anterior inferior cerebellar artery. A vestibular schwannoma located in the meatus would likely affect the facial nerve and result in facial weakness. The vagus and glossopharyngeal nerves exit the skull via the jugular foramen (along with the accessory nerve). The cerebellar arteries originate within the skull and distribute to structures within the skull. (p. 42)

7. Answer **C**:   The lingual gyrus is the lower bank of the calcarine sulcus; the upper (cuneus) and lower banks of this sulcus are the location of the primary visual cortex. The precuneus is the medial aspect of the parietal lobe, and the angular gyrus is a portion of the inferior parietal lobule on the lateral aspect of the hemisphere. The cingulate and parahippocampal gyri are located on the medial aspect of the hemisphere and are parts of the limbic lobe. (p. 13–15, 28)

8. Answer **A**:   The cerebral aqueduct is about 1.5–2.0 mm in diameter, and connects the third ventricle with the fourth ventricle. When this part of the ventricular system appears in a sagittal MRI, the plane of the scan is at the midline. Neither the interventricular foramen nor the superior colliculus are on the midline. Both the interpeduncular fossa and the corpus callosum are on the midline, but extend off the midline well beyond the width of the cerebral aqueduct. (p. 28–31, 49, 50, 52)

9. Answer **D**:   Trauma may cause epidural hemorrhage, subdural hemorrhage, or subarachnoid hemorrhage. Acute subdural hemorrhage/hematoma will appear white in CT and will usually present as a comparatively thin but long defect. Epidural hemorrhage will usually be seen as a shorter but thicker lesion and may appear loculated (have some sort of internal structure). The structure (shape) of this lesion does not conform to hemorrhage into the substance of the brain (brain parenchyma), into the subarachnoid space (or cisterns), and certainly not to hemorrhage into the ventricles. (p. 46, 48, 51)

10. Answer **A**:   The only portion of the ventricular system that does not contain choroid plexus is the cerebral aqueduct. The choroid plexus in the lateral ventricle is continuous from the inferior horn into the atrium and into the body of the ventricle, and through the interventricular foramen with the choroid plexus located along the roof of the third ventricle. There is a tuft of choroid plexus in the fourth ventricle, a small part of which extends into the lateral recess and through the lateral foramen (of Luschka) into the subarachnoid space at the cerebellopontine angle. (p. 52–53)

11. Answer **E**:   Branches of the superior cerebellar artery are most frequently involved in cases of trigeminal neuralgia that are presumably of vascular origin. The posterior cerebral artery and its larger branches serve the midbrain-diencephalic junction or join the medial surface of the hemisphere. The basilar artery serves the basilar pons and the anterior inferior cerebellar artery serves the caudal midbrain, inner ear, and the inferior surface of the cerebellar surface. The basal vein drains the medial portions of the hemisphere and passes through the ambient cistern to enter the great cerebral vein (of Galen). (p. 41)

12. Answer **C**:   The afferent limb of the corneal reflex is via the ophthalmic division of the trigeminal nerve (V); the cell body of origin is in the trigeminal ganglion and the central terminations in the pars caudalis of the spinal trigeminal nucleus. The efferent limb originates in the motor nucleus of the facial nerve (VII) and distributes to the facial muscles around the eye. None of the other choices contains fibers related to the corneal reflex. (p. 42)

13. Answer **B**:   The callosomarginal artery, a branch of the anterior cerebral artery, serves the medial aspect of the superior frontal gyrus and that portion of this gyrus on the superior and lateral aspects of the hemisphere. M_4 segments of the middle cerebral artery serve the lateral aspects of the hemisphere; P_4 segments of the posterior cerebral artery serve the medial aspects of the hemisphere caudal to the parietooccipital sulcus, and the angular artery (an M_4 branch) serves the angular gyrus of the inferior parietal lobule. The lenticulostriate arteries are branches of M_1 that serve internal structures of the hemisphere. (p. 17, 29)

14. Answer **B**:   The limbic lobe, consisting primarily of the cingulate gyrus and the parahippocampal gyrus, is located on the most

medial aspect of the hemisphere; the cingulate gyrus is located immediately adjacent to the corpus callosum. None of the other lobes of the cerebral cortex borders directly on the corpus callosum. (p. 13, 28)

15. Answer **B**: The inferior frontal gyrus consists of the pars orbitalis (Brodmann area 47), pars triangularis (area 45), and pars opercularis (area 44). A lesion located primarily in areas 44 and 45 in the dominant hemisphere will result in a nonfluent (Broca) aphasia. The supramarginal (area 40) and angular (area 39) gyri represent what is called the Wernicke area, and the middle frontal gyrus contains areas 6 and 8. The lateral one-third of the precentral gyrus is the face area of the somatomotor cortex. (p. 14)

16. Answer **A**: Areas 3, 1, 2 collectively represent the primary somatosensory cortex. Area 4 is the primary somatomotor cortex, area 17 the primary visual cortex, and area 22 the primary auditory cortex. Area 40 is in the supramarginal gyrus, a large part of which is called the Wernicke area. (p. 14)

17. Answer **D**: The body is represented in the somatomotor cortex (precentral gyrus, anterior paracentral gyrus) in the following pattern: the face in about the lateral one-third of the precentral gyrus above the lateral sulcus; the hand and upper extremity in about its middle third; and the trunk and hip in about its medial third. The lower extremity and foot are represented in the anterior paracentral gyrus. Caudal portions of the middle frontal gyrus are the location of the frontal eye field. (p. 15)

18. Answer **C**: The L4-L5 interspace is commonly used for a lumbar puncture. The L3-L4 space may also be used. Levels T12 to L2-L3 are too high. Because the caudal end of the spinal cord (the conus medullaris) may be as low as L2 in some individuals, levels T12-L1 to L2-L3 are not used, as this would most likely result in damage to the spinal cord. The S1-S2 vertebrae are fused so there is no intervertebral space through which a needle can pass. Furthermore, the dural sac ends at about S2. (p. 12)

19. Answer **B**: The oculomotor nerve (III) exits from the medial aspect of the midbrain into the interpeduncular fossa/cistern. It traverses this space, courses through the lateral wall of the cavernous sinus to eventually enter (along with the trochlear [IV] and abducens [VI] nerves) the superior orbital fissure. Cranial nerves IV, VI, and V_1 (the ophthalmic portion of the trigeminal nerve), along with III, pass through the cavernous sinus. Cranial nerve II (optic) is quite rostral to the interpeduncular fossa. (p. 24, 30, 40)

20. Answer **D**: A lesion in area 44 (the pars opercularis) that spreads will affect the lower portions of the precentral gyrus in which the face is represented. This will result in weakness of facial muscles, accompanied by other cranial nerve deficits. The cortical areas for hearing and vision are far separated from area 44. Also, a lesion in the primary auditory cortex will not result in a hearing loss in one ear. The hand area of the sensory cortex and the upper extremity area of the motor cortex are not adjacent to Brodmann area 44. (p. 14)

21. Answer **D**: The superficial middle cerebral vein is located on the surface of the cerebral hemisphere in the immediate vicinity of the lateral sulcus and, of the choices, is the most likely candidate. The deep middle cerebral vein is located on the surface of the insular lobe. The inferior sagittal sinus primarily drains the medial aspect of the hemisphere immediately superior to the corpus callosum. The internal cerebral vein (to the great cerebral vein) drains the internal parts of the hemisphere; the ophthalmic vein connects the orbit with the cavernous sinus; and the superior petrosal sinus connects the cavernous sinus with the sigmoid sinus at its junction with the transverse sinus. (p. 19, 23, 29)

22. Answer **A**: As they descend in the dural sac from their origin from the spinal cord to their exit at their respective intervertebral foramen, the anterior and posterior roots form the cauda equina. The conus medullaris is the most caudal end of the spinal cord, and the filum terminale internum is the strand of pia that extends from the conus caudally to attach to the inner aspect of the dural sac at about S2. The denticulate ligament anchors the spinal cord laterally to the inner surface of the dural sac, and the filum terminale externum anchors the dural sac caudally to the inner aspect of the coccyx. (p. 12, 85, 87)

23. Answer **B**: The primary somatomotor cortex consists of the precentral gyrus and the anterior paracentral gyrus; area 4 is found in these structures. Areas 3, 1, and 2 are the primary somatosensory cortex; areas 5 and 7 make up the superior parietal lobule and the precuneus; and area 6 is located rostral to area 4. Portions of area 6 in the caudal region of the middle frontal gyrus are the frontal eye field. (p. 15)

24. Answer **A**: In this patient, the meningioma is located in the falx cerebri and is impinging on the anterior paracentral gyrus correlating with her motor deficit. The lower extremity is represented in the anterior paracentral gyrus (somatomotor) and in the posterior paracentral gyrus (somatosensory). The precentral gyrus contains the motor representation for the face (lateral part) and the trunk and hip (medial part). The postcentral gyrus is part of the somatosensory cortex. (p. 15)

25. Answer **D**: The M_4 segments of the middle cerebral artery serve the lateral aspect of the cerebral hemisphere. The named M_4 vessels that serve the pre- and postcentral gyri (hemorrhage into approximately the lower two-thirds of these gyri explain the motor and sensory deficits) are the precentral branches (prerolandic), central branches (Rolandic branches), and anterior parietal branches. The M_2 segment serves the insular cortex, and the M_3 segment serves the inner surface of the frontal, parietal, and temporal opercula. The A_1 segment serves hypothalamic structures, the subcallosal and septal areas, and adjacent structures. P_4 serves the medial aspect of the occipital lobe (visual cortex). (p. 19, 29)

26. Answer **E**: The uncus is a small elevation at the rostral and medial aspect of the parahippocampal gyrus adjacent to the crus cerebri of the midbrain. In addition to the catastrophic effect of decerebration, herniation of the uncus may also affect corticospinal and corticonuclear (corticobulbar) fibers in the crus cerebri and the root of the oculomotor nerve. None of the other areas of the forebrain listed as choices is related to uncal herniation. (p. 20, 22)

27. Answer **E**: The P_4 segments of the posterior cerebral artery consist of the parieto-occipital and calcarine branches; the latter being located in the calcarine sulcus and a primary blood supply to the primary visual cortex. M_3 and M_4 segments of the middle cerebral are located, respectively, on the inner aspect of the frontal, parietal, and temporal opercula and on the lateral aspect of the cere-

bral hemisphere. The P$_2$ segment of the posterior cerebral artery is located just distal to the posterior communicating–posterior cerebral intersection and gives rise to medial and lateral posterior choroidal and to thalamogeniculate arteries. The A$_1$ segment is located between the internal carotid and anterior communicating artery and gives rise to branches that serve anterior hypothalamic structures, septal areas, and the optic chiasm. (p. 21, 29)

28. Answer **B**: The glomus choroideum is found in the atrium of the lateral ventricle. This part of the choroid plexus is rostrally continuous with that in the body of the lateral ventricle and continuous anteroinferiorly with that in the temporal horn. The roof of the third ventricle has a small portion of choroid plexus that is continuous with that in the body of the ventricle via the interventricular foramen. The anterior horn contains no choroid plexus. (p. 52)

29. Answer **E**: Trauma is the most common cause of subarachnoid hemorrhage (SAH). The most common cause of spontaneous (also called nontraumatic) SAH is bleeding from a ruptured aneurysm (about 75% of all spontaneous cases). Bleeding from an arteriovenous malformation (AVM) is an infrequent cause of SAH (about 5% of cases), and bleeding from brain tumors into the subarachnoid space is rare. Meningiomas are usually slow-growing tumors that may have a rich vascular supply but rarely hemorrhage spontaneously. (p. 46)

30. Answer **D**: The prepontine cistern is located external to the basilar pons and contains the abducens nerve, basilar artery, origin of the anterior inferior cerebellar artery, and small perforating arteries and veins. The ambient cistern is located on the lateral aspect of the midbrain and contains the trochlear nerve and several major arteries. The premedullary cistern is located at the anterior surface of the medulla and contains the anterior spinal artery. The inferior cerebellopontine cistern contains the glossopharyngeal, vagus, and accessory nerves. The superior cerebellopontine cistern contains the trigeminal, facial, and vestibulocochlear nerves plus a short segment of the trochlear nerve. (p. 50, 51)

31. Answer **B**: Lenticulostriate arteries, also called the lateral striate arteries, originate from the M$_1$ segment of the middle cerebral artery and serve much of the lenticular nucleus and adjacent parts of the internal capsule. A$_1$ branches serve the anterior hypothalamus and optic chiasm, and M$_2$ branches serve the insular cortex. The P$_1$ and P$_2$ segments give rise to many small perforating branches and to the thalamoperforating and quadrigeminal arteries (P$_1$), medial and lateral posterior choroidal arteries, and the thalamogeniculate artery (P$_2$). (p. 25, 49, 242)

32. Answer **A**: The gyrus rectus is located on the inferior and medial aspect of the frontal lobe. It is separated from the orbital gyri by the olfactory sulcus in which the olfactory bulb and tract is located. None of the other lobes has a direct relationship to the gyrus rectus. (p. 20, 22)

33. Answer **B**: The optic tract lies immediately on the surface of the crus cerebri, a relationship frequently seen in MRI. The fact that this patient has a right-sided weakness of the extremities specifies that the lesion is in the left crus cerebri. The bilateral visual deficits correlate with damage to the left optic tract. Lesions of the left basilar pons and pyramid would result in a right-sided weakness but no visual deficits. A lesion in the right optic nerve would result in blindness in that eye but no weakness of the extremities. (p. 20, 26, 40, 220–221)

34. Answer **E**: Cerebrospinal fluid in the ventricles, and throughout the subarachnoid space, appears very white in T$_2$-weighted MRI images. Structures located in, or traversing the subarachnoid space (such as vessels or cranial nerve roots, including the oculomotor nerve) appear grey to black against a white background. (p. 46–47, 49, 51, 54)

35. Answer **A**: Cerebrospinal fluid, and other fluids, appear black in T1-weighted MRI images. Consequently, the ventricles, and more obvious parts of the subarachnoid space, appear black. Changes in ventricular shape (i.e., enlargement, midline shift), or obliterated sulci, or even subarachnoid space, most likely represent a potentially serious clinical issue. (p. 2–4, 33 as one example)

36. Answer **E**: Patients who experience rupture of an intracranial aneurysm frequently complain of an intense, sudden headache ("the most horrible headache I have ever had"). Acute blood in the subarachnoid space will appear white to very white on CT. This will contrast with the medium grey of the brain and the black of cerebrospinal fluid (CSF) in the ventricles. The degree of white may vary somewhat, based on the relative concentration of blood, from very white (concentrated blood) to white (mostly blood, some CSF), to very light grey (mixture of blood and CSF). (p. 46–47, 51)

37. Answer **C**: The hypoglossal nerve exits the medulla via the preolivary sulcus of the medulla immediately (and laterally) adjacent to the pyramid. The abducens nerve exits in line with the preolivary sulcus, but, at the caudal edge of the pons, and the trigeminal nerve exits the lateral aspect of the pons. The vagus nerve exits the lateral aspect of the medulla via the postolivary sulcus, and the facial nerve in line with this sulcus, but at the pons-medulla junction. (p. 24, 44)

38. Answer **E**: Approximately one-half of cases of bacterial meningitis in adults are caused by *S. pneumoniae*. *E. coli* and *L. monocytogenes* are causative agents in neonates and children, although the latter (*L. monocytogenes*) is present in less than 10% of cases. While *H. influenzae* was a major cause of bacterial meningitis in children, the use of a vaccine has reduced this bacterium as a causative agent to well under 10% of cases. *H. simplex* is a virus. (p. 46)

39. Answer **D**: The trochlear nerve exits the posterior (dorsal) aspect of the brainstem just caudal to the inferior colliculus and passes around the lateral aspect of the midbrain in the ambient cistern, en route to its exit from the skull via the superior orbital fissure. The abducens nerve exits at the caudal edge of the pons in line with the preolivary fissure, and the hypoglossal exits from the medulla via this fissure. The trigeminal nerve exits the lateral aspect of the pons, and the vestibulocochlear nerve exits at the most lateral aspect of the pons-medulla junction. (p. 26, 33, 34)

40. Answer **B**: As it exits the anterior (ventral) surface of the midbrain, the oculomotor nerve passes between the superior cerebellar artery (which is caudal to the nerve root) and the P$_1$ segment of the posterior cerebral artery (which is rostral to the nerve root). The trigeminal root is adjacent to more distal portions of the superior cerebellar artery; the labyrinthine artery accompanies the vestibulocochlear nerve as it enters the internal acoustic meatus; and the ophthalmic artery accompanies the optic nerve along part of its extent. The abducens nerve passes rostrally adjacent to the basilar artery in the prepontine cistern. (p. 25, 39, 40)

41. Answer **D**: The rostral edge of the striae medullares (of the fourth ventricle) is regarded as the border between the pontine and medullary portions of the fourth ventricle. These fibers pass from the median fissure in the floor of the ventricle laterally into the lateral recess where they arch up into the cerebellum. The facial colliculus and median eminence are located in the floor of the pontine portion of the ventricle, and the vagal and hypoglossal trigones are found in the medial floor of the medullary portion of the fourth ventricle. (p. 34, 35, 36)

42. Answer **D**: The primary fissure is the deepest fissure in the cerebellum and it separates the anterior lobe from the posterior lobe and extends from the vermis to the lateral cerebellar margin. The posterolateral fissure is located between the flocculonodular lobe and the posterior lobe. The horizontal, secondary, and posterior superior fissures are all located within the posterior lobe. (p. 32, 33)

43. Answer **C**: The tonsil of the cerebellum is found on the caudal and inferior aspect of the cerebellar hemisphere, adjacent to the midline and immediately posterior (dorsal) to the medulla. The cisterna magna is located in this area. Sudden tonsillar herniation may compress the medulla and damage respiratory and cardiac centers resulting in sudden death. The tonsil herniates downward through the foramen magnum. Consequently, no other part of the brainstem is directly affected. (p. 32, 44)

44. Answer **A**: A CT is a fast method, does not require sedation of young patients, and shows bone fractures and acute intracranial blood in detail. MRI (T1- and T2-weighted) does not show acute blood or bone fracture to advantage, takes much longer to do, and may require sedation in a child. Enhanced MRI is uniquely useful for tumors, and PET is useful in identifying metabolic activity of brain tissue, not anatomic detail. (p. 4–6)

45. Answer **B**: The long and short gyri (gyri longi et breves) are components of the insular lobe. This lobe is located deep to the lateral sulcus, has a central sulcus that separates the short gyri (rostral to this sulcus) from the long gyri (caudal to this sulcus). The cortex of the insular lobe is separated from the adjacent frontal, parietal, and temporal opercula by the circular sulcus of the insula. None of the other lobes has gyri that are specifically named long and short gyri. (p. 13, 45, 56)

46. Answer **C**: The glossopharyngeal nerve contains the afferent limb of the gag reflex and, through its innervation of the stylopharyngeus muscle, is an important part of the efferent limb of this reflex. The nucleus ambiguus, the location of the motor neurons serving the stylopharyngeus, also contributes to the innervation of muscle served by the vagus nerve and, therefore, to the efferent limb of the gag reflex. The trigeminal and facial nerves participate in the afferent and efferent limbs (respectively) of the corneal reflex. The accessory nerve innervates the ipsilateral trapezius and sternocleidomastoid muscles, and the hypoglossal nerve innervates the ipsilateral genioglossus muscle. (p. 24, 43)

Review and Study Questions for Chapters 3 and 4

1. A 47-year-old woman presents with signs of increased intracranial pressure (vomiting, headache, lethargy). MRI shows a large tumor invading the head of the caudate nucleus, the rostral portion of the putamen and involving a fiber bundle located between these two structures. This fiber bundle is most likely the
   - (A) anterior commissure
   - (B) anterior limb of the internal capsule
   - (C) column of the fornix
   - (D) external capsule
   - (E) posterior limb of the internal capsule

2. A 76-year-old woman is diagnosed as having "probable" Alzheimer's disease based on a steady decline in cognitive function. It is likely that this woman has cell dropout in the nucleus accumbens. Which of the following most specifically describes the location of this cell group?
   - (A) At the junction of the caudate head and putamen
   - (B) At the junction of the pallidum and putamen
   - (C) At the junction of the pallidum and substantia nigra
   - (D) In the anterior wall of the temporal horn
   - (E) Internal to the uncus

3. Which of the following structures is located in the medial wall of the temporal horn of the lateral ventricle and, if severely damaged, may result in memory deficits?
   - (A) Amygdaloid complex
   - (B) Calcar avis
   - (C) Hippocampus
   - (D) Pulvinar
   - (E) Tail of the caudate

4. Which of the following represents the fibers that fan out from the internal capsule into the white matter of the hemisphere?
   - (A) Cingulum
   - (B) Corona radiata
   - (C) Genu of the corpus callosum
   - (D) Superior longitudinal fasciculus
   - (E) Uncinate fasciculus

5. The lamina of white matter located immediately internal to the cortex of the insula is the:
   - (A) Arcuate fasciculus
   - (B) External capsule
   - (C) Extreme capsule
   - (D) Internal capsule
   - (E) Tapetum

6. A 48-year-old man presents with a movement disorder (chorea) and mental deterioration. MRI shows the loss of a structure in the wall of the anterior horn of the lateral ventricle. Which of the following is most likely lost in this patient?
   - (A) Anterior thalamic nucleus
   - (B) Body of the caudate nucleus
   - (C) Column of the fornix
   - (D) Dorsomedial nucleus
   - (E) Head of the caudate nucleus

7. A 76-year-old man presents with a resting tremor, bradykinesia, and stooped posture. These observations suggest loss of a prominent population of cells in the brain. Which of the following structures is most likely affected in this patient?

   ○ (A)   Lateral cerebellar nucleus
   ○ (B)   Locus ceruleus
   ○ (C)   Red nucleus
   ○ (D)   Substantia nigra
   ○ (E)   Subthalamic nucleus

8. Which of the following represents the larger, more laterally located portion of the basal nuclei (also called the basal ganglia)?

   ○ (A)   Caudate nucleus
   ○ (B)   Globus pallidus
   ○ (C)   Putamen
   ○ (D)   Subthalamic nucleus
   ○ (E)   Substantia nigra

9. The MRI of a 59-year-old woman shows a large arteriovenous malformation (AVM) located between the lenticular nucleus and the dorsal thalamus. Based on its location, this AVM most likely involves which of the following structures?

   ○ (A)   Anterior limb of the internal capsule
   ○ (B)   Crus cerebri
   ○ (C)   External capsule
   ○ (D)   Posterior limb of the internal capsule
   ○ (E)   Retrolenticular limb of the internal capsule

10. A 29-year-old man is brought to the emergency department with a severe and persistent headache. MRI shows a large tumor of the pineal gland. Based on its location, this pineal lesion would most likely impinge on which of the following structures?

    ○ (A)   Anterior thalamic nucleus
    ○ (B)   Body of the caudate nucleus
    ○ (C)   Globus pallidus
    ○ (D)   Pulvinar nucleus(i)
    ○ (E)   Ventral posteromedial nucleus

11. The hippocampal commissure contains fibers from one hippocampal formation that cross the midline to distribute to targets on the opposite side of the hemisphere. Which of the following structures is directly adjacent to this commissure?

    ○ (A)   Body of the corpus callosum
    ○ (B)   Genu of the corpus callosum
    ○ (C)   Splenium of the corpus callosum
    ○ (D)   Spiral fibers of the hippocampus
    ○ (E)   Precommissural fornix

12. An 85-year-old woman is brought to the emergency department by her family because she suddenly became confused and lethargic. CT shows a hemorrhage into the medial and lateral geniculate bodies. Which of the following structures would also likely be involved in this lesion due to its apposition to the geniculate bodies?

    ○ (A)   Anterior thalamic nucleus
    ○ (B)   Rostral dorsomedial nucleus
    ○ (C)   Globus pallidus
    ○ (D)   Pulvinar nucleus(i)
    ○ (E)   Subthalamic nucleus

13. A 29-year-old woman presents with neurologic deficits that wax and wane over time suggestive of multiple sclerosis. MRI (especially T2-weighted) shows small, demyelinated areas at several locations in her brain, one of these being the mammillothalamic tract. Which of the following structures is most intimately associated with this tract?

    ○ (A)   Anterior thalamic nucleus
    ○ (B)   Centromedian nucleus
    ○ (C)   Dorsomedial nucleus
    ○ (D)   Ventral anterior thalamic nucleus
    ○ (E)   Ventral lateral thalamic nucleus

14. Which of the following structures is a primary target of the optic tract as it passes caudally from the optic chiasm?

    ○ (A)   Lateral geniculate nucleus
    ○ (B)   Mammillary body
    ○ (C)   Medial geniculate nucleus
    ○ (D)   Pulvinar
    ○ (E)   Ventral posterolateral nucleus

15. An 82-year-old man presents with a severe motor deficit (resting tremor) and dementia. The former correlates with degenerative changes in the putamen and globus pallidus and the latter with degenerative changes in the ventral striatum and ventral pallidum. Which of the following structures separates these two areas in the basal forebrain?

    ○ (A)   Anterior commissure
    ○ (B)   Lamina terminalis
    ○ (C)   Massa intermedia
    ○ (D)   Posterior commissure
    ○ (E)   Septum pellucidum

16. A 23-year-old man is brought to the emergency department by emergency medical personnel after an automobile collision. CT shows bilateral damage to the temporal pole and the uncus. Which of the following structures is also most likely damaged in this patient?

    ○ (A)   Amygdaloid complex
    ○ (B)   Anterior thalamic nucleus
    ○ (C)   Cingulum
    ○ (D)   Gracile nucleus
    ○ (E)   Hippocampal formation

17. The optic radiations are closely associated with which of the following spaces?

    ○ (A)   Anterior horn of the lateral ventricle
    ○ (B)   Body of the lateral ventricle
    ○ (C)   Cisterns adjacent to the midbrain
    ○ (D)   Posterior horn of the lateral ventricle
    ○ (E)   Third ventricle

18. A 31-year-old man presents with ill-defined neurologic complaints (persistently tired, headache, confusion). CT shows an arteriovenous malformation occupying most of the dorsomedial nucleus (DM) of the thalamus. Which of the following structures separates the DM from the lateral thalamic nuclei and encompasses the centromedial nucleus?

    ○ (A)   Ansa lenticularis
    ○ (B)   External medullary lamina
    ○ (C)   Internal medullary lamina
    ○ (D)   Lamina terminalis
    ○ (E)   Stria medullaris thalami

19. A 48-year-old woman presents with violent, flailing movements of her left upper extremity. CT shows a small hemorrhage in the subthalamic nucleus. Which of the following structures is located directly adjacent to the subthalamic nucleus?

○ (A)   Centromedian nucleus
○ (B)   Globus pallidus
○ (C)   Medial geniculate nucleus
○ (D)   Putamen
○ (E)   Substantia nigra

20. Which of the following structures is located immediately caudal to the anterior commissure and appears as a distinct black spot in a T2-weighted axial MRI?

○ (A)   Anterior limb of internal capsule
○ (B)   Column of the fornix
○ (C)   Crus of the fornix
○ (D)   Lenticular fasciculus
○ (E)   Mammillothalamic tract

Answers for Chapters 3 and 4

1. Answer **B**:   The anterior limb of the internal capsule is insinuated between the head of the caudate nucleus and the rostral aspect of the lenticular nucleus, mostly the putamen. The posterior limb is between the lenticular nucleus and the thalamus; the column of the fornix is rostromedial to the interventricular foramen; and the anterior commissure traverses the midline at the level of the genu of the internal capsule. The external capsule is a thin sheet of white matter lateral to the lenticular nucleus and medial to the claustrum. (p. 64–65, 76–77)

2. Answer **A**:   The nucleus accumbens is located in the rostral and basal forebrain at the point where the head of the caudate is continuous with the putamen. The amygdaloid nucleus is located internal to the uncus and in the anterior wall of the temporal horn. The pallidum (globus pallidus) and the substantia nigra do not have a continuum with the nucleus accumbens. (p. 64, 78)

3. Answer **C**:   The hippocampal formation, commonly called the hippocampus, is located in the medial wall of the temporal (inferior) horn of the lateral ventricle. Damage to the hippocampus may result in memory problems. The amygdaloid complex is located in the rostral wall of the temporal horn, the tail of the caudate in its lateral wall, and the calcar avis (also called the calcarine spur, a ridge in the wall of the posterior horn indicating the depth of the calcarine sulcus) is in the medial wall of the posterior horn of the lateral ventricle. The pulvinar is part of the diencephalon. (p. 58, 68–71)

4. Answer **B**:   The corona radiata (radiating crown) are those fibers of the internal capsule that fan out in all directions from its superior edge. These fibers contain a variety of fibers traveling to and from the cerebral cortex. The superior longitudinal and uncinate fasciculi are organized bundles of corticocortical fibers on the ipsilateral side, and the cingulum is a fiber bundle located internal to the cingulate cortex. The fibers of the genu of the corpus callosum contain corticocortical fibers that pass between the cerebral hemispheres. (p. 57, 65–69)

5. Answer **C**:   The layer of white matter located internal to the insular cortex, and external to the claustrum, is the extreme capsule. The external capsule is found between the claustrum and the putamen, and the internal capsule is a large bundle of fibers located primarily between the lenticular nucleus on one side and the head of the caudate and the diencephalon on the other side. The tapetum is located in the lateral wall of the posterior horn of the lateral ventricle. Arcuate fasciculi are small bundles of fibers passing between gyri. (p. 65, 67–68, 77)

6. Answer **E**:   The large bulge in the lateral wall of the anterior horn of the lateral ventricle is the head of the caudate nucleus. The position of the interventricular foramen represents the point at which the head of the caudate becomes the body of the caudate. The dorsomedial nucleus borders on the third ventricle; the anterior thalamic nucleus is located at the rostral end of the diencephalon and is caudomedial to the interventricular foramen; and the column of the fornix is rostromedial to this foramen. (p. 64–65, 76)

7. Answer **D**:   These deficits are characteristic of Parkinson's disease and are directly correlated with loss of the dopamine (and melanin)-containing cells of the substantia nigra of the midbrain. The locus (nucleus) ceruleus, also called the nucleus pigmentosus pontis, also contains cells with melanin, but loss of these cells does not cause motor deficits. The other choices do not contain pigmented cells, but damage to these structures does cause a different series of motor deficits. (p. 68–69, 78)

8. Answer **C**:   The putamen is the most lateral part of the basal nuclei; taken together, the putamen and the globus pallidus comprise the lenticular nucleus. The caudate nucleus, specifically its head and body portions, is located medial to the internal capsule. While the subthalamic nucleus and the substantia nigra function in concert with the basal nuclei, these structures are medially located and are not part of the basal nuclei. (p. 65–68, 76)

9. Answer **D**:   The posterior limb of the internal capsule, containing important cortical afferent and efferent fibers, is located between the lenticular nucleus and the dorsal thalamus. Damage to this structure may result in sensory and/or motor deficits on the opposite side of the body. The anterior limb is located between the head of the caudate and the putamen, while the retrolenticular limb is found caudal to the lenticular nucleus. The crus cerebri is on the inferolateral aspect of the midbrain. The external capsule is lateral to the putamen. (p. 67–69, 76–77)

10. Answer **D**:   The pineal gland is located in the quadrigeminal cistern, superior to the colliculi, and between the pulvinar nuclei of the thalamus. At this location, the lesion would potentially involve the colliculi and pulvinar. The other thalamic nuclei are not adjacent to the pineal, the globus pallidus is lateral to the posterior limb of the internal capsule, and the body of the caudate is located in the lateral wall of the body of the lateral ventricle. (p. 71)

11. Answer **C**:   The hippocampal commissure is located immediately inferior to the splenium of the corpus callosum; the crossing of these fibers takes place at this point. Other parts of the corpus callosum are not related to the hippocampal commissure, and the spiral fibers of the hippocampus are bundles within the hippocampal formation in the temporal lobe. Some of the fibers in the hippocampal commissure enter the precommissural fornix, but by no means all. (p. 72)

12. Answer **D**:   The geniculate bodies are tucked-up under the caudal and inferior aspect of the pulvinar. The groove between the medial geniculate body and the pulvinar contains the brachium of the superior colliculus. The geniculate bodies and the pulvinar have a common blood supply from the thalamogeniculate artery, a branch of P$_2$. None of the other choices have a close apposition with the geniculate bodies. The anterior thalamic, rostral dorsomedial, and subthalamic nuclei do not share a common blood supply with the pulvinar. (p. 58–59, 70)

13. Answer **A**:   The mammillothalamic tract extends from the mammillary bodies to the anterior nucleus of the thalamus; the cells of origin are in the mammillary nuclei and the axons terminate in the anterior nucleus. This tract is frequently visible in axial T2-weighted MRI. The ventral anterior nucleus is laterally adjacent to the mammillothalamic tract, but does not receive input therefrom. The other choices are nuclei located more caudally in the diencephalon. (p. 67, 77)

14. Answer **A**:   Many of the fibers contained in the optic tract terminate in the lateral geniculate nucleus. Some of these fibers bypass this nucleus to traverse the brachium of the superior colliculus and a few enter the suprachiasmatic nucleus. The medial geniculate nucleus receives input via the brachium of the inferior colliculus (auditory); the pulvinar has interconnections with the visual cortex and superior colliculus; and the ventral posterolateral nucleus receives input from the anterolateral system and the medical lemniscus. The mammillary body is located rostral to the interpeduncular fossa and medial to the optic tract. (p. 58, 59)

15. Answer **A**:   The anterior commissure, as it passes laterally from the midline, separates the dorsal basal nuclei (putamen and globus pallidus) from the ventral striatum and ventral pallidum. The posterior commissure is located at the caudal aspect of the third ventricle just above the opening of the cerebral aqueduct, and the Massa intermedia bridges the third ventricle in about 80% of individuals. The rostral wall of the third ventricle is formed by the lamina terminalis and the septum pellucidum forms the medial wall of the anterior horn of the lateral ventricle. (p. 65, 152–153)

16. Answer **A**:   The amygdaloid complex is located immediately internal to the uncus. Bilateral damage to rostral portions of the temporal lobe may include the amygdala and result in a constellation of deficits known as the Klüver-Bucy syndrome. The hippocampal formation is internal to the cortex of the parahippocampal gyrus, and the anterior thalamic nucleus is internal to the anterior thalamic tubercle. The cingulate gyrus overlies the longitudinally oriented fibers of the cingulum and the gracile tubercle is the external elevation formed by the gracile nucleus. (p. 58–59, 65–66, 78, 170)

17. Answer **D**:   The optic radiations are located in the lateral wall of the posterior horn of the lateral ventricle as they pass through the retrolenticular limb of the internal capsule from the lateral geniculate nucleus to the primary visual cortex. A thin layer of white matter, the tapetum, separates the optic radiations from the wall of the ventricle. The cisterns at the midbrain on the basal aspect of the hemisphere contain the optic tract. The other ventricular spaces listed have no direct relationship to the optic radiations. (p. 71–72, 77, 138–141, 162)

18. Answer **C**:   The internal medullary lamina is a vertically oriented sheet of fibers that extends from the rostral portion of the thalamus caudally to surround the centromedian nucleus; this nucleus is frequently referred to as "in" the internal medullary lamina due to its position. This lamina separates the dorsomedial nucleus from the laterally adjacent ventral anterior, ventral lateral, and ventral posterolateral nuclei. The external medullary lamina is located between the thalamus and the posterior limb of the internal capsule, and the lamina terminalis is the rostral wall of the third ventricle. The stria medullaris is a small bundle of fibers passing rostrocaudally along the upper medial edge of the thalamus from the general location of the interventricular foramen to the habenula, and the ansa lenticularis contains pallidothalamic fibers. (p. 68–69, 76, 144–149, 162)

19. Answer **E**:   The subthalamic nucleus is separated from the substantia nigra by only a thin layer of myelinated fibers; these two structures are directly adjacent to each other. Damage to the subthalamic nucleus gives rise to hemiballistic movements (described in this question) while loss of cells in the substantia nigra results in the motor deficits seen in Parkinson's disease. The putamen, globus pallidus, and the medial geniculate nucleus are all lateral to the internal capsule; the subthalamic nucleus is medial. The centromedial nucleus is separated from the subthalamic nucleus by other thalamic nuclei. (p. 68–69, 148–149)

20. Answer **B**:   The column of the fornix is that portion of this fiber bundle that arches around the rostromedial end of the thalamus. As it does so, the column joins its counterpart on the opposite side and "leans against" the anterior commissure. The column of the fornix also signifies, in cross section or axial planes, the laterally adjacent interventricular foramen and genu of the internal capsule. The mammillothalamic tract is located caudal to the fornix, and the crus of the fornix is found along the midline superior to the thalamus. The anterior limb of the internal capsule is found between the head of the caudate nucleus and the lenticular nucleus (mainly the putamen). The lenticular fasciculus contains pallidothalamic fibers and traverses the posterior limb of the internal capsule en route to the dorsal thalamus. (p. 31, 77, 163–164)

Review and Study Questions for Chapter 5

1. A 16-year-old boy is brought to the emergency department following a diving accident at a local quarry. The examination reveals a bilateral loss of motor and sensory function in the trunk and lower extremities. At 36 hours after the accident the boy is able to dorsiflex his toes, barely move his right lower extremity at the knee, and is able to perceive pinprick stimulation of the perianal skin (sacral sparing). Which of the following most specifically describes the spinal cord lesion in this patient?

   ○ (A) Central cord
   ○ (B) Complete
   ○ (C) Hemisection
   ○ (D) Incomplete
   ○ (E) Large syringomyelia

2. A 54-year-old morbidly obese and hypertensive man is brought to the emergency department after experiencing sudden onset of weakness of his left upper and lower extremities. CT shows an infarcted area in the medulla. Damage to which of the following tracts or fiber bundles of the medulla would most likely explain this deficit?

- ○ (A) Anterolateral system
- ○ (B) Corticospinal fibers
- ○ (C) Medial lemniscus
- ○ (D) Rubrospinal tract
- ○ (E) Vestibulospinal fibers

3. A 78-year-old healthy, active woman experiences a sudden weakness of her right upper extremity during an angiogram to determine the patency of her carotid bifurcation. The immediate examination reveals weakness of both extremities on the right and a partial loss of vision in both eyes (homonymous hemianopsia). These observations suggest an embolic stroke resulting in a lesion involving motor and visual structures. The infarcted area in CT points to the occlusion of one vessel. Which of the following vessels is most likely occluded?

- ○ (A) Anterior cerebral artery
- ○ (B) Anterior choroidal artery
- ○ (C) Ophthalmic artery
- ○ (D) Lateral posterior choroidal artery
- ○ (E) Posterior cerebral artery (P3 and P4 segments)

4. A 69-year-old man is brought to the emergency department by his wife after complaining of a bad headache and becoming stuporous. CT shows a hemorrhage into the head of the caudate nucleus that has ruptured into the anterior horn of the lateral ventricle. This hemorrhage has most likely originated from which of the following vessels?

- ○ (A) Anterior choroidal artery (branch of internal carotid)
- ○ (B) Lenticulostriate branches (of M1)
- ○ (C) Medial posterior choroidal artery (branch of P2)
- ○ (D) Medial striate artery (branch of A2)
- ○ (E) Thalamoperforating artery(ies)

Questions 5 and 6 are based on the following patient.

A 23-year-old man is brought to the emergency department from the site of an automobile collision. The neurologic examination reveals weakness of the right lower extremity and a loss of pain and thermal sensations on the left side beginning at the level of the umbilicus. CT shows a fracture of the vertebral column with displacement of bone fragments into the vertebral canal.

5. Damage to which of the following tracts would correlate with weakness of the lower extremity in this man?

- ○ (A) Left lateral corticospinal tract
- ○ (B) Reticulospinal fibers on the right
- ○ (C) Right lateral corticospinal tract
- ○ (D) Right rubrospinal tract
- ○ (E) Vestibulospinal fibers on the right

6. Which of the following represents the most likely level of damage to the spinal cord resulting from the fracture to the vertebral column in this man?

- ○ (A) T6 on the left
- ○ (B) T8 on the left
- ○ (C) T8 on the right
- ○ (D) T10 on the left
- ○ (E) T10 on the right

7. The artery of Adamkiewicz is an especially large spinal medullary artery supplementing the arterial blood supply to the spinal cord. Which of the following represents the most consistent location of this vessel?

- ○ (A) At C7–C8 on the left
- ○ (B) At L5–S1 on the left
- ○ (C) At L5–S1 on the right
- ○ (D) At T6–T7 on the right
- ○ (E) At T12–L1 on the left

8. The CT of a 73-year-old woman shows an infarcted area in the rostral portions of the dorsomedial nucleus, the anterior nucleus, and the ventral anterior nucleus. Which of the following arteries supply blood to this area of the brain?

- ○ (A) Anterior choroidal
- ○ (B) Lateral striate (lenticulostriate)
- ○ (C) Medial striate
- ○ (D) Thalamogeniculate
- ○ (E) Thalamoperforating

9. Which of the following structures is insinuated between the external and extreme capsules and is functionally related to the insular cortex?

- ○ (A) Claustrum
- ○ (B) External medullary lamina
- ○ (C) Lamina terminalis
- ○ (D) Putamen
- ○ (E) Stria terminalis

10. An 83-year-old man is brought to the emergency department by his daughter, who explains that her father started having "fits". The examination reveals an alert, otherwise healthy, man who frequently has uncontrollable flailing movements of his left arm. Which of the following structures is most likely involved in this lesion?

- ○ (A) Cerebellar cortex plus nuclei
- ○ (B) Lenticular nucleus
- ○ (C) Subthalamic nucleus
- ○ (D) Ventral lateral nucleus
- ○ (E) Ventral posterolateral nucleus

11. A 17-year-old girl presents with a bilateral loss of pain and thermal sensations at the base of the neck (C3 dermatome) and extending over the upper extremity and down to the level of the nipple (C4 to T4 dermatomes). MRI shows a cavitation in the spinal cord at these levels. Damage to which of the following structures would most likely explain this deficit?

- ○ (A) Anterior white commissure
- ○ (B) Left anterolateral system
- ○ (C) Medial longitudinal fasciculus
- ○ (D) Posterior columns
- ○ (E) Right anterolateral system

12. Which of the following structures is located within the territory of the medulla that is served by the anterior spinal artery?

   ○ (A)   Anterolateral system
   ○ (B)   Gracile fasciculus
   ○ (C)   Medial lemniscus
   ○ (D)   Rubrospinal tract
   ○ (E)   Spinal trigeminal tract

13. A 59-year-old man complains to his family physician that he has trouble chewing. The examination reveals a weakness of masticatory muscles on the left side. Which of the following nuclei is specifically related to the deficit seen in this man?

   ○ (A)   Left facial motor
   ○ (B)   Left hypoglossal
   ○ (C)   Left trigeminal motor
   ○ (D)   Right facial motor
   ○ (E)   Right trigeminal motor

14. A 15-year-old boy with signs of increased intracranial pressure (stupor, vomiting, headache) is referred to a neurologist. The examination reveals a paralysis of upward gaze, and MRI shows a large tumor of the pineal gland. Damage to which of the following structures would be most specifically related to the gaze deficit?

   ○ (A)   Exit of the trochlear nerve
   ○ (B)   Inferior colliculus
   ○ (C)   Occlusion of the great cerebral vein
   ○ (D)   Posterior commissure
   ○ (E)   Superior colliculus

15. A 61-year-old man is brought to the emergency department after a fall from his garage roof. The examination reveals a hemiplegia on the left, a loss of vibratory sense on the left, and a loss of pain and thermal sensation on the right side involving the upper and lower extremities. These deficits are characteristically seen in which of the following syndromes?

   ○ (A)   Benedikt
   ○ (B)   Brown-Séquard
   ○ (C)   Claude
   ○ (D)   Wallenberg
   ○ (E)   Weber

16. Based on their relative locations in the spinal cord, which of the following tracts or fiber bundles would most likely be involved in a lesion located in the immediate vicinity of the lateral corticospinal tract?

   ○ (A)   Anterolateral system
   ○ (B)   Anterior spinocerebellar tract
   ○ (C)   Gracile fasciculus
   ○ (D)   Medial longitudinal fasciculus
   ○ (E)   Rubrospinal tract

17. A 92-year-old woman is brought to the emergency department by her caregiver. The woman had suddenly become drowsy and confused. The examination revealed no cranial nerve deficits and age-normal motor function, but a loss of pain, thermal, vibratory, and discriminative touch sensations on one side of the body excluding the head. CT shows a small infarcted area. Which of the following structures is the most likely location of this lesion?

   ○ (A)   Anterolateral system
   ○ (B)   Medial geniculate nucleus
   ○ (C)   Subthalamic nucleus
   ○ (D)   Ventral posterolateral nucleus
   ○ (E)   Ventral posteromedial nucleus

18. In its location immediately internal to the anterior spinocerebellar tract, which of the following fiber bundles would most likely be damaged in a lesion to this area of the spinal cord?

   ○ (A)   Anterolateral system
   ○ (B)   Anterior corticospinal tract
   ○ (C)   Anterior white commissure
   ○ (D)   Cuneate fasciculus
   ○ (E)   Lateral corticospinal tract

19. A 37-year-old man is brought to the emergency department with a severe head injury. Within a few hours he is decerebrate (upper and lower extremities extended) and comatose. The extension of his extremities indicates a dominant input to extensor motor neurons through vestibulospinal and reticulospinal fibers/tracts. Which of the following most specifically describes the position of these activated fibers within the spinal cord?

   ○ (A)   Anterolateral area (area of anterolateral system)
   ○ (B)   Posterolateral area (area of lateral corticospinal tract)
   ○ (C)   Posterior columns
   ○ (D)   Posterolateral (dorsolateral) tract
   ○ (E)   Intermediate zone

Question 20 and 21 are based on the following patient.

A 71-year-old woman presents to her family physician with the complaint that "food dribbles out of my mouth when I eat". The examination reveals a unilateral weakness of muscles around the eye (palpebral fissure) and the opening of the mouth (oral fissure). She also has a loss of pain and thermal sensations on the opposite side of the body excluding the head. CT shows an infarcted area in the lateral portion of the pontine tegmentum.

20. Damage to which of the following nuclei would most likely explain the muscle weakness experienced by this woman?

   ○ (A)   Abducens
   ○ (B)   Arcuate
   ○ (C)   Facial motor
   ○ (D)   Hypoglossal
   ○ (E)   Trigeminal motor

21. The loss of pain and thermal sensations experienced by this woman would most likely correlate with a lesion involving which of the following structures?

   ○ (A)   Anterior (ventral) trigeminothalamic tract
   ○ (B)   Anterolateral system
   ○ (C)   Lateral lemniscus
   ○ (D)   Medial lemniscus
   ○ (E)   Spinal trigeminal tract

22. A 77-year-old woman is discovered slumped on the floor in the grocery store; emergency medical personnel transport her to a local hospital. The examination reveals a drowsy somewhat stuporous woman who is difficult to arouse. CT shows a large hemorrhage within the brain medial to the internal medullary lamina. Which of the following structures is most likely involved in this lesion?

   ○ (A) Anterior thalamic nucleus
   ○ (B) Dorsomedial nucleus
   ○ (C) Globus pallidus
   ○ (D) Ventral lateral and anterior nuclei
   ○ (E) Ventral posterolateral nucleus

23. A 78-year-old man presents with deficits suggesting an occlusion of the posterior spinal artery at spinal cord levels C4-T2. Which of the following structures are in the territory served by this vessel at these levels?

   ○ (A) Anterolateral system
   ○ (B) Cuneate fasciculus
   ○ (C) Gracile nucleus
   ○ (D) Lateral corticospinal tract
   ○ (E) Medial longitudinal fasciculus

24. Based partially on their embryological origin from a common group of cells, which of the following combinations of structures appear to be the same shade of grey in a T1- weighted MRI?

   ○ (A) Dorsomedial nucleus and Globus pallidus
   ○ (B) Globus pallidus and Caudate
   ○ (C) Globus pallidus and Putamen
   ○ (D) Putamen and Caudate nucleus
   ○ (E) Putamen and Pulvinar

25. Which of the following portions of the trigeminal nuclear complex is found in lateral areas of the brainstem between the level of the obex and the spinal cord-medulla junction and is the source of trigeminothalamic fibers conveying pain and thermal information originating from the face and oral cavity?

   ○ (A) Mesencephalic nucleus
   ○ (B) Principal sensory nucleus
   ○ (C) Spinal trigeminal nucleus, pars caudalis
   ○ (D) Spinal trigeminal nucleus, pars interpolaris
   ○ (E) Spinal trigeminal nucleus, pars oralis

26. Which of the following structures is located within the territory served by branches of the posterior inferior cerebellar artery (commonly called PICA by clinicians)?

   ○ (A) Corticospinal fibers
   ○ (B) Hypoglossal root
   ○ (C) Medial lemniscus
   ○ (D) Nucleus raphe magnus
   ○ (E) Solitary nucleus

27. Space-occupying lesions within the posterior cranial fossa, or events that increase pressure within this infratentorial region, may result in herniation of a portion of the cerebellum through the foramen magnum. Which of the following parts of the cerebellum is most likely involved in this event?

   ○ (A) Anterior lobe
   ○ (B) Flocculus
   ○ (C) Nodulus
   ○ (D) Simple lobule
   ○ (E) Tonsil

28. A 67-year-old woman is brought to the emergency department. She is stuporous and has signs that suggest a lesion in the brainstem; CT confirms this. Her right pupil is constricted (small) when compared with the left. Damage to which of the following tracts or fiber bundles in the pons or medulla would most likely explain this observation?

   ○ (A) Anterolateral system
   ○ (B) Hypothalamospinal fibers
   ○ (C) Medial longitudinal fasciculus
   ○ (D) Reticulospinal fibers
   ○ (E) Vestibulospinal fibers

29. In addition to the medial and lateral geniculate nuclei, which of the following structures is also served by the thalamogeniculate artery, a branch of P_2?

   ○ (A) Anterior thalamic nucleus
   ○ (B) Globus pallidus
   ○ (C) Pulvinar nucleus(i)
   ○ (D) Substantia nigra
   ○ (E) Ventral anterior thalamic nucleus

30. A 71-year- old man is brought to the emergency department by his wife. She explains that he suddenly became weak in his left lower extremity. She immediately rushed him to the hospital, a trip of about 20 minutes. The examination reveals an alert man who is obese and hypertensive. He has no cranial nerve deficits, is slightly weak on his left side, and has no sensory deficits. Within 2 hours the weakness has disappeared. An MRI obtained the following day shows no lesions. Which of the following most specifically describes this man's medical experience?

   ○ (A) Central cord syndrome
   ○ (B) Small embolic stroke
   ○ (C) Small hemorrhagic stroke
   ○ (D) Syringobulbia
   ○ (E) Transient ischemic attack

Questions 31 and 32 are based on the following patient.

A 41-year-old man is brought to the emergency department after an accident at a construction site. The examination reveals a weakness (hemiplegia) and a loss of vibratory sensation and discriminative touch all on the left lower extremity, and a loss of pain and thermal sensations on the right lower extremity. CT shows a fracture of the vertebral column adjacent to the T8 level of the spinal cord.

31. Damage to which of the following fiber bundles or tracts would most likely explain the loss of vibratory sensation in this man?

   ○ (A) Anterolateral system on the right
   ○ (B) Cuneate fasciculus on the left
   ○ (C) Cuneate fasciculus on the right
   ○ (D) Gracile fasciculus on the left
   ○ (E) Gracile fasciculus on the right

32. The loss of pain and thermal sensation in this man reflects damage to which of the following fiber bundles or tracts?

   ○ (A) Anterolateral system on the left
   ○ (B) Anterolateral system on the right
   ○ (C) Cuneate fasciculus on the left
   ○ (D) Gracile fasciculus on the left
   ○ (E) Posterior spinocerebellar tract on the left

33. Which of the following is the prominent population of melanin-containing cells located immediately internal to the crus cerebri? The loss of these cells may result in motor deficits.
    - (A) Locus ceruleus
    - (B) Pontine nuclei
    - (C) Red nucleus
    - (D) Reticular formation
    - (E) Substantia nigra

34. Which of the following structures receives visceral sensory input and is located immediately inferior to the medial and spinal vestibular nuclei at medullary levels?
    - (A) Cochlear nuclei
    - (B) Inferior salivatory nucleus
    - (C) Nucleus ambiguus
    - (D) Spinal trigeminal nucleus
    - (E) Solitary nucleus

35. Which of the following groups of visceromotor (autonomic) cell bodies is located lateral to the abducens nucleus, directly adjacent to the exiting fibers of the facial nerve, and sends its axons out of the brainstem via this cranial nerve?
    - (A) Dorsal motor nucleus
    - (B) Edinger-Westphal nucleus
    - (C) Inferior salivatory nucleus
    - (D) Intermediolateral cell column
    - (E) Superior salivatory nucleus

36. A 56-year-old woman presents to her family physician with persistent headache and nausea. MRI shows a tumor in the fourth ventricle impinging on the facial colliculus. Which of the following nuclei is found immediately internal to this elevation?
    - (A) Abducens
    - (B) Facial
    - (C) Hypoglossal
    - (D) Trigeminal
    - (E) Vestibular

Questions 37 through 39 are based on the following patient.

An 88-year-old man is brought to the emergency department by his daughter. She indicates that he complained of weakness of his "arm" and "leg" (upper and lower extremities) on the right side and of "seeing two of everything" (double vision—diplopia). CT shows an infarcted area in the medial area of the pons at the pons-medulla junction. The infarcted area is consistent with the vascular territory served by paramedian branches of the basilar artery.

37. Weakness of the extremities on the right can be explained by damage to which of the following structures?
    - (A) Corticospinal fibers on the left
    - (B) Corticospinal fibers on the right
    - (C) Middle cerebellar peduncle on the left
    - (D) Rubrospinal fibers on the left
    - (E) Rubrospinal fibers on the right

38. The diplopia (double vision) this man is having is most likely the result of damage to which of the following structures?
    - (A) Abducens nerve root
    - (B) Facial nerve root
    - (C) Oculomotor nerve root
    - (D) Optic nerve
    - (E) Trochlear nerve or root

39. Recognizing that this patient's lesion involves the territory served by paramedian branches of the basilar artery, which of the following structures is also most likely included in the area of infarction?
    - (A) Anterolateral system
    - (B) Facial motor nucleus
    - (C) Hypoglossal nucleus
    - (D) Medial lemniscus
    - (E) Spinal trigeminal tract

40. A 77-year-old man presents with a weakness of his right upper and lower extremities and he is unable to abduct his left eye on attempted gaze to the left. Which of the following most specifically describes this deficit?
    - (A) Alternating hemianesthesia
    - (B) Hemihypesthesia
    - (C) Inferior alternating hemiplegia
    - (D) Middle alternating hemiplegia
    - (E) Superior alternating hemiplegia

41. In axial MRI which of the following structures is an important landmark that separates the third ventricle (rostral to this point) from the quadrigeminal cistern (caudal to this point)?
    - (A) Lamina terminalis
    - (B) Habenular nucleus
    - (C) Massa intermedia
    - (D) Pulvinar
    - (E) Superior colliculus

42. A 77-year-old woman presents with deficits that suggest a lesion involving long tracts and a cranial nerve. CT shows an infarct in the region served by the penetrating branches of the basilar bifurcation. Which of the following structures is most likely located in this vascular territory?
    - (A) Abducens nerve
    - (B) Anterolateral system
    - (C) Corticospinal fibers in pyramid
    - (D) Medial lemniscus
    - (E) Red nucleus

Questions 43 through 46 are based on the following patient.

A 69-year-old man is brought to the emergency department with the complaint of a sudden loss of sensation. The history reveals that the man is overweight, hypertensive, and does not regularly take medication. When the man speaks his voice is gravely and hoarse. The examination further reveals a loss of pain and thermal sensations on the right side of his body and on the left side of his face. CT shows an infarcted area in the medulla.

43. Damage to which of the following structures would most likely explain the man's hoarse, gravely voice?
    - (A) Facial nucleus
    - (B) Gracile nucleus
    - (C) Hypoglossal nucleus
    - (D) Nucleus ambiguus
    - (E) Spinal trigeminal nucleus

44. Injury to which of the following structures in this man is most specifically related to the loss of pain and thermal sensations on the body below the neck?

   ○ (A) Anterolateral system
   ○ (B) Cuneate fasciculus
   ○ (C) Gracile fasciculus
   ○ (D) Medial lemniscus
   ○ (E) Spinal trigeminal tract

45. Damage to which of the following structures would most specifically explain the loss of pain and thermal sensations on the man's face?

   ○ (A) Anterolateral system
   ○ (B) Medial lemniscus
   ○ (C) Medial longitudinal fasciculus
   ○ (D) Solitary tract
   ○ (E) Spinal trigeminal tract

46. The CT shows an infarcted area in the medulla in this man. Based on the deficits described, and the corresponding structures involved, which of the following vessels is most likely occluded?

   ○ (A) Anterior spinal artery
   ○ (B) Posterior spinal artery
   ○ (C) Posterior inferior cerebellar artery
   ○ (D) Anterior inferior cerebellar artery
   ○ (E) Penetrating branches of the vertebral artery

47. A 77-year-old man presents with an ataxic gait. There are no other deficits. CT shows an infarcted area in the medulla in the territory served by the posterior inferior cerebellar artery. Damage to which of the following structures would most likely explain the symptoms experienced by this man?

   ○ (A) Anterolateral system
   ○ (B) Corticospinal tract
   ○ (C) Nucleus ambiguus
   ○ (D) Restiform body
   ○ (E) Vestibular nuclei

48. Which of the following cranial nerve nuclei is located in the anterior (ventral or inferior) and medial portion of the periaqueductal grey at the cross-sectional level of the superior colliculus?

   ○ (A) Abducens
   ○ (B) Mesencephalic
   ○ (C) Oculomotor
   ○ (D) Trigeminal motor
   ○ (E) Trochlear

49. A 53-year-old woman presents with motor deficits that the examining neurologist describes as a superior alternating hemiplegia. Which of the following cranial nerve roots is most likely involved in this lesion?

   ○ (A) Abducens
   ○ (B) Hypoglossal
   ○ (C) Oculomotor
   ○ (D) Trigeminal
   ○ (E) Trochlear

50. An 82-year-old woman presents to the emergency department with difficulty swallowing (dysphagia). Which of the following nuclei of the medulla contain motor neurons that innervate muscles involved in swallowing?

   ○ (A) Dorsal motor vagal
   ○ (B) Hypoglossal
   ○ (C) Inferior salivatory
   ○ (D) Medial vestibular
   ○ (E) Nucleus ambiguus

Questions 51 through 53 are based on the following patient.

A 73-year-old man is brought to the emergency department after losing consciousness at his home. CT shows a hemorrhage into the right hemisphere. The man regains consciousness, but is not fully alert. After 3–4 days the man begins to rapidly deteriorate: his pupils are large (dilated) and respond slowly to light, eye movement becomes restricted, there is weakness in the extremities on the left side, and the man becomes comatose. Repeat CT shows an uncal herniation.

51. Based on its location, which of the following parts of the brainstem is most likely to be directly affected by uncal herniation, especially in the early stages?

   ○ (A) Diencephalon/thalamus
   ○ (B) Mesencephalon/midbrain
   ○ (C) Myelencephalon/medulla
   ○ (D) Pons and cerebellum
   ○ (E) Pons only

52. Damage to corticospinal fibers in which of the following locations would most likely explain the weakness in his extremities?

   ○ (A) Left basilar pons
   ○ (B) Left crus cerebri
   ○ (C) Right basilar pons
   ○ (D) Right crus cerebri
   ○ (E) Right posterior limb of the internal capsule

53. The dilated, and slowly responsive, pupils in this man are most likely explained by damage to fibers in which of the following?

   ○ (A) Abducens nerve
   ○ (B) Corticonuclear fibers in the crus
   ○ (C) Oculomotor nerve
   ○ (D) Optic nerve
   ○ (E) Sympathetic fibers on cerebral vessels

54. The sagittal MRI of a 26-year-old man shows a dark shadow in the midbrain tegmentum on the midline at the cross-sectional level of the inferior colliculus. Which of the following structures does this dark area represent?

   ○ (A) Central portions of the red nucleus
   ○ (B) Compact and reticular parts of the substantia nigra
   ○ (C) Decussation of the superior cerebellar peduncle
   ○ (D) Decussation of trigeminothalamic fibers
   ○ (E) Motor (pyramidal) decussation

55. The CT of a 39-year-old man with untreated hypertension shows a small hemorrhage in the brainstem. This lesion encompasses the brachium of the inferior colliculus and the brain substance immediately internal to this structure. Which of the following structures is also most likely involved in this lesion?

   ○ (A) Anterolateral system
   ○ (B) Central tegmental tract
   ○ (C) Corticospinal fibers
   ○ (D) Mesencephalic tract
   ○ (E) Oculomotor nerve

56. A 69-year-old man complains of difficulty walking. The examination reveals no weakness, but does reveal a loss of discriminative touch and vibratory sense on the left lower extremity. MRI shows a small infarcted area in the midbrain. Which of the following structures is most likely involved in the infarcted area?

   ○ (A) Anterolateral system
   ○ (B) Corticospinal fibers
   ○ (C) Lateral part of the medial lemniscus
   ○ (D) Medial part of the medial lemniscus
   ○ (E) Rubrospinal fibers

57. Which of the following nuclei containing visceromotor (autonomic) cell bodies is located immediately inferior to the medial vestibular nucleus, medial to the solitary tract and nucleus, and has axons that exit the brainstem on the glossopharyngeal nerve?

   ○ (A) Dorsal motor nucleus
   ○ (B) Edinger-Westphal nucleus
   ○ (C) Inferior salivatory nucleus
   ○ (D) Intermediolateral cell column
   ○ (E) Superior salivatory nucleus

58. An 81-year-old woman is brought to the emergency department by her adult grandson. He explains that during dinner she slumped off of her chair, did not lose consciousness, but had trouble speaking. The examination reveals weakness of the upper and lower extremities on the left and deviation of the tongue to the right on protrusion. Which of the following most specifically describes this deficit in this elderly patient?

   ○ (A) Alternating hemianesthesia
   ○ (B) Hemihypesthesia
   ○ (C) Inferior alternating hemiplegia
   ○ (D) Middle alternating hemiplegia
   ○ (E) Superior alternating hemiplegia

Questions 59 and 60 are based on the following patient.

A 79-year-old woman is brought to the emergency department after a fall in her home from which she was unable to get up. The examination reveals a deviation of the tongue to the left on protrusion, a pronounced weakness of the right upper and lower extremities, and a loss of position and vibratory sense and discriminative touch on the right side of the body below the neck. CT shows an infarcted area in the medulla.

59. Which of the following represents the best localizing sign in this patient?

   ○ (A) Deviation of the tongue
   ○ (B) Motor loss on lower extremity
   ○ (C) Motor loss on upper extremity
   ○ (D) Sensory loss on lower extremity
   ○ (E) Sensory loss on upper extremity

60. Damage to which of the following tracts or fiber bundles would most likely give rise to the sensory deficits experienced by this patient?

   ○ (A) Anterolateral system
   ○ (B) Medial lemniscus
   ○ (C) Medial longitudinal fasciculus
   ○ (D) Solitary tract
   ○ (E) Spinal trigeminal tract

61. The MRI of a 12-year-old boy reveals a cavity within the medulla. Which of the following terms most specifically describes this condition?

   ○ (A) Brown-Séquard syndrome
   ○ (B) Central cord syndrome
   ○ (C) Hydromyelia
   ○ (D) Syringobulbia
   ○ (E) Syringomyelia

62. Which of the following cell groups within the white matter of the cerebellum characteristically appears as a long undulating line, looking somewhat like the principle olivary nucleus in the medulla?

   ○ (A) Dentate nucleus
   ○ (B) Emboliform nucleus
   ○ (C) Fastigial nucleus
   ○ (D) Globose nucleus
   ○ (E) Red nucleus

Answers for Chapter 5

1. Answer **D**:   Although this patient initially presented with complete motor and sensory losses, some function had returned by 36 hours; in this case the lesion is classified as an incomplete lesion of the spinal cord. Patients with no return of function at 24+ hours and no sacral sparing have suffered a lesion classified as complete and it is unlikely that they will recover useful neurologic function. In a central cord and a large syringomyelia there is sparing of posterior column sensations and in a hemisection the loss of motor function is unilateral. (p. 94–95)

2. Answer **B**:   A medullary lesion that results in weakness of the extremities on one side indicates involvement of the corticospinal fibers located in the pyramid on the contralateral side; these fibers largely cross in the pyramidal (motor) decussation. Rubrospinal and vestibulospinal fibers influence the activity of spinal motor neurons, but isolated lesions of these fibers would not result in a unilateral weakness of upper and lower extremities. The anterolateral system and the medial lemniscus are sensory tracts. (p. 98–108, 110–111)

3. Answer **B**:   The anterior choroidal artery serves the optic tract (homonymous hemianopsia) and the inferior portions of the posterior limb of the internal capsule (weakness of the extremities). The ophthalmic artery, via its central retinal branch, serves the retina; the anterior cerebral artery serves the lower extremity areas of the motor and sensory cortices; and distal segments of the posterior cerebral artery serve the medial temporal cortex and the visual cortex. The lateral posterior choroidal artery serves the choroid plexus in the lateral ventricle and some adjacent structures. (p. 21, 25, 29, 35, 158–159)

4. Answer **D**:   The head of the caudate nucleus is located in the lateral wall of the anterior horn of the lateral ventricle and receives its blood supply from the medial striate artery (also called the artery of Heubner). This vessel also serves much of the anterior limb of the internal capsule. The lenticulostriate arteries serve a large part of the lenticular nucleus and portions of the surrounding internal capsule, and thalamoperforating arteries serve anterior portions of the dorsal thalamus. The anterior choroidal artery provides blood supply to inferior portions of the internal capsule, optic tract, and structures in the medial portions of the temporal lobe. The medial posterior choroidal artery serves choroid plexus in the lateral and third ventricles and adjacent areas of the lateral midbrain and caudomedial thalamus. (p. 154–158)

5. Answer **C**:   In this patient the weakness of the right lower extremity is related to a lesion of lateral corticospinal tract fibers on the right side of the spinal cord. The left corticospinal tract serves the left side of the spinal cord and the left lower extremity. Rubrospinal, reticulospinal, and vestibulospinal fibers influence the activity of spinal motor neurons; however, the deficits related to corticospinal tract damage (significant weakness) will dominate over the lack of excitation to flexor or extensor motor neurons in the spinal cord via these tracts. (p. 86–88, 94)

6. Answer **C**:   The loss of pain and thermal sensations beginning at the level of the umbilicus (T10 dermatome) on the left side results from damage to fibers of the anterolateral system at about the T8 level on the right. These fibers ascend 1 to 2 levels as they cross the midline. Damage at the T6 level would result in a loss beginning at the T8 level on the contralateral side and damage at the T10 level would result in a loss beginning at about the T12 level. (p. 88–89, 94)

7. Answer **E**:   The artery of Adamkiewicz is usually located at the T12-L1 spinal cord levels and is more frequently (about 65% of the time) seen on the left side. The other cord levels listed may have small spinal medullary arteries but not the large diameter vessel characteristic of Adamkiewicz. (p. 94)

8. Answer **E**:   The thalamoperforating arteries serve the more rostral portions of the dorsal thalamus. These vessels may originate as a single trunk or as several vessels from the P_1 segment of the posterior cerebral artery. The anterior choroidal artery serves the optic tract, inferior portions of the internal capsule, choroid plexus in the temporal horn, and structures in the medial region of the temporal lobe. The thalamogeniculate artery supplies blood to the caudal thalamus, the medial striate arteries to the head of the caudate nucleus, and the lateral striate arteries to much of the lenticular nucleus. (p. 25, 158–159)

9. Answer **A**:   The claustrum is the thin layer of grey matter that is located between the extreme and external capsules. It is generally regarded as being functionally related to the insular cortex. The external medullary lamina is found at the interface of the lateral portions of the thalamus with the internal capsule and the lamina terminalis is the thin structure forming the rostral wall of the third ventricle. The putamen is located medial to the external capsule and lateral to the globus pallidus and the stria terminalis is a fiber bundle in the groove between the body of the caudate nucleus and the dorsal thalamus. (p. 144–153, 162)

10. Answer **C**:   Wild flailing movements of the extremities, especially the upper, are hemiballistic movements (hemiballismus); these are characteristic of a lesion in the subthalamic nucleus. Damage to the cerebellar cortex and nuclei and the lenticular nucleus will result in motor deficits, but these are usually described as involving tremor, ataxia, and related motor problems. The ventral lateral nucleus is a thalamic relay center for motor information and the ventral posterolateral nucleus is a sensory relay nucleus. Lesions of these nuclei will result in motor (but not hemiballismus) and sensory deficits. (p. 146–149, 158)

11. Answer **A**:   Fibers conveying pain and thermal sensations cross the midline in the anterior white commissure. Consequently, a lesion of this structure, as in syringomyelia, would result in a bilateral loss of these sensations, reflecting the levels of the syrinx. Damage to fibers of the anterolateral system results in a loss of these sensations on the contralateral side and the posterior columns convey proprioception, discriminative touch, and vibratory sense. The medial longitudinal fasciculus does not contain fibers conveying sensory input. (p. 90–91, 94)

12. Answer **C**:   The anterior spinal artery serves the medial portion of the medulla, an area that encompasses the medial lemniscus, exiting roots of the hypoglossal nerve, and the corticospinal fibers in the pyramid. The anterolateral system, spinal trigeminal tract, and rubrospinal tract are in the territory of the posterior inferior cerebellar artery (commonly called PICA by clinicians). The posterior spinal artery in the caudal medulla and spinal cord serves the gracile fasciculus. (p. 110–111)

13. Answer **C**:   The masticatory muscles receive their motor innervation via the motor neurons located in the trigeminal motor nucleus on the ipsilateral side; this excludes the right trigeminal nucleus. Facial motor neurons innervate the muscles of facial expression on the ipsilateral side and the hypoglossal nucleus innervates the ipsilateral side of the tongue. (p. 120–121, 124)

14. Answer **E**:   A pineal tumor impinging on the superior colliculus may result in a paralysis of upward gaze (Parinaud syndrome). The inferior colliculus is related to the auditory system, trochlear fibers innervate the ipsilateral superior oblique muscle, and the posterior commissure contains fibers related to the pupillary light pathway. Occlusion of the great cerebral vein may cause serious neurologic deficits but not specifically a paralysis of upward gaze. (p. 136)

15. Answer **B**:   Alternating sensory losses accompanied by a motor deficit on the same side as the loss of vibratory sensation are characteristics of the Brown-Séquard syndrome (also commonly called a spinal cord hemisection). The Wallenberg syndrome is seen in lesions of the medulla, and the Benedikt, Claude, and Weber syndromes are seen in lesions of the midbrain. In these brainstem syndromes there are usually characteristic cranial nerve and long tract signs and symptoms. (p. 90–91, 94, 110, 136)

16. Answer **E**:   The rubrospinal tract lies immediately anterior (ventral) to, and partially overlaps with, the lateral corticospinal tract. The anterolateral system is in the anterolateral area of the spinal cord and is spatially separated from the lateral corticospinal tract. The gracile fasciculus is in the posterior columns, the medial longitudinal fasciculus is in the ventral funiculus, and the anterior spinocerebellar tract is located on the anterolateral surface of the spinal cord. (p. 90–91, 94–95, 100)

17. Answer **D**:   The ventral posterolateral nucleus of the thalamus receives the pathways (medial lemniscus and anterolateral system) that relay the information lost as a result of the lesion in this woman. The ventral posteromedial nucleus relays comparable information from the face and the medial geniculate nucleus is related to the auditory system. Lesions in the subthalamic nucleus result in hemiballismus. The anterolateral system relays pain and thermal sense; this is only part of the sensory deficits experienced by this woman. (p. 142, 158–159)

18. Answer **A**:   The anterolateral system is located internal to the position of the anterior spinocerebellar tract; damage to this area of the spinal cord would most likely result in a loss of pain and thermal sensations on the contralateral side of the body below the lesion. The lateral corticospinal tract is located internal to the posterior spinocerebellar tract, the anterior white commissure and the anterior corticospinal tract are located in the anterior funiculus of the cord, and the cuneate fasciculus is in the posterior column medial to the posterior horn at upper thoracic and cervical levels. (p. 88–91, 95)

19. Answer **A**:   Reticulospinal fibers (medial and lateral) and lateral vestibulospinal fibers are found predominately in the anterolateral area of the spinal cord; medial vestibulospinal fibers are located in the medial longitudinal fasciculus. In the decerebrate patient, the descending influence of rubrospinal fibers on spinal flexor motor neurons is removed, and descending influence on extensor motor neurons is predominant. The posterior columns, posterolateral area of the cord, and the posterolateral tract do not contain vestibulospinal or reticulospinal fibers. The intermediate zone, a part of the spinal cord grey matter, contains some of the terminals of these fibers but not the descending tracts in toto. (p. 86, 88, 90, 95)

20. Answer **C**:   Weakness of the muscles of the face, particularly when upper and lower portions of the face are involved, indicate a lesion of either the facial motor nucleus or the exiting fibers of the facial nerve; both are located in the lateral pontine tegmentum at caudal levels. The hypoglossal nucleus innervates muscles of the tongue, the trigeminal nucleus innervates masticatory muscles, and the abducens nucleus innervates the lateral rectus muscle, all on the ipsilateral side. The arcuate nucleus is a group of cells located on the surface of the pyramid. (p.106, 116–120, 124)

21. Answer **B**:   The fibers of the anterolateral system are located in the lateral portion of the pontine tegmentum anterior (ventral) to the facial motor nucleus; these fibers convey pain and thermal inputs. The spinal trigeminal tract and the anterior trigeminothalamic tract also convey pain and thermal input but from the ipsilateral and contralateral sides of the face, respectively. The lateral lemniscus is auditory in function and the medial lemniscus conveys proprioception, vibratory sense, and discriminative touch. (p. 116–120, 124)

22. Answer **B**:   The dorsomedial nucleus is located medial to the internal medullary lamina and, through its connections, one if its functions is to participate in arousal of the cerebral cortex. The other choices are in (anterior nucleus) or lateral to the internal medullary lamina, or, in the case of the globus pallidus, lateral to the internal capsule. (p. 144–149)

23. Answer **B**:   Penetrating branches of the posterior spinal artery serve the posterior columns (gracile and cuneate fasciculi) of the spinal cord at all levels. Branches of the posterior spinal artery also serve the gracile nucleus, but this structure is in the medulla, not in the spinal cord. The lateral corticospinal tract and the anterolateral system are served by the arterial vasocorona on the surface of the cord and the internal branches of the anterior spinal artery. The medial longitudinal fasciculus is in the territory of the anterior spinal artery. (p. 95, 111)

24. Answer **D**:   The putamen and the caudate nucleus originate from the same group of developing neurons, are collectively referred to as the neostriatum, and appear in the same shade of grey in a T1-weighted MRI. In general, the globus pallidus and pulvinar are distinctly lighter than the putamen and the dorsomedial nucleus frequently appears dark in a shade of grey distinctly different from that of the globus pallidus. (p. 151, 153, 155, 162)

25. Answer **C**:   The pars caudalis portion of the spinal trigeminal nucleus is located in the lateral medulla adjacent to the spinal trigeminal tract in cross-sectional levels between the obex and the C1 level of the spinal cord. This portion of the spinal trigeminal nucleus is responsible for relaying pain and thermal information originating from the face and oral cavity on one side to the ventral posteromedial nucleus on the contralateral side. The pars interpolaris is found at levels between the obex and the rostral end of the hypoglossal nucleus and the pars oralis between the interpolaris and the principal sensory nucleus. The principal sensory nucleus is in the pons and the mesencephalic nucleus is in the midbrain. (p. 98–106, 120, 130)

26. Answer **E**:   The solitary nucleus receives general visceral afferent (GVA) and special visceral afferent information (SVA, this input is taste) and is located in the region of the medulla served by posterior inferior cerebellar artery. All of the other choices are in the territory served by the anterior spinal artery. (p. 111)

27. Answer **E**:   The tonsil of the cerebellum is located close to the midline and immediately above the medulla: its position relative to the cerebellum is caudal, medial, and inferior. Tonsillar herniation may compress the medulla, and if sudden, may result in death. The other portions of the cerebellum do not herniate. (p. 110, 123)

28. Answer **B**:   In addition to other signs or symptoms, lesions in lateral areas of the brainstem may also interrupt hypothalamospinal fibers descending from the hypothalamus to the intermediolateral cell column in upper thoracic levels of the spinal cord. In this case the patient may present with a Horner syndrome, part of which is a small (constricted) pupil. In addition, the affected pupil may react slowly to reduced light. The anterolateral system conveys somatosensory input and fibers of the medial longitudinal fasciculus (originating from the medulla) are primarily descending to spinal cord levels. Reticulospinal and vestibulospinal tracts influence spinal motor neurons. (p. 124)

29. Answer **C**:   The pulvinar, geniculate nuclei, ventral posteromedial and posterolateral nuclei, centromedian, and some other adjacent nuclei are served by the thalamogeniculate artery. The anterior and ventral anterior thalamic nuclei receive their blood supply from thalamoperforating arteries, the substantia nigra via branches of P_1 and P_2, and globus pallidus from the lenticulostriate branches of M1. (p. 140–141, 158–159)

30. Answer **E**:   The short-term loss of function, frequently involving a specific part of the body, is characteristic of a transient ischemic attack (commonly called a TIA). The follow-up MRI shows no lesion because there has been no permanent damage. TIAs are caused by a brief period of inadequate perfusion of a localized region of the nervous system; recovery is usually rapid and complete. However, TIAs, especially if repeated, may be indicative of an impending stroke. Hemorrhagic strokes frequently result in some type of permanent deficit, and the central cord syndrome has bilateral deficits. A small embolic stroke would be visible on the follow-up MRI, and in this patient would have resulted in a persistent deficit. Syringobulbia may include long tract signs as well as cranial nerve signs. (p.158)

31. Answer **D**:   Damage to the gracile fasciculus on the left (at the T8 level this is the only part of the posterior columns present) accounts for the loss of vibratory sensation (and discriminative touch). Injury to the gracile fasciculus on the right would result is this type of deficit on the right side. The level of the cord damage is caudal to the cuneate fasciculi and the anterolateral system conveys pain and thermal sensations. (p. 86, 88, 90, 94)

32. Answer **A**:   The loss of pain and thermal sensations on the right side of the body correlates with a lesion involving the anterolateral system on the left side of the spinal cord. A lesion of the right anterolateral system would result in a left-sided deficit. The gracile and cuneate fasciculi convey discriminative touch, vibratory sensation, and proprioception. The posterior spinocerebellar tract conveys similar information, but it is not perceived/recognized as such (consciously) by the brain. (p. 88, 90, 94)

33. Answer **E**:   The substantia nigra contains a large population of melanin-containing cells, is located in the midbrain just internal to the crus cerebri, and the loss of these cells gives rise to the motor deficits characteristic of Parkinson disease. The neurotransmitter associated with these cells is dopamine. The reticular formation is in the core of the brainstem and the pontine nuclei are in the basilar pons; neither of these contain cells with melanin. The red nucleus is in the midbrain, but its reddish tone is related to a rich vascular supply, not to cells containing a pigment. (p. 128–133)

34. Answer **E**:   The solitary nucleus is located immediately inferior (ventral) to the medial and spinal vestibular nuclei and is the only nucleus in the choices to receive a general visceral afferent (GVA) and special visceral afferent (SVA-taste) input. The inferior salivatory nucleus and the nucleus ambiguus are visceromotor (general visceral efferent [GVE] and special visceral efferent [SVE], respectively) and the spinal trigeminal and cochlear nuclei are sensory (general somatic afferent [GSA] and special somatic afferent [SSA], respectively). (p. 104, 106, 174–175)

35. Answer **E**:   The superior salivatory nucleus lies adjacent to the exiting fibers of the facial nerve in a position just lateral to the abducens nucleus in caudal levels of the pons. The preganglionic axons originating from these cells distribute on peripheral branches of the facial nerve. The dorsal motor and inferior salivatory nuclei are in the medulla and associated, respectively, with the vagus and glossopharyngeal nerves. The Edinger-Westphal nucleus is related to the oculomotor nucleus and the intermediolateral cell column is located primarily in thoracic levels of the spinal cord. (p.116, 203)

36. Answer **A**:   The facial colliculus is an elevation in the floor of the fourth ventricle located medial to the sulcus limitans and formed by the underlying abducens nucleus and fibers (internal genu) originating from the facial nucleus. The vestibular area, indicating the position of the vestibular nuclei, is lateral to the sulcus limitans and the hypoglossal nucleus is internal to the hypoglossal trigone in the medial floor of the ventricle in the medulla. The trigeminal and facial nuclei are located in the pontine tegmentum and do not border on the ventricular space. (p. 34–36, 114–117)

37. Answer **A**:   In this case the weakness of the upper and lower extremities on the right reflects damage to corticospinal fibers on the left side of the basilar pons. A lesion of these fibers on the right side of the pons would produce a left-sided weakness. Rubrospinal fibers are not located in the territory of paramedian branches of the basilar artery. Also, lesions of rubrospinal fibers and of the middle cerebellar peduncle do not cause weakness but may cause other types of motor deficits. (p. 24, 116, 124, 190–191)

38. Answer **A**:   The exiting fibers of the abducens nerve (on the left) are in the territory of the paramedian branches of the basilar artery and are laterally adjacent to corticospinal fibers in the basilar pons. Diplopia may result from lesions of the oculomotor and trochlear nerves, but these structures are not in the domain of the paramedian basilar branches. A lesion of the optic nerve results in blindness in that eye and damage to the facial root does not affect eye movement but may cause a loss of view of the external world if the palpebral fissure is closed due to facial muscle weakness. (p. 24, 116, 124)

39. Answer **D**:   At caudal pontine levels most, if not all, of the medial lemniscus is located within the territory served by paramedian branches of the basilar artery. Penetrating branches of the anterior spinal artery serve the hypoglossal nucleus. The other choices are generally in the territories of short or long circumferential branches of the basilar artery. (p. 124–125)

40. Answer **D**:   Weakness of the extremities accompanied by paralysis of the lateral rectus muscle (innervated by the abducens nerve) on the contralateral side indicates a lesion in the caudal and medial pons involving the abducens nerve root and corticospinal fibers. This is a middle alternating hemiplegia. Inferior alternating hemiplegia specifies involvement of the hypoglossal root and the pyramid, and superior alternating hemiplegia indicates damage to the oculomotor root and the crus cerebri. Alternating (or alternate) hemianesthesia and hemihypesthesia are sensory losses. (p. 116, 124)

41. Answer **B**:   The prominent elevation formed on the caudal and medial wall of the third ventricle, at the general level of the posterior commissure, represents the location of the habenular nucleus. This is an excellent landmark to use in axial MRI when designating the separation between the third ventricle (rostral to this point on the midline) and the quadrigeminal cistern (caudal to this point). The pulvinar is lateral to the quadrigeminal cistern, the lamina terminalis forms the rostral wall of the third ventricle, and the massa intermedia bridges the space of the third ventricle. When present (in about 80% of patients) the Massa intermedia appears as a shadow in T2-weighted MRI bridging the third ventricle. The superior colliculus is a mesencephalic structure found in the quadrigeminal cistern. (p. 76, 138–143, 162)

42. Answer **E**:   The red nucleus, exiting fibers of the oculomotor nerve, portions of the corticospinal fibers in the crus cerebri, and a number of other medially located structures are found in the territory of the penetrating branches of the basilar bifurcation. The paramedian branches of the basilar artery and the corticospinal fibers in the pyramid serve the abducens nerve by branches of the anterior spinal artery. The anterolateral system and the medial lemniscus are mainly, if not entirely, in the region of the midbrain served by branches of the quadrigeminal and posterior medial choroidal arteries. (p. 137)

43. Answer **D**:   The vocalis muscle (this muscle is actually the medial portion of the thyroarytenoid muscle) is innervated, via the vagus nerve, by motor neurons located in the nucleus ambiguus. The gracile nucleus conveys sensory input from the body and the spinal trigeminal nucleus relays sensory input from the face. The hypoglossal nucleus is motor to the tongue and the facial nucleus is motor to the muscles of facial expression. (p. 100–106, 110)

44. Answer **A**:   Fibers comprising the anterolateral system convey pain and thermal sensations from the body, excluding the face. These fibers are located in lateral portions of the medulla adjacent to the spinal trigeminal tract; this latter tract relays pain and thermal sensations from the face. The gracile and cuneate fasciculi convey proprioception, discriminative touch, and vibratory sense in the spinal cord and the medial lemniscus conveys this same information from the medulla to the dorsal thalamus. (p. 100, 102, 104, 106, 110)

45. Answer **E**:   The loss of pain and thermal sensations on one side of the face correlates with damage to the spinal trigeminal tract; in this case the loss is ipsilateral to the lesion. The anterolateral system relays pain and thermal sensations from the contralateral side of the body, the solitary tract conveys visceral sensory input (especially taste), and the medial lemniscus contains fibers relaying information related to position sense and discriminative touch. The medial longitudinal fasciculus does not contain sensory fibers. (p. 100–108, 110)

46. Answer **C**:   The posterior inferior cerebellar artery (commonly called PICA by clinicians) serves the posterolateral portion of the medulla, which encompasses the anterolateral system, spinal trigeminal tract, and nucleus ambiguus. The anterior and medial areas of the medulla (containing the pyramid, medial lemniscus, and hypoglossal nucleus/nerve) are served by the anterior spinal artery and the anterolateral area of the medulla (the region of the olivary nuclei) is served by penetrating branches of the vertebral artery. The posterior spinal artery serves the posterior column nuclei in the medulla and the anterior inferior cerebellar artery (commonly called AICA) serves caudal portions of the pons and cerebellum. (p. 111)

47. Answer **D**:   The restiform body is a large fiber bundle located in the posterolateral area of the medulla in the region served by posterior inferior cerebellar artery (PICA). This structure contains a variety of cerebellar afferent fibers including those of the posterior spinocerebellar tract. Damage to the vestibular nuclei will result in a tendency to fall to the ipsilateral side but will also produce diplopia (double vision) and nausea; symptoms not experienced by this patient. The anterolateral system is sensory, the nucleus ambiguus is motor to muscles of the throat (including the vocalis), and the corticospinal tract is not in the PICA territory. (p. 104, 106, 110–111)

48. Answer **C**:   The oculomotor nucleus (containing general somatic efferent [GSE] cell bodies), along with the Edinger-Westphal (containing general visceral efferent [GVE] cell bodies) nucleus, is found in the most anterior and medial portion of the periaqueductal grey at the superior colliculus level. The trochlear nucleus is found at a comparable position, but at the cross-sectional level of the inferior colliculus. The mesencephalic nucleus is found in the lateral area of the periaqueductal grey, and the trigeminal and abducens nuclei are located in the pons. (p. 130–133, 201)

49. Answer **C**:   A superior alternating (or alternate) hemiplegia is characterized by a loss of most eye movement (damage to oculomotor nerve fibers) on the ipsilateral side and weakness of the upper and lower extremities (damage to corticospinal fibers in the crus cerebri) on the contralateral side. The abducens nerve is the cranial nerve involved in a middle alternating hemiplegia and the hypoglossal is that nerve involved in an inferior alternating hemiplegia. The trigeminal nerve innervates the muscles of mastication and the trochlear nerve innervates the superior oblique muscle. (p. 132, 136, 200)

50. Answer **E**:   Motor neurons in the nucleus ambiguus innervate, primarily through the vagus nerve, the muscles of the throat that move a bolus of food from the oral cavity to the esophagus. The tongue, via the hypoglossal nucleus and nerve, may move food around in the mouth and toward the back of the oral cavity, but the actual act of swallowing is through the action of pharyngeal and laryngeal musculature. The dorsal motor vagal and inferior salivatory nuclei are both visceromotor (autonomic) nuclei, and the medial vestibular nucleus is involved in the regulation of eye movement and in balance and equilibrium. (p. 100–106, 110)

51. Answer **B**:   The uncus is at the rostral and medial aspect of the parahippocampal gyrus, and, in this position, is directly adjacent to the anterolateral aspect of the midbrain. The diencephalon is rostral to this point and the medulla, the most caudal part of the brainstem, is located in the posterior fossa. Late stages of uncal herniation may, but not always, result in damage to the rostral pons; this is especially so if the patient becomes decerebrate. The cerebellum is not involved in uncal herniation. (p. 20, 22, 24, 38, 78, 136)

52. Answer **D**:   Uncal herniation compresses the lateral portion of the brainstem, eventually resulting in compression of the corticospinal fibers in the crus cerebri. Weakness on the patient's left side indicates damage to corticospinal fibers in the right crus. In situations of significant shift of the midbrain due to the herniation, the contralateral crus may also be damaged resulting in bilateral weakness. While all other choices contain corticospinal fibers, none of these areas are directly involved in uncal herniation. (p, 136)

53. Answer **C**:   The root of the oculomotor nerve conveys GSE fibers to four of the six major extraocular muscles and GVE parasympathetic preganglionic fibers to the ciliary ganglion from which postganglionic fibers travel to the sphincter muscle of the iris. Pressure on the oculomotor root, as in uncal herniation, will usually compress the smaller diameter, and more superficially located GVE fibers first. Optic nerve damage results in blindness in that eye, injury to sympathetic fibers to the eye results in constriction of the pupil, and an abducens root injury results in an inability to abduct that eye. A lesion of corticonuclear fibers in the crus results primarily in motor deficits related to the facial, hypoglossal, and accessory nerves. (p. 136, 201, 221)

54. Answer **C**:   The decussation of the superior cerebellar peduncle is a prominent fiber bundle located in the tegmentum of the midbrain directly on the midline at the level of the inferior colliculus. This bundle is made up of cerebellar efferent fibers. The red nucleus is located in the midbrain tegmentum, but not on the midline. Decussating trigeminothalamic fibers are found in the medulla and do not form a visible structure on the midline. The motor decussation is a compact bundle on the midline, but it is in the medulla, not the midbrain. The main parts of the substantia nigra are in the midbrain, are seen in sagittal MRI, but they are definitely not on the midline. (p. 128, 163, 211)

55. Answer **A**:   The anterolateral system is located just internal to the brachium of the inferior colliculus in the lateral portions of the midbrain tegmentum. This tract conveys pain and thermal sensations from the contralateral side of the body excluding the face. Corticospinal fibers are located in the crus cerebri, the mesencephalic tract at the lateral edge of the periaqueductal (central) grey, and the central tegmental tract is, as its name indicates, in the central part of the tegmentum. Oculomotor fibers within the midbrain leave the nucleus, arch through the tegmentum, and exit on the medial surface of the basis pedunculi into the interpeduncular cistern. (p. 128–131)

56. Answer **C**:   Fibers conveying discriminative touch, vibratory sensations, and proprioception are located in the lateral lemniscus; those from the contralateral upper extremity are medial while those from the contralateral lower extremity are lateral. This man has difficulty walking due to a lesion of fibers conveying position sense from the lower extremity, not due to a lesion influencing descending fibers passing to spinal motor neurons. Fibers of the anterolateral system convey pain and thermal sensation. Rubrospinal and corticospinal are motor in function; however this man has no weakness. (p. 126–132, 178–179)

57. Answer **C**:   The inferior salivatory nucleus is located in the rostral medulla, medial to the solitary tract and nuclei and inferior to the medial vestibular nucleus. Preganglionic axons that originate from these cells distribute on branches of the glossopharyngeal nerve. The dorsal motor nucleus is in the medulla, its axons travel on the vagus nerve. The superior salivatory nucleus is in the caudal pons and is associated with the facial nerve. Cells of the Edinger-Westphal nucleus are associated with the oculomotor nucleus of the midbrain and the intermediolateral cell column is located primarily in thoracic levels of the spinal cord. (p. 106, 203)

58. Answer **C**:   Weakness of the extremities accompanied by paralysis of muscles on the contralateral side of the tongue (seen as a deviation of the tongue to that side on protrusion) indicates a lesion in the medulla involving the corticospinal fibers in the pyramid and the exiting hypoglossal roots. This is an inferior alternating hemiplegia. Middle alternating hemiplegia refers to a lesion of the pontine corticospinal fibers and the root of the abducens nerve, and superior alternating hemiplegia specifies damage to the oculomotor root and crus cerebri. Alternating (alternate) hemianesthesia and hemihypesthesia are sensory losses. (p. 102, 110)

59. Answer **A**:   The deviation of the tongue to the left on attempted protrusion is the best localizing sign in this woman. This is especially the case when the deviation of the tongue is seen in concert with the motor and sensory losses described for this patient. This clearly indicates a lesion in the medial medulla encompassing the corticospinal fibers, medial lemniscus, and exiting fibers on the hypoglossal nerve. Motor and sensory losses, without the cranial nerve sign, could suggest a lesion at several different levels of the neuraxis. (p. 83, 110–111)

60. Answer **B**:   All of the sensory deficits seen in this woman reflect a lesion in the medial lemniscus, which is located in the medial medulla in the territory of the anterior spinal artery. The anterolateral system and the spinal trigeminal tract convey pain and thermal sensations from the body (sans face) and face, respectively. The solitary tract is made up of the central processes of viscerosensory fibers and the medial longitudinal fasciculus at this level contains descending fibers that influence spinal motor neurons. (p. 100–108, 110–111)

61. Answer **D**:   Syringobulbia is a cavitation within the medulla. A cavitation in this location may communicate with a cavity in cervical levels of the spinal cord (syringomyelia). Hydromyelia refers to a cavity of the spinal cord that is lined with ependymal cells. The central cord and Brown-Séquard syndromes are lesions of the spinal cord that give rise to characteristic motor and sensory losses. (p. 110)

62. Answer **A**:   The dentate nucleus appears as a long thin undulating line within the white matter core of the cerebellar hemisphere. It is frequently described as having the three-dimensional shape of a crumpled bag with its hilus (the opening of the bag) directed rostromedially. The other cerebellar nuclei (fastigial, globose, emboliform) are small clumps of cells, and the red nucleus is found in the midbrain, not in the cerebellum. (p. 112–115)

Review and Study Questions for Chapter 6

1. The MRI of a 66-year-old man shows a tumor 2.0 cm in diameter located in the lateral wall of the atrium of the lateral ventricle. Which of the following structures does this lesion most likely damage?

   ○ (A) Corticonuclear (corticobulbar) fibers
   ○ (B) Corticospinal fibers
   ○ (C) Optic radiations
   ○ (D) Pulvinar nucleus
   ○ (E) Splenium of the corpus callosum

2. Which of the following structures is clearly seen in coronal and axial brain slices, and in many MRIs, in planes extending from the midline laterally through the basal nuclei?

   ○ (A) Anterior commissure
   ○ (B) Column of the fornix
   ○ (C) Genu of the internal capsule
   ○ (D) Optic chiasm
   ○ (E) Posterior commissure

3. The MRI of a 49-year-old woman with movement and personality disorders and with cognitive dysfunction shows a large anterior horn of the lateral ventricle. The attending physician suspects that her disease has resulted in loss of brain tissue in the lateral wall of the anterior horn. A loss of which of the following structures would result in this portion of the ventricular system being enlarged?

○ (A)   Body of the caudate nucleus
○ (B)   Head of the caudate nucleus
○ (C)   Lenticular nucleus
○ (D)   Pulvinar nucleus (i)
○ (E)   Septum pellucidum and fornix

4. The axial MRI of a 54-year-old man shows an arteriovenous malformation located between the thalamus and the lenticular nucleus. Which of the following structures is probably most affected by this malformation?

○ (A)   Anterior commissure
○ (B)   Anterior limb of the internal capsule
○ (C)   Extreme capsule
○ (D)   Retrolenticular limb of the internal capsule
○ (E)   Posterior limb of the internal capsule

5. In a sagittal MRI, and in a sagittal brain slice, both taken just off the midline (2–4 mm), which of the following structures would be clearly evident immediately caudal to the anterior commissure?

○ (A)   Column of the fornix
○ (B)   Lamina terminalis
○ (C)   Mammillothalamic tract
○ (D)   Optic chiasm
○ (E)   Precommissural fornix

6. The coronal MRI of a 15-year-old boy shows a 2.0 cm-diameter tumor in the rostral tip of the temporal (inferior) horn of the lateral ventricle. It is possibly arising from the choroid plexus in this area of the ventricle. In addition to the hippocampus, this tumor is most likely impinging on which of the following structures?

○ (A)   Amygdaloid nucleus
○ (B)   Body of the caudate nucleus
○ (C)   Hypothalamus
○ (D)   Optic radiations
○ (E)   Putamen

7. Which of the following structures is located immediately internal to the crus cerebri and appears as a dark shade of grey (hypointense) in a sagittal T1-weighted MRI?

○ (A)   Brachium of the inferior colliculus
○ (B)   Periaqueductal grey
○ (C)   Pretectal area
○ (D)   Red nucleus
○ (E)   Substantia nigra

8. An 81-year-old man is brought to the emergency department following a fall while walking in the park. The examination reveals mild confusion and memory loss, but no obvious motor or sensory deficits. MRI shows an old infarct in the territory of the thalamus served by the thalamoperforating artery. Which of the following nuclei is most likely involved in this lesion?

○ (A)   Centromedian
○ (B)   Medial geniculate
○ (C)   Ventral anterior
○ (D)   Ventral posterolateral
○ (E)   Ventral posteromedial

9. Which of the following nuclei is located within the internal medullary lamina and may be visible in an axial MRI in either T1- or T2-weighted images?

○ (A)   Centromedian
○ (B)   Dorsomedial
○ (C)   Pulvinar
○ (D)   Ventral anterior
○ (E)   Ventral lateral

10. The sagittal MRI of a 23-year-old woman shows a mass in the right interventricular foramen (possibly a colloid cyst); the right lateral ventricle is enlarged. Based on its location, this mass is most likely impinging on which of the following structures?

○ (A)   Anterior nucleus of thalamus
○ (B)   Posterior limb of internal capsule
○ (C)   Habenular nucleus
○ (D)   Head of caudate nucleus
○ (E)   Lamina terminalis

11. The sagittal MRI of a 42-year-old woman taken adjacent to the midline shows a round structure immediately rostral to the interpeduncular fossa on the inferior surface of the hemisphere. Which of the following most likely represents this elevation?

○ (A)   Anterior commissure
○ (B)   Basilar pons
○ (C)   Lamina terminalis
○ (D)   Mammillary body
○ (E)   Optic chiasm

12. Which of the following structures is located immediately inferior to the pulvinar and, in the sagittal plane (MRI or brain section), forms a distinct elevation immediately adjacent to the lateral aspect of the crus cerebri?

○ (A)   Mammillary nuclei
○ (B)   Medial geniculate nucleus
○ (C)   Optic tract
○ (D)   Subthalamic nucleus
○ (E)   Uncus

Answers for Chapter 6

1. Answer **C**:   The optic radiations are located in the lateral wall of the atrium of the lateral ventricle, represent projections from the lateral geniculate nucleus to the calcarine cortex, pass through the retrolenticular limb of the internal capsule, and are separated from the ventricular space by a thin layer of fibers called the tapetum. The pulvinar and splenium are located rostromedial and medial, respectively, to the atrium. Corticonuclear and corticospinal fibers are found in the genu, and the posterior limb of the internal capsule within the hemisphere. (p. 76, 77, 138, 162)

2. Answer **A**:   The anterior commissure is a mediolaterally oriented bundle of fibers that crosses the midline and extends laterally, immediately inferior to the basal nuclei. In sagittal section, or in a sagittal MRI, this bundle can be followed into planes of the hemisphere that include the most lateral portions of the thalamus and the lenticular nucleus. The column of the fornix and optic chiasm are located immediately adjacent to the midline. The posterior commissure is located at the caudal aspect of the third ventricle and immediately

superior to the opening of the cerebral aqueduct. The genu of the internal capsule is medial to the lenticular nucleus and rostrolateral to the anterior nucleus of the thalamus. (p. 163, 165, 167, 169, 171)

3. Answer **B**:   The head of the caudate nucleus forms a prominent bulge in the lateral wall of the anterior horn of the lateral ventricle. In Huntington's disease, this elevation disappears, and the wall of the ventricle may become concave laterally; the result being an enlarged anterior horn (hydrocephalus *ex vacuo*). The body of the caudate is located in the lateral wall of the body of the lateral ventricle. The lenticular nucleus lies within the hemisphere and does not border on any ventricular space. The septum and the fornix are located in the medial wall of the ventricle, and the pulvinar borders on the superior cistern. (p. 75, 76, 152–156, 162)

4. Answer **E**:   The posterior limb of the internal capsule is located between the lenticular nucleus, which is lateral, and the thalamus, which is medial. This large fiber bundle contains thalamocortical projections related to motor and sensory function and descending corticospinal fibers. The anterior limb of the internal capsule is located between the head of the caudate and the lenticular nucleus, and the retrolenticular limb is found caudal to the lenticular nucleus. The anterior commissure is in the rostroventral portion of the hemisphere, and the extreme capsule is immediately internal to the insular cortex. (p. 162, 164, 166)

5. Answer **A**:   The column of the fornix, commonly called the postcommissural fornix, lies caudal to, and against, the anterior commissure as it arches around the interventricular foramen and the anterior tubercle of the thalamus. The precommissural fornix is a diffuse bundle of fibers rostral to the anterior commissure, and the mammillothalamic tract is located between the mammillary body and the anterior nucleus of the thalamus. The lamina terminalis and the optic chiasm are inferior to the anterior commissure. (p. 163)

6. Answer **A**:   The amygdaloid nucleus is in the rostral wall of the temporal horn of the lateral ventricle. In this position the amygdala is separated from the rostral tip of the hippocampus (the hippocampus occupies the medial and inferior wall of the temporal horn) by a narrow space of the ventricle. The optic radiations are in the lateral wall of the temporal horn, but are quite caudal to its rostral tip. The other choices do not have direct structural relationship to the rostral portions of the temporal horn. (p. 170, 171)

7. Answer **E**:   The substantia nigra is located internal to the crus cerebri and, in T1-weighted MRI, appears a darker shade of grey (hypointense) than does the crus. The red nucleus and the periaqueductal grey are located in the midbrain, but do not border on the crus cerebri. The brachium of the inferior colliculus is found on the lateral surface of the midbrain, and the pretectal area is adjacent to the cerebral aqueduct at the midbrain-diencephalic junction. (p. 165, 167)

8. Answer **C**:   The ventral anterior nucleus is located in the rostral portions of the thalamus, is in the territory of the thalamoperforating artery, and projects to large regions of the frontal lobe. An occlusion of the vessels serving this portion of the thalamus may result in a decreased level of alertness. The other choices are in caudal regions of the thalamus, are not in the territory served by the thalamoperforating artery, and, with the exception of the centromedian nucleus, do not relate to the cortex of the frontal lobe. (p. 159, 162, 164)

9. Answer **A**:   The centromedian nucleus is found within the internal medullary lamina in a position just rostral to the pulvinar. The ventral anterior and ventral lateral nuclei are lateral to the internal medullary lamina, the dorsomedial nucleus is medial to this lamina, and the pulvinar is the large nucleus forming the caudal part of the dorsal thalamus. (p. 76, 142–143, 162, 164)

10. Answer **A**:   The interventricular foramen is the space formed between the column of the fornix (located somewhat rostromedially) and the anterior nucleus of the thalamus (located somewhat caudolaterally). The anterior nucleus is located internal to the anterior tubercle of the thalamus. The head of the caudate is found in the lateral wall of the anterior horn of the lateral ventricle, and the posterior limb is located in the hemisphere between the thalamus and the lenticular nucleus. The lamina terminalis extends from the anterior commissure inferiority to the upper edge of the optic chiasm. The habenula is a small elevation in the caudal and medial wall of the third ventricle. (p. 76, 162, 164)

11. Answer **D**:   The mammillary body forms an obvious elevation on the inferior aspect of the hemisphere rostral to the interpeduncular fossa/cistern; this small bulge is clearly evident in MRI. The optic chiasm and the basilar pons are both on the inferior aspect of the brain at the midline. The former is rostral to the infundibulum (and the mammillary body) and the latter is caudal to the interpeduncular fossa. The lamina terminalis forms the rostral end of the third ventricle and the anterior commissure is adjacent to the column of the fornix. (p. 31, 163, 170)

12. Answer **B**:   The medial and lateral geniculate nuclei are located inferior to the pulvinar, and form elevations on the surface of the dorsal thalamus; the medial geniculate is adjacent to the lateral edge of the crus cerebri. The subthalamic nucleus is located internally, the mammillary nuclei (medial and lateral) are on the inferior aspect of the thalamus, and the uncus is on the medial portion on the temporal pole. The optic tract lies on the surface of the crus cerebri, but it does not form a distinct elevation on the brain surface inferior to the pulvinar; rather, it has a structural relationship to the lateral geniculate nucleus. (p. 26, 59, 169)

Review and Study Questions for Chapter 7

1. A 15-year-old boy is brought to the emergency department after an accident on his father's farm. The examination reveals weakness of the left lower extremity, but no frank paralysis. There is a loss of pinprick sensation on the right side beginning at the T8 dermatome (about half way between the nipple and umbilicus), and dorsiflexion of the great toe in response to plantar stimulation. Based on this examination, which of the following represents the most likely approximate location of this lesion?

○ (A) T6 on the left side
○ (B) T6 on the right side
○ (C) T8 on the left side
○ (D) T8 on the right side
○ (E) T10 on the left side

2. A 47-year-old man is transported to the emergency department from the site of an automobile collision. The examination reveals a paralysis of both lower extremities. Which of the following most specifically identifies this clinical picture?

  ○ (A) Alternating hemiplegia
  ○ (B) Hemiplegia
  ○ (C) Monoplegia
  ○ (D) Quadriplegia
  ○ (E) Paraplegia

3. A 68-year-old woman presents with a complaint of difficulty swallowing. Which of the following most specifically identifies this condition in this patient?

  ○ (A) Dysarthria
  ○ (B) Dysmetria
  ○ (C) Dysphagia
  ○ (D) Dyspnea
  ○ (E) Dysdiadochokinesia

4. A 37-year-old man presents to his family physician with a complaint of pain on his face. The examination shows that gentle stimulation of the cheek and corner of the mouth precipitates a severe, sharp, lancinating pain. A consulting neurologist orders an MRI (T2-weighted), which reveals a vascular loop that appears to be pressing on the trigeminal root proximal to the ganglion. Which of the following vessels is most likely involved?

  ○ (A) Anterior inferior cerebellar artery
  ○ (B) Posterior cerebral artery
  ○ (C) Posterior inferior cerebellar artery
  ○ (D) Quadrigeminal artery
  ○ (E) Superior cerebellar artery

5. Which of the following brainstem structures receives input from the frontal eye field (in the caudal part of the middle frontal gyrus, areas 6 and 8) and is regarded as a vertical gaze center?

  ○ (A) Abducens nucleus
  ○ (B) Edinger-Westphal nucleus
  ○ (C) Oculomotor nucleus
  ○ (D) Paramedian pontine reticular formation (PPRF)
  ○ (E) Rostral interstitial nucleus of the medial longitudinal fasciculus (MLF)

6. A newborn girl baby is unable to suckle. The examination reveals that muscles around the oral cavity and of the cheek are poorly developed or absent. A failure in proper development of which of the following structures would most likely contribute to this problem for this baby?

  ○ (A) Head mesoderm
  ○ (B) Pharyngeal arch 1
  ○ (C) Pharyngeal arch 2
  ○ (D) Pharyngeal arch 3
  ○ (E) Pharyngeal arch 4

7. Which of the following neurotransmitters is associated with hypothalamic fibers that project to the cerebellar cortex (hypothalamocerebellar fibers)?

  ○ (A) Gamma aminobutyric acid
  ○ (B) Glutamate
  ○ (C) Histamine
  ○ (D) Noradrenalin
  ○ (E) Serotonin

Questions 8 through 9 are based on the following patient.

A 62-year-old woman presents with tremor and ataxia on the right side of the body excluding the head, and with a loss of most eye movement on the left; the woman's eye is rotated slightly down and out at rest. The left pupil is dilated. There are no sensory losses on her face or body.

8. Based on the deficits seen in this woman, which of the following represents the most likely location of the causative lesion?

  ○ (A) Cerebellum on the left
  ○ (B) Cerebellum on the right
  ○ (C) Midbrain on the left
  ○ (D) Midbrain on the right
  ○ (E) Rostral pons on the right

9. The dilated pupil in this woman is most likely a result of which of the following?

  ○ (A) Intact parasympathetic fibers on the left
  ○ (B) Intact parasympathetic fibers on the right
  ○ (C) Intact sympathetic fibers on the left
  ○ (D) Intact sympathetic fibers on the right
  ○ (E) Interrupted hypothalamospinal fibers on the left

10. Which of the following nuclei are the primary target of cerebellar efferent fibers that arise in the dentate, emboliform, and globose nuclei on the left side?

  ○ (A) Ventral anterior nucleus on the right
  ○ (B) Ventral lateral nucleus on the left
  ○ (C) Ventral lateral nucleus on the right
  ○ (D) Ventral posterolateral nucleus on the left
  ○ (E) Ventral posterolateral nucleus on the right

11. A 22-year-old man presents to his family physician with motor deficits. The examination reveals that the man has jerky up-down movements of his upper extremities especially noticeable in his hands when his arms are extended. Which of the following most specifically designate this abnormal movement?

  ○ (A) Akinesia
  ○ (B) Asterixis
  ○ (C) Dystonia
  ○ (D) Intention tremor
  ○ (E) Resting tremor

12. A 59-year-old man is brought to his family physician by his wife. He complains of frequent and severe headaches. His wife states that he does not seem to understand what she is saying when she talks to him. The examination reveals that the man can speak fluently and clearly, can read notes written on paper, can hear noise, but has great difficulty understanding or interpreting sounds. MRI shows a tumor in the temporal lobe. This man is most likely suffering from which of the following?

  ○ (A) Agnosia
  ○ (B) Agraphia
  ○ (C) Alexia
  ○ (D) Aphasia
  ○ (E) Aphonia

13. A 47-year-old man is brought to the emergency department by lo-cal law enforcement personnel. The man is thin, undernourished, somnolent, and clearly intoxicated. Other indicators, such as a lack of personal hygiene, suggest that the man's condition has been long-term. When the physician asks the man his name and where he lives the man give a nonsensical response. This man is most likely suffering from which of the following?

   ○ (A) Broca aphasia
   ○ (B) Klüver-Bucy syndrome
   ○ (C) Korsakoff syndrome
   ○ (D) Munchausen syndrome
   ○ (E) Pick disease

Questions 14 through 15 are based on the following patient.

A 69-year-old man is diagnosed with dysarthria. The history reveals that the man has had this problem for several weeks. MRI shows an in-farcted area in the brainstem on the right side.

14. Damage to which of the following structures would most likely explain this deficit in this man?

   ○ (A) Cuneate nucleus
   ○ (B) Nucleus ambiguus
   ○ (C) Solitary tract and nuclei
   ○ (D) Spinal trigeminal tract
   ○ (E) Vestibular nuclei

15. Assuming that the infarcted area in the brain of this man is the re-sult of a vascular occlusion, which of the following arteries is most likely involved?

   ○ (A) Anterior inferior cerebellar
   ○ (B) Labyrinthine
   ○ (C) Posterior inferior cerebellar
   ○ (D) Posterior spinal
   ○ (E) Superior cerebellar

16. Which of the following neurotransmitters is associated with the cells in the somatomotor cortex that project to the spinal cord as corticospinal fibers?

   ○ (A) Acetylcholine
   ○ (B) Dopamine
   ○ (C) Gamma aminobutyric acid
   ○ (D) Glutamate
   ○ (E) Serotonin

17. A 77-year-old woman presents with a loss of pain and thermal sen-sations on the right side of her face and on the left side of her body. Which of the following most specifically describe this deficit in this woman?

   ○ (A) Alternating hemianesthesia
   ○ (B) Epidural anesthesia
   ○ (C) Facial hemiplegia
   ○ (D) Hemifacial spasm
   ○ (E) Superior alternating hemiplegia

18. During a busy day in the emergency department, the neurology resident sees three patients with brainstem lesions. The first is an 83-year-old woman with a lesion in the territory of the midbrain served by the quadrigeminal and lateral posterior choroidal arter-ies. The second is a 68-year-old man with a posterior inferior cere-bellar artery (lateral medullary or Wallenberg) syndrome. The third is a 47-year-old woman with a presumptive glioblastoma multiforme invading the mid- to lateral portions of the pontine tegmentum and adjacent portions of the middle cerebellar pedun-cle. Which of the following would most likely be seen in all three patients assuming a thorough neurologic examination?

   ○ (A) Claude syndrome
   ○ (B) Contralateral hemiplegia
   ○ (C) Facial hemiplegia
   ○ (D) Horner syndrome
   ○ (E) Medial medullary syndrome

19. Which of the following structures serves as an important landmark in the placement of the intentional division of the spinal cord (myelotomy) in an anterolateral cordotomy?

   ○ (A) Anterior median sulcus
   ○ (B) Anterolateral sulcus
   ○ (C) Denticulate ligament
   ○ (D) Posterior intermediate sulcus
   ○ (E) Posterolateral sulcus

20. A 17-year-old boy is brought to the emergency department from a high school football game. The examination reveals a loss of vi-bratory sensation and discriminative touch on the left lower ex-tremity and to the level of the umbilicus. CT shows a vertebral fracture with bone displacement into the vertebral canal. Which of the following indicates the most likely level of damage to the spinal cord in this boy?

   ○ (A) T7–8 on the left
   ○ (B) T10 on the left
   ○ (C) T12 on the left
   ○ (D) T8–9 on the right
   ○ (E) T10 on the right

21. During the neurologic examination of a 52-year-old man, the physician decides to test the gag reflex. Which of the following dif-ficulties does this man have that would cause the physician to de-cide to test this particular reflex?

   ○ (A) Dysgeusia
   ○ (B) Dysmetria
   ○ (C) Dysphagia
   ○ (D) Dyspnea
   ○ (E) Gustatory agnosia

22. A 57-year-old woman presents with the main complaint of diffi-culty speaking. The examination reveals that the woman's tongue deviates to the right on attempted protrusion. When she says "Ah" her soft palate elevates slightly on the left and the uvula deviates to the same side. This combination of deficits would most likely indicate a small lesion in which of the following?

   ○ (A) Crus cerebri on the right
   ○ (B) Genu of the internal capsule on the left
   ○ (C) Genu of the internal capsule on the right
   ○ (D) Lateral medulla on the right
   ○ (E) Medial medulla on the right

23. A 36 year-old-woman is diagnosed with myasthenia gravis. Which of the following deficits are seen first in about one-half of patients with this disease and is present in most at some time during its course?
    - ○ (A) Diplopia
    - ○ (B) Dysmetria
    - ○ (C) Lower extremity weakness
    - ○ (D) Tremor
    - ○ (E) Upper extremity weakness

Questions 24 through 26 are based on the following patient.

An 80-year-old woman is brought to the emergency department from an assisted care facility. The woman, who is in a wheelchair, complains of not feeling well, of numbness on her face, and of being hoarse, although she claims not to have a cold. The examination reveals a loss of pain and thermal sensations on the right side of her face and on the left side of her body. CT shows an infarcted area in the lateral portion of the medulla.

24. A lesion of which of the following structures in this woman would explain the loss of pain and thermal sensations on her body excluding the head?
    - ○ (A) Anterolateral system on the left
    - ○ (B) Anterolateral system on the right
    - ○ (C) Medial lemniscus on the left
    - ○ (D) Spinal trigeminal nucleus on the left
    - ○ (E) Spinal trigeminal tract on the left

25. The hoarseness in this woman is most likely due to which of the following?
    - ○ (A) Lesion of the facial nucleus
    - ○ (B) Lesion of the hypoglossal nucleus/nerve
    - ○ (C) Lesion of the nucleus ambiguus
    - ○ (D) Lesion of the spinal trigeminal tract
    - ○ (E) Lesion of the trigeminal nucleus

26. Assuming this woman suffered a vascular occlusion, which of the following vessels is most likely involved?
    - ○ (A) Anterior inferior cerebellar artery
    - ○ (B) Anterior spinal artery
    - ○ (C) Posterior inferior cerebellar artery
    - ○ (D) Posterior spinal artery
    - ○ (E) Superior cerebellar artery

27. In the course of a neurologic examination of a 23-year-old man, the physician places her index finger on the midline of the mandible and taps it with a percussion hammer stimulating the afferent limb of the jaw (jaw-jerk) reflex. Collateral fibers from which of the following brainstem nuclei enter the trigeminal motor nucleus to initiate the motor response?
    - ○ (A) Hypoglossal
    - ○ (B) Mesencephalic
    - ○ (C) Principal sensory
    - ○ (D) Spinal trigeminal, pars caudalis
    - ○ (E) Spinal trigeminal, pars interpolaris

28. A 45-year-old-man is brought to his family physician by his wife. The man's main complaint is that he feels "real dizzy" and a little nauseated. The examination reveals that the man has a disease of his semicircular canals. While sitting still the man perceives that his body is actually moving around the room. Which of the following most specifically describes this condition?
    - ○ (A) Ataxia
    - ○ (B) Hysterical vertigo
    - ○ (C) Nystagmus
    - ○ (D) Objective vertigo
    - ○ (E) Subjective vertigo

Questions 29 and 30 are based on the following patient.

A 37-year-old-man is brought to the emergency department from the site of an automobile collision. He was unrestrained and, as a result, has extensive injuries to his face and head. CT shows numerous fractures of the facial bones and skull and blood in the rostral areas of the frontal lobes and in the rostral 3–4 cm of the temporal lobes, bilaterally. After several weeks of recovery the man is moved to a long-term care facility. His behavior is characterized by (1) difficulty recognizing sounds such as music or words; (2) a propensity to place inappropriate objects in his mouth; (3) a tendency to eat excessively or to eat non-food items such as the leaves on the plant in his room; and (4) a tendency to touch his genitalia.

29. Which of the following most specifically describes the tendency of this man to eat excessively?
    - ○ (A) Aphagia
    - ○ (B) Dysphagia
    - ○ (C) Dyspnea
    - ○ (D) Hyperorality
    - ○ (E) Hyperphagia

30. Based on the totality of this man's deficits he is most likely suffering from which of the following?
    - ○ (A) Klüver-Bucy syndrome
    - ○ (B) Korsakoff syndrome
    - ○ (C) Senile dementia
    - ○ (D) Wallenberg syndrome
    - ○ (E) Wernicke aphasia

31. A 31-year-old woman is examined by an otolaryngologist pursuant to her complaint of hearing difficulties. The physician places a tuning fork against the woman's mastoid bone until she no longer perceives sound, then moves the prongs to her external ear where a faint sound is again heard. This maneuver is best described as:
    - ○ (A) A negative (abnormal) Rinne test
    - ○ (B) A normal Binet test
    - ○ (C) A normal Weber test
    - ○ (D) A positive (normal) Rinne test
    - ○ (E) Weber test localizing to the deaf side

32. A 64-year-old man is brought to a rural health clinic by a neighbor. The history reveals that the man is a recluse, lives by himself, and does not regularly visit a physician. The examination reveals that the man has difficulty walking, chorea and dystonia, and is suffering dementia. The neighbor believes that the man's father died from a similar disease. A tentative diagnosis of Huntington's disease is made. Absence of which of the following structures in an MRI of this man would be consistent with this diagnosis?

    ○ (A)   Anterior lobe of cerebellum
    ○ (B)   Head of the caudate
    ○ (C)   Lateral thalamic nuclei
    ○ (D)   Substantia nigra
    ○ (E)   Subthalamic nucleus

33. A 23-year-old man is brought to the emergency department from an accident at a construction site. CT shows a fracture of the left mastoid bone with total disruption of the stylomastoid foramen. Which of the following deficits would most likely be seen in this man?

    ○ (A)   Alternating hemianesthesia
    ○ (B)   Alternating hemiplegia
    ○ (C)   Central seven
    ○ (D)   Facial hemiplegia
    ○ (E)   Hemifacial spasm

34. Cell bodies located in which of the following ganglia of the head supply postganglionic fibers to the parotid gland?

    ○ (A)   Ciliary
    ○ (B)   Intramural
    ○ (C)   Otic
    ○ (D)   Pterygopalatine
    ○ (E)   Submandibular

Questions 35 and 36 are based on the following patient.

A 23-year-old man is brought to the emergency department from the site of an automobile collision. CT shows fractures of the facial bones and evidence of bilateral trauma to the temporal lobes (blood in the substance of the brain).

35. As this man recovers, which of the following deficits is most likely to be the most obvious in this man?

    ○ (A)   A bilateral sensory loss in the lower body
    ○ (B)   A loss of immediate and short-term memory
    ○ (C)   A loss of long-term (remote) memory
    ○ (D)   Dementia
    ○ (E)   Dysphagia and dysarthria

36. Assuming that this man has also sustained bilateral injury to the Meyer-Archambault loop, which of the following deficits would this man also most likely have?

    ○ (A)   Bitemporal hemianopsia
    ○ (B)   Bilateral inferior quadrantanopia
    ○ (C)   Bilateral superior quadrantanopia
    ○ (D)   Left superior quadrantanopia
    ○ (E)   Right superior quadrantanopia

37. A 59-year-old man, who is a family physician, confides in a neurology colleague that he believes he has early stage Parkinson's disease. The neurologic examination reveals a slight resting tremor of the left hand, a slow gait, and a lack of the normal range of facial expression for this man. Which of the following is the most likely location of the degenerative changes at this stage of this physician's disease?

    ○ (A)   Bilateral substantia nigra
    ○ (B)   Left globus pallidus
    ○ (C)   Left substantia nigra
    ○ (D)   Right globus pallidus
    ○ (E)   Right substantia nigra

38. A 14-year-old boy is brought to the emergency department after an accident on his BMX bicycle. The examination reveals that the boy has severe facial injuries. Craniofacial CT shows fracture of facial bones and probable crushing of the structures traversing the superior orbital fissure. Damage to which of the following structures passing through this fissure would result in diplopia when attempting to look down and in?

    ○ (A)   Abducens nerve
    ○ (B)   Oculomotor nerve
    ○ (C)   Ophthalmic nerve
    ○ (D)   Ophthalmic vein
    ○ (E)   Trochlear nerve

Questions 39 through 41 are based on the following patient.

A 67-year-old man is brought to the emergency department by his wife. She explains that he fell suddenly, could not get up, and complained of feeling sick. The examination revealed a left-sided weakness of the upper and lower extremities, a lack of most movement of the right eye, and a dilated pupil on the right. MRI shows an infarcted area in the brainstem.

39. The weakness of this man's extremities is explained by damage to the axons of cell bodies that are located in which of the following regions of the brain?

    ○ (A)   Left somatomotor cortex
    ○ (B)   Right anterior paracentral gyrus
    ○ (C)   Right crus cerebri
    ○ (D)   Right precentral gyrus
    ○ (E)   Right somatomotor cortex

40. This man's dilated pupil is due to damage to which of the following fiber populations?

    ○ (A)   Preganglionic fibers from the Edinger-Westphal nucleus
    ○ (B)   Preganglionic fibers from the inferior salivatory nucleus
    ○ (C)   Postganglionic fibers from the ciliary ganglion
    ○ (D)   Postganglionic fibers from the geniculate ganglion
    ○ (E)   Postganglionic fibers from the superior cervical ganglion

41. Which of the following descriptive phrases best describes the constellation of signs and symptoms seen in the man?

    ○ (A)   Alternating hemianesthesia
    ○ (B)   Brown-Séquard syndrome
    ○ (C)   Inferior alternating hemiplegia
    ○ (D)   Middle alternating hemiplegia
    ○ (E)   Superior alternating hemiplegia

42. Which of the following structures contains the cell bodies of origin for fibers conveying taste information from the anterior two-thirds of the tongue?

   ○ (A) Ciliary ganglion
   ○ (B) Geniculate ganglion
   ○ (C) Superior ganglion of the vagus nerve
   ○ (D) Superior ganglion of the glossopharyngeal nerve
   ○ (E) Trigeminal ganglion

43. During a screening neurologic examination of a 39-year-old man, the physician taps the supraorbital ridge, stimulating the supraorbital nerve, and elicits a motor response. Which of the following most likely represents the motor response in this man?

   ○ (A) Constriction of the masticatory muscles
   ○ (B) Constriction of the orbicularis oculi muscle
   ○ (C) Constriction of the pupil
   ○ (D) Dilation of the pupil
   ○ (E) Horizontal nystagmus

44. A 67-year-old man has a bilateral anterolateral cordotomy at T10 for intractable pelvic pain. Four months after this procedure the man begins to experience pain sensations. Which of the following would most likely explain this apparent recurrence of pain in this man?

   ○ (A) Activation of postsynaptic posterior column and spinocervicothalamic pathways
   ○ (B) Activation of recurrent corticospinal fibers
   ○ (C) Activation of spinoreticular-reticulothalamic-thalamo-cortical pathways
   ○ (D) Regeneration of anterolateral system fibers in the spinal cord
   ○ (E) Regeneration of anterolateral system fibers into the posterior column system

45. An 84-year-old woman presents to her physician with the complaint of difficulty walking. The examination reveals that the woman has an unsteady gait and tends to forcibly slap her feet to the floor as she walks. She has no other deficits. The physician concludes that the woman has sensory ataxia. Degenerative changes in which of the following would most likely explain this deficit?

   ○ (A) Anterolateral system fibers
   ○ (B) Corticospinal fibers
   ○ (C) Posterior column fibers
   ○ (D) Posterior root fibers
   ○ (E) Vestibulospinal and reticulospinal fibers

Questions 46 through 48 are based on the following patient.

A 70-year-old woman is brought to the emergency department by her daughter after becoming ill during a trip to the mall. The woman is conscious but lethargic, and she has trouble speaking and swallowing. The examination reveals a loss of pain and thermal sensation on the left side of the face and a hoarse gravely voice (as if the woman has a sore throat). Movements of the extremities are normal for the woman's age, but she has a loss of pain and thermal sensations on the right side of her body. The corneal reflex is absent on the left side. MRI shows an infarcted area in the brainstem.

46. The facial sensory deficits experienced by this woman are explained by a lesion to the axons of cell bodies located in which of the following structures?

   ○ (A) Anterior trigeminothalamic fibers on the left
   ○ (B) Left trigeminal ganglion
   ○ (C) Principal sensory nucleus on the left
   ○ (D) Right trigeminal ganglion
   ○ (E) Spinal trigeminal nucleus on the right

47. The loss of pain and thermal sensations experienced by this woman on the right side of her body (excluding the face) is most likely the result of damage to which of the following structures?

   ○ (A) Anterolateral system fibers on the left
   ○ (B) Anterolateral system fibers on the right
   ○ (C) Anterior trigeminothalamic fibers on the left
   ○ (D) Medial lemniscus on the left
   ○ (E) Medial lemniscus on the right

48. Taking into account all the deficits experienced by this woman, which of the following characterizes the syndrome, and the side, in this patient?

   ○ (A) Benedikt syndrome on the left
   ○ (B) Lateral medullary syndrome on the left
   ○ (C) Lateral medullary syndrome on the right
   ○ (D) Parinaud syndrome (bilateral)
   ○ (E) Weber syndrome on the right

49. A 17-year-old boy from a poor rural community is diagnosed with hepatolenticular degeneration (Wilson's disease). Which of the following is accumulating in certain tissues of his body and producing health problems?

   ○ (A) Arsenic
   ○ (B) Copper
   ○ (C) Lead
   ○ (D) Magnesium
   ○ (E) Mercury

50. Which of the following represents the location of the postganglionic fibers that influence the dilator pupillae muscle of the iris on the ipsilateral side?

   ○ (A) Ciliary ganglion
   ○ (B) Edinger-Westphal nucleus
   ○ (C) Hypothalamus
   ○ (D) Intermediolateral cell column
   ○ (E) Superior cervical ganglion

51. A 37-year-old man presents with vertigo, nystagmus, ataxia, and hearing loss in his right ear. MRI shows a tumor in the cerebellopontine angle. A biopsy specimen of this tumor indicates that this mass most likely originated from myelin-forming cells on the root of the vestibulocochlear nerve. Which of the following terms most correctly identifies this tumor?

   ○ (A) Acoustic neuroma
   ○ (B) Ependymoma
   ○ (C) Glioblastoma multiforme
   ○ (D) Meningioma
   ○ (E) Vestibular schwannoma

52. An inherited (autosomal recessive) disorder may appear early in the teenage years. These patients have degenerative changes in the spinocerebellar tracts, posterior columns, corticospinal fibers, cerebellar cortex, and at select places in the brainstem. The symptoms of these patients may include ataxia, paralysis, dysarthria, and other clinical manifestations. This constellation of deficits is most characteristically seen in which of the following?

    ○ (A) Friedreich ataxia
    ○ (B) Huntington disease
    ○ (C) Olivopontocerebellar degeneration (atrophy)
    ○ (D) Parkinson disease
    ○ (E) Wallenberg syndrome

53. A 45-year-old man complains to his family physician that there seems to be something wrong with his mouth. The examination reveals a weakness of the masticatory muscles, a deviation of the jaw to the left on closure, and a sensory loss on the same side of the lower jaw. MRI shows a tumor, presumably a trigeminal schwannoma, in the foramen ovale. Compression of which of the following structures would most likely be the cause of the deficits experienced by this man?

    ○ (A) Maxillary and mandibular nerves and motor fibers on the left
    ○ (B) Motor fibers and mandibular nerve on the left
    ○ (C) Motor fibers and mandibular nerve on the right
    ○ (D) Motor fibers and maxillary nerve on the left
    ○ (E) Motor fibers and maxillary nerve on the right

54. A 49-year-old man visits his ophthalmologist with what the man interprets as "trouble seeing". The history reveals that the man had a sudden event a few days before in which he felt sick and was nauseated. The man said his trouble "seeing" started after this sudden sickness. The examination reveals a loss of abduction and adduction of the right eye and a loss of adduction of the left eye. MRI confirms an infarcted area in the caudal and medial pontine tegmentum. Which of the following most specifically identifies this man's clinical problem?

    ○ (A) Horizontal gaze palsy
    ○ (B) Internuclear ophthalmoplegia
    ○ (C) One-and-a-half syndrome
    ○ (D) Parinaud syndrome
    ○ (E) Vertical gaze palsy

55. Collaterals of ascending anterior (ventral) trigeminothalamic fibers that contribute to the vomiting reflex would most likely project into which of the following brainstem structures?

    ○ (A) Dorsal motor vagal nucleus
    ○ (B) Facial nucleus
    ○ (C) Nucleus ambiguus
    ○ (D) Superior salivatory nucleus
    ○ (E) Trigeminal motor nucleus

56. The topographical arrangement of fibers in the medial lemniscus at mid-olivary levels is such that the sensory information being conveyed by those fibers located most anterior (ventral) in this bundle will eventually terminate in which of the following structures?

    ○ (A) Anterior paracentral gyrus
    ○ (B) Lateral one-third of the postcentral gyrus
    ○ (C) Medial one-third of the postcentral gyrus
    ○ (D) Middle one-third of the postcentral gyrus
    ○ (E) Posterior paracentral gyrus

57. An 11-year-old girl is brought to the family physician by her mother. The mother explains that the girl has been complaining that her hands and arms "feel funny". In fact, the mother states that the girl cut her little finger, but did not realize it until she saw blood. The examination reveals a bilateral loss of pain and thermal sensation on the upper extremities and shoulder. Which of the following is the most likely cause of this deficit in this girl?

    ○ (A) Brown-Séquard syndrome
    ○ (B) Posterior inferior cerebellar artery syndrome
    ○ (C) Tabes dorsalis
    ○ (D) Syringobulbia
    ○ (E) Syringomyelia

58. A 57-year-old obese man is brought to the emergency department by his wife. The examination reveals that cranial nerve function is normal but the man has bilateral weakness of his lower extremities. He has no sensory deficits. MRI shows a small infarcted area in the general region of the cervical spinal cord-medulla junction. Which of the following represents the most likely location of this lesion?

    ○ (A) Caudal part of the pyramidal decussation
    ○ (B) Lateral corticospinal tract on the left
    ○ (C) Pyramids bilaterally
    ○ (D) Pyramid on the right
    ○ (E) Rostral part of the pyramidal decussation

Questions 59 through 61 are based on the following patient.

A 34-year-old woman presents with the complaint of seeing "two of everything" (diplopia). The history reveals that the woman becomes tired during the workday to the point where she frequently must leave her workplace early. The woman said that her vision problems appeared first, and later she noticed that, when she drank, it would "go down the wrong pipe". The examination reveals weakness of the ocular muscle, difficulty in swallowing (dysphagia), and mild weakness of the upper extremities. Sensation is normal. Further laboratory tests indicate that the woman has a neurotransmitter disease.

59. Based on the history and symptoms experienced by this woman, which of the following is the most likely cause of her medical condition?

    ○ (A) Amyotrophic lateral sclerosis
    ○ (B) Huntington disease
    ○ (C) Myasthenia gravis
    ○ (D) Multiple sclerosis
    ○ (E) Parkinson disease

60. Which of the following represents the most likely location of the neurotransmitter dysfunction in this woman?

    ○ (A) At the termination of corticonuclear fibers
    ○ (B) At the termination of corticospinal fibers
    ○ (C) At the neuromuscular junction
    ○ (D) Within the basal nuclei
    ○ (E) Within the cerebellum

61. Which of the following represents the neurotransmitter most likely affected in this woman?

    ○ (A) Acetylcholine
    ○ (B) Dopamine
    ○ (C) Glutamate
    ○ (D) GABA
    ○ (E) Serotonin

62. A 39-year-old woman complains to her family physician that "sometimes I see two of everything, but not always". The examination reveals that the woman can abduct both eyes and can adduct her left eye but cannot adduct her right eye. All other eye movement is normal. MRI shows a small lesion suggesting an area of demyelination in the pons. Which of the following represents the most likely location of this lesion?

- ○ (A)   Left abducens nucleus
- ○ (B)   Left medial longitudinal fasciculus
- ○ (C)   Right abducens nucleus
- ○ (D)   Right medial longitudinal fasciculus
- ○ (E)   Right PPRF

63. A 20-year-old man is brought to the emergency department from the site of a motorcycle accident. The examination reveals multiple head injuries and a broken humerus. Cranial CT shows a basal skull fracture extending through the jugular foramen. Assuming that the nerve or nerves that traverse this opening are damaged, which of the following deficits would most likely be seen in this man?

- ○ (A)   Deviation of the tongue to the injured side on protrusion
- ○ (B)   Diplopia and ptosis
- ○ (C)   Drooping and difficulty elevating the shoulder
- ○ (D)   Drooping of the face on the ipsilateral side
- ○ (E)   Loss of the efferent limb of the corneal reflex

64. A 17-year-old boy is brought to the pediatrician by his mother. The examination reveals that the boy has rigidity, athetoid movements (athetosis), and difficulty speaking. His ophthalmologist reports that the boy has a greenish-brown ring at the corneoscleral margin. This boy is most likely suffering from which of the following?

- ○ (A)   Huntington disease
- ○ (B)   Parkinson disease
- ○ (C)   Pick disease
- ○ (D)   Sydenham chorea
- ○ (E)   Wilson disease

65. A 32-year-old woman complains to her gynecologist that her breasts are tender and a white fluid issues from her nipples. The examination reveals that the woman is not pregnant (she had her ovaries removed at age 28 resultant to a diagnosis of ovarian cancer), that a milky substance can be expressed from her nipples, and that she has a visual field deficit. MRI shows a tumor impinging on the midline portion of the optic chiasm. Based on the position of this tumor which of the following visual deficits would most likely be seen in this woman?

- ○ (A)   Bitemporal hemianopsia
- ○ (B)   Left homonymous hemianopsia
- ○ (C)   Left superior quadrantanopia
- ○ (D)   Right homonymous hemianopsia
- ○ (E)   Right superior quadrantanopia

66. Which of the following portions of the cerebellum have a close structural and functional relationship with the vestibular apparatus and the vestibular nuclei?

- ○ (A)   Dentate nucleus and interposed nuclei
- ○ (B)   Dentate nucleus only
- ○ (C)   Fastigial nucleus and flocculonodular lobe
- ○ (D)   Hemisphere of the posterior lobe
- ○ (E)   Interposed nuclei and hemisphere of the anterior lobe

67. A 17-year-old boy presents with the major complaint that he is having trouble playing baseball on the high school varsity team. The examination reveals a healthy, well-nurtured, athletic boy with normal motor and sensory function. The visual examination reveals a superior right quadrantanopia. MRI shows a small lesion in a position consistent with the visual field loss. Which of the following represents the most likely location of the lesion in this boy?

- ○ (A)   Crossing fibers in the optic chiasm
- ○ (B)   Lower portions of the optic radiations in the left temporal lobe
- ○ (C)   Lower portions of the optic radiations in the right temporal lobe
- ○ (D)   Upper portions of the optic radiations in the left parietal lobe
- ○ (E)   Upper portions of the optic radiations in the right parietal lobe

68. A 68-year-old man is brought to the emergency department by his daughter. She explains that he unexpectedly began to have sudden movements of his left "arm". The examination reveals a slender man with hypertension and with periodic, uncontrollable flailing movements of his left upper extremity suggestive of hemiballismus. Assuming this to result from a vascular occlusion, MRI would most likely show an infarction in which of the following structures?

- ○ (A)   Left substantia nigra
- ○ (B)   Left subthalamic nucleus
- ○ (C)   Right motor cortex
- ○ (D)   Right substantia nigra
- ○ (E)   Right subthalamic nucleus

Questions 69 through 72 are based on the following patient.

A 67-year-old man visits his family physician with the complaint that he is not able to "do things like I used to". The examination reveals that the man is not able to perform rapid alternating movements with his left upper extremity, and is not able to touch his left index finger to his nose because of a tremor that worsens as the finger approaches the nose. He is able to do these movements on the right. When he walks, he is unsteady with a tendency to fall to the left. He has no sensory deficits.

69. Which of the following terms specifically designates the inability of this man to perform rapid alternating movements?

- ○ (A)   Dysarthria
- ○ (B)   Dysdiadochokinesia
- ○ (C)   Dysmetria
- ○ (D)   Intention tremor
- ○ (E)   Resting tremor

70. Which of the following terms specifically designates this man's inability to touch his nose with his index finger?

- ○ (A)   Dysmetria
- ○ (B)   Intention tremor
- ○ (C)   Rebound phenomenon
- ○ (D)   Resting tremor
- ○ (E)   Static tremor

71. The MRI of this man shows an infarcted area in the brain. Based on the deficits this man is experiencing, which of the following represents the most likely location of this lesion?

    ○ (A) Basal nuclei on the left side
    ○ (B) Basal nuclei on the right side
    ○ (C) Cerebellar cortex and nuclei on the left side
    ○ (D) Cerebellar cortex and nuclei on the right side
    ○ (E) Midbrain on the right side

72. Assuming this lesion to be the result of the occlusion of an artery, which of the following is the most likely candidate?

    ○ (A) Left anterior inferior cerebellar artery
    ○ (B) Left superior cerebellar artery
    ○ (C) Lenticulostriate arteries on the left
    ○ (D) Right anterior inferior cerebellar artery
    ○ (E) Right superior cerebellar artery

73. A 61-year-old woman complains to her family physician that the muscles of her face sometimes twitch. The examination reveals that the woman has irregular and intermittent contractions of facial muscles; sometimes these are painful. MRI shows an aberrant loop of an artery that appears to be compressing the facial nerve root. Which of the following is most likely the offending vessel in this case?

    ○ (A) Anterior inferior cerebellar artery
    ○ (B) Anterior spinal artery
    ○ (C) Posterior inferior cerebellar artery
    ○ (D) Posterior spinal artery
    ○ (E) Superior cerebellar artery

74. An 81-year-old man presents with a loss of pain, thermal sensations, discriminative touch, and vibratory sense on the right side of his body excluding his head. CT shows a comparatively small infarct representing the territory of one vessel. Based on the positions and relationships of the pathways conveying the sensations lost in this man, which of the following represents the most likely location of this lesion?

    ○ (A) Caudal pons
    ○ (B) Midbrain
    ○ (C) Mid-medulla
    ○ (D) Rostral medulla
    ○ (E) Upper cervical spinal cord

75. The MRI of a 70-year-old man shows an infarcted area in the medial medulla at a mid-olivary level on the left. This correlates with a loss of position sense from the man's upper right extremity. Which of the following represents the location of the cell bodies of origin of those fibers damaged in this patient in the medulla?

    ○ (A) Cuneate nucleus on the left
    ○ (B) Cuneate nucleus on the right
    ○ (C) Gracile nucleus on the left
    ○ (D) Gracile nucleus on the right
    ○ (E) Posterior root ganglia on the left

76. A 39-year-old woman presents with sustained and oscillating muscle contractions that have twisted her trunk and extremities into unusual and abnormal postures. This woman is most likely suffering from which of the following?

    ○ (A) Dysarthria
    ○ (B) Dysmetria
    ○ (C) Dysphagia
    ○ (D) Dyspnea
    ○ (E) Dystonia

77. A 21-year-old man is brought to the emergency department from the scene of an automobile collision. He has a compound fracture of the humerus, a fractured tibia, various cuts and bruises, and significant facial trauma. Cranial CT shows fractures of the bones of the face and orbit on the left, and a total collapse of the optic canal on that side with probable transection of the optic nerve. Following an initial recovery period, which of the following would most likely be seen during an ophthalmologic examination?

    ○ (A) A loss of both the direct and consensual pupillary response when the light is shown in the right eye
    ○ (B) A loss of only the consensual pupillary response when the light is shown in the right eye
    ○ (C) A loss of the direct but not the consensual pupillary response when a light is shown in the left eye
    ○ (D) Direct and consensual pupillary responses are intact when light is shown in the left eye
    ○ (E) Direct and consensual pupillary responses are intact when light is shown in the right eye

78. A 27-year-old man presents with athetosis (athetoid movements), rigidity, and dysarthria. He also has a flapping tremor. The man has an obvious greenish-brown ring at the corneoscleral margin. A tentative diagnosis of advanced Wilson disease is made. MRI showing which of the following would provide further, if not conclusive evidence, of this disease?

    ○ (A) Atrophy of gyri of the frontal and temporal lobes
    ○ (B) Degeneration and cavitation of the putamen
    ○ (C) Lacunae in the thalamus and internal capsule
    ○ (D) Loss of cells in the substantia nigra
    ○ (E) Loss of the caudate nucleus

79. A 77-year-old man complains to his family physician that he is having trouble picking up his coffee cup, shaving with a safety razor, and picking up the checkers when playing with his grandson. The examination reveals that the man is unable to control the distance, power, or accuracy of a movement as the movement is taking place. He undershoots or overshoots that target. Which of the following most specifically describes this condition?

    ○ (A) Bradykinesia
    ○ (B) Dysarthria
    ○ (C) Dysdiadochokinesia
    ○ (D) Dysmetria
    ○ (E) Dysphagia

Questions 80 through 82 are based on the following patient.

A 70-year-old woman is brought to the emergency department by members of the volunteer fire department of a small town. She primarily complains of weakness. The examination reveals a hemiplegia involving the left upper and lower extremities, sensory losses (pain, thermal sensations, and proprioception) on the left side of the body and face, and a visual deficit in both eyes. MRI shows an area of infarction consistent with the territory served by the anterior choroidal artery.

80. Which of the following visual deficits is seen in this woman?

   ○ (A)   Left homonymous hemianopsia
   ○ (B)   Left nasal hemianopsia
   ○ (C)   Left superior quadrantanopia
   ○ (D)   Right homonymous hemianopsia
   ○ (E)   Right superior quadrantanopia

81. Which of the following most specifically identifies the pattern of sensory deficits experienced by this woman?

   ○ (A)   Alternating hemianesthesia
   ○ (B)   Hemianesthesia
   ○ (C)   Paresthesia
   ○ (D)   Sensory level
   ○ (E)   Superior alternating hemiplegia

82. The weakness of the extremities in this woman is most likely due to damage to which of the following?

   ○ (A)   Corticospinal fibers on the left
   ○ (B)   Corticospinal fibers on the right
   ○ (C)   Somatomotor cortex on the right
   ○ (D)   Thalamocortical fibers to motor cortex on the right
   ○ (E)   Thalamocortical fibers to sensory cortex on the right

83. A 16-year-old boy is brought to the family physician by his mother. The mother explains that her son is having trouble in school even though he is a hard worker and is well behaved. The examination reveals that the boy has a sensorineural hearing loss in his right ear. He has no other deficits. Which of the following represents the most likely location of the lesion in this boy?

   ○ (A)   Auditory cortex
   ○ (B)   Cochlea
   ○ (C)   External ear
   ○ (D)   Inferior colliculus
   ○ (E)   Middle ear

84. Which of the following laminae of the lateral geniculate nucleus receive input from the contralateral retina?

   ○ (A)   1, 2
   ○ (B)   1, 3, 5
   ○ (C)   1, 4, 6
   ○ (D)   2, 3, 5
   ○ (E)   3, 4, 5, 6

85. A 12-year-old girl is brought to the pediatrician by her mother who explains that the girl has started to "act funny". The history reveals that the girl was treated for a hemolytic streptococcus infection 4 weeks before the appearance of her symptoms; the mother states that the girl has had this problem for 3 weeks. The examination reveals a well-nurtured girl with brisk, flowing, and irregular movements of her face, neck, and upper extremities. This girl is most likely suffering from which of the following?

   ○ (A)   Huntington disease
   ○ (B)   Parkinson disease
   ○ (C)   Senile chorea
   ○ (D)   Sydenham chorea
   ○ (E)   Weber syndrome

Answers for Chapter 7

1. Answer **A**:   The combination of weakness on one side (corticospinal involvement) and a loss of pain sensation on the opposite side specifies components of a Brown-Séquard syndrome. The motor loss is ipsilateral to the damage and the sensory loss is contralateral; second order fibers conveying pain information cross in the anterior white commissure ascending one to two spinal segments in the process. In this patient, the lesion is on the left side at about the T6 level; this explains the loss of pain sensation on the right beginning at the T8 dermatome level. Lesions at T8 or T10 would result in a loss of pain sensation beginning, respectively, at dermatome levels T10 or T12 on the contralateral side. (p. 180–181)

2. Answer **E**:   The paralysis of both lower extremities is paraplegia. Monoplegia specifies paralysis of one extremity, hemiplegia of both extremities on the same side, and quadriplegia of all four extremities. An alternating hemiplegia is the combination of a motor cranial nerve deficit on one side and a hemiplegia on the contralateral side; this is a brainstem lesion not a spinal cord lesion. (p. 190–193)

3. Answer **C**:   While the causes of swallowing difficulties may be central or peripheral (and multiple), this particular problem is called dysphagia. Dysmetria is an inability to control the distance or power of a movement and is commonly seen in cerebellar disease. Dysarthria is difficulty in speaking, and dyspnea is a difficulty in breathing; the latter is usually associated with diseases of the lungs or heart. Dysdiadochokinesia, an inability to perform rapid alternating movements, is seen most commonly in cerebellar disease. (p. 190, 202)

4. Answer **E**:   One possible cause of trigeminal neuralgia (tic douloureux) is compression of the trigeminal root by the superior cerebellar artery or its main branches; surgical relocation of the aberrant vessel (neurovascular decompression) relieves the symptoms. Hemifacial spasm may be caused by compression of the facial nerve by the anterior inferior cerebellar artery (commonly called AICA). The other choices do not cause trigeminal neuralgia and are not a principal cause of cranial nerve dysfunction via root compression. (p. 41, 184–185)

5. Answer **E**:   The rostral interstitial nucleus of the medial longitudinal fasciculus receives cortical input from the frontal eye field on the ipsilateral side and projects to the ipsilateral (heavy) and contralateral (light) oculomotor and trochlear nuclei. This nucleus is regarded as the vertical gaze center. The paramedian pontine reticular formation is the horizontal gaze center. The oculomotor and abducens nuclei do not receive direct input from the frontal eye field and the Edinger-Westphal is a visceromotor nucleus containing preganglionic parasympathetic cell bodies. (p. 192–193)

6. Answer **C**:   The absence of, or the aberrant development of, muscle around the oral cavity and over the cheek (muscles of facial expression, innervated by the facial [VII] nerve) indicate a failure of proper differentiation of the second (2nd) pharyngeal arch. Arch 2 also gives rise to the stapedius, buccinator, stylohyoid, platysma, and posterior belly of the digastric. Mesoderm of the head outside of the pharyngeal arches gives rise to the extraocular muscles and muscles of the tongue. The muscles of mastication

(plus the tensor tympani, tensor veli palati, mylohyoid, anterior belly of the digastric) arise from arch 1, the stylopharyngeus from arch 3, and striated muscles of the pharynx, larynx, and upper esophagus from arch 4. (p. 202–203)

7. Answer **C**:   Hypothalamocerebellar fibers that project to the cerebellar nuclei and cortex contain histamine. GABA is found in several neurons that are located in the cerebellar cortex, and in Purkinje cells glutamate is found in many pontocerebellar fibers and in granule cells of the cerebellar cortex; and noradrenalin is found in ceruleocerebellar fibers. Serotonin is found in cells of the reticular formation and in some raphe cells that project to the cerebellum. (p. 206–207)

8. Answer **C**:   The best localizing sign in this patient is the paucity of eye movement and dilated pupil on the left; this indicates a lesion of the midbrain on the left at the level of the exiting oculomotor fibers. The red nucleus is found at the same level and, more importantly, immediately lateral to the red nucleus is a compact bundle of cerebellothalamic fibers. The ataxia and tremor are related primarily to damage to these cerebellar efferent fibers. The motor deficit is contralateral to the lesion because the corticospinal fibers, through which the deficit is expressed, cross at the motor (pyramidal) decussation. Lesions at the other choices would not result in a paucity of eye movement and are, therefore, not potential candidates. (p. 132–133, 208–211)

9. Answer **C**:   The lesion on the exiting oculomotor fibers (on the left) damages the preganglionic fibers from the Edinger-Westphal nucleus and removes their influence on the pupil. Consequently, the intact postganglionic sympathetic fibers from the ipsilateral superior cervical ganglion predominate, and the pupil dilates. Choices on the right are on the incorrect side. Damage to hypothalamospinal fibers would remove sympathetic influence at the intermediolateral cell column, and the pupil would constrict (parasympathetic domination). (p. 200–201, 208–211, 220–221)

10. Answer **C**:   Cerebellar efferent fibers exit the cerebellum via the superior cerebellar peduncle, cross in its decussation, and terminate primarily in the ventral lateral nucleus (VL). Consequently, the cerebellar nuclei on the left project to the right VL. The ventral anterior nucleus does not receive significant cerebellar input. While the ventral posterolateral nucleus receives a limited amount of cerebellar input, its major role is the relay of somatosensory information to the primary somatosensory cortex (postcentral gyrus). (p. 210–211)

11. Answer **B**:   The jerking movements of the upper extremity (asterixis) are also called a flapping tremor and are seen in patients with hepatolenticular degeneration (Wilson disease). Akinesia is lack of movement. Resting tremor is seen in patients with disease of the basal nuclei, such as Parkinson disease, and an intention tremor is a characteristic of patients with cerebellar lesions. Dystonia is the result of sustained muscle contractions that twist the extremities, trunk, and neck into distorted and abnormal postures. (p. 214–215)

12. Answer **A**:   This man is unable to recognize or comprehend the meaning of sounds; although he is able to hear sounds, he is not able to put meaning to the sounds; this man is suffering from auditory agnosia. Agraphia is the inability to write in a person with no paralysis, and alexia is the inability to comprehend the mean-

ing of written or printed words. Aphonia is a loss of the voice frequently due to disease of, or injury to, the larynx. Aphasia is seen in individuals with a lesion in the dominant hemisphere, and is manifest as an inability to comprehend the meaning of spoken, written, or various other types of input. (p. 226–227)

13. Answer **C**:   The Korsakoff syndrome is a constellation of deficits the include memory loss, confabulation, amnesia, and dementia that is seen in chronic alcoholics; the manifestations are related, in part, to excessive alcohol consumption and malnutrition. Therapeutic doses of thiamine are used to treat this disease. Broca aphasia (nonfluent or expressive aphasia) results from lesions in the dominant hemisphere. The Klüver-Bucy syndrome is related to bilateral lesions to the amygdaloid complex, and Pick disease is dementia related to atrophy of the frontal and temporal lobes. Munchausen syndrome is the fabrication or feigning of illness or disease to gain attention or control. (p. 232–233)

14. Answer **B**:   Cell bodies in the nucleus ambiguus innervate muscles of the pharynx and larynx, including what is commonly called the vocalis muscle. A lesion of this nucleus is one cause of dysarthria. The solitary tract and nuclei are concerned with visceral afferent information including taste, and the spinal trigeminal tract is made the central processes of primary sensory fibers conveying general somatic afferent (GSA) information from the ipsilateral side of the face and oral cavity. Proprioceptive information from the ipsilateral upper extremity is transmitted via the cuneate nucleus; the vestibular nuclei are related to balance, equilibrium, and control of eye movement. (p. 202–203)

15. Answer **C**:   The area of the brainstem that contains the nucleus ambiguus is served by branches of the posterior inferior cerebellar artery (PICA). Occlusion of this vessel usually gives rise to the PICA (lateral medullary or Wallenberg) syndrome. The anterior inferior cerebellar artery (AICA) serves the lateral and inferior cerebellar surface and the superior cerebellar artery serves the superior surface and much of the cerebellar nuclei. The labyrinthine artery, a branch of AICA, serves the inner ear. The posterior spinal artery serves the posterior columns and their nuclei. (p. 110–111, 202–203)

16. Answer **D**:   Glutamate is found in many efferent fibers of the cerebral cortex including those of the corticospinal tract. Consequently, there are many glutaminergic terminals in the spinal cord. Acetylcholine is found at many central nervous system (CNS) sites and at the neuromuscular junction, and dopamine is found mainly in cells of the substantia nigra-pars compacta and in their nigrostriatal terminals. Gamma aminobutyric acid (GAMA) is an inhibitory neurotransmitter and is found in many interneurons in the CNS. Serotonin is found in CNS areas such as the hypothalamus, basal nuclei, and the raphe nuclei. (p. 190)

17. Answer **A**:   The loss of sensation on one side of the face and the opposite side of the body is an alternating hemianesthesia (also called an alternate hemianesthesia or a crossed hemianesthesia). Epidural anesthesia refers to anesthesia resultant to injection of an appropriate agent into the epidural space. The other choices are motor abnormalities. (p. 180–181, 186–187)

18. Answer **D**:   Lesions in the lateral portions of the brainstem damage descending projections from the hypothalamus to the ipsilateral intermediolateral cell column at spinal levels T1-T4, these be-

ing the hypothalamospinal fibers. The result is Horner syndrome on the side ipsilateral to the lesion. Horner syndrome may also be seen following cervical spinal cord lesions. A contralateral hemiplegia is not seen in lesions in lateral areas of the brainstem. The other choices are syndromes or deficits specific to medial brainstem areas or to only a particular level. (p. 110, 124, 136, 220–221)

19. Answer **C**:   The denticulate ligament is located on the lateral aspect of the spinal cord at a midpoint in the posterior-anterior extent of the spinal cord. The anterolateral system, the tract divided in the anterolateral cordotomy, is located in the anterolateral portion of the spinal cord just inferior to the position of the denticulate ligament. The posterolateral sulcus is the entrance point for sensory fibers of the posterior roots; the anterolateral sulcus is the exit point for motor fibers of the anterior root; and the posterior intermediate sulcus separates the gracile and cuneate fasciculi. The anterior median sulcus is located on the anterior midline and contains the anterior spinal artery. (p. 182–183)

20. Answer **B**:   Damage to the gracile fasciculus on the left at T10, the level of the umbilicus, will result in the deficits experienced by this boy. The gracile fasciculus contains uncrossed ascending fibers conveying vibratory sensation, discriminative touch, and proprioception; consequently, the deficits will be seen beginning at the level of the lesion and extending caudally on the same side. These fibers are the central processes of primary sensory neurons whose cell bodies are located in the ipsilateral posterior root ganglion. The other choices are either on the wrong side (right) or at the wrong level. (p. 178–179)

21. Answer **C**:   The gag reflex is not regularly tested. However, in patients with dysphagia (difficulty swallowing) or dysarthria (difficulty speaking), the gag reflex should be evaluated. Dysmetria is a movement disorder associated with cerebellar lesions; dysgeusia is the perception of an abnormal taste or of a tastant when there is none; and dyspnea is difficulty breathing, usually associated with disease of the lung or heart. Gustatory agnosia is the inability to recognize food or distinguish between different food items. (p. 186–187)

22. Answer **B**:   The combination of a deviation of the tongue to one side (right) and the uvula to the opposite side (left) indicates a lesion in the genu of the internal capsule on the left involving corticonuclear (corticobulbar) fibers. Corticonuclear fibers to the hypoglossal nucleus are crossed and the tongue deviates toward the weak side on protrusion. These fibers to the nucleus ambiguus are also crossed resulting in weakness of the contralateral side of the palate. However, on attempted phonation (say "Ah"), the strong side of the palate will contract and elevate, and the uvula will deviate to the intact side (opposite to the tongue). Lesions in the right genu would result in deficits on the opposite sides. Lesions in the medial medulla on the right would include the tongue, exclude the uvula but also show a left-sided hemiplegia. Lesions of the right lateral medulla could include the uvula, but exclude the tongue. A lesion in the crus would include a number of additional deficits and would have to be on the left, not the right. (p. 192–193)

23. Answer **A**:   Deficits of eye movement (resulting in diplopia and ptosis) are seen first in about 50% of all patients with myasthenia gravis and are eventually seen in approximately 85% of all patients

with this disease. Weakness of the extremities may be seen, but this almost always follows ocular movement disorders. Dysmetria is most commonly seen in cerebellar disease and may be present in patients with lesions involving corticospinal fibers. Tremor is commonly seen in diseases or lesions of the basal nuclei and the cerebellum. (p. 200–201)

24. Answer **B**:   The lesion in this woman is in the medulla, and the sensory loss on the body (excluding the head) is on her left side; a lesion in the medulla on the right side, involving fibers of the anterolateral system (ALS), accounts for this sensory deficit. A lesion of the ALS on the left side of the medulla would result in sensory deficits on the right side of the body. The spinal trigeminal tract and nucleus convey pain and thermal sensations from the ipsilateral side (right side in this case) of the face, and the medial lemniscus conveys vibratory and discriminative touch sensations from the contralateral side of the body. (p. 180–181, 184–185)

25. Answer **C**:   The woman is hoarse because the lesion involves the region of the medulla that includes the nucleus ambiguus. These motor neurons serve, via the glossopharyngeal (IX) and vagus (X) nerves, the muscles of the larynx and pharynx, including the medial portion of the thyroarytenoid, also called the vocalis muscle. Paralysis of the vocalis on one side will cause hoarseness of the voice. Hypoglossal nucleus or nerve, or facial nucleus lesions may cause difficulty with speech but not hoarseness. The spinal trigeminal tract conveys sensory input from the ipsilateral side of the face. There are no historical or examination findings to support a diagnosis of upper respiratory viral findings (cold or flu). (p. 180–181, 202–203)

26. Answer **C**:   The posterior inferior cerebellar artery (PICA) serves the lateral area of the medulla that contains the anterolateral system, spinal trigeminal tract (loss of pain and thermal sensations from the ipsilateral side of the face), and the nucleus ambiguus. Many patients that present with a PICA (Wallenberg or lateral medullary) syndrome also have involvement of the vertebral artery on that side. The posterior spinal artery serves the posterior column nuclei in the medulla, and the anterior spinal artery serves the pyramid, medial lemniscus, and exiting roots of the hypoglossal nerve. The anterior inferior cerebellar artery and the superior cerebellar artery distribute to the pons and midbrain, respectively, plus significant portions of the cerebellum. (p. 110–111, 180)

27. Answer **B**:   The mesencephalic nucleus, a part of the trigeminal complex, has peripheral processes attached to neuromuscular spindles in the masticatory muscles, unipolar cell bodies in the rostral pons and midbrain, and central collaterals that distribute bilaterally to the trigeminal motor nucleus. Through these connections, stretching of the spindle initiates a motor response. The principal sensory and spinal trigeminal nuclei relay touch and pain/thermal sensations respectively. The hypoglossal nucleus is motor to the ipsilateral side of the tongue. (p. 184–185)

28. Answer **E**:   The patient's perception that his body is moving around the room when he is actually sitting or laying still is subjective vertigo. Objective vertigo is the perception, on the part of the patient, that he is still and objects in the room are moving. As its name clearly implies, hysterical vertigo is a psychosomatic disorder. Nystagmus is abnormal rhythmic movements of the eyes, usually with fast and slow components. Ataxia is an inability to co-

ordinate muscle activity resulting in an unsteady gait or other un-coordinated movements. (p. 228–229)

29. Answer **E**: Excessive eating (gluttony), which may include a propensity to attempt to eat things not considered food items, is hyperphagia. Dysphagia is difficulty in swallowing, and aphagia is the inability to eat. Hyperorality is the tendency to put items in the mouth or to appear to be examining objects by placing them in the oral cavity. Dyspnea is difficulty breathing. (p. 234–235)

30. Answer **A**: The constellation of deficits experienced by this man is characteristic of the Klüver-Bucy syndrome; this may be seen following bilateral damage to the temporal poles that includes the amygdaloid complex. The Korsakoff syndrome is seen, for example, in chronic alcoholics, and senile dementia is a loss of cognitive and intellectual function associated with neurodegenerative diseases of the elderly (such as Alzheimer). Wernicke (receptive or fluent) aphasia is seen in patients with a lesion in the area of the inferior parietal lobule, and the Wallenberg syndrome results from a lesion in the medulla characterized by alternating hemisensory losses and, depending on the extent of the damage, other deficits. (p. 234–235)

31. Answer **D**: Hearing a sound in the ipsilateral ear with the application of a tuning fork to the mastoid bone (actually the mastoid process of the temporal bone), and then hearing the sound again at the external ear by moving the prongs to the external ear after the sound disappears at the mastoid is a normal Rinne test. In a negative Rinne test, the sound is not heard at the external meatus after it has disappeared from touching the mastoid. In a normal Weber test, sound is heard equally in both ears with application of a tuning fork to the midline of the forehead. A localizing Weber test indicates that sound is heard in the normal ear, but not in the ear with disease or lesion. The Binet is an intelligence test. (p. 226–227)

32. Answer **B**: In Huntington disease, especially in advanced stages, there is a loss of the caudate nucleus and ex vacuo enlargement of the ventricles. The most obvious portion of the caudate missing in MRI coronal or axial planes is the head. The anterior lobe of the cerebellum is diminished in size in alcoholic cerebellar degeneration, but not so in Huntington disease. Lesions of the subthalamic nucleus result in hemiballismus, and degenerative changes in the substantia nigra result in the motor deficits seen in Parkinson disease. One of the main responsibilities of the lateral thalamic nuclei is to convey input to the somatomotor and somatosensory cortices. (p. 214–215)

33. Answer **D**: The paralysis of facial muscles on one side of the face (left in this case) with no paralysis of the extremities is a facial hemiplegia; this is also commonly known as Bell palsy or facial palsy. Hemifacial spasms are irregular contractions of the facial muscles, and a central seven refers to paralysis of muscles on the lower half of the face contralateral to a lesion in the genu of the internal capsule. Alternating hemiplegia describes a motor loss related to a cranial nerve on one side of the head and motor deficits of the extremities on the contralateral side of the body. A similar pattern of sensory losses is called an alternating hemianesthesia. (p. 202–203)

34. Answer **C**: The otic ganglion receives preganglionic parasympathetic fibers from the inferior salivatory nucleus (associated with the glossopharyngeal [IX] nerve) and sends postganglionic fibers to the parotid gland. The ciliary receives from the Edinger-Westphal nucleus and sends to the pupil; the pterygopalatine and submandibular receives from the superior salivatory nucleus (associated with the facial [VII] nerve) and send, to the lacrimal, submandibular, and sublingual glands, respectively. Intramural ganglia are located in the gut and receive input from the dorsal motor vagal nucleus. (p. 202–203)

35. Answer **B**: Bilateral damage to the temporal lobes, as in an automobile collision, may result in damage to the hippocampus. While remote memory, the ability to recall events that happened years or decades ago, is intact, the man will have difficulty "remembering" recent or immediate events. That is, he will find it difficult, if not impossible, to turn a new experience into longer-term memory (something that can be recalled in its proper context at a later time). Dysphagia (difficulty swallowing) and dysarthria (difficulty speaking) are deficits usually seen in brainstem lesions. Bilateral sensory losses of the lower portion of the body could be seen with bilateral damage to the posterior paracentral gyri (falcine meningioma) or to the anterior white commissure of the spinal cord. Dementia is a multiregional symptom that usually involves several areas of the brain, cortical as well as subcortical. (p. 232–233)

36. Answer **C**: The Meyer-Archambault loop is composed of optic radiation fibers that loop through the temporal lobe; these fibers, on each side, convey visual input from the contralateral superior quadrant of the visual field. Consequently, a bilateral lesion of these fibers results as a bilateral superior quadrantanopia. Bilateral inferior quadrantanopia is seen in bilateral lesions that would involve the superior portion of the optic radiations. Right or left superior quadrantanopia is seen in cases of unilateral damage to, respectively, the left or right Meyer-Archambault loop. A bitemporal hemianopsia results in a lesion of the optic chiasm. (p. 220, 223)

37. Answer **E**: Degenerative changes in the dopamine-containing cells of the substantia nigra pars compacta on the right side correlate with a left-sided tremor. The altered message through the lenticular nucleus and thalamus and on to the motor cortex on the side of the degenerative changes will result in tremor on the opposite (right) side via altered messages traveling down the corticospinal tract. The initial symptoms of Parkinson disease appear on one side in about 80% of patients and extend to bilateral involvement as the disease progresses. Bilateral changes in the substantia nigra correlate with bilateral deficits. The globus pallidus does not receive direct nigral input but rather input via a nigro-striatal-striatopallidal circuit. (p. 214–215)

38. Answer **E**: Damage to the trochlear nerve will cause diplopia on gaze inward and downward on the side of the injury. Abducens damage will result in an inability to look laterally on the side of the lesion, and oculomotor injury will result in the loss of most eye movement on that side; the eye will be deviated slightly down and out. The ophthalmic nerve is sensory. (p. 200–201)

39. Answer **E**: The combination of eye movement disorders and a contralateral hemiplegia localizes this lesion to the midbrain on the side of the ocular deficits (right side). This also specifies that corticospinal fibers on the right (in the crus) are damaged, and places the location of the cells of origin for these fibers in the somato-motor cortex on the right side. The right crus contains the axons

of these fibers but not the neuronal cell bodies. The left somato-motor cortex influences the right extremities. The right precentral gyrus does not contain cells projecting to the left lumbosacral spinal cord (left lower extremity), and the right anterior paracentral gyrus does not contain the cells that project to the left cervical spinal cord (left upper extremity). (p. 15, 190–193)

40. Answer **A:** The lesion in this man is central (brainstem) and involves the IIIrd nerve. Consequently, the damage is to the preganglionic parasympathetic fibers in the root of the oculomotor (III) nerve; this removes the parasympathetic influence (pupil constriction) that originates from the Edinger-Westphal nucleus. Fibers from the superior cervical ganglion are intact, hence the dilated pupil. Fibers from the geniculate ganglion and inferior salivatory nucleus distribute on the facial (VII) and glossopharyngeal (IX) nerves respectively. Postganglionic fibers from the ciliary ganglion, while involved in this pathway, are not damaged in this lesion. (p. 200–201)

41. Answer **E:** The loss of most eye movement on one side (oculomotor nerve root involvement) coupled with a paralysis of the extremities on the contralateral side is a superior alternating hemiplegia (this is also Weber syndrome): *superior* because it is the most rostral of three; *alternating* because it is a cranial nerve on one side and the extremities on the other; and *hemiplegia* because one-half of the body below the head is involved. A middle alternating hemiplegia involves the abducens (VI) nerve root and adjacent corticospinal fibers, and an inferior alternating hemiplegia involves the hypoglossal (XII) nerve root and corticospinal fibers in the pyramid. Alternating hemianesthesia is a sensory loss, and a Brown-Séquard syndrome is a spinal cord lesion with no cranial nerve deficits. (p. 200–201)

42. Answer **B:** Taste fibers (special visceral afferent, SVA) that serve the anterior two-thirds of the tongue on the ipsilateral side are conveyed on the facial nerve and have their cell bodies of origin in the geniculate ganglion. The trigeminal ganglion contains cell bodies that convey general sensation (general somatic afferent, GSA), and the ciliary ganglion contains visceromotor cell bodies (general visceral efferent GVE, postganglionic, parasympathetic). The superior ganglion of the glossopharyngeal contains cell bodies for taste from the posterior one-third of the tongue, and the superior ganglion of the vagus nerve contains cell bodies for taste from the root of the tongue. (p. 187)

43. Answer **B:** Stimulation of the supraorbital nerve (Vth nerve, afferent limb of the supraorbital reflex) results in contraction of the orbicularis oculi muscle (VIIth nerve, efferent limb of the supraorbital reflex). Changes in pupil size relate to the third nerve, the pupillary light reflex, and the distribution of postganglionic fibers from the superior cervical ganglion. Contraction of masticatory muscles is seen in the jaw-jerk reflex, and nystagmus usually results from cerebellum or brainstem lesions or disease of the vestibular apparatus. (p. 184–185, 202–203)

44. Answer **A:** Fibers in the postsynaptic posterior column and in the spinocervicothalamic pathways are spared in an anterolateral cordotomy. These pathways originate from those laminae of the posterior horn that also contribute to the anterolateral system. It is possible that these pathways remodel to transmit pain and thermal sensations in the absence of the normal anterolateral system (ALS) pathway. Regeneration to a functional state probably does

not normally take place in the human nervous system; spinoreticular fibers are in the divided ALS; and corticospinal fibers function in the motor sphere. (p. 182–183)

45. Answer **C:** The ataxia seen in patients with lesions of posterior column fibers is due to the loss of proprioceptive input and the resultant inability of the patient to accurately judge the relative position of the extremity. Thus, the extremity is forcibly slapped to the floor partially in an attempt to "create" the missing input. Anterolateral system fibers convey pain and thermal sensations, and posterior root fibers convey these sensations plus those related to the posterior columns. Corticospinal, vestibulospinal, and reticulospinal fibers function in the motor sphere. (p. 178–179)

46. Answer **B:** The axons of cell bodies located in the left trigeminal ganglion collect inside the brainstem to form the spinal trigeminal tract on the left (this tract is made up of the central processes of primary sensory fibers on the trigeminal [V] nerve). A lesion of these fibers on the left side of the medulla will result in a loss of pain and thermal sensations on the left side of the face. Lesions of the right trigeminal ganglion, trigeminothalamic fibers on the left, and the right spinal trigeminal nucleus would all result in pain and thermal losses on the right side of the face. The principal sensory nucleus conveys touch information. (p. 184–185)

47. Answer **A:** Recognizing that this woman has a sensory loss on the left side of her face, damage to fibers of the anterolateral system on the left correlates with the loss of pain and thermal sensations on the right side of her body. These anterolateral system (ALS) fibers cross in the spinal cord within about two levels of where they enter. Lesions of ALS on the right would result in a left-sided deficit on the body. Damage to anterior trigeminothalamic fibers on the left would produce a corresponding right-sided deficit on the face. The medial lemniscus conveys vibratory, discriminative touch, and proprioceptive sensations. (p. 180–181, 184–185)

48. Answer **B:** This patient has a lateral medullary syndrome (also commonly called a posterior inferior cerebellar artery, or PICA syndrome) on the left; this correlates with the left-sided sensory loss on the face and right-sided sensory loss on the body. A lateral medullary lesion on the right would result in the same deficits, but on the opposite sides. The Parinaud, Weber, and Benedikt syndromes are all associated with lesions in the midbrain. (p. 180–181, 184–185, see also p. 136)

49. Answer **B:** Wilson disease (hepatolenticular degeneration) is an inherited error of copper metabolism. Plasma levels of copper are decreased; urinary levels are increased; and copper accumulates in the liver, lenticular nuclei, and kidneys. Wilson disease can be treated by reducing the level of dietary copper and administering a copper-chelating agent. Maintenance can be achieved by taking zinc, and treatment must be life-long. Ingestion of the other choices can cause serious illness and death. However, none of these is the causative agent in hepatolenticular degeneration. (p. 214–215)

50. Answer **E:** The dilator pupillae muscle of the iris is innervated by postganglionic sympathetic fibers whose cell bodies of origin are located in the ipsilateral superior cervical ganglion. Preganglionic sympathetic cell bodies are found in the intermediolateral cell column. Preganglionic parasympathetic cell bodies are found

in the Edinger-Westphal nucleus; axons of these cells terminate in the ciliary ganglion, which, in turn, innervates the sphincter pupillae muscle of the iris. The hypothalamus is the origin of hypothalamospinal fibers that project to the intermediolateral cell column. (p. 220–21)

51. Answer **E:**   The deficits described for the man are consistent with a tumor on the root of the vestibulocochlear (VIII) nerve; these are correctly called a vestibular schwannoma because they arise from the Schwann cells on the root of the vestibular portion of the VIIIth nerve. Acoustic neuroma is an earlier, and now incorrect, designation for this lesion. Meningiomas arise primarily from the arachnoid layer, ependymomas from the cells lining the ventricular spaces, and a glioblastoma multiforme arises from astrocytes within the substance of the brain. (p. 228–229)

52. Answer **A:**   This inherited disease is Friedreich ataxia; it initially appears in children in the age range of 8–15 years and has the characteristic deficits described. Huntington disease is inherited, but appears in adults; olivopontocerebellar atrophy is an autosomal dominant disease and gives rise to a different set of deficits. The cause of Parkinson disease is unclear, but it is probably not inherited; the Wallenberg syndrome is a brainstem lesion resulting from a vascular occlusion. (p. 204–205)

53. Answer **B:**   A tumor in the foramen would damage the motor root of the trigeminal nerve and the mandibular root (sensory) of the Vth nerve. In this patient, the jaw deviates to the left and the sensory loss is on the left; this indicates that the tumor is on the left. The deviation of the jaw to the left is due to the action of the intact pterygoid muscles on the right (unlesioned side). Motor fibers on the trigeminal (V) nerve travel in association with the mandibular root and through the foramen ovale. Maxillary fibers are sensory for the upper jaw and cheek area of the face. (p. 202–203)

54. Answer **C:**   The loss of abduction and adduction in one eye and of adduction in the opposite eye (the one-and-a-half syndrome) indicates a lesion in the area of the paramedian pontine reticular formation and abducens nucleus (in this case on the right side) and the adjacent medial longitudinal fasciculus (MLF). The lesion damages the ipsilateral abducens motor neurons, internuclear neurons passing to the contralateral MLF, and internuclear axons in the ipsilateral MLF coming from the contralateral abducens nucleus. Parinaud syndrome is a paralysis of upward gaze, and gaze palsies tend to be toward one side and may result from cortical lesions. Internuclear ophthalmoplegia is a deficit of medial gaze in one eye, assuming a one-sided lesion. (p. 192–193)

55. Answer **A:**   Anterior trigeminothalamic collaterals that project into the dorsal motor nucleus of the vagus are an important link in the reflex pathway for vomiting. The superior salivatory nucleus is involved in the tearing or lacrimal reflex, the nucleus ambiguus in the sneezing reflex, and the facial nucleus in the corneal reflex. Collaterals of primary afferent fibers to the mesencephalic nucleus that branch to enter the trigeminal motor nucleus mediate the jaw reflex. (p. 184–184)

56. Answer **E:**   The most anterior (ventral) portion of the medial lemniscus at mid-olivary levels contains second order fibers conveying discriminative touch, vibratory sense, and proprioception from the contralateral lower extremity. These axons will terminate in the lateral parts of the ventral posterolateral nucleus and, from there, be relayed to the posterior paracentral gyrus (the lower extremity area of the primary somatomotor cortex). The postcentral gyrus is the primary sensory cortex for the face (approximately the lateral one-third), upper extremity (middle one-third), and the trunk (medial). The anterior paracentral gyrus is the somatomotor cortex for the lower extremity. (p. 179–180)

57. Answer **E:**   Syringomyelia is a cavitation in central areas of the spinal cord that results in damage to fibers conveying pain and thermal sensation as they cross the midline in the anterior white commissure. The loss is bilateral since fibers from both sides are damaged as they cross. Tabes dorsalis presents as posterior column deficits and lancinating pain; syringobulbia (cavitation within the brainstem) may have long tract signs and cranial nerve deficits; and PICA syndrome characteristically has alternating sensory losses (one side of face, opposite side of body). The Brown-Séquard syndrome has both sensory (anterolateral system and posterior column) and motor (corticospinal) deficits. (p. 180–181)

58. Answer **A:**   There are basically only two areas where a relatively restricted lesion would result in weakness of both lower extremities. One is in caudal parts of the pyramidal decussation (damage to decussating corticospinal fibers traveling to the lumbosacral cord levels), and the other would be a lesion in the falx cerebri (such as a meningioma) damaging the lower extremity areas on the somatomotor cortex bilaterally. Decussating fibers in the rostral part of the pyramidal decussation terminate in cervical levels of the spinal cord. Damage to either the pyramid or the lateral corticospinal tract would result in a hemiplegia (pyramid-contralateral, lateral corticospinal tract-ipsilateral). Damage to the pyramids bilaterally would result in quadriplegia. (p. 190–191)

59. Answer **C:**   The fatigability (progressive weakness), involvement of ocular muscles initially, followed by other muscle weakness, is characteristic of myasthenia gravis. Amyotrophic lateral sclerosis is an inherited disease that affects spinal and/or brainstem motor neurons and may result in upper or lower motor neuron symptoms; this disease is usually fatal within a few years. Multiple sclerosis is a demyelinating disease; Parkinson and Huntington diseases are neurodegenerative conditions that eventually have a dementia component. (p.190, 202)

60. Answer **C:**   The history and the combination of signs and symptoms seen in this woman indicate a probable diagnosis of myasthenia gravis and, consequently, a neurotransmitter disease at the neuromuscular junction. Damage to corticospinal and corticonuclear terminals and to synaptic contacts within the basal nuclei and the cerebellum would result in motor deficits but not in the pattern seen in this woman. (p. 190, 202)

61. Answer **A:**   The neurotransmitter at the neuromuscular junction is acetylcholine; a blockage of postsynaptic nicotinic acetylcholine receptors is the cause of the motor deficits characteristically seen in patients with myasthenia gravis. A loss of dopamine results in Parkinson disease, motor deficits that are not seen in this woman. Glutamate and GABA are found in many pathways involved in motor function but are not located at the neuromuscular junction. Serotonin is found in pathways related to the basal nuclei, raphe nuclei, and the hypothalamus. (p. 190, 202)

62. **Answer D:**   A lesion in the medial longitudinal fasciculus (MLF) on the right interrupts axons of the interneurons that arise from the left abducens nucleus and pass to oculomotor motor neurons on the right innervating the medial rectus muscle (internuclear ophthalmoplegia). Damage to the abducens nucleus will indeed destroy these interneurons, but will also result in an inability to abduct the eye on the ipsilateral side. Injury to the MLF on the left would result in an inability to adduct the left eye, and a lesion in the PPRF would most likely produce a bilateral horizontal gaze palsy. (p. 192–193, 200–201)

63. **Answer C:**   A fracture through the jugular foramen would potentially damage the glossopharyngeal (IX), vagus (X), and spinal accessory (XI) nerves. The major observable deficit would be a loss of the efferent limb of the gag reflex and a paralysis of the ipsilateral trapezius and sternocleidomastoid muscles (drooping of the shoulder, difficulty elevating the shoulder especially against resistance, difficulty turning the head to the contralateral side). Involvement of facial muscles would suggest damage to the internal acoustic or stylomastoid foramina; this would also be the case for the efferent limb of the corneal reflex. Diplopia and ptosis would suggest injury to the superior orbital fissure, as all three nerves controlling ocular movement traverse this space. The hypoglossal nerve (which supplies muscles of the tongue) passes through the hypoglossal canal. (p. 200–201)

64. **Answer E:**   The constellation of signs and symptoms experienced by this boy are characteristic of Wilson disease, also called hepatolenticular degeneration. These may include movement disorders, tremor, the Kayser-Fleischer ring at the corneoscleral margin, and eventual cirrhosis of the liver. Huntington and Parkinson diseases are predominately motor problems in the early stages and Pick disease is a degenerative disease of the cerebral cortex affecting mainly the frontal and temporal lobes; dementia is the primary deficit. Sydenham chorea is seen in children following an infection with hemolytic streptococcus; after treatment for the infection, the choreiform movements usually resolve. (p. 214–215)

65. **Answer A:**   A tumor impinging on the midline of the optic chiasm would damage crossing fibers from both eyes that are coming from the nasal retinae and would reflect a loss of all, or part of both temporal retinal fields. Between 60% and 70% of pituitary adenomas are prolactin-secreting tumors. Right or left homonymous hemianopsia (the nasal visual field of one eye and the temporal visual field of the other eye) are seen following lesions of, respectively, the left and right optic tracts. Quadrantanopsias result from lesions in the optic radiations. (p. 220–221)

66. **Answer C:**   The flocculonodular lobe and the fastigial nucleus receive input from the vestibular apparatus (primary vestibulocerebellar fibers) and from the vestibular nuclei (secondary vestibulocerebellar fibers). In turn, the Purkinje cells of the flocculonodular cortex and cells of the fastigial nucleus project to the vestibular nuclei as cerebellar corticovestibular and cerebellar efferent fibers, respectively. While other areas of the cerebellar cortex may have a small projection to the vestibular nuclei, this is not significant compared to that of the flocculonodular lobe. (p. 228–229)

67. **Answer B:**   Quadrantanopia, a loss of approximately one quarter (a quadrant) of the visual field, is seen in lesions in the optic radiations (geniculocalcarine radiations). The visual loss is in the visual field contralateral to the side of the lesion. Lesions in the lower portions of the radiations result in deficits in the contralateral superior quadrants, while lesions in the upper portions of the radiations result in deficits in the contralateral lower quadrants. Consequently, in this boy (with a superior right quadrantanopia), the lesion is in the lower portions of the optic radiations in the left temporal lobe (Meyer-Archambault loop). The lesion in the chiasm would result in a bitemporal hemianopsia. (p. 220–223)

68. **Answer E:**   Hemiballismus is the result of a lesion largely confined to the subthalamic nucleus on the side contralateral to the deficit. These movements are violent, flinging, unpredictable, and uncontrollable. The abnormal movements are contralateral to the lesion because the expression of the lesion is through the corticospinal tract. Lesions in the left subthalamic nucleus would result in a right-sided problem. Damage in the motor cortex would be seen as a contralateral weakness, and cell loss in the substantia nigra would result in motor deficits characteristic of Parkinson disease (resting tremor, bradykinesia, stooped posture, festinating gait). (p. 216–217)

69. **Answer B:**   The inability to perform a rapid alternating movement, such as pronating and supinating the hand on the knee, is dysdiadochokinesia. This is one of several cardinal signs of cerebellar disease or stroke. Dysmetria is an inability to judge power, distance, and accuracy during a movement, and dysarthria is difficulty speaking. A resting tremor is seen in diseases of the basal nuclei, and an intention tremor is seen in cerebellar lesions. (p. 208–211)

70. **Answer B:**   The tremor that worsens as this man attempts to bring his index finger to his nose is called an intention tremor, sometimes referred to as a kinetic tremor. This type of tremor is one cardinal sign of cerebellar lesions. A resting tremor is seen in diseases of the basal nuclei and a static tremor (postural tremor) is seen in the trunk and extremities in a static position. Dysmetria is an inability to judge distance, power, or accuracy during a movement. The rebound phenomenon is an inability of agonist and antagonist muscles to rapidly adapt to changes in load. (p. 208–211)

71. **Answer C:**   The signs and symptoms in this man clearly indicate a lesion in the cerebellum on the left side. The cerebellar nuclei on the left (lesion side) project to the contralateral thalamus (right) and from here to motor cortical areas (also right). The motor cortex projects, via the corticospinal tract and its decussation, back to the side of the body, excluding the head, on which the lesion is located (left cerebellum). The motor expression of the cerebellar deficit is through the corticospinal tract. The man's left-sided deficits are not consistent with a right cerebellar lesion, and the deficits are not consistent with a midbrain lesion. Lesions of the basal nuclei would result in a different set of motor disorders. (p. 208–211)

72. **Answer B:**   The superior cerebellar artery serves the cortex on the superior surface of the cerebellum and most of the cerebellar nuclei on the same side; in this case, it is the left artery. The anterior inferior cerebellar artery serves the cortex on the lateral inferior surface of the cerebellum and a small caudal tip of the dentate nucleus. A lesion that involves primarily the cerebellar cortex will not result in long-term deficits. A lesion that involves cortex plus nuclei or primarily nuclei, especially in an older patient (as in this

man), is likely to result in long-term deficits. The lenticulostriate arteries serve the basal nuclei. (p. 208–211)

73. Answer **A**: One cause of hemifacial spasm (intermittent and abnormal contractions of the facial muscles) is compression of the facial root by a loop of the anterior inferior cerebellar artery, or perhaps one of its larger branches. Aberrant loops of the superior cerebellar artery may compress the trigeminal root (trigeminal neuralgia), and the posterior inferior cerebellar artery serves the lateral medulla and medial regions of the cerebellum. The anterior and posterior spinal arteries serve areas of the medulla. (p. 202–203)

74. Answer **B**: The anterolateral system and the medial lemniscus are adjacent to each other in lateral portions of the midbrain and are served largely by the same vessel(s), these being penetrating branches of the quadrigeminal artery. This area may also receive some blood supply from the posterior choroidal arteries. Throughout the spinal cord, medulla, and into about the mid- to more rostral pons, these fiber bundles are spatially separated from each other and have separate blood supplies. (p. 137, 178–181)

75. Answer **B**: Fibers in the left medial lemniscus conveying position sense from the right upper extremity originate from cell bodies located in the right cuneate nucleus. These cuneate neurons give rise to axons that form the internal arcuate fibers that arch towards the midline, cross, and collect to form the contralateral medial lemniscus. The left cuneate nucleus sends axons to the right medial lemniscus, and the gracile nucleus (right or left) conveys information from the lower extremity. Posterior root ganglia neurons project to the gracile or cuneate nuclei. (p. 178–179)

76. Answer **E**: Dystonia is a movement disorder characterized by abnormal, sometimes intermittent, but frequently sustained, contractions of the muscles of the trunk and extremities that force the body into a twisted posture. Dystonia may be seen in patients with diseases of the basal nuclei. Dysmetria is the inability to judge the distance and trajectory of a movement. Dyspnea is difficulty breathing; this may result from heart and/or lung disorders as well as from neurologic disorders. Dysphagia is difficulty swallowing, and dysarthria is difficulty speaking. (p. 124–215)

77. Answer **E**: Transection of the optic nerve (on the left in this man) eliminates the afferent limb of the pupillary light reflex, but the efferent limb, via the oculomotor nerve, is intact. Consequently, there is a loss of both the direct response (in the blind eye) and the consensual response (in the good eye) when light is shined in the blind eye, because the afferent limb is eliminated and no input is getting to the center from which the efferent limb originates. On the other hand, light shined into the good eye (right in this man) results in a direct pupillary response (in the good eye) and a consensual pupillary response in the blind eye because the efferent limb of this reflex is not damaged for the blind eye. Other combinations of responses may occur as a result of lesions in other portions of the nervous system. (p. 220–221)

78. Answer **B**: In addition to the motor deficits characteristic of this disease, MRI would reveal a spongy degeneration (with cavitations) of the lenticular nucleus most noticeable in the putamen. There may also be a spongy degeneration in areas of the cerebral cortex. Atrophy of frontal and temporal lobe gyri is seen in Pick disease; loss of nigral cells is characteristic of Parkinson disease; and loss of the caudate nucleus (especially noticeable as absence of

its head) is seen in Huntington disease. Lacunae are usually seen in patients who have had small strokes. (p. 214–215)

79. Answer **D**: The inability of this man to control the distance, power, and accuracy of a movement is dysmetria; this is characteristically seen in cerebellar lesions. Dysphagia is difficulty swallowing, and dysarthria is difficulty speaking. The inability to perform rapid alternating movements is dysdiadochokinesia, and bradykinesia is a slowness to initiate movement. The latter is characteristic of individuals with disease of the basal nuclei. (p. 208–211)

80. Answer **A**: The territory served by the anterior choroidal artery includes the optic tract, inferior portions of the posterior limb of the internal capsule, thalamocortical radiations within the posterior limb, and structures in the temporal lobe. The left-sided deficits indicate a lesion on the right side. A lesion of the right optic tract results in a loss of vision in the opposite (left) visual fields; this being the temporal visual field of the left eye and the nasal visual field of the right eye (left homonymous hemianopsia). This constellation of deficits is known as the anterior choroidal artery syndrome. Quadrantanopia specifies a lesion in a portion of the optic radiations, and a nasal hemianopsia indicates a small lesion in the lateral aspect of the optic chiasm on one side. (p. 158–159, 220–223)

81. Answer **B**: This woman has sensory losses on the left side of her body and face that include pain/thermal sensations and the general category of proprioception (discriminative touch, vibratory and position sense); this is a hemianesthesia, a loss of sensation on one side of the body. This is a result of damage to thalamocortical fibers projecting from the ventral posteromedial and ventral posterolateral thalamic nuclei to the somatosensory cortex. Alternating hemianesthesia refers to a sensory loss on one side of the face and on the contralateral side of the body. A sensory level is a characteristic of lesions in the spinal cord, and paresthesia refers to an abnormal spontaneous sensation not a loss. A superior alternating hemiplegia is a motor deficit. (p. 158–159, 178–181, 220–223)

82. Answer **B**: The corticospinal fibers traversing the inferior portions of the posterior limb of the internal capsule are damaged by an occlusion of the anterior choroidal artery; a left-sided deficit correlates with a lesion on the right side, especially when taking into consideration the concurrent visual loss. Damage to corticospinal fibers on the left would result in a right-sided deficit. The somatomotor cortex is not involved in the lesion. While thalamocortical fibers are certainly damaged in this lesion, the deficits related to corticospinal fiber involvement predominate. (p. 190–191)

83. Answer **B**: Sensorineural hearing loss, also called nerve deafness, results from lesions or diseases that involve the cochlea or the cochlear portion of the vestibulocochlear nerve. Obstructions of the external ear or diseases of the middle ear result in conductive deafness (conductive hearing loss). Lesions in the inferior colliculus, auditory cortex, or other areas within the brain may result in difficulty localizing, interpreting, or understanding sound but do not result in total deafness in one ear. (p. 226–227)

84. Answer **C**: Laminae 1, 4, and 6 receive input from the ganglion cells in the contralateral retina. Laminae 2, 3, and 5 receive an ipsilateral input; laminae 1 and 2 are the magnocellular layers of the

lateral geniculate nucleus; and laminae 3, 4, 5, and 6 are its parvocellular layers. (p. 222)

85. Answer **D**:   Sydenham chorea is a disease of childhood thought to be an autoimmune disorder seen in children as a sequel to a hemolytic streptococcus infection. In most children the disease is self-limiting and the patient recovers with no permanent deficits. Huntington disease, Parkinson disease, and senile chorea present with motor deficits that partially resemble those seen in this girl but these are diseases of adults or the elderly. Weber syndrome (a superior alternating hemiplegia) is a motor deficit involving the oculomotor nerve on one side and the corticospinal tract on the opposite side. (p. 214–215)

Review and Study Questions for Chapter 8

1. Which of the following arteries is generally found in the area of the cingulate sulcus and has branches that serve the lower extremity areas of the somatomotor and somatosensory cortex?

   - ○ (A)   Callosomarginal
   - ○ (B)   Frontopolar
   - ○ (C)   Internal parietal
   - ○ (D)   Parietooccipital
   - ○ (E)   Pericallosal

2. A 44-year-old woman presents to her family physician with intermittent headache and the complaint that she can't see in her left eye. The examination reveals that the woman is blind in her left eye. When a light is shined into her left eye there is no direct or consensual pupillary light reflex. Magnetic resonance angiography (MRA) shows a large aneurysm at the origin of the ophthalmic artery. Which of the following represents the usual point of origin of this vessel?

   - ○ (A)   Cavernous part of the internal carotid artery
   - ○ (B)   Cerebral part of the internal carotid artery
   - ○ (C)   First segment (A1) of the anterior cerebral artery
   - ○ (D)   First segment (M1) of the middle cerebral artery
   - ○ (E)   Petrous part of the internal carotid artery

3. The venous phase of an angiogram of a 52-year-old man suggests a small tumor at what the neuroradiologist refers to as the venous angle. Which of the following points most specifically describes the position of the venous angle?

   - ○ (A)   Where the internal cerebral vein meets the great cerebral vein
   - ○ (B)   Where the superficial middle cerebral vein meets the cavernous sinus
   - ○ (C)   Where the thalamostriate vein turns to form the internal cerebral vein
   - ○ (D)   Where the transverse sinus turns to form the sigmoid sinus
   - ○ (E)   Where the vein of Labbé meets the vein of Trolard

4. The superficial middle cerebral vein forms a direct anastomotic junction with which of the following venous structures on the lateral aspect of the cerebral hemisphere?

   - ○ (A)   Cavernous sinus
   - ○ (B)   Confluence of sinuses
   - ○ (C)   Superior sagittal sinus
   - ○ (D)   Transverse sinus
   - ○ (E)   Veins of Labbé and Trolard

5. The coronal MRI of a 69-year-old man reveals an infarcted area in the region of the cerebral hemisphere lateral to the internal capsule but internal to the insular cortex. A comparison of coronal and sagittal MRI suggests that the vessels involved are branches of the middle cerebral artery. Which of the following branches or segments of the middle cerebral artery are most likely involved in this man?

   - ○ (A)   Anterior and polar temporal branches
   - ○ (B)   Insular branches
   - ○ (C)   Lenticulostriate branches
   - ○ (D)   Opercular segment
   - ○ (E)   Uncal artery

6. The anterior and middle cerebral arteries are the terminal branches of which of the following vascular trunks?

   - ○ (A)   Basilar artery
   - ○ (B)   Cavernous part of the internal carotid
   - ○ (C)   Cerebral part of the internal carotid
   - ○ (D)   External carotid artery
   - ○ (E)   Petrous part of the internal carotid

7. The superior sagittal sinus, straight sinus, and transverse sinuses converge at which of the following landmarks?

   - ○ (A)   Clivus
   - ○ (B)   Confluens sinuum
   - ○ (C)   Great cerebral vein
   - ○ (D)   Jugular foramen
   - ○ (E)   Venous angle

8. A 47-year-old woman is brought to the emergency department by her husband. She has a severe headache, nausea, and is somnolent. The examination reveals that the woman is hypertensive and has papilledema. MRI shows evidence of cerebral edema, bilateral infarcted areas in the thalamus, and a large sinus thrombosis that is blocking the egress of blood through the vascular system. This thrombus is most likely located in which of the following venous structures?

   - ○ (A)   Inferior sagittal sinus
   - ○ (B)   Left sigmoid sinus
   - ○ (C)   Right transverse sinus
   - ○ (D)   Straight sinus
   - ○ (E)   Superior sagittal sinus

9. A 39-year-old man presents to his family physician with a complaint of difficulty swallowing. The history reveals that the man has had severe recurring headaches over the last 5 days and suffered several bouts of vomiting. The examination confirms the difficulty swallowing, and reveals that the man's voice is hoarse and gravely, and that he is unable to elevate his left shoulder against resistance. MRI shows a dural sinus thrombosis. Based on this man's deficits, which of the following represents the most likely location of this thrombus?

   ○ (A) Left cavernous sinus
   ○ (B) Left jugular bulb
   ○ (C) Left transverse sinus
   ○ (D) Right jugular bulb
   ○ (E) Straight sinus

10. Which of the following vessels forms a characteristic loop in the cisterna magna that is prominent on lateral angiograms and, in the process, supplies blood to the choroid plexus of the fourth ventricle?

   ○ (A) Anterior inferior cerebellar artery
   ○ (B) Posterior inferior cerebellar artery
   ○ (C) Posterior spinal artery
   ○ (D) Superior cerebellar artery
   ○ (E) Vertebral artery

11. The MRI of a 42-year-old man shows a small tumor in the choroid plexus of the third ventricle. Angiogram and MRA suggest that this tumor contains numerous vascular loops. Which of the following represents the blood supply to this portion of the choroid plexus?

   ○ (A) Anterior choroidal artery
   ○ (B) Choroidal branches of AICA
   ○ (C) Choroidal branches of PICA
   ○ (D) Lateral posterior choroidal artery
   ○ (E) Medial posterior choroidal artery

12. The angiogram of a 56-year-old woman shows an aneurysm originating from the lateral aspect of the basilar bifurcation and extending into the space between the posterior cerebral and superior cerebellar arteries. Based on the structure(s) located at this point, which of the following deficits would most likely be seen in this woman?

   ○ (A) Constriction of the ipsilateral pupil
   ○ (B) Inability to look down and out with the ipsilateral eye
   ○ (C) Inability to look laterally with the ipsilateral eye
   ○ (D) Inability to look up, down, or medially with the ipsilateral eye
   ○ (E) Loss of pain and thermal sensation from the ipsilateral side of the face

13. The position of the posterior communicating artery, as frequently seen in MRA, is an important landmark that specifies the intersection of which of the following?

   ○ (A) A1 and A2 segments
   ○ (B) M1 and M2 segments
   ○ (C) M2 and M3 segments
   ○ (D) P1 and P2 segments
   ○ (E) P2 and P3 segments

14. A 16-year-old boy with developmental delay has been followed since birth by a pediatric neurologist. A recent MRA is done in which major arteries and venous sinuses are visualized. It is concluded that the pattern of the boy's venous sinuses is essentially normal. Which of the following describes the usual pattern of the superior sagittal sinus at the confluence of sinuses?

   ○ (A) Always drains equally into the right and left transverse sinuses
   ○ (B) Always drains into the left transverse sinus
   ○ (C) Always drains into the right transverse sinus
   ○ (D) Usually drains into the left transverse sinus
   ○ (E) Usually drains into the right transverse sinus

Answers for Chapter 8

1. Answer **A**:   The callosomarginal artery lies generally in the region of the cingulate sulcus and gives rise to branches (paracentral branches) that distribute to the anterior and posterior paracentral gyri. The pericallosal artery is located immediately superior to the corpus callosum and the frontopolar artery serves the medial aspect of the frontal lobe. The internal parietal arteries are the terminal branches of the pericallosal artery; these vessels distribute to the medial portion of the parietal lobe, the precuneus. The parietooccipital artery is one of the terminal branches (part of P4) of the posterior cerebral artery. (p. 29, 240)

2. Answer **B**:   In most instances (approximately 80–85%), the ophthalmic artery originates from the cerebral portion of the internal carotid artery just as this parent vessel leaves the cavernous sinus and passes through the dura. In a small percentage of cases the ophthalmic artery may originate from other locations on the internal carotid artery, including its cavernous portion. This vessel does not originate from the petrous portion of the internal carotid or from anterior or middle cerebral arteries. (p. 25, 240)

3. Answer **C**:   The point at which the thalamostriate vein (also called the superior thalamostriate vein at this position) abruptly turns 180° to form the internal cerebral vein is called the venous angle. This angle is located immediately caudal to the position of the interventricular foramen and is, therefore, an important landmark. The thalamostriate vein is located in the groove between the thalamus and the caudate nucleus. At the superior aspect of the thalamus, this vein is the superior thalamostriate vein, and, on the inferior surface, it is called the inferior thalamostriate vein. None of the other choices is involved in the formation of the venous angle. (p. 241)

4. Answer **E**:   The superficial middle cerebral vein is a comparatively obvious venous structure on the lateral surface of the hemisphere that communicates directly with the veins of Trolard (to the superior sagittal sinus) and Labbé (to the transverse sinus). The superficial middle cerebral vein also communicates with the cavernous sinus, but this sinus in not on the lateral aspect of the hemisphere as specified in the question. The other choices do not receive venous blood directly from the superficial middle cerebral vein. (p. 19, 241)

5. Answer **C**:   The position of this lesion is in that portion of the hemisphere occupied by the lenticular nucleus; the lenticulostri-

ate branches of the M1 segment of the middle cerebral artery serve this structure. The uncal, anterior, and polar temporal branches originate from the M1 segment but do not serve structures in the area of the hemisphere described. Insular branches (M2) and opercular branches (M3) serve cortical structures. (p. 25, 242)

6. Answer **C**:   As the internal carotid artery exits the cavernous sinus, it becomes the cerebral part of the internal carotid and, after giving rise to three important small branches (ophthalmic, anterior choroidal, posterior communicating), bifurcates into the anterior and middle cerebral arteries. These two cerebral vessels are the terminal branches of the cerebral part of the internal carotid artery. In approximately 70–75% of specimens, the anterior cerebral artery is the smaller of these two terminal branches. None of the other choices gives rise to the anterior and middle cerebral arteries. (p. 242)

7. Answer **B**:   The superior sagittal sinus, straight sinus, the two transverse, and the occipital sinus (when present) converge at the confluence of sinuses (confluens sinuum), which is located internal to the external occipital protuberance. The venous angle is the junction of the thalamostriate and the internal cerebral veins, and the great cerebral vein (of Galen) receives the internal cerebral veins and several smaller veins including the basal vein (of Rosenthal) and empties into the straight sinus. The jugular foramen contains the transition from the sigmoid sinus to the internal jugular vein and the terminus of the inferior petrosal sinus. The clivus is composed mainly of the basal part of the occipital bone; this is the location of the basilar plexus. (p. 19. 23, 243–245)

8. Answer **D**:   A key observation in this woman is the bilateral infarcted areas in the thalamus. The straight sinus receives venous flow from both internal cerebral veins; a blockage of flow through the straight sinus would adversely affect both thalami. Such a lesion would also cause potential damage to the medial temporal lobe due to the disruption of flow through the basal vein (of Rosenthal). None of the other choices receives venous drainage directly from the thalamus. (p. 29, 248, 250)

9. Answer **B**:   The deficits experienced by this man (difficulty swallowing, hoarseness, inability to elevate the left shoulder against resistance) point to damage to the glossopharyngeal (IXth), vagus (Xth), and spinal accessory (XIth) nerves or to their roots. All three of these cranial nerves exit the jugular foramen along with the continuity of the sigmoid sinus with the internal jugular vein (jugular bulb or bulb of the jugular vein). In this case, the venous thrombosis is at the left jugular bulb and impinging on these three cranial nerve roots. Dural sinus thrombosis of the other choices

may cause certain deficits, but not those experienced by this man. (p. 244, 250)

10. Answer **B**:   The posterior inferior cerebellar artery (commonly called PICA) originates from the vertebral artery, courses around the lateral aspect of the medulla, loops sharply into the space of the cisterna magna (giving off small branches to the choroid plexus in the fourth ventricle), then joins the inferior and medial surface of the cerebellum. None of the other choices forms prominent vascular structures in the cisterna magna or serves the choroid plexus of the fourth ventricle. (p. 246)

11. Answer **E**:   The medial posterior choroidal artery originates from the P2 segment of the posterior cerebral artery, arches around the midbrain, and enters the caudal end of the third ventricle. The anterior choroidal artery serves the choroid plexus in the temporal horn, and the lateral posterior choroidal artery serves the glomus choroideum and extends into the plexi of the temporal horn and the body of the ventricle. These patterns may be somewhat variable. Choroidal branches of anterior inferior cerebellar artery (AICA) serve the choroid plexus extending through the foramen of Luschka, and these branches from the posterior inferior cerebellar artery (PICA) serve the plexus within the fourth ventricle. (p. 251)

12. Answer **D**:   The oculomotor nerve (III) is located between the posterior cerebral and superior cerebellar arteries and may be damaged by aneurysms at this location. Most eye movement would be lost (the trochlear (IV) and abducens (VI) nerves are intact) and the ipsilateral pupil would be dilated, not constricted. Sensation from the face is carried on the trigeminal nerve. Movement deficits related to injury to the IVth nerve (looking down and out) or the VIth nerve (looking laterally) are not affected. (p. 39, 40, 247, 252)

13. Answer **D**:   The posterior communicating artery originates from the cerebral part of the internal carotid artery and courses caudally to join the posterior cerebral artery (PCA). The part of the PCA medial to this intersection is the P1 segment and the part of the PCA immediately lateral to this junction is the P2 segment. Important branches arise from both of these parts of the PCA. None of the other choices have any direct relationship to the points of origin of the posterior communicating artery. (p. 25, 247, 249)

14. Answer **E**:   The drainage pattern of the superior sagittal sinus at the confluence of sinuses is variable, including about equal to both transverse sinuses or mainly to the right or to the left. However, the usual pattern is for the superior sagittal sinus to drain predominately into the right transverse sinus. (p. 245)

Sources and Suggested Readings

AbuRahma A, Bergan JJ. Noninvasive Vascular Diagnosis. London: Springer-Verlag, 2000.

Afifi AK, Bergman RA. Functional Neuroanatomy, Text and Atlas. New York: McGraw-Hill, 1998.

Airaksinen MS, Panula P. The histaminergic system in the guinea pig central nervous system: An immunocytochemical mapping study using an antiserum against histamine. J Comp Neurol 1988;273:163–186.

Airaksinen MS, Flugge G, Fuchs E, Panula P. Histaminergic system in the tree shrew brain. J Comp Neurol 1989;286:289–310.

Aminoff MJ, Greenberg DA, Simon RP. Clincial Neurology, 3rd ed. Stanford, CT: Appleton & Lange, 1996.

Anderson KD, Reiner A. Extensive co-occurrence of substance P and dynorphin in striatal projection neurons: An evolutionarily conserved feature of basal ganglia organization. J Comp Neurol 1990; 295:339–369.

Angevine JB, Mancall EL, Yakovlev PI. The Human Cerebellum: An Atlas of Gross Topography in Serial Sections. Boston: Little, Brown, 1961.

Beckstead RM, Morse JR, Norgren R. The nucleus of the solitary tract in the monkey: Projections to the thalamus and brain stem nuclei. J Comp Neurol 1980;190:259–282.

Benarroch EE, Westmoreland BF, Daube JR, Reagan TJ, Sandok BA. Medical Neuroscience, An Approach to Anatomy, Pathology, and Physiology by Systems and Levels, 4th Ed. Baltimore: Lippincott Williams & Wilkins, 1999.

Bishop GA, Ho RH, King JS. Localization of immunoreactivity in the opossum cerebellum. J Comp Neurol 1985;235:301–321.

Bobillier P, Seguin S, Petitjean F, Salvert D, Touret M, Jouvert M. The raphe nuclei of the cat brainstem: A topographical atlas of their efferent projections as revealed by autoradiography. Brain Res 1976; 113:449–486.

Brodal A. Neurological Anatomy in Relation to Clinical Medicine, 3rd ed. New York: Oxford University Press, 1981.

Brodal P. The Central Nervous System: Structure and Function. 2nd ed. New York: Oxford University Press, 1998.

Broman J, Blomqvist A. Substance P-like immunoreactivity in the lateral cervical nucleus of the owl monkey (Aotus trivirgatus): A comparison with the cat and rat. J Comp Neurol 1989;289:111–117.

Broman J, Westman J, Ottersen OP. Spinocervical tract terminals are enriched in glutamate-like immunoreactivity: An anterograde transport-quantitative immunogold study in the cat. Neurosci Abstr 1989;15:941.

Brown AG. Organization in the Spinal Cord. Berlin: Springer-Verlag, 1981.

Buisseret-Delmas C, Batini C, Compoint C, Daniel H, Menetrey D. The GABAergic neurones of the cerebellar nuclei: Projection to the caudal inferior olive and to the bulbar reticular formation. In: P Strata (ed). The Olivocerebellar System in Motor Control. (also Exp Brain Res Ser 17:108–110). New York: Springer-Verlag, 1989.

Burt AM. Textbook of Neuroanatomy. Philadelphia: WB Saunders Co, 1993.

Cassini P, Ho RH, Martin GF. The brainstem origin of enkephalin- and substance-P-like immunoreactive axons in the spinal cord of the North American opossum. Brain Behav Evol 1989;34:212–222.

Clemente CD. Anatomy: A Regional Atlas of the Human Body, 3rd ed. Baltimore: Urban & Schwarzenberg, 1987.

Council of Biology Editions Style Manual Committee. Scientific Style and Format—The CBE Manual for Authors, Editors, and Publishers, 6th Ed. Cambridge: Cambridge University Press, 1994.

Craig AD, Jr, Sailer S, Kniffki K-D. Organization of anterogradely labeled spinocervical tract terminations in the lateral cervical nucleus of the cat. J Comp Neurol 1987;263:214–222.

Craig AD, Jr, Tapper DN. Lateral cervical nucleus in the cat: Functional organization and characteristics. J Neurophysiol 1978;41:1511–1534.

Crosby EC, Humphrey T, Lauer EW. Correlative Anatomy of the Nervous System. New York: Macmillan, 1962.

DeArmond SJ, Fusco MM, Dewev MM. Structure of the Human Brain: A Photographic Atlas, 3rd ed. New York: Oxford University Press, 1989.

deGroot J. Correlative Neuroanatomy of Computed Tomography and Magnetic Resonance Imaging. Philadelphia: Lea & Febiger, 1984.

DeLacalle S, Hersh LB, Saper CB. Cholinergic innervation of the human cerebellum. J Comp Neurol 1993;328:364–376.

Dietrichs E, Haines DE. Interconnections between hypothalamus and cerebellum. Anat Embryol 1989;179:207–220.

Donaghy M. Neurology. New York: Oxford, 1997.

Dublin AB, Dublin WB. Atlas of Neuroanatomy with Radiologic Correlation and Pathologic Illustration. St. Louis: Warren H. Green Inc., 1982.

Duus P. Topical Diagnosis in Neurology: Anatomy, Physiology, Signs, Symptons, 2nd ed. Stuttgart: Georg Thieme Verlag, 1989.

Duvernoy HM. The Human Brain Stem and Cerebellum, Surface, Structure, Vascularization, and Three-Dimensional Sectional Anatomy with MRI. Wein: Springer-Verlag, 1995.

England MA, Wakely J. Color Atlas of the Brain and Spinal Cord. St. Louis: Mosby Year Book, 1991.

Federative Committee on Anatomical Terminology. Terminologia Anatomica. Stuttgart and New York: Thieme, 1998.

Fischer HW, Ketonen L. Radiographic Neuroanatomy: A Working Atlas. New York: McGraw-Hill, 1991.

Fix JD. Atlas of the Human Brain and Spinal Cord. Rockville, MD: Aspen Publishers, 1987.

Gasser RF. Personal communication, 1989.

Gasser RF. Atlas of Human Embryos. New York: Harper & Row, 1975.

Giesler GJ, Jr, Bjorkeland M, Xu Q, Grant G. Organization of the spinocervicothalamic pathway in the rat. J Comp Neurol 1989;268: 223–233.

Gilman S, Winans SS. Manter and Gatz's Essentials of Clinical Neuroanatomy and Neurophysiology, 10th ed. Philadelphia: FA Davis Company, 2003.

Giuffrida R, Rustioni A. Glutamate and aspartate immunoreactivity in corticospinal neurons of rats. J Comp Neurol 1989;288:154–164.

Gluhbegovic N, Williams TH. The Human Brain: A Photographic Guide. Hagerstown, MD: Harper & Row, 1980.

Greenberg MS. Handbook of Neurosurgery, 5th Ed. New York: Thieme, 2001.

Groenewegen HJ, Berendse HW. Connections of the subthalamic nucleus with ventral striatopallidal parts of the basal ganglia in the rat. J Comp Neurol 1990;294:607–622.

Haines DE (ed). Fundamental Neuroscience, 2nd Edition. Philadelphia: Churchill Livingstone/Elsevier Science, 2002.

Haines DE, Dietrichs E. On the organization of interconnections between the cerebellum and hypothalamus. In: JS King (ed), New Concepts in Cerebellar Neurobiology, pp. 113–149. New York: Alan R. Liss, 1987.

Haines DE, May PJ, Dietrichs E. Neuronal connections between the cerebellar nuclei and hypothalamus in Macaca fascicularis: Cerebellovisceral circuits. J Comp Neurol 1990;299:106–122.

Hamilton WJ, Mossman HW. Human Embryology, 4th ed. Baltimore: Williams & Wilkins, 1972.

Heimer L. The Human Brain and Spinal Cord: Functional Neuroanatomy and Dissection Guide. New York: Springer-Verlag, 1995.

Herbert H, Saper CB. Cholecystokinin-, galamin-, and corticotropin-releasing factor-like immunoreactive projections from the nucleus of the solitary tract to the parabrachial nucleus in the rat. J Comp Neurol 1990;293:581–598.

Huang X-F, Törk I, Paxinos G. Dorsal motor nucleus of the vagus nerve: A cyto-and chemoarchitectonic study in the human. J Comp Neurol 1993;330:158–182.

Iverson MA et al. American Medical Association Manual of Style—A Guide for Authors and Editors, 9th Ed. Baltimore: Williams & Wilkins, 1998.

Jackson GD, Duncan JS. MRI Neuroanatomy: A New Angle on the Brain. New York: Churchill Livingstone, 1996.

Jennes L, Traurig HH, Conn PM. Atlas of the Human Brain. Philadelphia: JB Lippincott Co, 1995.

Jones SL, Light AR. Serotoninergic medullary raphespinal projection to the lumbar spinal cord in the rat: A retrograde immunohistochemical study. J Comp Neurol 1992;322:599–610.

Kandel ER, Schwartz JH, Jessell TM. Principles of Neural Sciences, 4th ed. McGraw-Hill: New York, 2000.

Keirman JA. Barr's The Human Nervous System: An Anatomical Viewpoint, 7th Ed. Philadelphia: Lippincott-Raven, 1998.

Kirkwood JR. Essentials of Neuroimaging. New York: Churchill Livingstone, 1990.

Krammer EB, Lischka MF, Egger TP, Reidl M, Gruber H. The motoneuronal organization of the spinal accessory nuclear complex. Adv Anat Embryol Cell Biol 1987;103:1–62.

Kretschmann H-J, Weinrich W. Cranial Neuroimaging and Clinical Neuroanatomy: Magnetic Resonance Imaging and Computed Tomography, 2nd ed. New York: Georg Thieme Verlag, 1993.

Larsell O, Jansen, J. The Comparative Anatomy and Histology of the Cerebellum: The Human Cerebellum, Cerebellar Connections, and Cerebellar Cortex. Minneapolis: University of Minnesota Press, 1972.

Leah J, Menetrey D, dePommery J. Neuropeptides in long ascending spinal tract cells in the rat: Evidence for parallel processing of ascending information. Neuroscience 1988;24:195–207.

Leblanc A. The Cranial Nerves: Anatomy Imaging Vascularization, 2nd ed. Berlin: Springer-Verlag, 1995.

Lechtenberg R. Synopsis of Neurology. Philadelphia: Lea & Febiger, 1991.

Lehéricy S, Hirsch EC, Cervera-Pierot P, Hersh LB, Bakchine S, Piette F, Duyckaerts C, Hauw J-J , Javoy-Agid F, Agid Y. Heterogeneity and selectivity of the degeneration of cholinergic neurons in the basal forebrain of patients with Alzheimer's disease. J Comp Neurol 1993;330:15–31.

Ljungdahl A, Hökfelt T, Nilsson G. Distribution of substance P-like immunoreactivity in the central nervous system of the rat I cell bodies and nerve terminals. Neuroscience 1978;3:861–943.

Lilly R, Cummings JL, Benson DF, Frankel M. The human Klüver-Bucy syndrome. Neurology 33:1141–1145, 1983.

Lu GW. Spinocervical tract-dorsal column postsynaptic neurons: A double-projection neuronal system. Somatosens Mot Res 1989;6: 445–454.

Lufkin R, Flannigan BD, Bentson IR, Wilson GH, Rauschning W, Hanafee W. Magnetic resonance imaging of the brainstem and cranial nerves. Surgical and Radiologic Anatomy 1986;8:49–66.

Magnusson KR, Clements JR, Larson AA, Madl JE, Beitz AJ. Localization of glutamate in trigeminothalamic projection neurons: A combined retrograde transport-immunohistochemical study. Somatosens Res 1987;4:177–190.

Mai J, Assheurer J, Paxinos G. Atlas of the Human Brain. New York: Academic Press, 1997.

Martin JH. Neuroanatomy: Text and Atlas, 2nd ed. Stanford, CT: Appleton & Lange, 1996.

Martin TJ, Corbett JJ. Neuro-Ophthalmology: The Requisites of Ophthalmology. St. Louis: Mosby, 2000.

McKusick VA. On the naming of clinical disorders, with particular reference to eponyms. Medicine 77:1–2 (1998a).

McKusick VA. Mendelian Inheritance in Man: A Catalog of Human Genes and Genetic Disorders. 12th edition. Baltimore: Johns Hopkins University Press, 1998b.

Mihailoff GA. Cerebellar nuclear projections from the basilar pontine nuclei and nucleus reticularis tegmenti pontis as demonstrated with PHA-L tracing in the rat. J Comp Neurol 1993;330:130–146.

Miller RA, Burack E. Atlas of the Central Nervous System in Man, 3rd ed. Baltimore: Williams & Wilkins, 1982.

Monaghan PL, Beitz AJ, Larson AA, Altschuler RA, Madl JE, Mullett MA. Immunocytochemical localization of glutamate-, glutaminase- and aspartate aminotransferase-like immunoreactivity in the rat deep cerebellar nuclei. Brain Res 1986;363:364–370.

Montemurro DG, Bruni JE. The Human Brain in Dissection, 2nd ed. New York: Oxford University Press, 1988.

Nahin RL. Immunocytochemical identification of long ascending, peptidergic lumbar spinal neurons terminating in either the medial or lateral thalamus in the rat. Brain Res 1988;443:345–349.

Nelson BJ, Mugnaini E. Origins of GABAergic inputs to the inferior olive. In: P Strata (ed), The Olivocerebellar System in Motor Control. (also Exp Brain Res Ser 17:86–107). New York: Springer-Verlag, 1989.

Newman DB, Hilleary SK, Ginsberg CY. Nuclear terminations of corticoreticular fiber systems in rats. Brain Behav Evol 1989;34:223–264.

Nicholls JG, Martin AR, Wallace BG. From Neuron to Brain, 3rd ed. Sunderland, MA: Sinauer Associates, Inc, 1992.

Nieuwenhuys R. Chemoarchitecture of the Brain. Berlin: Springer-Verlag, 1985.

Nieuwenhuys R, Voogd J, van Huijzen C. The Central Nervous System: A Synopsis and Atlas, 3rd ed. Berlin: Springer-Verlag, 1988.

Noback CR, Strominger NL, Demarest RJ. The Human Nervous System, Structure and Function, 5th ed. Baltimore: Williams & Wilkins, 1996.

Nolte J. The Human Brain: An Introduction to its Functional Anatomy, 5th ed. St. Louis: CV Mosby, 2002.

Nolte J, Angevine JB. The Human Brain in Photographs and Diagrams. St. Louis: CV Mosby, 1995.

Nudo RJ, Sutherland DP, Masterton RB. Inter- and intra-laminar distribution of tectospinal neurons in 23 mammals. Brain Behav Evol 1993;42:1–23.

Olszewski J, Baxter D. Cytoarchitecture of the Human Brain Stem, 2nd ed. Basel: S. Karger, 1982.

Pansky B, Allen DJ, Budd GC. Review of Neuroscience, 2nd ed. New York: Macmillan Publishing Company, 1988.

Parent A. Carpenters Human Neuroanatomy, 9th ed. Baltimore: Williams & Wilkins, 1996.

Parent A, DeBellefeuille L. The pallidointralaminar and pallidonigral projections in primate as studied by retrograde double-labeling method. Brain Res 1983;278:11–27.

Platzer W (ed). Pernkopf Atlas of Topographic and Applied Human Anatomy, 3rd ed. Volume I, Head and Neck. Baltimore: Urban & Schwarzenberg, 1989.

Poritsky R. Neuroanatomical Pathways. Philadelphia: WB Saunders Co, 1984.

Rasmussen AT. Atlas of Cross Section Anatomy of the Brain: Guide to the Study of the Morphology and Fiber Tracts of the Human Brain. New York: Blakiston Division, McGraw-Hill Book Company, Inc, 1951.

Reddy VK, Cassini P, Ho RH, Martin GF. Origins and terminations of bulbospinal axons that contain serotonin and either enkephalin or substance P in the North American opossum. J Comp Neurol 1990;294:96–108.

Reddy VK, Fung SJ, Zhuo H, Barnes CD. Localization of enkephalinergic neurons in the dorsolateral pontine tegmentum projecting to the spinal cord of the cat. J Comp Neurol 1990;291:195–202.

Rhoton AL, Jr. The posterior cranial fossa: Microsurgical anatomy and surgical approaches. Neurosurgery 2000; 47 (Supplement); S7–S297.

Rhoton AL, Jr. The supratentorial cranial space: Microsurgical anatomy and surgical approaches. Neurosurgery 2002; 51 (Supplement); S1–S410.

Rosenberg RN. Neurology, Volume 5 of The Science and Practice of Clinical Medicine, JM Dietschy, Editor-in-Chief. New York: Grune & Stratton, 1980.

Rowland LP (ed.). Merritt's Textbook of Neurology, 10th ed. Baltimore: Lippincott Williams & Wilkins, 2000.

Rustioni A. Non-primary afferents to the nucleus gracilis from the lumbar cord of the cat. Brain Res 1973;51:81–95.

Rustioni A. Non-primary afferents to the cuneate nucleus in the brachial dorsal funiculus of the cat. Brain Res 1974;75:247–259.

Rustioni A, Kaufman AB. Identification of cells of origin of non-primary afferents to the dorsal column nuclei of the cat. Exp Brain Res 1977;27:1–14.

Salt TE, Hill RG. Neurotransmitter candidates of somatosensory primary afferent fibres. Neuroscience 1983;10:1083–1103.

Schnitzlein HN, Hartley EW, Murtagh FR, Grundy L, Fargher JT. Computed Tomography of the Head and Spine: A Photographic Color Atlas of CT, Gross, and Microscopic Anatomy. Baltimore: Urban & Schwarzenberg, 1983.

Schnitzlein HN, Murtagh FR. Imaging Anatomy of the Head and Spine: A Photographic Color Atlas of MRI, CT, Gross, and Microscopic Anatomy in Axial, Coronal, and Sagittal Planes, 2nd ed. Baltimore: Urban & Schwarzenberg, 1990.

Schwedtfeger WK, Buhl EH, Germroth P. Disynaptic olfactory input to the hippocampus mediated by stellate cells in the entorhinal cortex. J Comp Neurol 1990;292:163–177.

Shepherd GM. Neurobiology, 3rd ed. New York: Oxford University Press, 1994.

Siegel G, Agranoff BW, Albers RW, Molinoff PB. Basic Neurochemistry, Molecular, Cellular, and Medical Aspects, 6th ed. Philadelphia: Lippincott-Raven, 1999.

Singer M, Yakovlev PI. The Human Brain in Sagittal Section. Springfield, IL: Charles C Thomas, 1964.

Smith CG. Serial Dissections of the Human Brain. Baltimore: Urban & Schwarzenberg, 1981.

Smith Y, Bolam JP. The output neurones and the dopaminergic neurones of the substantia nigra receive a GABA-containing input from the globus pallidus in the rat. J Comp Neurol 1990;296:47–64.

Smith Y, Hazrati L-N, Parent A. Efferent projections of the subthalamic nucleus in the squirrel monkey as studied by the PHA-L anterograde tracing method. J Comp Neurol 1990;294:306–323.

Strata P (ed). The Olivocerebellar System in Motor Control. Berlin: Springer-Verlag, 1989.

Sugiura K, Robinson GA, Stuart DG. Illustrated Guide to the Central Nervous System. St. Louis: Ishiyaku EuroAmerica, Inc, 1989.

Swash M, Oxburgy J (eds). Clinical Neurology, volumes 1 and 2. New York: Churchill Livingstone, 1991.

Tatu L, Moulin T, Bogousslavsky J, Duvernoy H. Arterial territories of human brain: Brainstem and cerebellum. Neurology 1996;47:1125–1135.

Terzian H, Ore GD. Syndrome of Klüver and Bucy reproduced in man by bilateral removal of the temporal lobes. Neurology 1955;5:373–380.

Tieman SB, Butler K, Neale JH. N-acetylaspartylglutamate: A neuropeptide in the human visual system. JAMA 1988;259:2020.

Victor M, Ropper AH. Adams and Victor's Principles of Neurology, 7th Ed. New York: McGraw-Hill, 2001.

Walker JJ, Bishop GA, Ho RH, King JS. Brainstem origin of serotonin- and enkephalin-immunoreactive afferents to the opossum's cerebellum. J Comp Neurol 1988;276:481–497.

Walton L. Essentials of Neurology, 6th ed. New York: Churchill Livingstone, 1989.

Watson C. Basic Human Neuroanatomy: An Introductory Atlas, 5th ed. Boston: Little, Brown, 1995.

Waxman SG, deGroot J. Correlative Neuroanatomy, 22nd ed. Norwalk, CT: Appleton & Lange, 1995.

Westlund KN, Carlton SM, Zhang D, Willis WD. Glutamate-immunoreactive terminals synapse on primate spinothalamic tract cells. J Comp Neurol 1992;322:519–527.

Wicke L. Atlas of Radiologic Anatomy, 3rd ed. Baltimore: Urban & Schwarzenberg, 1982.

Willard FH. Medical Neuroanatomy: A Problem-Oriented Manual with Annotated Atlas. Philadelphia: JB Lippincott Co, 1993.

Willis WD, Jr. The Pain System: The Neural Basis of Nociceptive Transmission in the Mammalian Nervous System, Volume 8, Pain and Headache. Basel: S Karger, 1985.

Willis WD, Grossman RG. Medical Neurobiology: Neuroanatomical and Neurophysiological Principles Basic to Clinical Neuroscience, 3rd ed. St. Louis: CV Mosby, 1981.

Witelson SF, Kigas DL. Sylvian fissure morphology and asymmetry in men and women: Bilateral differences in relation to handedness in men. J Comp Neurol 1992;323:326–340.

Woolsey TA, Hanaway J, Gado MH: The Brain Atlas: A Visual Guide to the Human Central Nervous System, 2nd Ed. Hoboken: Wiley, 2003.

Yasargil MG. Microneurosurgery I Microsurgical Anatomy of the Basal Cisterns and Vessels of the Brain, Diagnostic Studies, General Operative Techniques and Pathological Considerations of the Intracranial Aneurysms. New York: Georg Thieme Verlag, 1984.

Zulegar S, Staubesand J. Atlas of the Central Nervous System in Sectional Planes. Baltimore: Urban & Schwarzenberg, 1977.

Index

Page numbers in *italics* denote illustrations; those followed by "Q" denote questions and those followed by "A" denote answers

A

Abdominal reflexes, loss of, 190
Abducens nerve
    anatomy of, *22–27, 37, 41–42, 114–115,*
        116, *116–117, 118–119, 125, 175,*
        200–201
    questions regarding, 257Q, 260A
    rostral portions of, 118
Abducens nucleus, *108–109,* 114, 116, *125, 163,*
    192–193, 200–201, 202–203,
    226–227, 228–229
Accessory cuneate nucleus, *100–101, 102–103,*
    104–105, 204–205
Accessory nerve, *24, 27, 35, 37, 175, 200–201*
Accessory nucleus, *98–99, 192–193, 200–201*
N-Acetylaspartylglutamate, 220, 222
Acetylcholine, 178, 190, 200, 202, 220, 234
Acute central cervical spinal cord syndrome, 94,
    180
Ageusia, 186
Agnosia, 178, 232, 234
Akinesia, 136, 158
Alcoholic cerebellar degeneration, 206
Alternating deficits, 83
Alternating hemianesthesia, 184, 186
Alternating hemiplegia
    description of, 190, 200
    questions regarding, 269Q, 275A
Alzheimer disease, 232, 234
Ambient cistern, *50–51*
Amiculum of olive, *102–103, 104–105, 106–107*
Ammon's horn, *232–233*
Amnesia, 234
Amnestic confabulatory syndrome, 232
Amygdalocortical fibers, *234–235*
Amygdalofugal pathway, *234–235*
Amygdaloid nuclear complex
    anatomy of, *52–53, 58–59, 66–67, 78,*
        146–147, 159, 169–171, 186–187,
        216–217, 232–233, 234–235
    blood supply to, *234–235*
    disorders of, 234
    lesions of, 234
    neurotransmitters, 234
Amygdaloid nucleus, *150–151, 152–153*
Amygdalonigral fibers, *216–217*
Amyotrophic lateral sclerosis, 190, 200, 202
Anesthesia dolorosa, 158
Aneurysm, carotid cavernous, 200
Angiography
    internal carotid artery, *240–243*
    magnetic resonance, *245*
    vertebral artery, *246*
Angular sulcus, *14, 18*
Anhidrosis, 220

Anosmia, 186
Ansa lenticularis, *142–143, 150–151, 165, 167,*
    216–217
Anterior cerebral artery
    anatomy of, *16–17, 21, 23, 29, 40, 154–155,*
        156–157
    angiogram of, *240, 242, 244, 248–250, 252*
    axial view of, *75, 78*
    branches of, *25, 27*
    callosomarginal branch of, *29, 240, 250*
    computed tomography of, *16*
    frontopolar branches of, *29*
    magnetic resonance imaging of, *20, 27, 38,*
        40, 78
    occlusion of, 158
    orbital branches of, *19, 21, 29*
    pericallosal branch of, *240, 250*
    questions regarding, 295Q, 296A
Anterior cerebral vein, *29*
Anterior choroidal artery
    anatomy of, *25, 159, 251*
    questions regarding, 286Q, 294A
Anterior choroidal artery syndrome, 158
Anterior cochlear nucleus, *106–107, 108–109,*
    112–113, 226–227
Anterior commissure
    anatomy of, *31, 65, 77, 142–143, 152–153,*
        163, 165–166, 167–169, 171,
        180–181, 182–183, 232–233,
        234–235
    questions regarding, 263Q, 265A, 276Q,
        277A
Anterior communicating artery
    anatomy of, *25, 38*
    angiogram of, *244*
Anterior corticospinal tract, *86, 88, 90, 92, 95,*
    98–99, 190–191
Anterior forceps, *74*
Anterior funiculus, *11*
Anterior hypothalamus, *234–235*
Anterior inferior cerebellar artery
    anatomy of, *23, 25, 27, 35, 37, 42*
    angiogram of, *244, 247, 251–252*
Anterior median artery, *11*
Anterior median fissure, *24, 81, 86, 88, 90*
Anterior medullary velum, *27, 31, 34–35, 37,*
    61, 204–205, 210–211
Anterior nucleus of thalamus, *66, 146–147,*
    148–149, 232–233
Anterior paracentral gyrus, *14–15, 28, 30,*
    190–191
Anterior perforated substance, *26, 59, 78,*
    152–153
Anterior quadrangular lobule, *32*
Anterior radicular artery, *11, 95*

Anterior root fibers, *86, 88*
Anterior spinal artery
    anatomy of, *10–11, 23, 25, 27, 37, 95*
    questions regarding, 266Q, 272A
    thrombosis of, 94
Anterior spinal medullary artery, *10, 95*
Anterior spinocerebellar tract
    anatomy of, *88, 90, 92, 98–99, 100–101,*
        102–103, 104–105, 106–107,
        108–109, 116–117, 118–119,
        120–121, 204–205
    questions regarding, 267Q, 272A
Anterior tegmental decussation, *130–131,*
    194–195, 196–197
Anterior temporal artery, *25*
Anterior tubercle, *75*
Anterior vertebral venous plexus, *23*
Anterior watershed infarcts, 158
Anterior white commissure (*see also* Anterior
    commissure)
    anatomy of, *88, 90*
    damage to, 94
Anterolateral cordotomy, 182, 280Q, 282Q,
    288A, 290A
Anterolateral sulcus, *90*
Anterolateral system
    anatomy of, *84, 86, 88, 90, 92, 95, 98–99,*
        100–101, 102–103, 104–105,
        106–107, 108–109, 111, 116–117,
        118–119, 122–123, 125, 126–127,
        128–129, 137, 178–179, 180–181,
        182–183, 184–185, 190–191,
        194–195, 202–203, 204–205,
        210–211, 226–227, 228–229
    blood supply to, *180–181*
    fibers of, 94
Aphasia, 234
Arachnoid mater, *10, 12, 47*
Arachnoid trabeculae, *47*
Arachnoid villus, *47, 243*
Arcuate nucleus, *100–101, 102–103, 104–105,*
    106–107, 108
Area postrema, *102–103*
Arnold-Chiari deformity, 208
Arteriovenous malformation, 94, 208, 262Q,
    264A, 276Q, 277A
Artery(ies)
    of Adamkiewicz
        description of, 11
        questions regarding, 266Q, 271A
    anterior cerebral
        anatomy of, *16–17, 21, 23, 29, 40,*
            154–155, 156–157
        angiogram of, *240, 242, 244, 248–250,*
            252

Artery(ies) (*Continued*)
  anterior cerebral (*Continued*)
    axial view of, *75, 78*
    branches of, *25, 27*
    callosomarginal branch of, *29, 240, 250*
    frontopolar branches of, *29*
    magnetic resonance imaging of, *20, 27, 38, 40, 78*
    occlusion of, 158
    orbital branches of, *19, 21, 29*
    pericallosal branch of, *240, 250*
    questions regarding, 295Q, 296A
  anterior choroidal
    anatomy of, *25, 159, 251*
    questions regarding, 286Q, 294A
  anterior communicating
    anatomy of, *25, 38*
    angiogram of, *244*
  anterior inferior cerebellar
    anatomy of, *23, 25, 27, 35, 37, 42*
    angiogram of, *244, 247, 251–252*
  anterior median, *11*
  anterior radicular, *11, 95*
  anterior spinal
    anatomy of, *10–11, 23, 25, 27, 37, 95*
    questions regarding, 266Q, 272A
    thrombosis of, 94
  anterior spinal medullary, *10, 95*
  anterior temporal, *25*
  basilar
    anatomy of, *23, 25, 37, 39, 41–42, 50, 79–81*
    angiogram of, *245–250, 252*
    questions regarding, 257Q, 260A, 269Q, 274A
  calcarine, *17, 249*
  common carotid, *252*
  external carotid, *252*
  internal carotid
    anatomy of, *23, 25, 27, 37, 39, 41*
    angiogram of, *240, 249–250, 252*
    cavernous part of, *240, 242, 245, 250, 252*
    cerebral part of, *240, 242, 245, 252*
    petrous part of, *240, 242, 245, 249, 252*
  labyrinthine
    anatomy of, *25, 27, 37*
    questions regarding, 254Q, 258A
  lateral posterior choroidal, *251*
  maxillary, *252*
  medial posterior choroidal, *159, 251*
  medial striate, *25, 251*
  middle cerebral
    anatomy of, *21, 23, 27, 39, 64–65, 154–155*
    angiogram of, *240, 242, 245, 248–249, 252*
    angular branches of, *19, 240*
    anterior branches of, *19*
    anterior temporal branches of, *19*
    branches of, *17, 19, 25*
    cortical branches of, *242*
    insular branches of, *242, 248–250*
    lenticulostriate branches of, *21, 23, 159, 242*
    magnetic resonance imaging of, *20, 27*
    middle temporal branches of, *19*
    occlusion of, 158
    orbitofrontal branches of, *19, 21*
    parietal branches of, *19, 240*
    posterior parietal branches of, *19*
    posterior temporal branches of, *19*
    prerolandic branches of, *19*
    questions regarding, 295Q, 296A
    rolandic branches of, *19*
  ophthalmic
    anatomy of, *25, 240, 249–250*
    questions regarding, 294Q, 296A
  orbitofrontal, *17*
  parietal, *17*
  polar temporal, *25*
  posterior cerebral
    anatomy of, *21, 27, 29, 37, 39–40, 67, 144–145*
    angiogram of, *244, 248–249, 251–252*
    anterior temporal branch of, *21, 29*
    branches of, *17, 27*
    calcarine branch of, *21, 29, 246, 249*
    cortical branches of, *27, 247*
    magnetic resonance imaging of, *27*
    parieto-occipital branch of, *21, 29, 246, 249*
    posterior temporal branch of, *21, 29*
    posteromedial branches of, *159*
    temporal branch of, *248*
    thalamogeniculate branches of, *159*
    thalamoperforating branches of, *159*
  posterior communicating
    anatomy of, *23, 25, 27, 37, 39*
    angiogram of, *246, 248–249, 251*
    questions regarding, 295Q, 297A
  posterior inferior cerebellar
    anatomy of, *23, 25, 27, 31, 35–37*
    angiogram of, *246–247, 251*
    branches of, *24*
    questions regarding, 267Q, 269Q, 273A–274A
  posterior spinal
    anatomy of, *10, 23, 25, 27, 35, 37, 95*
    questions regarding, 267Q, 273A
  posterior spinal medullary, *10, 95*
  quadrigeminal
    anatomy of, *25, 27, 35, 37*
    questions regarding, 254Q, 258A
  Rolandic, *17*
  segmental, *95*
  spinal
    anterior, *10–11*
    posterior, *10*
  spinal medullary
    anterior, *10*
    posterior, *10*
  sulcal, *95*
  superior cerebellar
    anatomy of, *23, 25, 27, 37, 39–41*
    angiogram of, *244, 246–249, 251–252*
    branches of, *35*
  temporal, *17*
  uncal, *25*
  vertebral
    anatomy of, *23, 25, 27, 37*
    angiogram of, *244–247, 249–252*
Ascending pain, 94
Aspartate, 196, 206, 210, 226
Astereognosis, 178
Asterixis, 214
Ataxia, 124
truncal, 178, 208, 228
Ataxia-telangiectasia, 206
Ataxic gait, 206, 228
Athetoid movements, 214
Auditory agnosia, 226, 232, 234
Auditory system
  pathways, *226–227*
  questions regarding, 281Q, 289A

B
Babinski reflex, 94
Babinski sign, 178, 190
Bacterial meningitis
  description of, 46
  questions regarding, 257Q, 261A
Basal ganglia, 158–159
Basal nuclei, 213–217
  of Meynert, *150–151, 152–153*
  questions regarding, 262Q, 264A, 276Q, 277A
Basal vein, *29, 241, 250*
Basal-lateral nuclei, *234–235*
Basilar artery
  anatomy of, *23, 25, 37, 39, 41–42, 50, 79–81*
  angiogram of, *245–250, 252*
  questions regarding, 257Q, 260A, 269Q, 274A
Basilar bifurcation
  anatomy of, *246*
  questions regarding, 295Q, 297A
Basilar plexus, *23*
Basilar pons, *22, 24–26, 30–33, 36, 38–42, 50, 54, 67–70, 79–81, 122–123, 125, 163, 165, 178–179, 190–191, 194–195, 200–201, 202–203, 210–211*
Bell palsy, 186, 202
Benedikt syndrome, 136
Bitemporal hemianopsia, 220
Biventer lobule, *32*
Body
  caudate nucleus, *52–53, 67–68, 70–71, 138–139, 140–141, 144–145, 146–147, 148–149, 159, 171*
  corpus callosum, *30, 53, 64–71, 74, 144–145, 146–147, 150–151, 154–155, 156–157, 165*
  fornix, *67–70, 140–141, 144–145, 146–147, 148–149, 159, 163, 165*
  juxtarestiform, *108–109, 114–115, 116–117, 208–209, 228–229*
  lateral geniculate, *26–27, 34–37, 58–59, 61*
  lateral ventricle, *52–53, 66–71, 74, 140–141, 144–145, 146–147*
  mammillary
    anatomy of, *20, 24–27, 31, 37–38, 40, 52–53, 59, 67, 78, 146–147, 159, 163, 170, 232–233*
    blood supply to, *232–233*
  medial geniculate, *26–27, 34–37, 58–59, 61*
  restiform, *27, 34–37, 43–44, 72, 81, 100–101, 102–103, 104–105, 108–109, 112–113, 114–115, 116–117, 178–179, 184–185, 186–187, 190–191, 194–195, 204–205, 206–207, 226–227, 228–229*
  thalamogeniculate, *27*
  trapezoid, *116–117, 118–119, 226–227*

Bradykinesia, 158, 214
Brain (see also specific anatomy)
    axial sections of, 74–81
    coronal sections of, 64–72
Brainstem
    blood supply to, 234–235
    circle of Willis, 25
    cranial nerve nuclei, 175
    dorsal view of, 34–35
    gliomas, 220
    lateral view of, 26–27, 36–37
    lesions of, 192
    median sagittal view of, 40
    questions regarding, 257Q, 261A, 270Q,
        275A, 278Q, 287A
    transverse section of, 126–127
    ventral view of, 22–25
Broca aphasia, 255Q–256Q, 259A
Brodmann areas, 255Q–256Q, 259A–260A
Brown-Sequard syndrome, 94, 204
Buccinator, 203

C
Calcar avis, 53, 58
Calcarine artery, 17, 249
Calcarine sulcus, 13, 28, 30, 53, 58, 171, 222
Calcitonin gene-related peptide, 180, 200, 202
Capsule
    external
        anatomy of, 56, 64–69, 77, 144–145,
            146–147, 148–149, 150–151,
            152–153, 154–155, 156–157, 159, 164
        questions regarding, 266Q, 271A
    extreme
        anatomy of, 64–68, 77, 144–145,
            146–147, 148–149, 150–151,
            152–153, 154–155, 156–157
        questions regarding, 266Q, 271A
    internal
        anatomy of, 35, 66, 176–177, 178–179,
            180–181, 184–185, 190–191,
            192–193, 206–207
        anterior limb of, 57, 64–65, 76–77,
            152–153, 154–155, 156–157, 159,
            162, 164, 166, 176–177, 206–207
        arteries to, 158–159
        genu of, 57, 76, 162, 176–177, 232–233
        posterior limb of, 57, 67–69, 76–77,
            142–143, 144–145, 146–147,
            148–149, 159, 162, 164, 166,
            176–177, 206–207
        questions regarding, 262Q, 263A
        retrolenticular limb of, 57, 70, 76–77,
            140–141, 159, 166, 206–207
        sublenticular limb of, 140–141, 206–207,
            226–227
Cardiac arrest, 110
Carotid cavernous aneurysms, 200
Cauda equina, 12, 47, 85, 87
Caudate nucleus
    axial view of, 74
    blood supply to, 214–215
    body of, 52–53, 67–68, 70–71, 138–139,
        140–141, 144–145, 146–147,
        148–149, 159, 171
    coronal view of, 138–139
    general images of, 61, 169, 176–177,
        214–215, 216–217, 234–235

head of, 52, 60, 64–65, 75–78, 152–153,
        154–155, 156–157, 162, 164,
        166–167, 265Q, 271A
    questions regarding, 262Q, 263A, 265Q,
        271A
    tail of, 52–53, 68–71, 75–78, 138–139,
        140–141, 144–145, 148–149, 159,
        162, 164, 168, 170
    veins of, 29
Cavernous sinus, 21, 23, 249
Central deafness, 226
Central gray, 98–99, 100–101, 120–121,
        122–123, 126–127, 128–129,
        130–131, 132–133, 134–135,
        140–141, 166, 210–211
Central midbrain syndrome, 136
Central nuclei, 234–235
Central sulcus, 13, 16, 19, 28, 30, 45, 56
Central tegmental tract, 102–103, 104–105,
        106–107, 108–109, 114–115,
        116–117, 118–119, 120–121,
        122–123, 126–127, 128–129,
        130–131, 132–133, 134–135,
        178–179
Centromedian nucleus of thalamus, 69, 76,
        142–143, 162, 164–167, 176–177,
        210–211, 216–217
Cerebellar corticonuclear fibers, 208–209
Cerebellar corticovestibular fibers, 228–229
Cerebellar efferent fibers, 210–211, 279Q, 287A
Cerebellar gait, 208
Cerebellar peduncle
    inferior, 32, 34–35, 61, 108–109, 114–115
    middle, 22, 24–27, 32–36, 61, 70–72, 80,
        118–119, 120–121, 122–123, 169,
        180–181, 206–207
    superior, 27, 32–37, 61, 70, 72, 78–79,
        114–115, 120–121, 122–123,
        206–207, 210–211
        brachium conjunctivum, 165, 167, 170
        decussation, 130–131, 163, 170,
            200–201, 210–211, 226–227,
            228–229
Cerebellar vermis, 42
Cerebellofugal fibers, 210
Cerebello-olivary fibers, 210–211
Cerebellorubral fibers, 132–133, 134–135,
        148–149, 210–211
Cerebellothalamic fibers, 132–133, 134–135,
        144–145, 148–149, 210–211
Cerebellum
    alcoholic degeneration of, 206
    anterior lobe of, 40–41, 79
    blood supply, 208–209
    caudal view of, 32
    general images of, 22, 25, 30, 39, 54, 78,
        204–205, 228–229
    inferior view of, 32
    lateral nucleus of, 209
    lateral view of, 33
    magnetic resonance imaging of, 20, 33
    median sagittal view of, 33
    nuclei, 204–205, 206–207, 208–209,
        228–229
    posterior lobe of, 79–81
    questions regarding, 258Q, 261A, 267Q,
        273A, 284Q, 292A
    rostral view of, 32–33

tonsil of
    anatomy of, 30, 42–44, 81, 112–113
    herniation of, 110
    ventral view of, 22–23
    white matter of, 271Q, 276A
Cerebral aqueduct, 20, 31, 40, 52, 70–71, 78,
        122–123, 126–127, 128–129,
        130–131, 134–135, 137
Cerebral artery
    anterior
        anatomy of, 16–17, 21, 23, 29, 40,
            154–155, 156–157
        angiogram of, 240, 242, 244, 248–250,
            252
        axial view of, 75, 78
        branches of, 25, 27
        callosomarginal branch of, 29, 240, 250
        computed tomography of, 16
        frontopolar branches of, 29
        magnetic resonance imaging of, 20, 27, 38,
            40, 78
        occlusion of, 158
        orbital branches of, 19, 21, 29
        pericallosal branch of, 240, 250
        questions regarding, 295Q, 296A
    middle
        anatomy of, 21, 23, 27, 39, 64–65,
            154–155
        angiogram of, 240, 242, 245, 248–249,
            252
        angular branches of, 19, 240
        anterior branches of, 19
        anterior temporal branches of, 19
        branches of, 17, 19, 25
        cortical branches of, 242
        insular branches of, 242, 248–250
        lenticulostriate branches of, 21, 23, 159,
            242
        magnetic resonance imaging of, 20, 27
        middle temporal branches of, 19
        occlusion of, 158
        orbitofrontal branches of, 19, 21
        parietal branches of, 19, 240
        posterior parietal branches of, 19
        posterior temporal branches of, 19
        prerolandic branches of, 19
        questions regarding, 295Q, 296A
        rolandic branches of, 19
    posterior
        anatomy of, 21, 27, 29, 37, 39–40, 67,
            144–145
        angiogram of, 244, 248–249, 251–252
        anterior temporal branch of, 21, 29
        branches of, 17, 27
        calcarine branch of, 21, 29, 246, 249
        cortical branches of, 27, 247
        magnetic resonance imaging of, 27
        parieto-occipital branch of, 21, 29, 246,
            249
        posterior temporal branch of, 21, 29
        posteromedial branches of, 159
        temporal branch of, 248
        thalamogeniculate branches of, 159
        thalamoperforating branches of, 159
Cerebral hemispheres
    arteries of, 16–17
    dorsal view of, 16–17
    inferior view of, 38–39

Cerebral hemispheres (*Continued*)
  lateral view of, *13–15*
  left
    dissection of, *58*
    lateral view of, *18, 45*
    magnetic resonance imaging of, *45*
    medial aspect of, *58*
  magnetic resonance imaging of, *27*
  medial view of, *13–15*
  midsagittal view of, *29*
  questions regarding, 257Q, 260A
  right
    dissection of, *56–57*
    lateral view of, *19, 56*
    magnetic resonance imaging of, *28, 30–31*
    midsagittal view of, *28, 30–31*
    sinuses of, *19*
  somatomotor cortex, *14*
  somatosensory cortex, *14*
  veins of, *17*
  ventral view of, *20–24, 58–59*
Cerebropontine fibers, *206–207*
Ceruleocerebellar fibers, *206–207*
Cervical dystonia, 214
Chiasmatic cistern, *50*
Chief sensory nucleus of trigeminal nerve, 120,
    167, 184–185, 204–205
Cholecystokinin, 180, 184, 186, 222, 226, 232
Chordoma, 202
Choreiform movements, 214
Choroid plexus, *24–25, 27, 31, 59–61,*
    112–113, 138–139, 140–141,
    144–145, 148–149, 150–151, 162,
    166, 170–171
  fourth ventricle, *35, 37, 251*
  inferior horn, *78*
  lateral ventricle, *35, 251*
  questions regarding, 255Q, 259A
  third ventricle, *37, 76, 251,* 295Q, 296A
Choroidal artery
  anterior
    anatomy of, *25, 159, 251*
    questions regarding, 286Q, 294A
  posterior
    anatomy of, *25, 27, 35, 37*
    angiogram of, *246*
    lateral, *251*
    medial, *159, 251*
Ciliary ganglion, *200–201, 220–221*
Cingulate gyrus
  anatomy of, *28, 30, 64, 75, 138–139,*
    144–145, 146–147, 150–151,
    152–153, 154–155, 232–233
  blood supply to, *232–233*
Cingulate sulcus
  anatomy of, *13, 28, 30, 176–177*
  questions regarding, 294Q, 296A
Cingulum, *58, 64, 138–139, 140–141, 144–145,*
    146–147, 152–153, 154–155,
    156–157, 232–233
Circle of Willis, *25*
Cistern(s)
  ambient, *50–51*
  anatomy of, *50*
  blood in, *51*
  chiasmatic, *50*
  crural, *50–51*
  dorsal cerebellomedullary, *52*

inferior cerebellopontine, *50*
interpeduncular, *50–51*
lamina terminalis, *50–51*
lumbar (*see* Lumbar cistern)
paracallosal, *50*
premedullary, *50*
prepontine, *50*
quadrigeminal (*see* Quadrigeminal cistern)
questions regarding, 257Q, 260A
superior, *138–139*
superior cerebellopontine, *50*
sylvian, *50–51*
Cisterna magna
  anatomy of, *50, 52*
  questions regarding, 295Q, 296A
Claude syndrome, 136, 196, 208
Claustrum, *64–69, 76–77, 144–145, 146–147,*
    148–149, 150–151, 152–153,
    154–155, 156–157, 162, 164, 166
Coccygeal ligament, *47*
Coccyx, *47*
Cochlea, *42*
Cochlear nerve, *106–107*
Cochlear nuclei
  anatomy of, *175, 226–227*
  anterior, *106–107, 108–109, 112–113,*
    226–227
  blood supply to, *226–227*
  posterior, *106–107, 111, 112–113, 169,*
    226–227
Cog wheel rigidity, 214
Collateral sulcus, *13, 20, 22*
Colliculus, *20, 32, 60*
  facial
    anatomy of, *34–35,* 114, *200–201*
    questions regarding, 268Q, 274A
  inferior
    anatomy of, *27, 31–34, 39, 50, 72, 78,*
      138–139, 163, 165, 167–168,
      210–211, 226–227, 228–229
    brachium of, *34–37, 61, 130–131,*
      132–133, 140–141, 168, 226–227
    central nucleus, *126–127*
    commissure, *126–127, 226–227*
    external nucleus, *126–127*
    pericentral nucleus, *126–127*
  superior
    anatomy of, *27, 31–32, 34–37, 39, 59, 71,*
      77, 128–129, 130–131, 132–133,
      163–167, 180–181, 194–195,
      196–197, 200–201, 210–211,
      216–217, 220–221, 226–227,
      228–229
    blood supply to, *220–221*
    brachium of, *34–35, 59, 61, 77, 128–129,*
      132–133, 134–135, 140–141, 164,
      169, 220–222
    commissure, *132–133*
Colloid cyst, *28*
Commissure
  anterior
    anatomy of, *31, 65, 77, 142–143,*
      152–153, 163, 165–166, 167–169,
      171, 180–181, 182–183, 232–233,
      234–235
    questions regarding, 263Q, 265A, 276Q,
      277A
  habenular, *142–143,* 164

hippocampal
  anatomy of, *72, 138–139, 162*
  questions regarding, 262Q, 264A
inferior colliculus, *126–127, 226–227*
posterior, *31, 52, 70, 134–135, 163,*
    220–221
superior colliculus, *132–133*
Common carotid artery, *252*
Complete spinal cord lesion, 94
Computed tomography
  advantages of, 3
  anterior cerebral artery region, *16*
  anterior horn, *54*
  basilar pons, *54*
  cerebellum, *54*
  contrast agents, 6
  description of, 3
  disadvantages of, 3
  fourth ventricle, *54*
  lateral ventricle
    anterior horn of, *54*
    atrium of, *54*
    posterior horn of, *54*
    temporal horn of, *54*
  pons-medulla junction, *54*
  subarachnoid hemorrhage findings, *3*
  tegmentum of the pons, *54*
  third ventricle, *54*
Computed tomography myelogram
  anterior root, *87, 89*
  cauda equina, *85, 87*
  lumbar cistern, *85*
  lumbar spinal cord, *87*
  posterior root, *87, 89, 93*
  sacral spinal cord, *85*
Conductive deafness, 226
Confluens of sinus
  anatomy of, *19, 21, 23, 29*
  angiogram of, *243–245, 250*
  questions regarding, 296Q, 297A
Conus medullaris, *47*
Cordotomy
  anterolateral, 182
  questions regarding, 280Q, 282Q, 288A,
    290A
Corneal reflex, 184, 202
Corona radiata, *57, 65–69, 74–75*
Corpus callosum
  anatomy of, *13, 39, 58, 60, 162*
  body of, *30, 53, 64–71, 74, 144–145,*
    146–147, 150–151, 154–155,
    156–157, 165
  genu of, *30, 52, 75–77, 163, 167, 232–233*
  magnetic resonance imaging of, *28*
  posterior vein of, *29*
  questions regarding, 255Q, 259A
  rostrum of, *30, 64, 156–157*
  splenium of, *30, 52–53, 59, 72, 75–77,*
    138–139, 163, 165, 167, 232–233
  sulcus of, *28, 30*
Cortex
  entorhinal, *232–233, 234–235*
  intermediate, *208–209*
  lateral, *208–209*
  medial frontal, *232–233*
  prepiriform, *234–235*
  retrosplenial, *232–233*
  vermal, *208–209*

Cortical nuclei, *234–235*

Corticoamygdaloid fibers, *234–235*

Corticohippocampal fibers, *232–233*

Corticonigral fibers, *130–131, 132–133,*
148–149, 216–217

Corticonuclear fibers, *132–133, 134–135,*
190–191, 192–193, 208–209

Corticoreticular fibers, *194–195*

Corticorubral fibers, *196–197*

Corticospinal fibers

anatomy of, *68, 79, 111, 116–117, 118–119,*
120–121, 122–123, 126–127,
128–129, 130–131, 132–133,
210–211, 216–217

degenerated, *97, 100–101, 102–103,*
104–105, 106–107, 108–109,
116–117, 118–119, 120–121,
122–123, 126–127, 128–129,
130–131, 132–133

questions regarding, 270Q, 275A

Corticospinal tracts

anatomy of, *190–191*

anterior, *86, 88, 90, 92, 95, 98–99*

injury to, 190

lateral, *84, 86, 88, 90, 92, 95, 111, 163,*
266Q, 272A

questions regarding, 266Q, 272A

Corticostriate fibers, *214–215*

Corticotectal fibers, *194–195*

Corticovestibular fibers, *208–209*

Cranial nerves

abducens

anatomy of, *22–27, 37, 41–42, 114–115,*
116, *116–117, 118–119, 125, 175,*
200–201

questions regarding, 257Q, 260A

rostral portions of, 118

accessory, *24, 27, 35, 37, 175, 200–201*

efferents, *200–203*

facial

anatomy of, *22–27, 37, 41–44, 108–109,*
114–115, 116, *118–119, 125, 167,*
202–203

internal genu, *116–117, 118–119*

questions regarding, 285Q, 293A

glossopharyngeal

angiogram of 106, *22, 24–25, 27, 35, 37,*
42–43, 81, *106–107, 202–203*

root of, 106

hypoglossal

anatomy of, *24, 27, 37, 42–44, 100–101,*
104–105, 111, 200–201

fascicles of, *100–101*

nuclei, 98, 100, 102, 104, 106, 108, 116,
120, 122, 126, 128, 130, 132, 134,
140, 142

oculomotor, *23–25, 27, 31, 37, 39–40, 67,*
130–131, 132–133, 137, 148–149,
163, 200–201, 220–221, 252

optic, *20, 23–26, 31, 38, 40, 58–59, 64, 163,*
220–221

questions regarding, 255Q, 257Q, 259A,
261A, 269Q, 275A

trigeminal, *23–25, 69, 80, 116–117, 122,*
202–203

anatomy of, *41*

chief sensory nucleus of, 120, *167,*
184–185

lesions of, 184, 202

mandibular division of, *184–185*

maxillary division of, *184–185*

motor nucleus of, 120

motor root, *26–27, 33, 36–37*

ophthalmic division of, *184–185*

pathways of, *184–185*

sensory root, *26–27, 33, 36–37, 41*

trochlear, *23–27, 33–37, 40, 72, 122,*
122–123, 125, 126–127, 138–139,
163, 175, 200–201

vagus

anatomy of, *22, 24, 27, 35, 37, 42–44, 81,*
104–105, 202–203

dorsal motor nucleus of, *100–101,*
102–103, 104–105, 111, 175,
202–203

vestibulocochlear

anatomy of, *22–27, 36–37, 41–42, 44, 81*

questions regarding, 283Q, 291A

Crossed deficits, 83

Crural cistern, *50–51*

Crus cerebri

anatomy of, *20, 24–27, 33–36, 38, 40–41,*
58–59, 68–69, 78, 126–127, 128–129,
130–131, 144–145, 148–149, 165,
167–170, 178–179, 180–181,
184–185, 190–191, 196–197,
200–201, 210–211, 220–221,
226–227

blood supply to, *214–215*

questions regarding, 268Q, 273A, 276Q,
277A

Cuneate fasciculus, *34–35, 88, 90, 92, 98–99,*
100–101, 102–103, 178–179,
182–183

Cuneate nucleus, *98–99, 100–101, 102–103,*
178–179, 182–183

Cuneate tubercle, *27, 35–37*

Cuneocerebellar fibers, *204–205*

Cuneus, *14, 28, 30*

D

Dandy-Walker syndrome, 208

Deafness, 226

Decerebrate rigidity, 194, 196

Decussation

anterior tegmental, *130–131, 194–195,*
196–197

medial, *111*

posterior tegmental, *130–131, 194–195,*
196–197

pyramids, *22, 24, 92, 98–99, 111*

sensory, 100

superior cerebellar peduncle, *130–131, 163,*
170, 200–201, 210–211, 226–227,
228–229

supraoptic, *150–151, 152–153*

Deep tendon reflexes, 94, 178

Dementia, 214, 232, 234

Dentate gyrus, *170–171, 232–233*

Dentate nucleus, *80, 112–113, 114–115, 169,*
171, 210–211

Denticulate ligament, *10, 47*

Diabetes mellitus, 200

Diagonal band of Broca, *152–153, 154–155*

Diencephalon

arteries to, *158–159*

general images of, *13, 176–177*

median sagittal view of, *40*

midsagittal view of, *29–30*

ventral view of, *22–24, 26*

Digastric, 203

Diplopia, 124, 190, 200, 268Q, 274A, 282Q,
290A

Discriminative touch

areas of, 98, 100, 102, 104, 106, 108, 116,
120, 122, 126, 128, 130, 132, 134,
140, 142

loss of, 124, 178

Disease

Alzheimer, 232, 234

Huntington, 214, 281Q, 289A

Parkinson's

description of, 158, 214

questions regarding, 282Q, 290A

Pick, 232, 234

Wilson

description of, 214

questions regarding, 283Q, 286Q, 291A,
293A

Dopamine, 214, 216

Dorsal accessory olivary nucleus, *206–207,*
210–211

Dorsal cerebellomedullary cistern, *52*

Dorsal column nuclei, 100

Dorsal motor nucleus of vagus, *100–101,*
102–103, 104–105, 111, 175,
202–203

Dorsal motor vagal nucleus, *234–235*

Dorsal thalamus, *31, 38–39, 53, 60*

Dorsal thoracic nucleus of Clarke, *88, 204–205*

Dorsal trigeminothalamic tract, *122–123,*
126–127, 128–129, 130–131,
132–133, 134–135, 184–185

Dorsolateral tract, *84, 86, 88, 90, 95*

Dorsolateral tract junction, *92*

Dorsomedial nucleus of thalamus

anatomy of, *67–69, 75–76, 144–145,*
146–147, 162–165, 167, 176–177

questions regarding, 263Q, 265A

Dura mater, *10, 12, 47*

Dynorphin, 214

Dysagusia, 110

Dysarthria, 186, 190, 200, 202, 206, 208, 214,
279Q, 288A

Dysdiadochokinesia, 208

Dyskinesia, 136

Dysmetria, 208

Dysosmia, 186

Dysphagia, 186, 190, 200, 202, 206, 214, 270Q,
275A, 278Q, 287A

Dyspnea, 110

Dystonia, 214

E

Echovirus, 208

Edinger-Westphal nucleus, 130, 132, *132–133,*
137, 175, 200–201, 210–211,
220–221

Embolic stroke, 265Q, 271A

Emboliform nucleus, *112–113, 114–115, 167,*
210–211

Embolization, 158

Embolus, 158

Enkephalin, 180, 186, 194, 214, 226, 232, 234

Enophthalmos, 220
Entorhinal cortex, *232–233, 234–235*
Ephapse, 184
Epidural hematoma, 46, *48*
Epidural space, *47*
Extensor plantar reflexes, 94
External capsule
  anatomy of, *56, 64–69, 77, 144–145, 146–147, 148–149, 150–151, 152–153, 154–155, 156–157, 159, 164*
  questions regarding, 266Q, 271A
External carotid artery, *252*
External medullary lamina, *140–141, 144–145, 146–147, 148–149, 171*
Extreme capsule
  anatomy of, *64–68, 77, 144–145, 146–147, 148–149, 150–151, 152–153, 154–155, 156–157*
  questions regarding, 266Q, 271A
Eye movements
  failure of, 136
  paralysis of, 136

F

Face, ipsilateral side of, 110
Facial colliculus
  anatomy of, *34–35,* 114, *200–201*
  questions regarding, 268Q, 274A
Facial hemiplegia, 202
Facial motor nucleus, 108, *114–115, 116–117, 118–119, 125, 175*
Facial muscles
  innervation of, 203
  paralysis of, 136
Facial nerve
  anatomy of, *22–27, 37, 41–44, 108–109, 114–115,* 116, *118–119, 125, 167, 202–203*
  internal genu, *116–117, 118–119*
  questions regarding, 285Q, 293A
Facial nucleus, 118, *165, 184–185, 192–193, 196–197, 202–203, 226–227*
Facial palsy, 228
  Bell, 186, 202
  central, 192
  ipsilateral, 202
Facial weakness, 190
Falx cerebri, *16*
Fasciculus
  cuneate, *34–35,* 88, 90, 92, *98–99, 100–101, 102–103, 178–179, 182–183*
  cuneatus, *11,* 95
  gracile, *34–35,* 84, 86, 88, 90, *98–99, 178–179, 182–183*
  gracilis, *11,* 95
  interfascicular, *90*
  lenticular, *144–145, 146–147, 148–149, 150–151, 165, 167, 169, 216–217*
  medial longitudinal
    anatomy of, *86,* 88, *90, 92, 95, 98–99, 100–101, 102–103, 104–105, 106–107,* 111, *112–113, 114–115, 116–117, 118–119, 120–121, 125, 126–127, 128–129, 130–131, 132–133, 134–135, 137, 163, 170, 178–179, 180–181, 190–191 194–195, 196–197, 200–201,*

202–203, 208–209, 210–211, 226–227, 228–229
    rostral interstitial nucleus of, 192, *192–193*
  occipitofrontal, *57*
  posterior longitudinal, *100–101, 102–103, 104–105, 106–107, 116–117, 120–121, 126–127, 128–129, 130–131, 132–133*
  subthalamic, *216–217*
  superior longitudinal, *56–57*
  thalamic, *142–143, 144–145, 146–147, 148–149, 165, 169, 210–211, 216–217*
  uncinate, *56–57*
Fasciculus cuneatus, *11, 95*
Fasciculus gracilis, *11, 95*
Fastigial nucleus, *112–113, 114–115, 163, 210–211*
Festinating gait, 158, 214
Fiber(s)
  amygdalocortical, *234–235*
  amygdalonigral, *216–217*
  anterior root, *86, 88*
  cerebellar corticovestibular, *228–229*
  cerebello-olivary, *210–211*
  cerebellorubral, *132–133, 134–135, 148–149, 210–211*
  cerebellothalamic, *132–133, 134–135, 144–145, 148–149, 210–211*
  cerebropontine, *206–207*
  ceruleocerebellar, *206–207*
  corticoamygdaloid, *234–235*
  corticohippocampal, *232–233*
  corticonigral, *130–131, 132–133, 148–149, 216–217*
  corticonuclear, *132–133, 134–135, 190–191, 192–193, 208–209*
  corticoreticular, *194–195*
  corticorubral, *196–197*
  corticospinal
    anatomy of, *68, 79,* 111, *116–117, 118–119, 120–121, 122–123, 126–127, 128–129, 130–131, 132–133, 210–211, 216–217*
    degenerated, *97, 100–101, 102–103, 104–105, 106–107, 108–109, 116–117, 118–119, 120–121, 122–123, 126–127, 128–129, 130–131, 132–133*
    questions regarding, 270Q, 275A
  corticostriate, *214–215*
  corticotectal, *194–195*
  corticovestibular, *208–209*
  cuneocerebellar, *204–205*
  frontopontine, *128–129, 130–131, 132–133, 206–207*
  hypoglossal, *102–103*
  hypothalamocerebellar
    anatomy of, *206–207*
    questions regarding, 278Q, 287A
  internal arcuate
    anatomy of, *100–101, 102–103,* 111, *178–179, 182–183*
    crossing of, 102
  medial division, *86*
  medullary reticulospinal, *86*
  nigroamygdaloid, *216–217*

nigrocollicular, *216–217*
nigrostriatal, *130–131, 132–133, 148–149, 214–215*
nigrosubthalamic, *216–217*
nigrotectal, *216–217*
nigrothalamic, *216–217*
nucleocortical, *208–209*
occipitopontine, *126–127, 128–129, 130–131, 132–133, 134–135, 206–207*
olivocerebellar, *102–103, 104–105, 106–107,* 167, *206–207*
pallidonigral, *130–131, 132–133, 148–149, 216–217*
parietopontine, *126–127, 128–129, 130–131, 132–133, 134–135, 206–207*
pontocerebellar, *116–117, 118–119, 120–121, 122–123, 126–127, 206–207*
posterior column, 94
propriospinal, *84, 86, 90, 92, 95*
raphecerebellar, *206–207*
raphespinal, *180–181*
raphestriatal, *214–215*
reticulocerebellar, *206–207*
reticulospinal, *98–99, 100–101, 106–107*
reticulothalamic, *180–181*
rostral spinocerebellar, *204–205*
secondary cochlear, *108–109*
spino-olivary, *88, 90, 92, 98–99*
spinoreticular, *180–181*
spinothalamic, *180–181*
striatonigral, *214–215*
striatopallidal, *214–215*
subthalamonigral, *216–217*
temporopontine, *126–127, 128–129, 130–131, 132–133, 134–135, 206–207*
thalamocortical, *210–211, 216–217*
thalamostriatal, *214–215*
ventral amygdalofugal, *150–151*
ventral trigeminothalamic
  anatomy of, *125, 137*
  questions regarding, 283Q, 291A
vestibulocerebellar
  primary, *228–229*
  secondary, *228–229*
vestibulospinal, *100–101*
Field of Forel, *167*
Filum terminale internum, *12, 47*
Finger-nose test, 208
Finger-to-finger test, 208
Fissure
  anterior median, *24, 81, 86, 88, 90*
  horizontal, *32*
  longitudinal, *16, 22*
  posterior superior, *32*
  posterolateral, *33*
  primary, *32–33*
  transverse cerebral, *61*
Flaccid paraplegia, 94
Flapping tremor, 214
Flexed posture, 214
Flocculonodular lobe, *204–205*
Flocculus, *22, 24, 32–33, 41, 43, 71, 208–209*
Foix-Alajouanine syndrome, 94
Foramen of Luschka, *36, 52, 251*

Forebrain
coronal section of, *138–139, 140–141, 144–145, 150–151, 152–153, 154–155, 156–157*
lesions of, 158
oblique section of, *142–143, 148–149*
vascular syndromes of, 158
Formation
hippocampal, *67–72, 76–78, 138–139, 140–141, 144–145, 159, 162, 164, 166, 168–171*
reticular, *122–123, 126–127, 128–129, 130–131, 180–181, 184–185, 210–211, 220–221, 226–227*
Fornix
anatomy of, *13, 27, 30–31, 37, 60–61, 134–135, 168, 176–177, 232–233, 234–235*
body of, *67–70, 140–141, 144–145, 146–147, 148–149, 159, 163, 165*
column of, *65–66, 76–77, 142–143, 150–151, 152–153, 162–164, 166*
crus of, *71–72, 75–77, 138–139, 159*
fimbria of, *70–71*
Fourth ventricle
choroid plexus of, *35, 37, 251*
floor of, *36*
general anatomy of, *22, 27, 31–33, 50, 52, 54, 72, 79–81, 111, 125, 165*
lateral recess of, *36, 42, 52, 54, 61, 112–113*
lateral ventricle of, *34*
magnetic resonance imaging of, *22*
questions regarding, 258Q, 261A, 268Q, 274A
rostral portion of, *39–40, 51*
striae medullares of, *34, 36, 106–107*
Foville syndrome, 190
Frenulum, *34, 61, 122–123*
Friedrich ataxia, 204
Frontal lobe, *38–39*
Frontal pole, *20, 22*
Frontopontine fibers, *128–129, 130–131, 132–133, 206–207*

G
Gag reflex, 186, 202, 258Q, 261A, 280Q, 288A
Gait
ataxic, 206, 228
festinating, 214
wide-based (cerebellar), 208
Gamma-aminobutyric acid, 186, 190, 196, 208, 210, 214, 216, 228, 232
Ganglion
basal, 158–159
ciliary, *200–201, 220–221*
otic, *202–203*
posterior root, *12, 178–179, 180–181, 182–183, 204–205*
pterygopalatine, *202–203*
spinal, *11*
spiral, *226–227*
submandibular, *202–203*
superior cervical, *220–221*
terminal, *202–203*
trigeminal, *41, 80*
vestibular, *228–229*
Gaze deficit, 266Q, 272A
Gaze palsy, 192

General somatic afferent, *174, 184–185*
General somatic efferent, *174*
General visceral afferent, *174–175, 186–187*
General visceral efferent, *174*
Geniculate bodies
lateral, *26–27, 34–37, 58–59, 61*
medial, *26–27, 34–37, 58–59, 61*
questions regarding, 262Q, 264A
Genioglossus, 201
Genu
corpus callosum, *30, 52, 75–77, 163, 167, 232–233*
facial nerve, *116–117, 118–119*
internal capsule, *57, 76, 162, 176–177, 232–233*
Gigantocellular reticular nucleus, *194–195*
Gland
lacrimal, 203
parotid, 203
pineal
anatomy of, *21, 31, 34–35, 52, 60, 71, 77, 134–135, 138–139, 232–233, 234–235*
questions regarding, 262Q, 264A
pituitary, *31*
sublingual, 203
submandibular, 203
Gliomas, 208, 220
brainstem, 220
Globose nucleus, *112–113, 114–115, 210–211*
Globus pallidus
anatomy of, *65–68, 76–77, 234–235*
blood supply, 216
efferents of, *216–217*
lateral segment of, *142–143, 144–145, 150–151, 152–153, 154–155, 164, 166, 169, 171, 176–177, 214–215, 216–217*
medial segment of, *142–143, 144–145, 150–151, 166, 169, 171, 176–177, 214–215, 216–217*
palleostriatum, *176–177*
Glomus
anatomy of, *61*
questions regarding, 256Q, 260A
Glossopharyngeal nerve
angiogram of 106, *22, 24–25, 27, 35, 37, 42–43, 81, 106–107, 202–203*
root of, 106
Glossopharyngeal neuralgia, 186
Glutamate, 180, 182, 190, 192, 194, 196, 204, 206, 210, 214, 226, 232, 234
Glycine, 216
Gracile fasciculus, *34–35, 84, 86, 88, 90, 92, 98–99, 178–179, 182–183*
Gracile lobule, *32*
Gracile nucleus, *98–99, 100–101, 102–103, 178–179, 182–183*
Gracile tubercle, *27, 35–37*
Great cerebral vein
anatomy of, *21, 29, 59*
angiogram of, *241, 248, 250*
Greater anastomotic vein, *17, 19*
Gyrus(i)
anterior paracentral, *14–15, 28, 30, 190–191*
breves, *45*
cingulate (*see* Cingulate gyrus)
dentate, *170–171, 232–233*

inferior frontal
pars opercularis, *14, 18*
pars orbitalis, *14, 18*
pars triangularis, *14, 18*
inferior temporal, *20*
insular, *56*
lingual, *14, 20, 28, 30*
longi, *45*
middle frontal, *16, 18, 45*
middle temporal, *18*
occipital, *16, 18, 20*
occipitotemporal, *20, 22, 28*
orbital, *20, 22, 156–157*
parahippocampal, *20, 22, 24, 28*
paraterminal, *28, 154–155*
postcentral, *45, 56, 178–179, 180–181*
posterior paracentral, *14–15, 28, 30, 178–179, 180–181*
precentral, *18, 56, 190–191*
questions regarding, 255Q–256Q, 258Q, 259A–261A
rectus, *20, 22, 24, 53, 156–157, 232–233*
subcallosal, *64, 77, 156–157*
superior frontal (*see* Superior frontal gyrus)
superior temporal, *18, 56*
supramarginal, *56*
transverse temporal, *45, 56, 60, 226–227*

H
Habenula, *31, 35, 60*
Habenular commissure, *142–143, 164*
Habenular nucleus, *76, 162–163*
Habenulopeduncular tract, *132–133, 134–135, 142–143*
Heel-to-shin test, 208
Hemiballismus, 158, 216
Hemifacial spasm, 202
Hemihypethesia, 158
Hemiparesis, 190
Hemiplegia, 158, 190, 196, 204
contralateral, 136, 158, 192
description of, 192, 200, 204
facial, 202
inferior alternating, 110, 200
middle alternating, 124, 200
questions regarding, 266Q, 269Q, 272A, 275A
superior alternating, 136, 200
Hemorrhage
magnetic resonance imaging of, *49*
spinal cord, 94
ventricular, *54*
Hereditary cerebellar ataxia, 206
Hereditary spinal ataxia, 204
Herniation
tonsillar, 110, 258Q, 261A
uncal, 136, 256Q, 260A
Herpes simplex encephalitis, 234
Herpes zoster, 184
Hiccups, 110
Hippocampal commissure
anatomy of, *72, 138–139, 162*
questions regarding, 262Q, 264A
Hippocampal formation, *67–72, 76–78, 138–139, 140–141, 144–145, 159, 162, 164, 166, 168–171*
Hippocampus
alveus of, *140–141, 144–145, 146–147*
blood supply to, *232–233*

Hippocampus (*Continued*)
  connections, *232–233*
  disorders of, 232
  fimbria of, *71, 76–77, 138–139, 140–141, 162, 166, 170–171*
  general images of, *58–59, 61, 148–149, 232–233*
  neurotransmitters, 232
  questions regarding, 276Q, 277A
  spiral fibers of, *58*
Hoarseness, 186
Homonymous hemianopsia, 158, 220
Homonymous inferior quadrantanopia, 220
Homonymous superior quadrantanopia, 220
Horizontal fissure, *32*
Horizontal gaze center, 192
Horizontal gaze palsy, 192
Horner syndrome, 220
Huntington disease, 214, 281Q, 289A
Hydrocephalus, 136
Hydromyelia, 94
Hyoglossus, 201
Hypacusis, 124
Hyperactive deep tendon reflexes, 94
Hyperacusis, 202
Hypermetamorphosis, 234
Hypermetria, 208
Hyperorality, 234
Hyperphagia, 234
Hyperreflexia, 190
Hypersexuality, 234
Hypoglossal fibers, *102–103*
Hypoglossal nerve
  anatomy of, *24, 27, 37, 42–44, 100–101, 104–105, 111, 200–201*
  fascicles of, *100–101*
Hypoglossal nucleus, 100, *100–101*, 102, *102–103, 104–105, 111, 163, 175, 184–185, 186–187, 192–193, 200–201, 202–203, 228–229*
Hypoglossal trigone, *34–36*
Hypokinesia, 158, 214, 216
Hypokinesias, 216
Hypometria, 208
Hypophonia, 214
Hypothalamic nuclei, *150–151*
Hypothalamic sulcus, *31*
Hypothalamocerebellar fibers
  anatomy of, *206–207*
  questions regarding, 278Q, 287A
Hypothalamus
  anatomy of, *27, 31, 40, 53, 66, 78, 134–135, 142–143, 159, 163, 165–166, 168, 170, 186–187, 206–207, 232–233, 234–235*
  anterior, *234–235*
  blood supply to, *232–233, 234–235*
  preoptic area of, *152–153*

I

Incomplete spinal cord lesion, 94
Indusium griseum
  lateral longitudinal stria of, *140–141, 144–145, 146–147, 150–151, 152–153*
  medial longitudinal stria of, *138–139, 144–145, 146–147, 150–151, 152–153, 154–155, 156–157*
Infarct, watershed, 158

Inferior alternating hemiplegia, 110, 200
Inferior anastomotic vein, *19, 241*
Inferior cerebellar peduncle, *32, 34–35, 61, 108–109, 114–115*
Inferior cerebellopontine cistern, *50*
Inferior cerebral veins, *19*
Inferior colliculus
  anatomy of, *27, 31–34, 39, 50, 72, 78, 138–139, 163, 165, 167–168, 210–211, 226–227, 228–229*
  brachium of, *34–37, 61, 130–131, 132–133, 140–141, 168, 226–227*
  central nucleus, *126–127*
  commissure, *126–127, 226–227*
  external nucleus, *126–127*
  pericentral nucleus, *126–127*
Inferior fovea, *34, 36*
Inferior frontal gyrus
  pars opercularis, *14, 18*
  pars orbitalis, *14, 18*
  pars triangularis, *14, 18*
Inferior frontal sulcus, *18*
Inferior medullary velum, *112–113*
Inferior olivary complex, *111*
Inferior parietal lobule, 14, *14*
Inferior petrosal sinus, *21, 23, 250*
Inferior pulvinar nucleus, *140–141*
Inferior sagittal sinus
  anatomy of, *21, 29*
  angiogram of, *243*
Inferior salivatory nucleus, *106–107, 175, 202–203*
Inferior semilunar lobule, *32*
Inferior temporal gyrus, *20*
Inferior vestibular nucleus, *104–105, 106–107, 112–113, 186–187, 196–197, 208–209, 210–211*
Infundibular recess, *31, 40*
Infundibulum, *20, 24–26, 31, 38, 58–59, 65*
Insula
  central sulcus of, *56*
  general images of, *64–69, 76–77, 150–151, 154–155, 164, 168*
  questions regarding, 262Q, 264A
Intention tremor, 208
Intercavernous sinus, *21, 23*
Interfascicular fasciculus, *90*
Intermediate cortex, *208–209*
Intermediate nerve, *24*
Intermediate zone, *84, 86, 90, 204–205*
Intermediolateral cell column, *88, 175, 220–221*
Internal arcuate fibers
  anatomy of, *100–101, 102–103, 111, 178–179, 182–183*
  crossing of, 102
Internal capsule
  anatomy of, *35, 66, 176–177, 178–179, 180–181, 184–185, 190–191, 192–193, 206–207*
  anterior limb of, *57, 64–65, 76–77, 152–153, 154–155, 156–157, 159, 162, 164, 166, 176–177, 206–207*
  arteries to, *158–159*
  genu of, *57, 76, 162, 176–177, 232–233*
  posterior limb of, *57, 67–69, 76–77, 142–143, 144–145, 146–147, 148–149, 159, 162, 164, 166, 176–177, 206–207*

  questions regarding, 262Q, 263A
  retrolenticular limb of, *57, 70, 76–77, 140–141, 159, 166, 206–207*
  sublenticular limb of, *140–141, 206–207, 226–227*
Internal carotid artery
  anatomy of, *23, 25, 27, 37, 39, 41*
  angiogram of, *240, 249–250, 252*
  cavernous part of, *240, 242, 245, 250, 252*
  cerebral part of, *240, 242, 245, 252*
  petrous part of, *240, 242, 245, 249, 252*
Internal cerebral vein
  anatomy of, *28–29, 31, 34*
  angiogram of, *241, 248, 250*
Internal jugular vein, *21, 23, 244, 250*
Internal medullary lamina
  anatomy of, *68–69, 76, 144–145, 146–147, 148–149*
  questions regarding, 267Q, 272A, 277Q, 278A
Internal occipital veins, *29*
Internuclear ophthalmoplegia, 192, 200, 228
Interparietal sulcus, *18*
Interpeduncular cistern, *50–51*
Interpeduncular fossa
  anatomy of, *20, 24, 31, 38–41, 67–69, 78, 128–129, 137*
  aneurysm of, 256Q, 259A
  questions regarding, 256Q, 259A
Interpeduncular nucleus, *128–129, 130–131*
Interstitial nucleus, *210–211*
Interventricular foramen, *31, 52, 60, 150–151*
Intervertebral ligament, *47*
Ipsilateral facial paralysis, 124

J

Jaw reflex, 184
Jugular bulb, *244*
Juxtarestiform body, *108–109, 114–115, 116–117, 208–209, 228–229*

K

Kayser-Fleischer ring, 214
Kinetic tremor, 208
Kluver-Bucy syndrome, 234
Korsakoff syndrome, 232

L

Labyrinthine artery
  anatomy of, *25, 27, 37*
  questions regarding, 254Q, 258A
Lacrimal gland, 203
Lacrimal reflex, 184
Lacunar strokes, 190, 192
Lamina
  external medullary, *140–141, 144–145, 146–147, 148–149, 171*
  internal medullary
    anatomy of, *68–69, 76, 144–145, 146–147, 148–149*
    questions regarding, 267Q, 272A, 277Q, 278A
Lamina terminalis, *31, 40, 52, 78, 166, 168, 170, 232–233, 234–235*
Lamina terminalis cistern, *50–51*
Lancinating pain, 178
Lateral cerebellar nucleus, *208–209*
Lateral cervical nucleus, *182–183*

Lateral cortex, *208–209*
Lateral corticospinal tract
    anatomy of, *84, 86, 88, 90, 92, 95, 111, 163, 190–191, 194–195, 196–197*
    questions regarding, 266Q, 272A
Lateral dorsal nucleus of thalamus, *159, 163, 165, 167*
Lateral geniculate body, *26–27, 34–37, 58–59, 61*
Lateral geniculate nucleus
    anatomy of, *70, 77–78, 132–133, 134–135, 140–141, 148–149, 159, 168, 171, 220–222, 226–227*
    blood supply to, *220–221*
    questions regarding, 286Q, 294A
Lateral hypothalamic area, *150–151, 234–235*
Lateral lacunae, *47*
Lateral lemniscus
    anatomy of, *116–117, 118–119, 120–121, 122–123, 125, 126–127, 137, 167, 170*
    blood supply to, *226–227*
    nucleus, *226–227*
Lateral longitudinal stria, *138–139, 144–145, 146–147, 150–151, 152–153, 154–155, 156–157*
Lateral medullary syndrome, *81*, 110, 186, 220
Lateral motor cell column, *175*
Lateral motor nuclei, *84, 86, 90*
Lateral nucleus
    basal-lateral nuclei, *234–235*
    of cerebellum, 209
    of pulvinar, *140–141, 142–143*
Lateral olfactory stria, *26, 152–153, 154–155*
Lateral pontine syndrome, 124, 206
Lateral posterior choroidal artery, *251*
Lateral rectus, 201
Lateral reticular nucleus, *100–101, 102–103, 104–105, 196–197, 206–207, 210–211*
Lateral sulcus, *13, 176–177*
Lateral thalamic nuclei, *75–77*
Lateral ventricle, *176–177*
    anterior horn of, *54, 60, 64, 75–76, 152–153, 154–155, 156–157, 165,* 262Q, 264A
    atrium of, *52–54, 75–77, 138–139, 166, 171,* 276Q, 277A
    body of, *52–53, 66–71, 74, 140–141, 144–145, 146–147*
    inferior horn of, *52–53, 58, 67–72, 78, 138–139, 140–141, 144–145, 146–147, 148–149, 170–171*
    posterior horn of, *52–53, 58, 72, 76–78*
    questions regarding, 276Q, 277A
    temporal horn of, *54,* 262Q, 263A
Lateral ventricular vein, *248*
Lateral vestibular nucleus
    anatomy of, *108–109, 114–115, 116–117, 196–197, 210–211, 228–229*
    questions regarding, 268Q, 273A
Lateral vestibulospinal tract, *86, 88, 90, 92, 196–197, 208–209, 228–229*
Lead pipe rigidity, 214
Left cerebral hemisphere
    dissection of, *58*
    lateral view of, *18, 45*
    magnetic resonance imaging of, *45*
    medial aspect of, *58*

Left inferior visual quadrant, *15*
Left superior visual quadrant, *15*
Legs, spastic weakness of, 178
Lemniscus
    lateral
        anatomy of, *116–117, 118–119, 120–121, 122–123, 125, 126–127, 137, 167, 170*
        blood supply to, *226–227*
        nucleus, *226–227*
    medial
        anatomy of, *79–81, 100–101, 102–103, 104–105, 106–107, 111, 120–121, 122–123, 126–127, 128–129, 132–133, 134–135, 163, 165, 167–168, 170, 178–179, 180–181, 182–183, 184–185, 190–191, 194–195, 196–197, 200–201, 202–203, 204–205, 206–207, 210–211, 220–221, 226–227, 228–229*
        questions regarding, 283Q, 291A
Lenticular fasciculus, *144–145, 146–147, 148–149, 150–151, 165, 167, 169, 216–217*
Lenticular nucleus, *57*
Lenticulostriate arteries
    anatomy of, *25*
    questions regarding, 257Q, 260A
Leptomeningitis, 46
Lesions
    amygdaloid nuclear complex, 234
    brainstem, 192
    forebrain, 158
    midbrain, 136
    pons, 284Q, 292A
    spinal cord, 94
    subthalamic nucleus, 158
    trigeminal nerve, 184, 202
    upper motor neuron, 190
Levator palpebrae, 201
Level of obex, *34, 102–103*
Limen insulae, *45*
Lingual gyrus, *14, 20, 28, 30*
Lobe
    cerebellum
        anterior, *40–41, 79*
        posterior, *79–81*
    flocculonodular, *204–205*
    frontal, *38–39*
    occipital, *79*
    temporal, *20, 38–39, 41, 45, 64, 79–80*
Lobule
    anterior quadrangular, *32*
    biventer, *32*
    gracile, *32*
    inferior parietal, 14, *14*
    inferior semilunar, *32*
    posterior quadrangular, *32*
    superior parietal, *16, 56*
    superior semilunar, *32*
Locus ceruleus, *122–123,* 184
Long insular gyri, *56*
Longitudinal fissure, *16, 22*
Lower back pain, 94
Lower extremity
    paralysis of, 94
    weakness of, 265Q, 271A

Lumbar cistern
    anatomy of, *47, 85*
    questions regarding, 256Q, 260A
Lumbar puncture
    description of, 12
    questions regarding, 256Q, 259A

M
Magnetic resonance angiography, *245*
Magnetic resonance imaging
    abducens nerve, *42*
    advantages of, 4
    ambient cistern, *50–51*
    amygdaloid nuclear complex, *66–67*
    anterior cerebral artery, *20, 27, 38, 40, 78*
    anterior commissure, *31, 65, 77*
    anterior communicating artery, *27, 38*
    anterior forceps, *74*
    anterior inferior cerebellar artery, *42*
    anterior median fissure, *81*
    anterior medullary velum, *31*
    anterior nucleus, 66
    anterior paracentral gyrus, *28, 30*
    basilar artery, *41–42, 50, 79–80*
    basilar pons, *22, 30–32, 38–42, 50, 67–68, 70, 79–80*
    bulb of eye, *38–39*
    calcarine sulcus, *28, 30*
    caudate nucleus, *74*
        body of, *69–71*
        head of, *64–66, 75–77*
    central sulcus, *18, 28, 30, 44*
        of the insula, *44*
    cerebellar hemisphere, *42*
    cerebellar lobules, *33*
    cerebellar tonsil, *42–44*
    cerebellar vermis, *42*
    cerebellum, *20, 22, 30, 39, 41–42, 44, 51, 78*
        anterior lobe of, *32, 40–41*
            hemisphere of, *79*
            vermis of, *79*
        posterior lobe of
            hemisphere of, *80–81*
            vermis of, *80–81*
        tonsil of, *30, 32, 42, 81*
    cerebral aqueduct, *20, 27, 31, 49, 70–71, 78*
    cingulate gyrus, *28, 30, 64*
    cingulate sulcus, *28, 30*
    cingulum, *64*
    cisterna magna, *50*
    claustrum, *64–66, 162*
    cochlea, *42*
    colliculi, *20*
    colloid cyst, *28*
    corona radiata, *65–68, 74–75*
    corpus callosum, *28, 39, 74*
        body of, *30, 64, 65, 66, 67–71*
        genu of, *30*
        rostrum of, *30, 64*
        splenium of, *30, 71–72, 76–77*
        sulcus of, *28, 30*
    crural cistern, *50–51*
    crus cerebri, *20, 27, 38, 40–41, 68–69, 78*
    cuneus, *28, 30*
    dentate nucleus, *80*
    description of, 3
    disadvantages of, 4

Magnetic resonance imaging (*Continued*)
  dorsal thalamus, *31, 38–39, 75*
  epidural hematoma, *48*
  external capsule, *64–67*
  extreme capsule, *64–67*
  facial nerve, *42*
  flocculus, *43*
  fornix, *30*
    body of, *31, 67–70*
    column of, *65–66, 76–77*
    crus of, *71–72, 77*
    fimbria of, *70–71*
  fourth ventricle, *22, 31–32, 39–40, 42, 50,*
    72, 79–81
  frontal lobe, *38–39, 49*
  globus pallidus, *65–68, 76–77*
  glossopharyngeal nerve, *43*
  gyri breves, *44*
  gyri longi, *44*
  gyrus rectus, *20, 22*
  habenular nucleus, *76*
  hemorrhage, *49*
  hippocampal commissure, *72*
  hippocampal formation, *67–71, 76–78*
  hippocampus, *66*
  hypoglossal nerve, *44*
  hypothalamus, *27, 31, 78*
  image types, *3*
  inferior cerebellopontine cistern, *50*
  inferior colliculus, *31–32, 39, 50, 72, 78*
  inferior frontal gyrus
    pars opercularis, *18*
    pars orbitalis, *18*
    pars triangularis, *18*
  inferior frontal sulcus, *18*
  infundibulum, *31, 38, 65*
  insula, *51, 64–68, 76–77*
  insular cortex, *50*
  internal capsule, *66, 75*
    anterior limb of, *64–65, 76–77, 162*
    genu of, *76, 162*
    posterior limb of, *67–69, 76–77, 162*
    retrolenticular limb of, *76*
  internal carotid artery, *39, 41*
  internal cerebral vein, *28, 31*
  internal medullary lamina, *68–69*
  interpeduncular cistern, *50–51*
  interpeduncular fossa, *20, 31, 38–41, 68–69,*
    78
  lamina terminalis cistern, *50–51*
  lateral geniculate nucleus, *70, 77*
  lateral medullary syndrome, *81*
  lateral sulcus, *18*
  lateral thalamic nuclei, *76–77*
  lateral ventricle, *75*
    anterior horn of, *64, 75–76*
    atrium of, *75–77*
    body of, *66–71, 74*
    inferior horn of, *67, 69–72, 78*
    posterior horn of, *72, 76–78*
  limen insulae, *44*
  lingual gyrus, *28, 30*
  mammillary body, *20, 31, 38, 40, 67, 78*
  mammillothalamic tract, *77*
  marginal sulcus, *28, 30*
  medial geniculate nucleus, *70, 77*
  medial lemniscus, *79*
  medulla, *30, 32, 44, 50, 71–72*

  midbrain, *32, 38, 40, 50–51*
  midbrain tegmentum, *30, 38, 40–41*
  middle cerebellar peduncle, *22, 41, 70–72,*
    80
  middle cerebral artery, *20, 65*
  middle frontal gyrus, *44*
  middle frontal sulcus, *18*
  middle temporal gyrus, *18*
  nucleus accumbens, *64*
  occipital gyri, *18*
  occipital lobe, *79*
  oculomotor nerve, *39–40*
  olfactory sulcus, *20, 22*
  olfactory tract, *64*
  olivary eminence, *43–44, 81*
  olive (inferior), *43*
  optic chiasm, *31, 38–39, 65*
  optic nerve, *38, 64*
  optic radiations, *72, 77*
  optic tract, *20, 38–40, 50, 66, 78*
  orbital gyri, *20, 22*
  paracallosal cistern, *50*
  paracentral sulcus, *28, 30*
  parieto-occipital sulcus, *28, 30*
  parolfactory gyri, *28*
  periaqueductal gray, *71*
  pineal, *31*
  pons-medulla junction, *42*
  pontine tegmentum, *30, 41–42, 79–80*
  postcentral gyrus, *44*
  postcentral sulcus, *18*
  posterior cerebral artery, *27, 39–40, 77*
  posterior communicating artery, *27*
  posterior forceps, *74*
  posterior lobe, *32*
  posterior paracentral gyrus, *28, 30*
  postolivary sulcus, *43–44, 81*
  precentral gyrus, *44*
  precentral sulcus, *18, 28*
  precuneus, *28, 30*
  premedullary cistern, *50*
  preolivary sulcus, *43–44, 81*
  prepontine cistern, *50*
  pretectal area, *70*
  pulvinar, *70–71, 76*
  putamen, *64–69, 76*
  pyramids, *41, 43–44, 72, 81*
  quadrigeminal cistern, *31, 50–51*
  questions regarding, *257Q, 261A, 276Q,*
    277A, 277Q, 278A
  radiofrequency pulse, *3*
  red nucleus, *27, 69, 77*
  restiform body, *43–44, 81*
  retroolivary (postolivary) sulcus, *43*
  semicircular canals, *42*
  septum, *65*
  septum pellucidum, *31, 74–75*
  subdural hematoma, *48*
  subdural hemorrhage, *50*
  substantia nigra, *68, 78*
  superior cerebellar artery, *39–41*
  superior cerebellar peduncle, *32, 72, 79*
  superior cerebellopontine cistern, *50*
  superior colliculus, *31–32, 39, 71, 77*
  superior frontal gyrus, *28, 30, 44*
  superior temporal gyrus, *18*
  superior temporal sulcus, *18*
  supraoptic recess, *51*

  Sylvian cistern, *50–51*
  T1, *3, 4, 267Q, 273A*
  T2, *3, 4*
  tapetum, *72, 77*
  temporal horn, *49, 51*
  temporal lobe, *20, 38–39, 41, 44, 64, 79*
  temporal pole, *22*
  tentorium cerebelli, *31, 51*
  thalamus
    anterior nucleus of, *67*
    anterior tubercle of, *66*
    dorsomedial nucleus of, *68–69, 76–77*
    ventral anterior nucleus of, *66–67*
    ventral lateral nucleus of, *68*
    ventral posterolateral nucleus of, *69*
  third ventricle, *41, 49, 51, 65–68, 76, 78*
  transverse temporal gyrus, *44*
  trigeminal ganglion, *41, 80*
  trigeminal nerve, *22, 41, 50, 69, 80*
  trochlear nerve, *40*
  uncus, *20, 38–39*
  vagus nerve, *43–44*
  ventral anterior nucleus, *66–67*
  vestibulocochlear nerve, *42*
Magnetic resonance venography, 250
Mammillary body
  anatomy of, *20, 24–27, 31, 37–38, 40,*
    52–53, 59, 67, 78, 146–147, 159, 163,
    170, 232–233
  blood supply to, *232–233*
Mammillotegmental tract, 232–233
Mammillothalamic tract
  anatomy of, *67, 77, 134–135, 142–143,*
    146–147, 148–149, 163–166, 168,
    232–233
  questions regarding, *263Q, 264A*
Marginal sulcus, *13, 28, 30*
Massa intermedia, *52–53, 60, 68, 77*
Masticatory muscles
  innervation of, 203
  paralysis of, *124, 202*
Maxillary artery, 252
Medial accessory olivary nucleus, *100–101,*
    102–103, 104–105, 106–107,
    206–207, 210–211
Medial cerebellar nucleus, 208–209
Medial decussation, 111
Medial division fibers, 86
Medial frontal cortex, 232–233
Medial geniculate body, *26–27, 34–37, 58–59,*
    61
Medial geniculate nucleus
  anatomy of, *70, 77, 130–131, 140–141, 159,*
    164, 166, 168–169, 220–222,
    226–227, 234–235
  blood supply to, 220–221
Medial lemniscus
  anatomy of, *79–81, 100–101, 102–103,*
    104–105, 106–107, 111, 120–121,
    122–123, 126–127, 128–129,
    132–133, 134–135, 163, 165,
    167–168, 170, 178–179, 180–181,
    182–183, 184–185, 190–191,
    194–195, 196–197, 200–201,
    202–203, 204–205, 206–207,
    210–211, 220–221, 226–227,
    228–229
  questions regarding, *283Q, 291A*

Medial longitudinal fasciculus
    anatomy of, *86, 88, 90, 92, 95, 98–99,*
        100–101, 102–103, 104–105,
        106–107, 111, 112–113, 114–115,
        116–117, 118–119, 120–121, 125,
        126–127, 128–129, 130–131,
        132–133, 134–135, 137, 163, 170,
        178–179, 180–181, 190–191 194–195,
        196–197, 200–201, 202–203,
        208–209, 210–211, 226–227, 228–229
    rostral interstitial nucleus of, *192, 192–193*
Medial longitudinal stria, *138–139, 140–141,*
        144–145, 146–147, 150–151,
        152–153, 154–155, 156–157
Medial medullary syndrome, 110, 178, 190, 200
Medial midbrain syndrome, 136
Medial motor cell column, *175*
Medial motor nuclei, *84, 86, 88, 90, 92, 98–99*
Medial nucleus, *140–141, 142–143, 234–235*
Medial olfactory stria, *26, 154–155*
Medial pontine syndrome, 124, 178
Medial posterior choroidal artery, *159, 251*
Medial striate artery, *25, 251*
Medial thalamic nuclei, *234–235*
Medial thalamus, *35, 232–233*
Medial vestibular nucleus
    anatomy of, *104–105, 106–107, 108–109,*
        112–113, 114–115, 116–117,
        186–187, 194–195, 196–197,
        208–209, 210–211, 228–229
    questions regarding, 268Q, 273A
Medial vestibulospinal tract, *196–197, 208–209,*
        228–229
Medulla
    anatomy of, *22, 30–33, 44, 71–72*
    blood supply, *206–207*
    infarction of, 285Q, 293A
    questions regarding, 265Q, 268Q–269Q,
        271A, 271Q, 273A–274A, 276A,
        285Q, 293A
    transverse section of, *98–107*
Medulla oblongata, *81, 175*
Medullary reticulospinal fibers, *86*
Medullary reticulospinal tract, *88, 90, 92*
Medulloblastoma, 208
Meninges
    cerebral, 46
    schematic diagram of, *47*
    spinal, 46
Meningiomas, 46, 202, 220
Meningitis, 46
Mesencephalic nucleus, *116–117, 118–119,*
        120–121, 122–123, 125, 126–127,
        128–129, 130–131, 132–133, 137,
        175, 184–185, 202–203, 204–205,
        228–229
Mesencephalic tract, *116–117, 118–119,*
        120–121, 122–123, 125, 126–127,
        128–129, 130–131, 132–133, 175
Mesencephalon, *176–177*
Metencephalon, *176–177*
Meyer-Archambault loop, 220, 281Q, 290A
Micrographia, 214
Micturition, 94
Midbrain
    anatomy of, *32–33, 38*
    arteries of, 136, *137, 210–211*
    blood supply to, *210–211, 220–221*

cranial nerve positions, *175*
    lesions of, 136
    questions regarding, 270Q, 275A
    transverse section of, *128–129, 130–131,*
        132–133
    vascular syndromes of, 136
Midbrain tegmentum
    anatomy of, *30, 38, 40–41,* 140
    blood supply to, *220–221*
    questions regarding, 270Q, 275A
Middle alternating hemiplegia, 124, 200
Middle cerebellar peduncle, *22, 24–27, 32–36,*
        61, 70–72, 80, 118–119, 120–121,
        122–123, 169, 180–181, 206–207
Middle cerebral artery
    anatomy of, *21, 23, 27, 39, 64–65, 154–155*
    angiogram of, *240, 242, 245, 248–249, 252*
    angular branches of, *19, 240*
    anterior branches of, *19*
    anterior temporal branches of, *19*
    branches of, *17, 19, 25*
    cortical branches of, *242*
    insular branches of, *242, 248–250*
    lenticulostriate branches of, *21, 23, 159, 242*
    magnetic resonance imaging of, *20, 27*
    middle temporal branches of, *19*
    occlusion of, 158
    orbitofrontal branches of, *19, 21*
    parietal branches of, *19, 240*
    posterior parietal branches of, *19*
    posterior temporal branches of, *19*
    prerolandic branches of, *19*
    questions regarding, 295Q, 296A
    rolandic branches of, *19*
Middle frontal gyrus, *16, 18, 45*
Middle temporal gyrus, *18*
Middle temporal sulcus, *18*
Midline thalamic nuclei, *234–235*
Millard-Gubler syndrome, 190
Miosis, 220
Monoplegia, 190
Motilin, 208
Motor deficits, 94
Motor nucleus of the trigeminal nerve, 120
Mucous membranes, 203
Multiple sclerosis, 184, 200
Muscle(s)
    buccinator, 203
    digastric, 203
    facial expression, 203
    genioglossus, 201
    hyoglossus, 201
    lateral rectus, 201
    levator palpebrae, 201
    masticatory, 203
    mylohyoid, 203
    oblique
        inferior, 201
        superior, 201
    pharyngeal, 203
    platysma, 203
    sphincter of iris, 201
    stapedius, 203
    sternocleidomastoid, 201
    styloglossus, 201
    stylohyoid, 203
    stylopharyngeus, 203
    superior rectus, 201

tensor tympani, 203
    tensor veli palatini, 203
    trapezius, 201
Myasthenia gravis
    description of, 190, 200, 202
    questions regarding, 280Q, 288A
Mydriasis, 196
Myelencephalon, *176–177*
Mylohyoid, 203

N
Nasal hemianopsia, 220
Nausea, 228
Nerve(s)
    abducens
        anatomy of, *22–27, 37, 41–42, 114–115,*
            116, *116–117, 118–119, 125, 175,*
            200–201
        questions regarding, 257Q, 260A
        rostral portions of, 118
    accessory, *24, 27, 35, 37, 175, 200–201*
    cochlear, *106–107*
    facial
        anatomy of, *22–27, 37, 41–44, 108–109,*
            114–115, 116, *118–119, 125, 167,*
            202–203
        internal genu, *116–117, 118–119*
        questions regarding, 285Q, 293A
    glossopharyngeal
        angiogram of 106, *22, 24–25, 27, 35, 37,*
            42–43, 81, 106–107, 202–203
        root of, 106
    hypoglossal
        anatomy of, *24, 27, 37, 42–44, 100–101,*
            104–105, 111, 200–201
        fascicles of, *100–101*
    nuclei, 98, 100, 102, 104, 106, 108, 116,
        120, 122, 126, 128, 130, 132, 134,
        140, 142
    oculomotor, *23–25, 27, 31, 37, 39–40, 67,*
        130–131, 132–133, 137, 148–149,
        163, 200–201, 220–221, 252
    optic, *20, 23–26, 31, 38, 40, 58–59, 64, 163,*
        220–221
    questions regarding, 255Q, 257Q, 259A,
        261A, 269Q, 275A
    trigeminal, *23–25, 69, 80, 116–117, 122,*
        202–203
        anatomy of, *41*
        chief sensory nucleus of, 120, *167,*
            184–185
        lesions of, 184, 202
        mandibular division of, *184–185*
        maxillary division of, *184–185*
        motor nucleus of, 120
        motor root, *26–27, 33, 36–37*
        ophthalmic division of, *184–185*
        pathways of, *184–185*
        sensory root, *26–27, 33, 36–37, 41*
    trochlear, *23–27, 33–37, 40, 72, 122,*
        122–123, 125, 126–127, 138–139,
        163, 175, 200–201
    vagus
        anatomy of, *22, 24, 27, 35, 37, 42–44, 81,*
            104–105, 202–203
        dorsal motor nucleus of, *100–101,*
            102–103, 104–105, 111, 175,
            202–203

Nerve(s) (*Continued*)
vestibulocochlear
anatomy of, *22–27, 36–37, 41–42, 44, 81*
questions regarding, 283Q, 291A
Nerve deafness, 226
Neural tube, 174
Neuralgia
glossopharyngeal, 186
trigeminal
description of, 41, 184, 202
questions regarding, 255Q, 259A
Neurotensin, 186, 234
Neurotransmitters (*see also specific neurotransmitter*)
N-acetylaspartylglutamate, 220, 222
acetylcholine, *178*, 190, 200, 202, 220, 234
aspartate, 196, 206, 210, 226
calcitonin gene-related peptide, 180, 200, 202
cholecystokinin, 180, 184, 186, 222, 226, 232
description of, 176
dopamine, 214, 216
dynorphin, 214
enkephalin, 180, 186, 194, 214, 226, 232, 234
gamma-aminobutyric acid, 186, 190, 196, 208, 210, 214, 216, 228, 232
glutamate, 180, 182, 190, 192, 194, 196, 204, 206, 210, 214, 226, 232, 234
glycine, 216
motilin, 208
neurotensin, 186, 234
questions regarding, 278Q, 284Q, 287A, 292A
serotonin, 180, 214, 216
somatostatin, 180, 186, 232, 234
substance P, 180, 182, 184, 186, 190, 194, 214, 234
taurine, 208
vasoactive intestinal polypeptide, 180, 234
Nigroamygdaloid fibers, *216–217*
Nigrocollicular fibers, *216–217*
Nigrostriatal fibers, *130–131, 132–133, 148–149, 214–215*
Nigrosubthalamic fibers, *216–217*
Nigrotectal fibers, *216–217*
Nigrothalamic fibers, *216–217*
Nodulus, *32*
Nucleocortical fibers, *208–209*
Nucleus(i)
abducens, *108–109*, 114, 116, *125, 163, 192–193, 200–201, 202–203, 226–227, 228–229*
accessory, *98–99, 192–193, 200–201*
accessory cuneate, *100–101, 102–103, 104–105, 204–205*
accumbens
anatomy of, *64, 78, 154–155, 232–233, 234–235*
questions regarding, 262Q, 263A
ambiguus, *100–101, 102–103, 104–105, 106–107, 111, 175, 186–187, 192–193, 202–203*
amygdaloid, *150–151, 152–153*
anterior cochlear, *106–107, 108–109, 112–113, 226–227*
anterior nucleus of thalamus, *66, 146–147, 148–149, 232–233*

arcuate, *100–101, 102–103, 104–105, 106–107,* 108
basal, 213–217
of Meynert, *150–151, 152–153*
questions regarding, 262Q, 264A, 276Q, 277A
basal-lateral, *234–235*
of Cajal, *134–135*
caudate
axial view of, *74*
blood supply to, *214–215*
body of, *52–53, 67–68, 70–71, 138–139, 140–141, 144–145, 146–147, 148–149, 159, 171*
coronal view of, *138–139*
general images of, *61, 169, 176–177, 214–215, 216–217, 234–235*
head of, *52, 60, 64–65, 75–78, 152–153, 154–155, 156–157, 162, 164, 166–167,* 265Q, 271A
questions regarding, 262Q, 263A, 265Q, 271A
tail of, *52–53, 68–71, 75–78, 138–139, 140–141, 144–145, 148–149, 159, 162, 164, 168, 170*
veins of, *29*
central, *234–235*
centralis, *122–123, 126–127, 234–235*
centromedian nucleus of thalamus, *69, 76, 142–143, 162, 164–167, 176–177, 210–211, 216–217*
cerebellum, *204–205, 206–207, 208–209, 228–229*
chief sensory nucleus of trigeminal nerve, 120, *167, 184–185, 204–205*
cochlear
anatomy of, *175, 226–227*
anterior, *106–107, 108–109, 112–113, 226–227*
blood supply to, *226–227*
posterior, *106–107, 111, 112–113, 169, 226–227*
coeruleus, *79, 120–121, 126–127, 206–207, 234–235*
cortical, *234–235*
cranial nerves, 98, 100, 102, 104, 106, 108, 116, 120, 122, 126, 128, 130, 132, 134, 140, 142
cuneate, *98–99, 100–101, 102–103, 178–179, 182–183*
cuneatus, 100, *165, 167*
of Darkschewitsch, *134–135, 180–181, 210–211*
dentate, *80, 112–113, 114–115, 169, 171, 210–211*
dorsal accessory olivary, *206–207, 210–211*
dorsal column, 100
dorsal motor nucleus of vagus nerve, *100–101, 102–103, 104–105, 111, 175, 202–203*
dorsal motor vagal, *234–235*
dorsal thoracic nucleus of Clarke, *88, 204–205*
dorsomedial nucleus of thalamus
anatomy of, *67–69, 75–76, 144–145, 146–147, 162–165, 167, 176–177*
questions regarding, 263Q, 265A
Edinger-Westphal, 130, 132, *132–133, 137, 175, 200–201, 210–211, 220–221*

emboliform, *112–113, 114–115, 167, 210–211*
facial, 118, *165, 184–185, 192–193, 196–197, 202–203, 226–227*
facial motor, 108, *114–115, 116–117, 118–119, 125, 175*
fastigial, *112–113, 114–115, 163, 210–211*
gigantocellular reticular, *194–195*
globose, *112–113, 114–115, 210–211*
gracile, *98–99, 100–101, 102–103, 178–179, 182–183*
gracilis, 100, *163, 165*
habenular, *76, 162–163*
hypoglossal, 100, *100–101,* 102, *102–103, 104–105, 111, 163, 175, 184–185, 186–187, 192–193, 200–201, 202–203, 228–229*
hypothalamic, *150–151*
inferior pulvinar, *140–141*
inferior salivatory, *106–107, 175, 202–203*
inferior vestibular, *104–105, 106–107, 112–113, 186–187, 196–197, 208–209, 210–211*
interpeduncular, *128–129, 130–131*
interstitial, *210–211*
lateral, *140–141, 142–143, 234–235*
lateral cerebellar, *208–209*
lateral cervical, *182–183*
lateral dorsal nucleus of thalamus, *159, 163, 165, 167*
lateral geniculate
anatomy of, *70, 77–78, 132–133, 134–135, 140–141, 148–149, 159, 168, 171, 220–222, 226–227*
blood supply to, *220–221*
questions regarding, 286Q, 294A
lateral motor, *84, 86, 90*
lateral nuclei (basal-lateral nuclei), *234–235*
lateral reticular, *100–101, 102–103, 104–105, 196–197, 206–207, 210–211*
lateral thalamic, *75–77*
lateral vestibular
anatomy of, *108–109, 114–115, 116–117, 196–197, 210–211, 228–229*
questions regarding, 268Q, 273A
lenticular, *57*
medial, *140–141, 142–143, 234–235*
medial accessory olivary, *100–101, 102–103, 104–105, 106–107, 206–207, 210–211*
medial cerebellar, *208–209*
medial geniculate
anatomy of, *70, 77, 130–131, 140–141, 159, 164, 166, 168–169, 220–222, 226–227, 234–235*
blood supply to, *220–221*
medial motor, *84, 86, 88, 90, 92, 98–99*
medial thalamic, *234–235*
medial vestibular
anatomy of, *104–105, 106–107, 108–109, 112–113, 114–115, 116–117, 186–187, 194–195, 196–197, 208–209, 210–211, 228–229*
questions regarding, 268Q, 273A
mesencephalic, *116–117, 118–119, 120–121, 122–123, 125, 126–127, 128–129, 130–131, 132–133, 137, 175,*

184–185, 202–203, 204–205, 228–229
midline thalamic, 234–235
motor nucleus of the trigeminal nerve, 120
oculomotor
    anatomy of, 130–131, 132–133, 137, 175, 192–193, 194–195, 196–197, 200–201, 210–211, 228–229
    blood supply to, 228–229
parabrachial, 186–187, 234–235
parafascicular, 234–235
paramedian reticular, 206–207
pedunculopontine, 216–217
peripeduncular, 132–133, 134–135
pontine, 108–109, 116–117, 118–119, 122–123, 126–127, 128–129, 206–207
pontobulbar, 106–107, 108–109
posterior accessory olivary, 102–103, 104–105, 106–107
posterior cochlear, 106–107, 111, 112–113, 169, 226–227
posterior thalamic, 158
posteromarginal, 84, 86, 88, 90
preoptic, 234–235
prepositus, 106–107, 111, 112–113
pretectal
    anatomy of, 134–135, 163, 220–221
    blood supply to, 220–221
principal olivary
    anatomy of, 100–101, 102–103, 104–105, 106–107, 108–109, 163, 165, 178–179, 190–191, 194–195, 200–201, 206–207, 210–211
    questions regarding, 271Q, 276A
principal sensory, 116–117, 118–119, 120–121, 175, 202–203, 204–205
proprius, 84, 86, 88, 90, 175
pulvinar, 35
raphe, 206–207, 214–215, 216–217
    dorsalis, 122–123, 126–127, 128–129, 180–181, 234–235
    magnus, 108–109, 116–117, 118–119, 180–181, 234–235
    obscurus, 102–103, 104–105, 106–107, 234–235
    pallidus, 106–107, 108–109, 234–235
    pontis, 120–121
red, 27, 59, 68–69, 77, 130–131, 134–135, 144–145, 148–149, 159, 163, 165, 167–168, 178–179, 180–181, 184–185, 190–191, 194–195, 196–197, 200–201, 206–207, 210–211, 220–221, 228–229
reticular, 194–195
reticulotegmental, 120–121, 206–207
salivatory, 186–187
septal, 152–153, 232–233, 234–235
solitary, 100–101, 102–103, 104–105, 106–107, 108–109, 111, 112–113, 116–117, 165, 175, 186–187, 228–229, 234–235
    cardiorespiratory portion of, 186–187
    gustatory portion of, 186–187
spinal accessory, 92
spinal cord, 175
spinal trigeminal, 102–103, 106–107, 111, 112–113, 114–115, 116–117,

118–119, 125, 175, 184–185, 202–203, 204–205
    gelatinosa portion of, 92, 98–99
    magnocellular portion of, 92, 98–99
    pars caudalis, 98–99, 100–101
    pars interpolaris, 102–103
    pars oralis, 106–107, 108–109, 112–113, 114–115, 116–117
spinal vestibular nucleus, 194–195
of the stria terminalis, 234–235
subthalamic
    anatomy of, 68, 77, 134–135, 142–143, 144–145, 146–147, 148–149, 159, 169, 176–177, 214–215, 216–217
    lesions of, 158
    questions regarding, 263Q, 265A
superior salivatory, 118–119, 175, 202–203
superior vestibular, 108–109, 114–115, 116–117, 118–119, 196–197, 208–209, 210–211
supramammillary, 232–233
supraoptic, 134–135, 152–153, 167
tegmental, 232–233
thalamic reticular, 144–145, 146–147, 148–149, 171
trapezoid, 116–117, 226–227
trigeminal, 125
trigeminal motor
    anatomy of, 116–117, 118–119, 120–121, 167, 175, 184–185, 192–193, 202–203, 204–205, 210–211
    questions regarding, 280Q, 289A
trochlear
    anatomy of, 128–129, 137, 140–141, 192–193, 200–201, 228–229
    blood supply to, 228–229
ventral anterior, 66–67, 75–76, 150–151, 162, 164–165, 167, 216–217
ventral lateral, 68, 76, 144–145, 162, 164, 166–167, 169, 171, 210–211, 216–217
ventral posterior thalamic nuclei, 77
ventral posterolateral nucleus of thalamus, 69, 76, 142–143, 162, 164, 166, 171, 176–177, 178–179, 180–181, 184–185, 210–211
ventral posteromedial nucleus of thalamus, 69, 142–143, 164, 166, 169, 176–177, 184–185, 186–187
ventromedial hypothalamic, 232–233, 234–235
vestibular
    anatomy of, 125, 175, 204–205
    blood supply, 208–209, 228–229
    disorders of, 228
    inferior, 104–105, 106–107, 112–113, 186–187, 196–197, 208–209, 210–211
    lateral, 108–109, 114–115, 116–117, 196–197, 210–211
    medial, 104–105, 106–107, 108–109, 112–113, 114–115, 116–117, 186–187, 194–195, 196–197, 208–209, 210–211
    neurotransmitters, 228
    questions regarding, 284Q, 292A
    spinal, 194–195

superior, 108–109, 114–115, 116–117, 118–119, 196–197, 208–209, 210–211
Nystagmus, 110, 136, 206, 208, 228

O
Obex, 34
    level of, 102, 102–103
Objective vertigo, 228
Occipital lobe, 79
Occipital pole, 20
Occipital sinus, 19, 23, 29
Occipitofrontal fasciculus, 57
Occipitopontine fibers, 126–127, 128–129, 130–131, 132–133, 134–135, 206–207
Occipitotemporal sulcus, 22
Oculomotor nerve, 23–25, 27, 31, 37, 39–40, 67, 130–131, 132–133, 137, 148–149, 163, 200–201, 220–221, 252
Oculomotor nucleus
    anatomy of, 130–131, 132–133, 137, 175, 192–193, 194–195, 196–197, 200–201, 210–211, 228–229
    blood supply to, 228–229
Olfactory bulb, 20, 22, 234–235
Olfactory sulcus, 20, 22, 156–157
Olfactory tract, 20, 22, 24–26, 59, 64, 156–157, 165
Olivary eminence, 22, 24–26, 42, 44, 81
Olive, 22, 24–26, 43, 102–103
    amiculum of, 102–103, 104–105, 106–107
    superior, 108–109, 116–117, 118–119, 120–121, 226–227
Olivocerebellar fibers, 102–103, 104–105, 106–107, 167, 206–207
Olivopontocerebellar degeneration, 206
Ondine's curse, 110
One-and-a-half syndrome, 192
Ophthalmic artery
    anatomy of, 25, 240, 249–250
    questions regarding, 294Q, 296A
Optic chiasm
    anatomy of, 20, 23, 25–26, 31, 38–39, 52, 58–59, 65, 154–155, 220–221, 232–233, 234–235
    questions regarding, 263Q, 264A
Optic nerve, 20, 23–26, 31, 38, 40, 58–59, 64, 163, 220–221
Optic radiations
    anatomy of, 57, 61, 72, 76–77, 138–139, 140–141, 162, 164, 166, 168, 170–171
    questions regarding, 263Q, 264A
Optic tract
    anatomy of, 20, 23–25, 27, 37, 39–40, 50, 58–59, 66–69, 78, 132–133, 134–135, 144–145, 146–147, 148–149, 150–151, 152–153, 165, 167–171, 220–221
    blood supply to, 220–221
    questions regarding, 257Q, 260A, 263Q, 264A
Orbital sulci, 22
Orbitofrontal artery, 17
Otic ganglion, 202–203
Otitis media, 226
Otosclerosis, 226

P

Pain
  intractable, 180, 182
  lancinating, 178
Pain sensation
  areas of, 98, 100, 102, 104, 106, 108, 116,
    120, 122, 126, 128, 130, 132, 134,
    140, 142
  loss of, 94, 110, 124, 158, 178
Palatal musculature weakness, 110
Pallidonigral fibers, *130–131, 132–133,
    148–149, 216–217*
Palsy
  Bell, 186, 202
  facial, 228
    Bell, 186, 202
    central, 192
    ipsilateral, 202
  gaze, 192
  horizontal gaze, 192
  vertical gaze, 192
Parabrachial nuclei, *186–187, 234–235*
Paracallosal cistern, *50*
Paracentral sulcus, *13, 28, 30*
Parafascicular nuclei, *234–235*
Parahippocampal gyrus, *20, 22, 24, 28*
Paralysis
  eye movement, 136
  facial muscles, 136
  ipsilateral facial, 94
  lower extremity, 94
  masticatory muscles, 124, 202
  upper extremity, 94
  upward gaze, 136
Paramedian pontine reticular formation,
    192–193
Paramedian reticular nuclei, *206–207*
Paraplegia, 94, 190
Paraterminal gyri, *28, 154–155*
Paresthesias, 180
Parietal artery, *17*
Parietooccipital sulcus, *13, 28, 30*
Parietopontine fibers, *126–127, 128–129,
    130–131, 132–133, 134–135,
    206–207*
Parinaud syndrome, 136, 192
Parkinson's disease
  description of, 158, 214
  questions regarding, 282Q, 290A
Parolfactory gyri, *28*
Parotid gland, 203
Pathways
  amygdalofugal, *234–235*
  auditory system, *226–227*
  pupillary, *220–221*
  solitary, *186–187*
  trigeminal nerve, *184–185*
  vestibular, *228–229*
  visual, *222–223*
Peduncle
  inferior cerebellar, *32, 34–35, 61, 108–109,
    114–115*
  middle cerebellar, *22, 24–27, 32–36, 61,
    70–72, 80, 118–119, 120–121,
    122–123, 169, 180–181, 206–207*
  superior cerebellar, *27, 32–37, 61, 70, 72,
    78–79, 114–115, 120–121, 122–123,
    206–207, 210–211*

brachium conjunctivum, *165, 167, 170*
  decussation, *130–131, 163, 170,
    200–201, 210–211, 226–227,
    228–229*
Pedunculopontine nucleus, *216–217*
Periaqueductal gray, *59, 70–71, 78, 122–123,
    128–129, 130–131, 132–133,
    134–135, 137, 140–141, 166,
    180–181, 210–211, 228–229,
    234–235*
Peripeduncular nucleus, *132–133, 134–135*
Pharyngeal musculature weakness, 110
Pia mater, 46, *47*
Pick disease, 232, 234
Pineal gland
  anatomy of, *21, 31, 34–35, 52, 60, 71, 77,
    134–135, 138–139, 232–233,
    234–235*
  questions regarding, 262Q, 264A
Pineal recess, *52*
Pituitary adenoma, 220
Pituitary gland, *31*
Placidity, 234
Platysma, 203
Polar temporal artery, *25*
Pole
  frontal, *20, 22*
  occipital, *20*
  temporal, *20, 22, 28*
Polyneuropathy, 200
Pons
  arteries of, 124, *125, 206–207*
  blood supply, 124, *125, 206–207*
  caudal, *116–117*
  cranial nerve positions, *175*
  lesions of, 284Q, 292A
  questions regarding, 268Q, 273A, 284Q,
    292A
  tegmentum of, *79–80*
  transverse section of, *114–115, 118–119,
    120–121, 122–123*
Pons-medulla junction, *54*
Pontine arteries, *25*
Pontine gliomas, 200
Pontine nuclei, *108–109, 116–117, 118–119,
    122–123, 126–127, 128–129,
    206–207*
Pontine syndrome, 124
Pontine tegmentum, *30, 41–42*
Pontobulbar nucleus, *106–107, 108–109*
Pontocerebellar fibers, *116–117, 118–119,
    120–121, 122–123, 126–127,
    206–207*
Pontoreticulospinal tract, *86, 88, 90, 92*
Postcentral gyrus, *45, 56, 178–179, 180–181*
Postcentral sulcus, *13–14, 16, 18*
Posterior accessory olivary nucleus, *102–103,
    104–105, 106–107*
Posterior cerebral artery
  anatomy of, *21, 27, 29, 37, 39–40, 67,
    144–145*
  angiogram of, *244, 248–249, 251–252*
  anterior temporal branch of, *21, 29*
  branches of, *17, 27*
  calcarine branch of, *21, 29, 246, 249*
  cortical branches of, *27, 247*
  magnetic resonance imaging of, *27*
  parieto-occipital branch of, *21, 29, 246, 249*

posterior temporal branch of, *21, 29*
  posteromedial branches of, *159*
  temporal branch of, *248*
  thalamogeniculate branches of, *159*
  thalamoperforating branches of, *159*
Posterior choroidal arteries
  anatomy of, *25, 27, 35, 37*
  angiogram of, *246*
Posterior cochlear nucleus, *106–107, 111,
    112–113, 169, 226–227*
Posterior column fibers, 94
Posterior column-medial lemniscus system,
    178–179
Posterior commissure, *31, 52, 70, 134–135, 163,
    220–221*
Posterior communicating artery
  anatomy of, *23, 25, 27, 37, 39*
  angiogram of, *246, 248–249, 251*
  questions regarding, 295Q, 297A
Posterior forceps, *74*
Posterior inferior cerebellar artery
  anatomy of, *23, 25, 27, 31, 35–37*
  angiogram of, *246–247, 251*
  branches of, *24*
  questions regarding, 267Q, 269Q,
    273A–274A
Posterior inferior cerebellar artery syndrome,
    180, 184, 186
Posterior intermediate sulcus, *11, 34, 88, 90, 92*
Posterior longitudinal fasciculus, *100–101,
    102–103, 104–105, 106–107,
    116–117, 120–121, 126–127,
    128–129, 130–131, 132–133*
Posterior median sulcus, *11, 34, 86, 88, 90, 92*
Posterior paracentral gyrus, *14–15, 28, 30,
    178–179, 180–181*
Posterior perforated substance, *26, 59*
Posterior quadrangular lobule, *32*
Posterior root ganglion, *12, 178–179, 180–181,
    182–183, 204–205*
Posterior spinal artery
  anatomy of, *10, 23, 25, 27, 35, 37, 95*
  questions regarding, 267Q, 273A
Posterior spinal medullary artery, *10, 95*
Posterior spinocerebellar tract, *88, 90, 92, 95,
    98–99, 100–101, 111, 204–205*
Posterior superior fissure, *32*
Posterior tegmental decussation, *130–131,
    194–195, 196–197*
Posterior thalamic nuclei, 158
Posterior watershed infarcts, 158
Posterolateral fissure, *33*
Posterolateral sulcus, *11, 34, 88, 90*
Posteromarginal nucleus, *84, 86, 88, 90*
Postolivary sulcus, *43–44*
Postsynaptic-posterior column system, *182–183*
Posture, stuped, 158
Precentral gyrus, *18, 56, 190–191*
Precentral sulcus, *14–16, 18, 28*
Precuneus, *28, 30*
Premedullary cistern, *50*
Preoccipital notch, *13, 18*
Preolivary sulcus
  anatomy of, *24, 26, 44, 81, 100–101,
    102–103*
  questions regarding, 257Q, 261A
Preoptic nucleus, *234–235*
Prepiriform cortex, *234–235*

Prepontine cistern, *50*
Prerubral field, *165*
Pretectal area, *70*
Pretectal nuclei
    anatomy of, *134–135, 163, 220–221*
    blood supply to, *220–221*
Primary fissure, *32–33*
Principal olivary nucleus
    anatomy of, *100–101, 102–103, 104–105,
        106–107, 108–109, 163, 165,
        178–179, 190–191, 194–195,
        200–201, 206–207, 210–211*
    questions regarding, *271Q, 276A*
Principal sensory nucleus, *116–117, 118–119,
        120–121, 175, 202–203, 204–205*
Proprioception/vibratory sense
    areas of, 98, 100, 102, 104, 106, 108, 116,
        120, 122, 126, 128, 130, 132, 134,
        140, 142
    loss of, 124, 158, 178
Propriospinal fibers, *84, 86, 90, 92, 95*
Pterygopalatine ganglion, *202–203*
Ptosis, 190, 200, 220
Pulvinar
    anatomy of, *59, 61, 70–71, 76–77*
    questions regarding, *277Q, 278A*
Pulvinar nuclear complex, *34, 134–135,
        140–141, 142–143, 162, 164–167,
        169, 171, 220–222, 226–227*
Pulvinar nucleus, *35*
Pupillary light reflex, 220
Pupillary pathways, *220–221*
Putamen
    anatomy of, *64–69, 76–77, 148–149,
        150–151, 152–153, 154–155,
        156–157, 162, 164, 166, 169, 171,
        176–177, 214–215, 216–217,
        234–235*
    blood supply to, *214–215*
Pyramids
    anatomy of, *24–26, 41–44, 70, 72, 81,
        98–99, 111, 163, 178–179, 180–181,
        190–191, 194–195, 196–197,
        200–201, 204–205, 206–207,
        228–229*
    decussation of, *22, 24, 92, 98–99, 111*

Q
Quadrantanopsia, *285Q, 293A*
Quadrigeminal artery
    anatomy of, *25, 27, 35, 37*
    questions regarding, *254Q, 258A*
Quadrigeminal cistern
    anatomy of, *31, 50–51*
    questions regarding, *269Q, 274A*
Quadriplegia, 94, 190

R
Radiofrequency pulse, 3
Raphe nuclei, *206–207, 214–215, 216–217*
    dorsalis, *122–123, 126–127, 128–129,
        180–181, 234–235*
    magnus, *108–109, 116–117, 118–119,
        180–181, 234–235*
    obscurus, *102–103, 104–105, 106–107,
        234–235*
    pallidus, *106–107, 108–109, 234–235*
    pontis, *120–121*

Raphecerebellar fibers, *206–207*
Raphespinal fibers, *180–181*
Raphestriatal fibers, *214–215*
Rebound phenomenon, 208
Recess
    infundibular, *31, 40, 170*
    lateral, of fourth, *36, 42, 52, 54, 61, 112–113*
    pineal, *52*
    supraoptic, *31, 40, 51, 65, 170*
    suprapineal, *31, 52, 61*
Red nucleus, *27, 59, 68–69, 77, 130–131,
        134–135, 144–145, 148–149, 159,
        163, 165, 167–168, 178–179,
        180–181, 184–185, 190–191,
        194–195, 196–197, 200–201,
        206–207, 210–211, 220–221,
        228–229*
Reflex
    abdominal, 190
    Babinski, 94
    corneal, 184, 202
    deep tendon, 94, 178
    extensor plantar, 94
    gag, 186, 202, 258Q, 261A, 280Q, 288A
    jaw, 184
    lacrimal, 184
    pupillary light, 220
    sneezing, 184
    supraorbital, 184
    tearing, 184
    trigeminofacial, 184
    vomiting, 184
Regional neurobiology, 173
Respiratory arrest, 110
Restiform body, *27, 34–37, 43–44, 72, 81,
        100–101, 102–103, 104–105,
        108–109, 112–113, 114–115,
        116–117, 178–179, 184–185,
        186–187, 190–191, 194–195,
        204–205, 206–207, 226–227,
        228–229*
Resting tremor, 158, 214
Reticular formation, *122–123, 126–127,
        128–129, 130–131, 180–181,
        184–185, 210–211, 220–221,
        226–227*
Reticular nuclei, *194–195*
Reticulocerebellar fibers, *206–207*
Reticulospinal fibers, *98–99, 100–101, 106–107*
Reticulospinal tract, *84, 95, 98–99, 194–195*
Reticulotegmental nucleus, *120–121, 206–207*
Reticulothalamic fibers, *180–181*
Retroolivary (postolivary) sulcus, *24, 26, 43, 81,
        100–101, 102–103*
Retrosplenial cortex, *232–233*
Rhinal sulcus, *28*
Right cerebral hemisphere
    dissection of, *56–57*
    lateral view of, *19, 56*
    magnetic resonance imaging of, *28, 30–31*
    midsagittal view of, *28, 30–31*
    sinuses of, *19*
Rigidity, 158, 214, 216
Rinne test, 226
Rolandic artery, *17*
Rolandic vein, *17, 19*
Rostral spinocerebellar fibers, *204–205*
Rubrospinal tract, *86, 88, 90, 92, 95, 98–99,*

        *100–101, 102–103, 104–105,
        106–107, 108–109, 111, 116–117,
        118–119, 120–121, 122–123,
        126–127, 128–129, 130–131,
        196–197, 210–211*

S
Salivatory nuclei, *186–187*
Secondary cochlear fibers, *108–109*
Segmental artery, *95*
Semicircular canals, *42*
Sensorineural hearing loss, 226
Sensory ataxia, 178
Sensory decussation, 100
Sensory loss
    complete, 158
    dissociated, 158
    pain sensation, 94, 110, 124, 158
    proprioception/vibratory sense, 124, 158
    temperature sensation, 94, 110, 124, 158
Septal nuclei, *152–153, 232–233, 234–235*
Septal veins, *29*
Septum, *30, 65, 67*
Septum pellucidum, *31, 60, 64, 74, 76,
        150–151, 152–153, 154–155,
        156–157, 159, 162, 164*
Serotonin, 180, 214, 216
Short insular gyri, *56*
Shuffling gait, 158
Sigmoid sinus
    anatomy of, *21, 23*
    angiogram of, *241, 243–245, 250*
Singultus, 110
Sinus
    cavernous, *21, 23, 249*
    confluens
        anatomy of, *19, 21, 23, 29*
        angiogram of, *243–245, 250*
        questions regarding, *296Q, 297A*
    inferior petrosal, *21, 23, 250*
    inferior sagittal
        anatomy of, *21, 29*
        angiogram of, *243*
    intercavernous, *21, 23*
    occipital, *19, 23, 29*
    right cerebral hemisphere, *19*
    sigmoid
        anatomy of, *21, 23*
        angiogram of, *241, 243–245, 250*
    sphenoparietal, *21, 23*
    straight
        anatomy of, *19, 21, 29*
        angiogram of, *241, 248, 250*
        questions regarding, *295Q, 296A*
    superior petrosal, *21, 23, 248*
    superior sagittal
        anatomy of, *17, 19, 29, 47*
        angiogram of, *241, 243–245, 248, 250*
        questions regarding, *295Q, 296A, 296Q,
            297A*
    transverse
        anatomy of, *19, 21, 23, 29, 47*
        angiogram of, *241, 243–245, 248, 250*
        questions regarding, *295Q, 296A*
Sinus confluens
    anatomy of, *19, 21, 23, 29*
    angiogram of, *243–245, 250*
    questions regarding, *296Q, 297A*

Sneezing reflex, 184
Solitary nuclei, *100–101, 102–103, 104–105, 106–107, 108–109, 111, 112–113, 116–117, 165, 175, 186–187, 228–229, 234–235*
    cardiorespiratory portion of, *186–187*
    gustatory portion of, *186–187*
Solitary pathways, *186–187*
Solitary tract, *100–101, 102–103, 104–105, 106–107, 108–109, 111, 112–113, 116–117, 165, 175, 186–187, 228–229*
Somatostatin, 180, 186, 232, 234
Spasmodic torticollis, 214
Spasticity, 190, 214
Special somatic afferent, *174*
Special somatic efferent, *174*
Special visceral afferent, *174, 186–187*
Sphenoparietal sinus, *21, 23*
Sphincter of iris, 201
Spinal accessory nucleus, *92*
Spinal artery
    anterior, *10–11*
    posterior, *10*
Spinal border cells, *204–205*
Spinal cord
    acute central cervical spinal cord syndrome, 94
    anterolateral cordotomy of, *280Q, 282Q, 288A, 290A*
    arteries of, *10–11*
    arteriovenous malformation in, 94
    blood supply to, 94, *95*
    C_1 level of, *92, 176–177*
    C_7 level of, *11, 90, 176–177*
    C_2–C_5 level of, *10, 176–177*
    coccygeal segment of, *12*
    computed tomography myelography of, *89, 91, 93*
    gray matter of, *84, 204*
    hemorrhage in, 94
    laminae I–IX, *84–91*
    laminae I–VIII, *180–181*
    laminae III–V, *178–179*
    laminae IV (III–VII), *182–183*
    laminae IV–IX, *190–191*
    laminae VI–VIII, *194–197*
    lesions of, 94
    lower thoracic, *12*
    lumbar, *12, 86–87, 176–177*
    magnetic resonance imaging of, *12*
    nuclei, *175*
    questions regarding, *266Q, 271A–272A, 280Q, 288A*
    sacral, *12, 85, 176–177*
    subacute combined degeneration of, 178
    thoracic, *12, 88, 176–177*
    transverse section of, *84*
    white matter of, *84*
Spinal cord injury, 94
Spinal ganglion, *11*
Spinal medullary artery
    anterior, *10*
    posterior, *10*
Spinal trigeminal nucleus, *102–103, 106–107, 111, 112–113, 114–115, 116–117, 118–119, 125, 175, 184–185, 202–203, 204–205*

gelatinosa portion of, *92, 98–99*
magnocellular portion of, *92, 98–99*
pars caudalis, *98–99, 100–101*
pars interpolaris, *102–103*
pars oralis, *106–107, 108–109, 112–113, 114–115, 116–117*
Spinal trigeminal tract, *92, 98–99, 102–103, 104–105, 106–107, 108–109, 111, 112–113, 116–117, 125, 184–185, 202–203, 204–205, 226–227, 228–229*
Spinal vestibular nucleus, *194–195*
Spinocerebellar tracts
    anterior, *88, 90, 92, 98–99, 100–101, 102–103, 104–105, 106–107, 108–109, 116–117, 118–119, 120–121, 204–205*
    blood supply to, 204
    disorders that affect, 204
    neurotransmitters, 204
    posterior, *88, 90, 92, 95, 98–99, 100–101, 111, 204–205*
Spino-olivary fibers, *88, 90, 92, 98–99*
Spinoreticular fibers, *180–181*
Spinotectal tract, *128–129, 130–131, 132–133*
Spinothalamic fibers, *180–181*
Spinothalamic tract, *128–129, 130–131, 132–133*
Spiral ganglion, *226–227*
Stapedius, 203
Static tremor, 208
Stereoagnosis, 178
Sternocleidomastoid, 201
Straight sinus
    anatomy of, *19, 21, 29*
    angiogram of, *241, 248, 250*
    questions regarding, *295Q, 296A*
Streptomycin, 226
Stria
    lateral longitudinal, *138–139, 144–145, 146–147, 150–151, 152–153, 154–155, 156–157*
    lateral olfactory, *26, 152–153, 154–155*
    medial longitudinal, *138–139, 140–141, 144–145, 146–147, 150–151, 152–153, 154–155, 156–157*
    medial olfactory, *26, 154–155*
Stria medullaris thalami, *31, 144–145, 146–147, 148–149, 163*
Stria terminalis, *53, 66–71, 74–76, 138–139, 140–141, 144–145, 146–147, 148–149, 152–153, 159, 162, 164, 168, 234–235*
Striae medullares of fourth ventricle, *34, 36, 106–107*
Striatal connections, *214–215*
Striatonigral fibers, *214–215*
Striatopallidal fibers, *214–215*
Stuped posture, 158
Styloglossus, 201
Stylohyoid, 203
Stylopharyngeus, 203
Subarachnoid hemorrhage, 46
Subarachnoid space
    anatomy of, *47*
    questions regarding, *256Q–257Q, 260A–261A*
Subcallosal gyrus, *64, 77, 156–157*

Subdural hematoma, 46, *48*
Subdural hemorrhage, *51*
Subiculum, *232–233, 234–235*
Subjective vertigo, 228
Sublingual gland, 203
Submandibular ganglion, *202–203*
Submandibular gland, 203
Substance P, 180, 182, 184, 186, 190, 194, 214, 234
Substantia gelatinosa, *84, 86, 88, 90, 175*
Substantia innominata, *234–235*
Substantia nigra, *20, 59, 68–69, 78, 144–145, 148–149, 159, 167, 169–170, 178–179, 190–191, 194–195, 206–207, 210–211, 220–221, 228–229*
    blood supply to, *214–215*
    connections, *216–217*
    pars compacta, *128–129, 130–131, 132–133, 214–215, 216–217, 234–235*
    pars reticulata, *130–131, 132–133, 214–215, 216–217*
Subthalamic fasciculus, *216–217*
Subthalamic nucleus
    anatomy of, *68, 77, 134–135, 142–143, 144–145, 146–147, 148–149, 159, 169, 176–177, 214–215, 216–217*
    lesions of, 158
    questions regarding, *263Q, 265A*
Subthalamonigral fibers, *216–217*
Sulcal artery, *95*
Sulcus(i)
    angular, *14, 18*
    anterolateral, *90*
    calcarine, *13, 28, 30, 53, 58, 171, 222*
    central, *13, 16, 19, 28, 30, 45, 56*
    central sulcus, *13, 16, 19, 28, 30, 45, 56*
    cingulate
        anatomy of, *13, 28, 30, 176–177*
        questions regarding, *294Q, 296A*
    collateral, *13, 20, 22*
    corpus callosum, *28, 30*
    hypothalamic, *31*
    inferior frontal, *18*
    interparietal, *18*
    lateral, *13, 176–177*
    limitans, *34, 36, 104–105, 174*
    marginal, *13, 28, 30*
    middle temporal, *18*
    occipitotemporal, *22*
    olfactory, *20, 22, 156–157*
    paracentral, *13, 28, 30*
    parietooccipital, *13, 28, 30*
    postcentral, *13–14, 16, 18*
    posterior intermediate, *11, 34, 88, 90, 92*
    posterior median, *11, 34, 86, 88, 90, 92*
    posterolateral, *11, 34, 88, 90*
    postolivary, *43–44*
    precentral, *14–16, 18, 28*
    preolivary (*see* Preolivary sulcus)
        anatomy of, *24, 26, 44, 81, 100–101, 102–103*
        questions regarding, *257Q, 261A*
    retroolivary (postolivary), *24, 26, 43, 81, 100–101, 102–103*
    rhinal, *28*
    superior frontal, *16, 18*
    superior temporal, *18, 56*
    supramarginal, *14, 16, 18*

Superficial cerebral veins, *241, 244, 250*
Superficial middle cerebral vein
    anatomy of, *241*
    questions regarding, 295Q, 296A
Superior alternating hemiplegia, 136, 200
Superior anastomotic vein, *241*
Superior cerebellar artery
    anatomy of, *23, 25, 27, 37, 39–41*
    angiogram of, *244, 246–249, 251–252*
    branches of, *35*
Superior cerebellar peduncle, *27, 32–37, 61, 70, 72, 78–79, 114–115, 120–121, 122–123, 206–207, 210–211*
    brachium conjunctivum, *165, 167, 170*
    decussation, *130–131, 163, 170, 200–201, 210–211, 226–227, 228–229*
Superior cerebellar veins, *21, 29*
Superior cerebellopontine cistern, *50*
Superior cerebral veins
    anatomy of, *17, 19*
    angiogram of, *241, 243*
Superior cervical ganglion, *220–221*
Superior cistern, *138–139*
Superior colliculus
    anatomy of, *27, 31–32, 34–37, 39, 59, 71, 77, 128–129, 130–131, 132–133, 163–167, 180–181, 194–195, 196–197, 200–201, 210–211, 216–217, 220–221, 226–227, 228–229*
    blood supply to, *220–221*
    brachium of, *34–35, 59, 61, 77, 128–129, 132–133, 134–135, 140–141, 164, 169, 220–222*
    commissure, *132–133*
Superior fovea, *34, 36*
Superior frontal gyrus
    anatomy of, *16, 18, 28, 30, 45*
    questions regarding, 255Q, 259A
Superior frontal sulcus, *16, 18*
Superior longitudinal fasciculus, *56–57*
Superior medullary velum, *108–109, 116–117, 118–119, 120–121, 125*
Superior middle cerebral vein, *19*
Superior olive, *108–109, 116–117, 118–119, 120–121, 226–227*
Superior ophthalmic vein, *23*
Superior parietal lobule, *16, 56*
Superior petrosal sinus, *21, 23, 248*
Superior sagittal sinus
    anatomy of, *17, 19, 29, 47*
    angiogram of, *241, 243–245, 248, 250*
    questions regarding, 295Q, 296A, 296Q, 297A
Superior salivatory nucleus, *118–119, 175, 202–203*
Superior semilunar lobule, *32*
Superior temporal gyrus, *18, 56*
Superior temporal sulcus, *18, 56*
Superior vestibular nucleus, *108–109, 114–115, 116–117, 118–119, 196–197, 208–209, 210–211*
Supramammillary nucleus, *232–233*
Supramarginal gyrus, *56*
Supramarginal sulcus, *14, 16, 18*
Supraoptic decussation, *150–151, 152–153*
Supraoptic nucleus, *134–135, 152–153, 167*
Supraoptic recess, *31, 40, 51, 65*

Supraorbital reflex, 184
Suprapineal recess, *31, 52, 61*
Sydenham chorea, 214
Sylvian cistern, *50–51*
Syndrome(s)
    acute central cervical spinal cord, 94, 180
    amnestic confabulatory, 232
    anterior choroidal artery, 158
    Benedikt, 136
    Brown-Sequard, 94, 204
    central midbrain, 136
    Claude, 136, 196, 208
    Dandy-Walker, 208
    Foix-Alajouanine, 94
    Foville, 190
    Horner, 220
    Kluver-Bucy, 234
    Korsakoff, 232
    lateral medullary, *81,* 110, 186, 220
    lateral pontine, 124, 206
    medial medullary, 110, 178, 190, 200
    medial midbrain, 136
    medial pontine, 124, 178
    Millard-Gubler, 190
    one-and-a-half, 192
    Parinaud, 136, 192
    pontine, 124
    posterior inferior cerebellar artery, 180, 184, 186
    thalamic, 178, 180
    Weber, 136, 190, 200
    Wernicke-Korsakoff, 232
Syringobulbia, 110, 200, 202
Syringomyelia, 94, 180
Syrinx, 94
System
    anterolateral
        anatomy of, *84, 86, 88, 90, 92, 95, 98–99, 100–101, 102–103, 104–105, 106–107, 108–109, 111, 116–117, 118–119, 122–123, 125, 126–127, 128–129, 137, 178–179, 180–181, 182–183, 184–185, 190–191, 194–195, 202–203, 204–205, 210–211, 226–227, 228–229*
        blood supply to, *180–181*
        fibers of, 94
    auditory
        pathways, *226–227*
        questions regarding, 281Q, 289A
    posterior column-medial lemniscus, *178–179*
    postsynaptic-posterior column, *182–183*

T

Tabes dorsalis, 178
Tachycardia, 110
Tachyphonia, 214
Tactile agnosia, 178, 232, 234
Tapetum, *52–53, 61, 72, 76–77, 138–139, 164*
Taurine, 208
Tearing reflex, 184
Tectospinal tract, *92, 98–99, 100–101, 102–103, 104–105, 106–107, 108–109, 112–113, 114–115, 116–117, 118–119, 120–121, 122–123, 126–127, 128–129, 194–195, 202–203*
Tectum, *52*

Tegmental nuclei, *232–233*
Tela choroidea, *34, 36, 112–113*
Telencephalon, *176–177*
Temperature sensation
    areas of, 98, 100, 102, 104, 106, 108, 116, 120, 122, 126, 128, 130, 132, 134, 140, 142
    loss of, 94, 110, 124, 158, 178
Temporal artery, *17*
Temporal cerebral veins, *19*
Temporal horn
    anatomy of, *59*
    questions regarding, 262Q, 263A
Temporal inferior horn, *61*
Temporal lobe, *20, 38–39, 41, 45, 64, 79–80*
Temporal pole, *20, 22, 28*
Temporomandibular joint, *184–185*
Temporopontine fibers, *126–127, 128–129, 130–131, 132–133, 134–135, 206–207*
Tensor tympani, 203
Tensor veli palatini, 203
Tentorium cerebelli, *31, 47, 51*
Terminal ganglion, *202–203*
Terminal vein, *66–71, 74–76*
Thalamic fasciculus, *142–143, 144–145, 146–147, 148–149, 165, 169, 210–211, 216–217*
Thalamic pain, 158
Thalamic reticular nucleus, *144–145, 146–147, 148–149, 171*
Thalamic syndrome, 178, 180
Thalamocortical fibers, *210–211, 216–217*
Thalamogeniculate arteries
    anatomy of, *35, 37*
    angiogram of, *246*
    questions regarding, 268Q, 273A
Thalamogeniculate body, *27*
Thalamoperforating arteries
    anatomy of, *246–247*
    questions regarding, 276Q, 277A
Thalamostriatal fibers, *214–215*
Thalamostriate vein, *241*
Thalamus
    anterior nucleus of, *60, 66–67, 75–76, 146–147, 148–149, 162–163, 165, 232–233*
    anterior tubercle of, *66*
    blood supply to, *234–235*
    centromedian nucleus of, *69, 76, 142–143, 162, 164–167, 176–177, 210–211, 216–217*
    dorsomedial nucleus of (*see* Dorsomedial nucleus of thalamus)
    emboliform nucleus of, *112–113, 114–115, 167*
    lateral dorsal nucleus of, *69, 144–145, 159, 163, 165, 167*
    ventral anterior nucleus of, *67, 75–76, 162, 164–165, 167, 216–217*
    ventral lateral nucleus of, *68, 76, 162, 164, 166–167, 169, 171, 210–211, 216–217*
    ventral posterolateral nucleus of, *69, 76, 142–143, 162, 164, 166, 171, 176–177, 178–179, 180–181, 184–185, 210–211*
    ventral posteromedial nucleus of, *69, 142–143, 164, 166, 169, 176–177, 184–185, 186–187*

Third ventricle
    anatomy of, *31, 41, 51, 54, 60, 65–66,*
        68–69, 77–78, 134–135, 148–149,
        150–151, 152–153
    choroid plexus, *37, 76, 251,* 295Q, 296A
    infundibular recess of, *170*
    questions regarding, 269Q, 274A
    supraoptic recess of, *170*
Thrombus, 158
Tic douloureux (*see* Trigeminal neuralgia)
Tinnitus, 202
Tongue muscles
    innervation of, 201
    weakness of, 110
Tonsil of cerebellum
    anatomy of, *30, 42–44, 81, 112–113*
    herniation of, 110
Tonsillar herniation
    description of, 110
    questions regarding, 258Q, 261A
Tract
    anterior corticospinal, *86, 88, 90, 92, 95,*
        98–99, 190–191
    anterior spinocerebellar
        anatomy of, *88, 90, 92, 98–99, 100–101,*
            102–103, 104–105, 106–107,
            108–109, 116–117, 118–119,
            120–121, 204–205
        questions regarding, 267Q, 272A
    central tegmental, *102–103, 104–105,*
        106–107, 108–109, 114–115,
        116–117, 118–119, 120–121,
        122–123, 126–127, 128–129,
        130–131, 132–133, 134–135,
        178–179
    corticospinal
        anatomy of, *190–191*
        anterior, *86, 88, 90, 92, 95, 98–99*
        injury to, 190
        lateral, *84, 86, 88, 90, 92, 95, 111, 163,*
            266Q, 272A
        questions regarding, 266Q, 272A
    dorsal trigeminothalamic, *122–123, 126–127,*
        128–129, 130–131, 132–133,
        134–135, 184–185
    dorsolateral, *84, 86, 88, 90, 92, 95*
    habenulopeduncular, *132–133, 134–135,*
        142–143
    lateral corticospinal
        anatomy of, *84, 86, 88, 90, 92, 95, 111,*
            163, 190–191, 194–195, 196–197
        questions regarding, 266Q, 272A
    lateral vestibulospinal, *86, 88, 90, 92,*
        196–197, 208–209, 228–229
    mammillotegmental, *232–233*
    mammillothalamic
        anatomy of, *67, 77, 134–135, 142–143,*
            146–147, 148–149, 163–166, 168,
            232–233
        questions regarding, 263Q, 264A
    medial vestibulospinal, *196–197, 208–209,*
        228–229
    medullary reticulospinal, *88, 90, 92*
    mesencephalic, *116–117, 118–119, 120–121,*
        122–123, 125, 126–127, 128–129,
        130–131, 132–133, 175
    olfactory, *20, 22, 24–26, 59, 64, 156–157,*
        165

optic
    anatomy of, *20, 23–25, 27, 37, 39–40, 50,*
        58–59, 66–69, 78, 132–133, 134–135,
        144–145, 146–147, 148–149, 150–151,
        152–153, 165, 167–171, 220–221
    blood supply to, *220–221*
    questions regarding, 257Q, 260A, 263Q,
        264A
    pontoreticulospinal, *86, 88, 90, 92*
    posterior spinocerebellar, *88, 90, 92, 95,*
        98–99, 100–101, 111, 204–205
    reticulospinal, *84, 95, 98–99, 194–195*
    rubrospinal, *86, 88, 90, 92, 95, 98–99,*
        100–101, 102–103, 104–105,
        106–107, 108–109, 111, 116–117,
        118–119, 120–121, 122–123,
        126–127, 128–129, 130–131,
        196–197, 210–211
    solitary, *100–101, 102–103, 104–105,*
        106–107, 108–109, 111, 112–113,
        116–117, 165, 175, 186–187,
        228–229
    spinal trigeminal, *92, 98–99, 102–103,*
        104–105, 106–107, 108–109, 111,
        112–113, 116–117, 125, 184–185,
        202–203, 204–205, 226–227,
        228–229
    spinocerebellar
        anterior, *88, 90, 92, 98–99, 100–101,*
            102–103, 104–105, 106–107,
            108–109, 116–117, 118–119,
            120–121, 204–205
        blood supply to, 204
        disorders that affect, 204
        neurotransmitters, 204
        posterior, *88, 90, 92, 95, 98–99,*
            100–101, 111, 204–205
    spinotectal, *128–129, 130–131, 132–133*
    spinothalamic, *128–129, 130–131, 132–133*
    tectospinal, *92, 98–99, 100–101, 102–103,*
        104–105, 106–107, 108–109,
        112–113, 114–115, 116–117,
        118–119, 120–121, 122–123,
        126–127, 128–129, 194–195,
        202–203
    ventral spinocerebellar, *210–211*
    ventral trigeminothalamic, *100–101,*
        102–103, 104–105, 106–107,
        108–109, 116–117, 118–119,
        120–121, 122–123, 126–127,
        128–129, 130–131, 132–133,
        134–135, 184–185
    vestibulospinal, *95, 98–99, 196–197*
Transient ischemic attack, 158
Transverse cerebral fissure, *61*
Transverse sinus
    anatomy of, *19, 21, 23, 29, 47*
    angiogram of, *241, 243–245, 248, 250*
    questions regarding, 295Q, 296A
Transverse temporal gyrus, *45, 56, 60, 226–227*
Trapezoid body, *116–117, 118–119, 226–227*
Trapezoid nuclei, *116–117, 226–227*
Tremor, 208, 214
    flapping, 214
    intention, 208
    kinetic, 208
    resting, 158, 214
    static, 208

Trigeminal ganglion, *41, 80*
Trigeminal motor nucleus
    anatomy of, *116–117, 118–119, 120–121,*
        167, 175, 184–185, 192–193,
        202–203, 204–205, 210–211
    questions regarding, 280Q, 289A
Trigeminal nerve, *23–25, 69, 80, 116–117, 122,*
    202–203
    anatomy of, *41*
    chief sensory nucleus of, 120, *167, 184–185*
    lesions of, 184, 202
    mandibular division of, *184–185*
    maxillary division of, *184–185*
    motor nucleus of, 120
    motor root, *26–27, 33, 36–37*
    ophthalmic division of, *184–185*
    pathways of, *184–185*
    sensory root, *26–27, 33, 36–37, 41*
Trigeminal neuralgia
    description of, 41, 184, 202
    questions regarding, 255Q, 259A
Trigeminal nuclei, *125*
Trigeminal tubercle, *34–36*
Trigeminofacial reflex, 184
Trochlear nerve, *23–27, 33–37, 40, 72, 122,*
    122–123, 125, 126–127, 138–139,
    163, 175, 200–201
Trochlear nucleus
    anatomy of, *128–129, 137, 140–141,*
        192–193, 200–201, 228–229
    blood supply to, *228–229*
Truncal ataxia, 208, 228
Tuber cinereum, *59*
Tuberculum cinereum, *35–36*
Tuberculum cuneatum, *34*
Tuberculum gracile, *34*

U
Uncal artery, *25*
Uncal herniation, 136, 256Q, 260A
Uncinate fasciculus, *56–57*
Uncus
    anatomy of, *20, 22, 24, 28, 38–39, 65, 78,*
        152–153
    herniation of, 136, 256Q, 260A
Unsteady gait, 228
Upper extremity paralysis, 94
Upper motor neuron lesion, 190
Upward gaze, paralysis of, 136
Urinary retention, 94

V
Vagal trigone, *34–36*
Vagus nerve
    anatomy of, *22, 24, 27, 35, 37, 42–44, 81,*
        104–105, 202–203
    dorsal motor nucleus of, *100–101, 102–103,*
        104–105, 111, 175, 202–203
Vasoactive intestinal polypeptide, 180, 234
Vein
    anterior cerebral, *29*
    basal, *29, 241, 250*
    great cerebral
        anatomy of, *21, 29, 59*
        angiogram of, *241, 248, 250*
    greater anastomotic, *17, 19*
    inferior anastomotic, *19, 241*
    inferior cerebral, *19*

internal cerebral
    anatomy of, *28–29, 31, 34*
    angiogram of, *241, 248, 250*
internal jugular, *21, 23, 244, 250*
internal occipital, *29*
of Labbé, *241, 250*
lateral ventricular, *248*
Rolandic, *17, 19*
septal, *29*
superficial cerebral, *241, 244, 250*
superficial middle cerebral
    anatomy of, *241*
    questions regarding, 295Q, 296A
superior anastomotic, *241*
superior cerebellar, *21, 29*
superior cerebral
    anatomy of, *17, 19*
    angiogram of, *241, 243*
superior middle cerebral, *19*
superior ophthalmic, *23*
temporal cerebral, *19*
terminal, *66–71, 74–76*
thalamostriate, *241*
Venous angle, *241,* 294Q, 296A
Ventral amygdalofugal fibers, *150–151*
Ventral anterior nucleus of thalamus, *66–67,*
        75–76, 150–151, 162, 164–165, 167,
        216–217
Ventral lateral nucleus of thalamus, *68, 76,*
        144–145, 162, 164, 166–167, 169,
        171, 210–211, 216–217
Ventral pallidum, *65*
Ventral posterior thalamic nuclei, *77*
Ventral posterolateral nucleus of thalamus, *69,*
        76, 142–143, 162, 164, 166, 171,
        176–177, 178–179, 180–181,
        184–185, 210–211
Ventral posteromedial nucleus of thalamus, *69,*
        142–143, 164, 166, 169, 176–177,
        184–185, 186–187
Ventral spinocerebellar tract, *210–211*
Ventral striatum, *65*
Ventral tegmental area, *234–235*
Ventral trigeminothalamic fibers
    anatomy of, *125, 137*
    questions regarding, 283Q, 291A
Ventral trigeminothalamic tract, *100–101,*
        102–103, 104–105, 106–107,
        108–109, 116–117, 118–119,
        120–121, 122–123, 126–127,
        128–129, 130–131, 132–133,
        134–135, 184–185
Ventricles
    dorsal view of, *52*
    fourth
        choroid plexus of, *35, 37, 251*
        floor of, *36*

general anatomy of, *22, 27, 31–33, 50, 52,*
        54, 72, 79–81, 111, 125, 165
    lateral recess of, *36, 42, 52, 54, 61,*
        112–113
    lateral ventricle of, *34*
    magnetic resonance imaging of, *22*
    questions regarding, 258Q, 261A, 268Q,
        274A
    rostral portion of, *39–40, 51*
    striae medullares of, *34, 36, 106–107*
    hemorrhages of, *54*
    lateral, *176–177*
        anterior horn of, *54, 60, 64, 75–76,*
            152–153, 154–155, 156–157, 165,
            262Q, 264A
        atrium of, *52–54, 75–77, 138–139, 166,*
            171, 276Q, 277A
        body of, *52–53, 66–71, 74, 140–141,*
            144–145, 146–147
        inferior horn of, *52–53, 58, 67–72, 78,*
            138–139, 140–141, 144–145,
            146–147, 148–149, 170–171
        posterior horn of, *52–53, 58, 72, 76–78*
        questions regarding, 276Q, 277A
        temporal horn of, *54,* 262Q, 263A
    lateral view of, *52–53*
    questions regarding, 255Q, 259A
    third
        anatomy of, *31, 41, 51, 54, 60, 65–66,*
            68–69, 77–78, 134–135, 148–149,
            150–151, 152–153
        choroid plexus, *37, 76, 251,* 295Q, 296A
        infundibular recess of, *170*
        questions regarding, 269Q, 274A
        supraoptic recess of, *170*
Ventromedial hypothalamic nuclei, *232–233,*
        234–235
Vermal cortex, *208–209*
Vermis, *32*
Vertebral artery
    anatomy of, *23, 25, 27, 37*
    angiogram of, *244–247, 249–252*
Vertical gaze center, *192*
Vertical gaze palsy, *192*
Vertigo, *202, 228*
Vestibular area, *34–36*
Vestibular ganglion, *228–229*
Vestibular nuclei
    anatomy of, *125, 175, 204–205*
    blood supply, *208–209, 228–229*
    disorders of, *228*
    inferior, *104–105, 106–107, 112–113,*
        186–187, 196–197, 208–209, 210–211
    lateral, *108–109, 114–115, 116–117,*
        196–197, 210–211
    medial, *104–105, 106–107, 108–109,*
        112–113, 114–115, 116–117,

        186–187, 194–195, 196–197,
        208–209, 210–211
    neurotransmitters, *228*
    questions regarding, 284Q, 292A
    spinal, *194–195*
    superior, *108–109, 114–115, 116–117,*
        118–119, 196–197, 208–209,
        210–211
Vestibular pathways, *228–229*
Vestibular schwannoma, *202, 226*
    illustration of, *249*
    questions regarding, 254Q-255Q, 258A
Vestibulocerebellar fibers
    primary, *228–229*
    secondary, *228–229*
Vestibulocochlear nerve
    anatomy of, *22–27, 36–37, 41–42, 44, 81*
    questions regarding, 283Q, 291A
Vestibulospinal fibers, *100–101*
Vestibulospinal tract, *95, 98–99, 196–197*
Vibratory sense
    areas of, *98, 100, 102, 104, 106, 108, 116,*
        120, 122, 126, 128, 130, 132, 134,
        140, 142
    loss of, *124, 178*
Viral meningitis, *46*
Visual agnosia, *232, 234*
Visual pathways, *222–223*
Vocal musculature weakness, *110*
Vomiting, *228*
Vomiting reflex, *184*

W

Wallerian degeneration, *96*
Watershed infarct, *158*
Weakness
    facial, *190*
    legs, *178*
    lower extremity, 265Q, 271A
    palatal musculature, *110*
    pharyngeal musculature, *110*
    spastic weakness of legs, *178*
    tongue muscles, *110*
    vocal musculature, *110*
Weber syndrome, *136, 190, 200*
Weber test, *226*
Wernicke-Korsakoff syndrome, *232*
White ramus communicans, *220–221*
Wilson disease
    description of, *214*
    questions regarding, 283Q, 286Q, 291A,
        293A

Z

Zona incerta, *142–143, 144–145, 146–147,*
        148–149, 169, 210–211, 214–215
Zone, intermediate, *84, 86, 90, 204–205*